WITHDRAWN
WRIGHT STATE UNIVERSITY LIBRARIES

ARRHYTHMIAS AND PACEMAKERS
Practical Management for Anesthesia and Critical Care Medicine

John L. Atlee, M.D.

*Professor
Department of Anesthesiology
Medical College of Wisconsin
Milwaukee, Wisconsin*

W.B. SAUNDERS COMPANY
A Division of Harcourt Brace & Company
Philadelphia London Toronto Montreal Sydney Tokyo

W.B. SAUNDERS COMPANY
A Division of Harcourt Brace & Company

The Curtis Center
Independence Square West
Philadelphia, Pennsylvania 19106

Library of Congress Catalog card number: 95–37106

ARRHYTHMIAS & PACEMAKERS   ISBN 0-7216-5580-6

Copyright © 1996, by W.B. Saunders Company

All rights reserved. No part of this publication may be reproduced or transmitted in any form or by any means, electronic or mechanical, including photocopy, recording, or any information storage and retrieval system, without permission from the publisher.

Printed in the United States of America

Last digit is the print number: 9   8   7   6   5   4   3   2   1

To

Barbara, Sarah and John Jr.

Preface

The heart can fail mechanically, electrically, or both. The literature in anesthesiology, cardiology and critical care is complete with numerous scholarly and practical works on the mechanical aspects of cardiac function and dysfunction. Similarly, there is a substantial literature on arrhythmias and pacemakers in the field of cardiology. Despite two editions of a previous comprehensive book by the author (1985, 1990)[1], there are no recent available works that succinctly address in a single volume mechanisms, diagnosis and management of cardiac electrical failure as pertains to anesthesia and critical care practice. This is an important deficiency. Cardiac electrical imbalance in anesthesia and critical care often does not have the same origin as that encountered by cardiologists (i.e., structural heart disease). Instead, electrical imbalance appears more related to drugs, autonomic and other imbalance, rather than to structural heart disease per se, the traditional focus of works in cardiology.

The author's previous book[1] was intended to be an authoritative, meticulously documented, complete source of information pertaining to perioperative cardiac arrhythmias, including their mechanisms, diagnosis, prevention and management. Such detailed information was compiled so that readers would not have to consult works in cardiology for the "why and wherefore," as well as stimulate further research. It is believed that both editions of the book achieved these goals, and a third edition with multiple contributors could appear around the end of this millennium. Nevertheless, I have been asked on more than one occasion whether I would consider writing a more succinct work focusing almost exclusively on the practical aspects of diagnosis and management.

Therefore, the purpose of this work is to provide in one volume the essential information pertaining to diagnosis and management of cardiac arrhythmias or pacemakers in perioperative and critical care settings. The book begins with a perspective on the problem of arrhythmias and patients with pacemakers, including historical aspects, significance and prevalence. The second chapter provides an overview of the current understanding of mechanisms for arrhythmias, and the third an overview of the causes for arrhythmias and common arrhythmic associations. The electrocardiographic (ECG) diagnosis of arrhythmias is discussed in Chapter 4. The final six chapters deal with various aspects of management. Antiarrhythmic and adjunct drugs are discussed in Chapter 5, which focuses more on those drugs that are suitable for parenteral administration. Chapter 6 introduces the subject of cardiac pacing. Chapter 7 and 8 deal with temporary pacing and permanent pacemakers/internal cardioverter-defibrillators, respectively. The final two chapters deal with recognition and management of supraventricular and ventricular arrhythmias, including tachycardia in patients with ventricular preexcitation and atrioventricular or fascicular heart block.

It is hoped that this volume will be useful to both physicians and non-physician medical personnel who manage patients with acute or chronic cardiac electrical imbalance, whether in anesthesia, post-anesthesia care, critical care or emergency medical circumstances.

John L. Atlee, M.D.
Milwaukee, Wisconsin

[1]Atlee, JL. Perioperative Cardiac Dysrhythmias. 2nd edition. Chicago. Year Book Medical Publishers. 1990. 443 pp.

Acknowledgment

A major concern when I undertook this work was whether I could ever assemble adequate ECG material for the illustrations. Not to worry! My colleagues in the Medical College of Wisconsin (MCW) Department of Anesthesiology supplied me with many useful stripchart recordings for rhythm disturbances commonly seen in preoperative holding areas, operating rooms, post-anesthesia recovery rooms, and surgical ICU's. Special thanks go to Saeed Dhamee, Alan Goldberg, Bill Campbell, Lourdes Burgos, Bob Kettler, Caridad Assidao, Mike Muzi, Quinn Hogan, Judy Kersten, Tim Olund, Ed Mathews, Chris Pattison and Nancy Bratanow. However, I also needed 12-lead ECG's. So, I turned to Karen Schuppie, who heads our preoperative anesthesia screening clinic. She found numerous good examples of arrhythmias and conduction disturbances for me, many of which appear in this book. Thank you Karen! Even so, I was still lacking examples of some rhythm disorders and ECG patterns. Therefore, I consulted several of my colleagues in MCW-Cardiology (Kiran Sagar, Ron Siegel, Bill Pochis), and was steered to Shankara Reddy (Marquette Electronics) and Mary Ann Gessell (MCW-Cardiology). A call to the MUSE system (an ECG archive) produced over a thousand ECG's, except that lacking was a good example of Osborn waves with hypothermia (ultimately borrowed). Thank you Shankara and Mary Ann! I acknowledge my computer software (McDraw™ II) for most of the schematics and flowcharts, except that some of the more complicated ones were prepared by Greg Diciaula and his staff of MCW Instructional Media. Thank you Greg! I am grateful for Microsoft™ Word 5.1 for chapter manuscript preparation, except for the "type 15 error" which destroyed the first manuscript for Chapter 3. This was "resurrected" from a scanned copy. I thank Julie Stubbe for assisting me with correspondence and permission letters, and for copying, collating and transmitting chapter manuscripts to W.B. Saunders. I wish to extend my sincere appreciation to several individuals at W.B. Saunders, with whom I have worked closely during preparation of this book: Avé McCracken, Acquisitions Editor; J. Matthew Harris, Editor Medical Books; Lesley Day, Medical Editor; and Joan Sinclair, Production Manager. I am most grateful to all these persons for their assistance and professional manner. However, I do especially want to thank Avé for her advice and constructive criticism during proposal development and early preparation of the book. Finally, I can't thank Barbara, Sarah and John Jr. enough for putting up with Dad on yet another of his book projects, but especially Barbara for tolerating my pre-dawn up-and-outs for most of 1994.

Contents

1 Perspectives on Arrhythmias and Pacemakers   1

2 Overview of Mechanisms for Arrhythmias   25

3 Arrhythmia Causes and Associations   59

4 Electrocardiographic Diagnosis of Cardiac Arrhythmias   105

5 Drug Treatment for Arrhythmias   154

6 Pacing and Cardiac Electroversion   205

7 Temporary Cardiac Pacing: Practical Aspects   247

8 Management of Patients with Pacemakers or ICD Devices   293

9 Recognition and Management of Supraventricular Arrhythmias   330

10 Recognition and Management of Arrhythmias Preexcitation, Ventricular Arrhythmias, and Heart Block   389

Index   449

Forewords

Over the past two decades, the work of John L. Atlee, III, M.D. has been synonymous with intraoperative arrhythmia recognition, the effects of general anesthetics on automaticity, and pacemaker technology. Most recently Dr. Atlee has focused on alternative pacing methods to facilitate the diagnosis and therapy of acute life threatening rhythm disturbances. There are few if any other clinician–investigators who are as well versed and qualified as Dr. Atlee to review and guide practitioners in the operating room and Intensive Care Unit (ICU) in the recognition and management of abnormalities in cardiac conduction.

Arrhythmias and Pacemakers briefly, yet comprehensively, describes normal cardiac conduction, mechanisms of arrhythmia production, diagnosis, and therapy of abnormal conduction. All too frequently, perioperative circumstances that are associated with life threatening arrhythmias may be misdiagnosed and approached with a cursory (and, at times inappropriate or deleterious) response. Dr. Atlee provides a solid foundation on which to approach such problems. He emphasizes the concept of proper identification of the type of rhythm disturbance and the need to recognize inconsequential alterations in cardiac conduction, potentially reversible causes such as light anesthesia or stress response to the ICU environment, and pharmacologic and nonpharmacologic modalities to treat significant arrhythmias. Furthermore, he reminds the reader of many crucial basic tenants, such as the fact that not all wide complex arrhythmias are ventricular in origin; not all ventricular ectopy requires therapy; and lidocaine is not a panacea.

The unique settings of the operating room and ICU present challenging and rapidly changing patient scenarios. In particular, the critically ill highly catabolic patient frequently has multiple pathophysiologic processes such as acid-base imbalance, hypo- or hyperthermia, electrolyte abnormalities, nutritional depletion, end-organ compromise, and unpredictable drug pharmacokinetics and dynamics. The later issues underline the need for careful assessment and drug therapy for significant arrhythmias in critically ill patients. The skill to approach life threatening cardiac dysfunction is a crucial one for all anesthesiologists and intensivists. To that end, *Arrhythmias and Pacemakers: Practical Management for Anesthesia and Critical Care*

Medicine serves practitioners well in a concise and contemporary manner.

Douglas B. Coursin, MD
Professor of Anesthesiology and Internal Medicine
Associate Director of the Trauma and Life Support Center

Dr. Atlee's new book is titled *Arrhythmias and Pacemakers: Practical Management for Anesthesia and Critical Care Medicine.* This title reflects the changes in content and orientation from his previous publications and is intended to bring a comprehensive yet practical approach to the diagnosis and treatment of disturbances in cardiac rhythm in perioperative and critical care settings.

This work deals with historical aspects of electrocardiography and cardiac arrhythmia detection as well as incidence and significance of disturbances in cardiac rhythm. Detailed descriptions of cardiac electrophysiology, mechanisms, and causes of arrhythmias are dealt with in early chapters while the latter chapters focus on practical aspects of diagnosis, treatment, and pertinent aspects of management in the perioperative period and in critical care units.

Dr. Atlee has provided two chapters dealing with pacing, including on the one hand, conventional pacing and cardiac electroversion while a separate chapter deals with many practical aspects of temporary cardiac pacing. In the past five years Dr. Atlee has developed a keen interest and innovative approaches to temporary cardiac pacing. Thus there has been a clear change in not only the arrangement of the book compared to his previous book but also in the content of some of the chapters.

The presentation of recognition and management of arrhythmias is divided into two chapters. Supraventricular Arrhythmias are presented in one chapter while Ventricular Arrhythmias and Heart Block are presented in a separate chapter. Dr. Atlee's own research has also involved development of models for supraventricular rhythm disturbances and reflects a significant move toward understanding the fundamental cellular basis for certain types of supraventricular arrhythmias.

Dr. Atlee has provided a style of presentation resulting in good readability and has produced a monograph more understandable for those who are less sophisticated in their background education and training. At the same time Dr. Atlee's book provides the most comprehensive overview of arrhythmias likely to be encountered in the perioperative and critical care setting with very complete yet practical approaches to diagnosis and management. He has approached this book with the same vigor and unflagging spirit that characterizes his approaches to the laboratory and clinical arena. His dedication to his work has provided an excellent example for younger staff and fellows seeking to increase their knowledge and skills in managing patients who have disturbances in cardiac rhythm. Changes in cardiac rhythm arising from intrinsic cardiac disease and its interaction with anesthetic drugs and adjuvants commonly used in surgical and critical care patients still present significant challenges to anesthesiologists and intensivists. Dr. Atlee's book provides the single most authoritative and comprehensive work in this area.

John P. Kampine, M.D., Ph.D.
Professor and Chairman
Department of Anesthesiology
Professor of Physiology
Medical College of Wisconsin

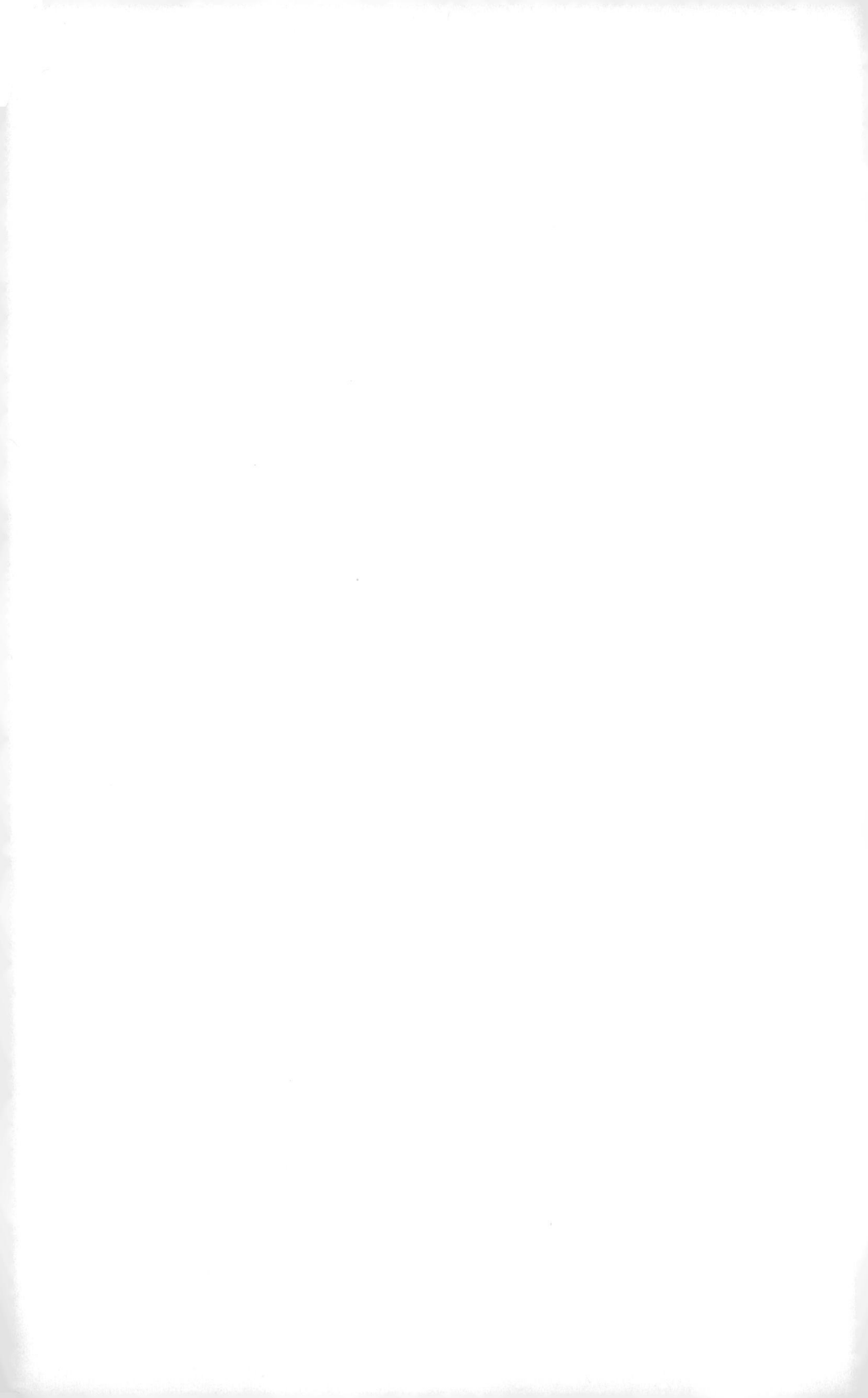

1

Perspectives on Arrhythmias and Pacemakers

Abbreviations Used in Chapter One	
AFIB-FLUT	Atrial fibrillation or flutter
AV	Atrioventricular
ECG	Electrocardiography
EEENT	Ear, eye, endocrine, nose, and throat
ICD	Internal (implantable) cardioverter-fibrillator
MI	Myocardial infarction
RV/LV	Right ventricular/left ventricular
VES/VT	Ventricular extrasystole/tachycardia
WPW	Wolff–Parkinson–White

TABLE 1-1 *Medical conditions that put patients at risk of symptomatic or malignant arrhythmias*

Myocardial ischemia, reperfusion injury, infarction
Congenital or acquired Q–T interval prolongation
Mitral valve prolapse ("mitral click") syndrome
Sinus node dysfunction; brady–tachy syndrome
WPW syndrome (preexcitation)
Disorders with autonomic nervous dysfunction
Myotonic dystrophy; muscular dystrophy
Cardiomyopathy; LV hypertrophy; RV dysplasia

The first recorded death under anesthesia is attributed to a cardiac arrhythmia—likely ventricular tachycardia followed by fibrillation [1]. These arrhythmias were probably the result of *sensitization,* the ability of some anesthetic drugs to facilitate ventricular arrhythmias with endogenous or exogenous catecholamines. Anesthetic sensitization has long been considered nearly synonymous with the problem of cardiac arrhythmias in relation to anesthesia and surgery, although other causes are recognized, too.[2,3] It is noteworthy that even today, sensitizing potential is apparently the only measure of arrhythmic potential obtained during preclinical testing of new anesthetic drugs. Cardiac electrophysiologic testing in relevant animal models has not been required. For example, no published reports of the cardiac electrophysiologic effects of desflurane or sevoflurane were found in a literature search performed in early 1995, and only one or two each for etomidate, midazolam, or propofol. Consequently, there is often little or no information on which to predict safety of anesthetic drugs in patients at risk of symptomatic or malignant arrhythmias (Table 1-1). This is surprising, given the substantial numbers of patients with the conditions listed in Table 1-1, and evidence that perioperative arrhythmias can have an adverse impact on anesthetic outcomes.[4,5]

Significance of Arrhythmia

The significance of a new or worsening cardiac arrhythmia within the context of anesthesia and critical care will depend on several factors, including the definition of arrhythmia, its electrocardiographic (ECG) appearance, the nature of the underlying physiologic imbalance, the patient's predisposition to life-threatening arrhythmias, and the hemodynamic impact of the arrhythmia. Each of these is discussed in more detail, below.

DEFINITION OF ARRHYTHMIA

The term *arrhythmia* requires both a morphologic and a physiologic definition. While arrhythmias are often considered dangerous based mainly on appearance (e.g., ventricular rhythm disturbances), lesser arrhythmias by appearance (e.g., atrioventricular [AV] junctional rhythm disturbances) may have an equally adverse circulatory impact.

From the etymological perspective, "arrhythmia" means *lack of* rhythm, with sinus rhythm implied. However, it could just as well mean *lack of any* rhythm, whether normal sinus or an abnormal rhythm. Lack of any rhythm, however, is equivalent to asystole, which most arrhythmias are not. This may be why some authors prefer to use the term *dysrhythmia.* "Dysrhythmia" means *abnormal* rhythm (i.e., any rhythm other than normal sinus rhythm), which conveys a more functional meaning. Nevertheless, arrhythmia is the preferred term in North America, and shall be used throughout this work. However, the definition of arrhythmia will be expanded to include both appearance and functional consequences, namely *any normal or abnormal heart rhythm at an inappropriate rate for the circumstance, without proper AV synchrony, or with ineffective atrial or ventricular contractions.* This definition, correctly, stresses the functional impact of arrhythmias. Therefore, a seemingly normal rhythm based on appearance could be abnormal for the circumstance, and therefore an "arrhythmia." Noncompensatory sinus tachycardia and disadvantageous bradycardia due to sinus node dysfunction fall into this category of "functional" arrhythmias because of their potentially adverse effects on circulatory homeostasis.

Such functional arrhythmias are usually not treated, but should be if they produce impaired hemodynamics. Conversely, frequent or multiform premature ventricular extrasystoles (VES) that have little circulatory impact are often treated based on their ominous appearance and presumed consequences, namely increased risk for ventricular tachycardia or fibrillation. While this may be true for patients with acute myocardial infarction (MI), it is not so in other circumstances (see Chapter 10). This has clinical relevance since there are potential dangers with drug treatment for arrhythmias (see below).

An expanded definition for arrhythmia emphasizes the three most important attributes of rhythm disturbances from a functional perspective: (1) *Rate*—what is the effective rate of the rhythm disturbance? While cardiac output is the product of heart rate and stroke volume, rates that are too high reduce diastolic time or produce ischemia, so

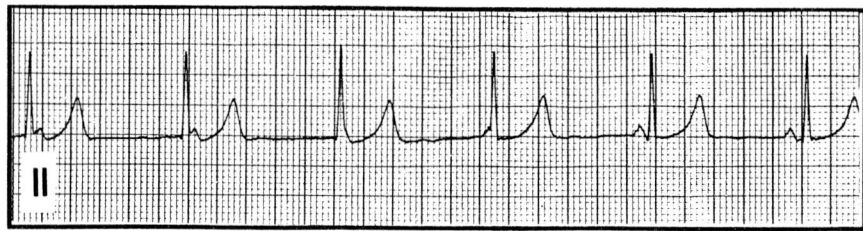

FIGURE 1-1 *AV junctional rhythm with isorhythmic AV dissociation. Note that P waves "march" in and out of the QRS complex, but bear no constant relation to it.*

that tachycardia is not compensatory or physiologic. (2) *AV synchrony*—is atrial transport function preserved? The importance of atrial contraction to ventricular filling increases with advancing age, and many cardiac disease processes are associated with diastolic dysfunction (see below). Thus, a seemingly benign rhythm disturbance, such as AV junctional rhythm with isorhythmic AV dissociation (Fig. 1-1), can produce significant hemodynamic compromise with ventricular diastolic dysfunction. (3) *Effective contractions*—are cardiac contractions orderly and effective? It is intuitively obvious that there must be a normal sequence of myocardial activation for effective atrial or ventricular systole. Arrhythmias and AV heart block often interfere with the normal sequence of myocardial activation, aside from their effects on heart rate or AV synchrony.

ELECTROCARDIOGRAPHIC APPEARANCE

We learn from our mistakes. So it is with "gut reaction" treatment of cardiac arrhythmias based on appearance and/or unfounded assumptions. Many will find it difficult to accept the notion that complex forms of VES (e.g., frequent, consecutive, multiform, R-on-T) do not necessarily portend malignant ventricular arrhythmias.[6,7] In fact, frequent or complex VES have only been shown to presage ventricular tachyarrhythmias in patients with acute MI.[8,9] While circumstance also supports such an association in patients with digitalis toxicity, catecholamine-anesthetic sensitization, reperfusion of ischemic myocardium, or previous infarction with severe left ventricular dysfunction,[1-3,8,9] this is by no means conclusive. The concern with aggressive drug treatment to suppress VES is that the drugs used may trigger new and potentially worse arrhythmias, a phenomenon termed *proarrhythmia*.[10,11] This was first exemplified by results of the Cardiac Arrhythmia Suppression Trials (CAST),[12,13] in which class IC antiar-

TABLE 1-2 *Types of imposed imbalance that can produce arrhythmias*

Sympathetic hyperactivity (pain)	Fluid or electrolyte derangements
Adverse drug effects; interactions	Caused by medical devices
Acid–base imbalance	Hypothermia; hyperthermia
Surgical traction reflexes	Hypocarbia or hypercarbia

rhythmic drugs (encainide, flecainide, and moricizine) were used to suppress asymptomatic VES because they might precipitate malignant ventricular arrhythmias and sudden death. However, use of these drugs actually increased mortality from ventricular arrhythmias, and cardiologists have rethought the wisdom of treatment based on unproven prognostic assumptions.[14,15] While the CAST findings do not necessarily apply to ventricular arrhythmias in the setting of anesthesia and critical care, they do challenge us to reconsider providing treatment based on assumptions as to prognosis as opposed to legitimate outcome data, especially since antiarrhythmic drugs may have adverse or proarrhythmic effects of their own.

NATURE OF UNDERLYING PHYSIOLOGIC IMBALANCE

New or more worrisome arrhythmias within the context of anesthesia and critical care, much as with sudden hyper- or hypotension and tachycardia, often signify imposed physiologic imbalance. This is true regardless of whether the patient has structural heart disease conducive to arrhythmias. Types of imposed imbalance that can cause new or worsening arrhythmias are listed in Table 1–2. Most of these are corrected without resorting to drugs or devices, which could further the imbalance. Importantly, removal of the imbalance often corrects the rhythm disturbance, or at least renders subsequent specific antiarrhythmic treatment more effective.

PREDISPOSITION TO LIFE-THREATENING ARRHYTHMIAS

It has already been stressed that multiform, R-on-T, or frequent VES do not necessarily set the stage for or trigger malignant ventricular tacharrhythmias, except with acute myocardial infarction (see above). However, there are two conditions that predispose the patient to potentially lethal tachyarrhythmias. One is acquired or congenital Q–T interval prolongation, in which patients are predisposed to episodes of

6 PERSPECTIVES ON ARRHYTHMIAS AND PACEMAKERS

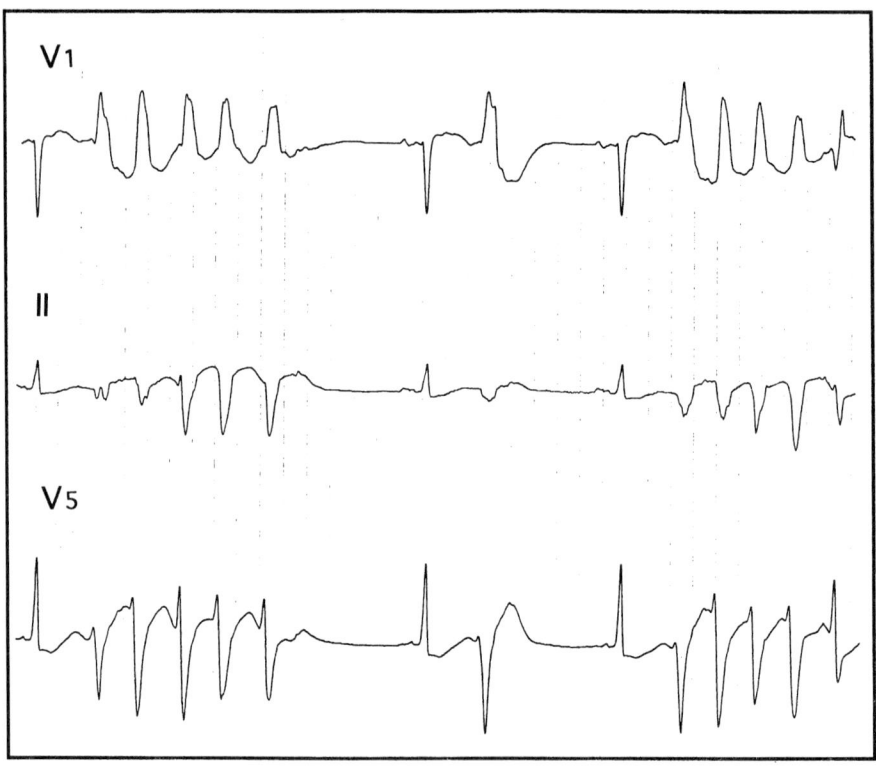

FIGURE 1-2 *Nonsustained torsades de pointes VT in a patient with Q-T interval prolongation.*

a fast, multiform ventricular tachycardia (VT) known as *torsades de points* (Fig. 1-2). Another is the Wolff–Parkinson–White (WPW) syndrome, in which patients have the capacity for more rapid than usual AV conduction during atrial flutter or fibrillation (Fig. 1-3). With either condition, extremely high ventricular rates ($\geq$ 200 beats/min) are possible. If tachycardia is sustained and prompt treatment is not provided, deterioration to ventricular fibrillation is probable.

HEMODYNAMIC IMPACT

Hemodynamics may be impaired by bradycardia, tachycardia, atrial transport dysfunction, ineffective contractions, or myocardial oxygen imbalance.

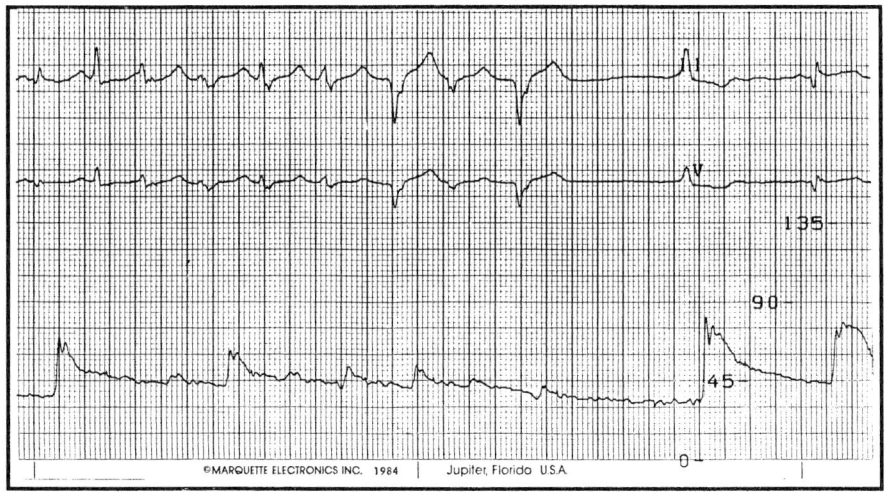

FIGURE 1-3 *Paroxysmal, fast atrial fibrillation with severe circulatory insufficiency in a patient with WPW syndrome. The ventricular rate in this patient exceeded 160 beats/min with some beats. Note that some beats during atrial fibrillation or sinus rhythm appear preexcited, while others with a more normal QRS complex do not.*

Bradycardia

Cardiac output is the product of heart rate and stroke volume. Stroke volume, in turn, is determined by changes in preload and contractility. Preload is affected by venous return, atrial systole, AV synchrony, AV valvular competence, and ventricular diastolic properties. However, with many types of end-stage heart disease, there may be little or no ability to adapt cardiac output to meet increased body needs by changes in stroke volume. If so, cardiac output is for all intents and purposes directly proportional to heart rate, provided there is no diastolic encroachment with heart rates that are too high. In such patients, bradycardia can be disastrous, regardless of whether the rhythm disturbance has a supraventricular or ventricular origin.

Tachycardia

With excessive heart rates, hemodynamics are compromised by a reduction in diastolic filling time (termed *diastolic encroachment*). Ventricular systole requires about 200 msec and most ventricular filling, except that due to atrial contraction, occurs over 150 to 200 msec.[16] Therefore, cardiac output is expected to decrease at rates exceeding 150 beats/min (cycle length ≤ 400 msec), even in patients without structural heart disease. Otherwise, tolerance of tachycardia by patients, as of bradycardia, depends on the nature of underlying heart disease. Patients with significant coronary stenoses or hypertrophic cardiomyopathy secondary to aortic stenosis or hypertension are least expected to tolerate tachycardia.

Atrial Transport Dysfunction

William Harvey was among the first to realize the importance of atrial systole when he wrote in the 17th century ". . .that the auricles beat, contract and *push* blood into the ventricles . . ."[17] However, knowledge of the importance of atrial contractions was not advanced until Gesell's work early in the 20th century.[18,19] Gesell demonstrated that properly timed atrial systoles augmented ventricular stroke volume by as much as 50 percent, and that randomly associated atrial and ventricular contractions would produce large beat-to-beat fluctuations in systolic blood pressure. Completely or incompletely dissociated atrial and ventricular contractions occur with AV heart block, atrial fibrillation, some atrial tachyarrhythmias, AV junctional rhythm disturbances, and ventricular rhythm disturbances. Loss of atrial transport function is expected to have the greatest adverse impact on circulatory function in patients with ventricular diastolic dysfunction. This is because impaired ventricular relaxation impedes early (rapid) diastolic filling, and reduced ventricular compliance slows passive filling, leaving the patient increasingly dependent on atrial systole. Indeed, the author has noted more than doubling of cardiac output by restoration of properly timed atrial systoles in patients with AV junctional rhythm presumed to have diastolic dysfunction.[20] Ventricular diastolic function can be impaired by advanced age and most cardiac disease processes,[21-24] as well as by available volatile anesthetics.[25]

Ineffective Contractions

Disorganized, ineffective contractions occur with atrial or ventricular fibrillation. With atrial fibrillation, and to a lesser extent flutter depending on the atrial rate, flow to the ventricles is passive. The effect of atrial fibrillation or flutter on cardiac output depends most on active and passive ventricular relaxation, since diastolic filling is passive. With ventricular fibrillation, wormlike contractions generate pressure insufficient to maintain vital organ perfusion. Atrial or ventricular contractions with polymorphic (multiform) atrial or ventricular tachycardia may be more or less effective, although the rate of tachycardia with diastolic encroachment becomes the most important determinant of tolerance of tachycardia.

TABLE 1-3 *Factors that affect myocardial oxygenation*

SUPPLY	DEMAND
Aortic diastolic pressure	Myocardial wall tension
LV end-diastolic pressure	Myocardial contractility
Coronary artery stenoses	Tachycardia

MYOCARDIAL OXYGEN IMBALANCE

Myocardial ischemia and hypoxia are important causes of cardiac arrhythmias. Factors affecting myocardial oxygenation in addition to arterial oxygen content are listed in Table 1-3. Arrhythmias could impact adversely on any of these to worsen arrhythmias. For example, exaggerated bradycardia might upset a favorable myocardial oxygen balance by reducing coronary perfusion pressure, the result of increased wall tension and end-diastolic pressure along with decreased aortic diastolic pressure. Perhaps a more important cause of myocardial ischemia, though, is the ventricular rate of tachycardia. High ventricular rates are particularly dangerous in patients with significant coronary stenoses. For example, sustained noncompensatory sinus tachycardia might be associated with myocardial ischemia, which in turn could lead to ventricular arrhythmias.

Incidence and Outcomes with Arrhythmias

VARIANCE IN REPORTED INCIDENCE

The reported incidence of perioperative cardiac arrhythmias depends to a great extent on the definition of arrhythmias, methods used for surveillance, and the patient population. If, for example, arrhythmia is defined as including all types of supraventricular rhythm disorders and continuous ECG surveillance is used, incidences of 60 to 80 percent will be reported.[1] Further, if only patients having cardiothoracic, intracranial, or major vascular surgery are included, the incidence of arrhythmias will be close to 100 percent. In contrast, with noncontinuous ECG surveillance, reported incidences are substantially lower (15 to 30 percent).[1] This reduced incidence is due to the fact that only consequential rhythm disturbances (Table 1-4) are detected and reported. Thus, while studies using continuous ECG monitoring report a higher overall incidence of arrhythmias than those using noncontinuous ECG monitoring, both types of studies should still report a similar incidence of consequential arrhythmias (Table 1-4).

TABLE 1-4 *Consequential sustained cardiac rhythm disturbances*

DISTURBANCE	CONSEQUENCE
Bradycardia ≤ 50 beats/min	Hypotension; facilitates bradycardia-dependent tachyarrhythmias
Tachycardia ≥ 150 beats/min	Hypotension caused by reduced diastolic time; myocardial ischemia
AFIB-FLUT with WPW syndrome	Circulatory collapse; rapidly deteriorate to ventricular fibrillation
Ventricular arrhythmias	Diastolic encroachment; loss of atrial systole; inherent instability

FACTORS THAT INCREASE INCIDENCE

Based on review of intraoperative arrhythmia incidence studies,[1] in which either continuous or noncontinuous ECG monitoring was used, some conclusions may be reached regarding positive arrhythmic associations. In addition to the predisposing cardiac conditions (Table 1-1) or imposed imbalances (Table 1-2) that may cause arrhythmias, the incidence of cardiac arrhythmias is expected to be higher in patients with any of the following conditions or circumstances: (1) significant cardiovascular or major systemic disease (e.g., coronary disease, hypertension, congestive heart failure, diabetes, morbid obesity, chronic obstructive pulmonary disease); (2) preexisting arrhythmias and conduction disturbances; (3) undergoing major vascular, cardiothoracic, or intracranial surgery; (4) during induction and emergence from general endotracheal anesthesia; (5) during tracheal intubation or with painful or stressful surgical manipulation; and (6) traction on hollow viscera and the oculocardiac reflex. Nevertheless, it is still uncertain whether the type of anesthesia (regional versus general) or contemporary agents used affects the overall incidence of perioperative arrhythmias. There is no question that older anesthetic agents, especially chloroform and cyclopropane, did affect the incidence of at least ventricular arrhythmias. A recent multicenter study reported an overall 70.2 percent incidence of perioperative tachycardia, bradycardia, and arrhythmias in 17,201 patients having general anesthesia (Fig. 1-4).[5] The breakdown by category of rhythm disturbance and anesthetic agent is shown in Figure 1-5. The incidence of tachycardia and ventricular arrhythmias was significantly higher in patients receiving isoflurane and halothane, respectively. Tachycardia and bradycardia were defined in this study as deviations of more than

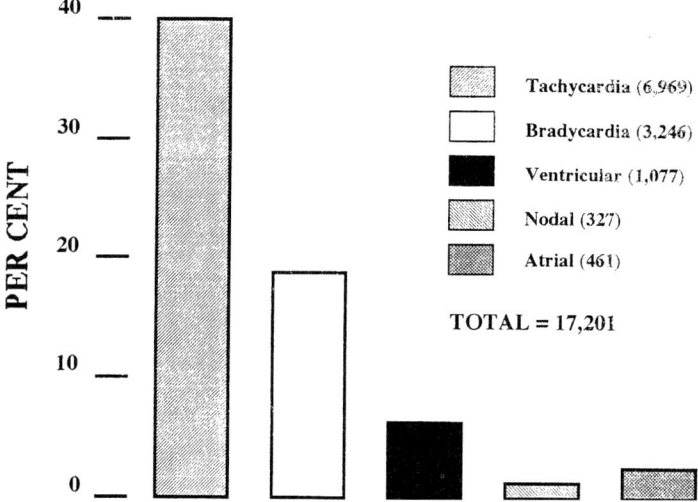

FIGURE 1-4 *Overall incidence of perioperative arrhythmias in the Multicenter Study of General Anesthesia (see text).*

20 percent from the value for heart rate recorded before induction of anesthesia, and the term *nodal rhythm* is synonymous with the term *AV junctional rhythm* used in this work.

INCIDENCE AND OUTCOMES

In a sequel to the report of the results of the Multicenter Study of General Anesthesia,[5] predictors of severe perioperative outcomes were determined.[4] Severity of outcomes from perioperative arrhythmias was coded 1 to 5 (Table 1–5), with major occurrences or death considered "severe" (code 3 to 5) adverse outcomes.[4] Absence of full recovery (Table 1–5) meant that treatment failed to fully reverse the condition, although the latter was not further defined. The percentage of patients with arrhythmias associated with severe adverse outcomes is shown for each anesthetic in Figure 1–6. Note that severe adverse outcomes related to tachycardia were more likely to occur in patients who had received isoflurane (1.3 percent incidence), and those related to ventricular arrhythmias were more likely in those who had received halothane (1.6 percent incidence). Significant ($P \leq 0.05$) predictors for severe outcomes from arrhythmias are shown in Table 1–6.[4]

12 PERSPECTIVES ON ARRHYTHMIAS AND PACEMAKERS

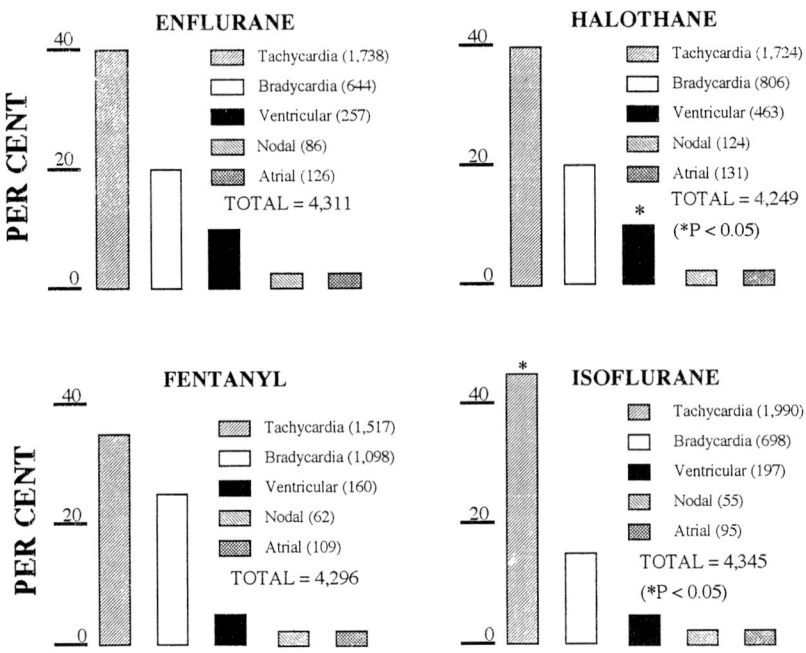

FIGURE 1-5 *Incidence of perioperative arrhythmias in patients receiving enflurane, fentanyl, halothane, or isoflurane in the Multicenter Study of General Anesthesia (see text).*

TABLE 1-5 *Outcomes in the Multicenter Study of General Anesthesia**

OUTCOME	DEFINITION
Code 1	Transient occurrence; no treatment; full recovery
Code 2	Minor occurrence; some treatment; full recovery
Code 3	Major occurrence; significant treatment; ± full recovery
Code 4	Major occurrence; cardiopulmonary resuscitation; ± full recovery
Code 5	Death

*SOURCE: Forrest et al.,[5] Appendix Form B, Anesthesiology 1990;72:262–268.

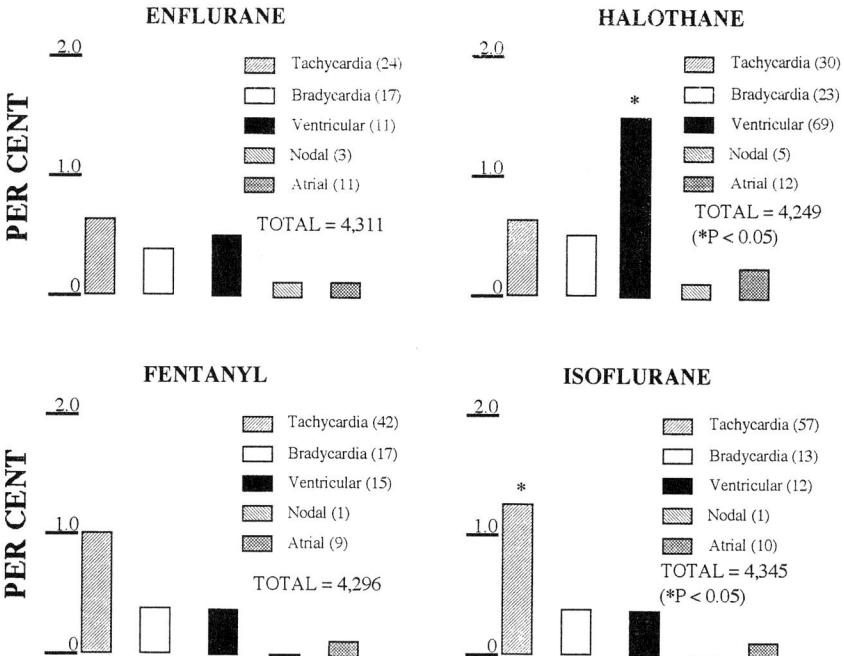

FIGURE 1-6 *Percentage of patients with severe outcomes (Table 1-5) related to arrhythmias, and receiving enflurane, fentanyl, halothane, or isoflurane in the Multicenter Study of General Anesthesia (see text).*

ESTIMATE OF ADVERSE OUTCOMES FROM PERIOPERATIVE ARRHYTHMIAS

Most patients (90.7 percent) in the Multicenter Study of General Anesthesia were ASA Physical Status 1 or 2,[5] yet there was an incidence of up to 1.6 percent of severe outcomes from bradycardia, tachycardia, or arrhythmias. While the Multicenter Study found a significant correlation only for ASA status 2–4 and severe outcomes from atrial arrhythmias (Table 1–6), the incidence of severe adverse outcomes from bradycardia, tachycardia, and other arrhythmias is also expected to be higher with advanced ASA status. It is not certain what the average ASA status of United States surgical patients is. Assuming that (1) the Multicenter Study included a representative surgical population, (2) approximately 25 million United States patients each year undergo surgery (Hospital Statistics—1992, American Hospital Association), (3) 60 percent of surgical patients receive

TABLE 1-6 *Significant predictors for bradycardia, tachycardia, or cardiac arrhythmias associated with severe outcomes*[*]

PREDICTOR	ARRHYTHMIA
Hypertension	Tachycardia; bradycardia
Myocardial ischemia	Ventricular arrhythmia; bradycardia
MI > 1 year	Tachycardia; ventricular arrhythmia
Ventricular arrhythmia	Ventricular arrhythmia
Gynecologic surgery	Tachycardia
Abdominal surgery	Tachycardia; ventricular arrhythmia
EEENT surgery	Tachycardia
Cardiovascular surgery	Tachycardia; ventricular/atrial arrhythmia
ASA status 2–4	Atrial arrhythmia
Smoking	Tachycardia
Study anesthetic[†]	Tachycardia; ventricular arrhythmias

*Based on data in the multicenter study of general anesthesia, III. Forrest et al.,[4] Anesthesiology 1992;76:3–15.
†Fentanyl, halothane, isoflurane.

some form of general anesthesia, and (4) there is a 1.6 percent risk of adverse outcomes from bradycardia, tachycardia, or arrhythmias, more than 200 thousand patients each year appear at risk of severe adverse outcomes from arrhythmias defined as bradycardia, tachycardia, or atrial, AV junctional (nodal), or ventricular rhythm disturbances.[4,5] This estimate might be conservative, since types of severe adverse outcomes[4,5] were not defined (Table 1–5). There are many possible types of adverse outcomes from cardiac arrhythmias (Table 1–7), and some of these may have been excluded. Thus, whether perioperative arrhythmias are considered from the perspective of incidence or potential for adverse outcomes, they do appear to represent a significant public health problem.

Pacemakers and Internal Cardioversion-Defibrillation Devices

HISTORICAL NOTES

The history of anesthesia and cardiac electrotherapy (i.e., pacing and cardioversion-defibrillation) are intertwined. The rising frequency of

TABLE 1-7 *Expanded list of possible adverse outcomes from cardiac arrhythmias*

ARRHYTHMIA	POSSIBLE ADVERSE OUTCOMES
Bradycardia	Reduction in vital organ or tissue perfusion causing stroke, myocardial infarction, splanchnic or renal damage, or death
Tachycardia	Myocardial ischemia and injury; reduction in cardiac output leading to permanent vital organ or tissue injury, or death
Atrial	Thromboembolic phenomena (AFIB-FLUT); otherwise, same as for bradycardia or tachycardia, including death
AV junctional	Reduction in cardiac output leading to permanent vital organ or tissue injury, or death
Ventricular	Myocardial ischemia and injury; reduction in cardiac output leading to permanent vital organ or tissue injury, or death
Arrhythmias in general	Added cost of treatment for arrhythmias or complications; risk of untoward effects from the treatment itself

operating room misadventrues following the introduction of chloroform anesthesia gave impetus to efforts at human electroresuscitation in hospital settings. Previous resuscitation attempts had been directed almost exclusively at victims of drowning or gas asphyxiation. Althaus in 1864 had demonstrated to members of the Royal Medical and Chirurgical Society of London that direct electrical shocks (termed "electropuncture") to the heart of two dogs could reverse arrest of the heart produced by chloroform.[26] Encouraged by similar successes in several dozen trials on sundry animals, Steiner performed electropuncture on a patient in Professor Bilroth's clinic in 1870. From Schechter:[26] "A young woman in whom chloroform narcosis was attempted promptly developed progressive syncope. All resuscitative measures were unsuccessful, including galvanism directed to the heart. Finally, a feeble current through an inserted needle proved effective. The excitability of the heart was soon reestablished."

The modern era of cardiac pacing and electroversion (i.e., DC cardioversion-defibrillation) had its inception in the early 1950s with the development of ventricular defibrillators and transcutaneous cardiac stimulation for Adams–Stokes syndrome (i.e., symptomatic bradycardia from heart block).[26,27] The high incidence of

AV heart block following open heart surgery for repair of valvular or congenital lesions provided the impetus for implantation of the first permanent (epicardial) pacemakers in 1958 by Senning and Elmqvist. Transvenous pacing leads were first used in 1962, demand pacing in 1963, and dual-chamber (AV sequential) pacing shortly thereafter. The pioneering work of Kouwenhoven and colleagues at Johns Hopkins in the early 1950s was the basis for later work by Mirowski, which led to the first successful animal testing in 1969 of internal (implantable) cardioverter-defibrillator (ICD) devices. However, ICD devices were not used in patients until 1980.

ELECTROTHERAPY VERSUS DRUGS FOR ARRHYTHMIAS

There are a number of potential disadvantages of drugs as treatment for cardiac arrhythmias, particularly in patients with severely impaired myocardial function. All antiarrhythmic drugs are direct or indirect cardiovascular depressants, in that they slow heart rate, impair conduction, depress myocardial contractility, cause arterial or venous vasodilation, or interfere with autonomic compensatory mechanisms. Disadvantages of antiarrhythmic drugs are summarized in Table 1-8.

In contrast, cardiac pacing and DC cardioversion-defibrillation have a number of advantages over drugs for treating arrhythmias (Table 1-9). This is not to say that electrotherapy will not on occasion fail to terminate or suppress arrhythmias, or initiate new ones.

TABLE 1-8 *Disadvantages of antiarrhythmic drugs*

Delayed onset of action	Variable duration of action
Difficult to titrate to effect	Unpleasant side effects
Adverse circulatory effects	Adverse drug interactions
Difficult to reverse effects	May cause proarrhythmia
Untoward bradycardia	Depress AV conduction

TABLE 1-9 *Advantages of electrotherapy for cardiac arrhythmias*

Immediate onset of action	Precise control of duration
Easier to titrate effects	Lacks side effects of drugs
Little effect on hemodynamics	No adverse drug interactions
Adverse effects easier to reverse	Less proarrhythmic potential

However, the practitioner has far more control over electrotherapy than is possible with drugs. Further, since drugs are frequently the cause of imbalance that provokes arrhythmias in perioperative and critical care settings, it would seem prudent to make more use of electrotherapy.

PREVALENCE

There were an estimated 500,000 or more patients with permanent (implanted) cardiac pacemakers in the United States in 1991, and this number had remained fairly constant over the previous decade.[28] The North American Society for Pacing and Electrophysiology (NASPE) estimated that in 1995, up to 100,000 new patients in the United States would receive pacemaker implants. Today, about half the patients receiving new pacemakers have them prescribed for symptomatic AV heart block,[29] with most of the remainder prescribed for symptomatic bradycardia due to sinus node dysfunction. One to two percent of patients have devices that are also programmed to terminate tachyarrhythmias, some with back-up cardioversion-defibrillation.[28]

The number of patients with ICD devices is more difficult to estimate, because the field is rapidly expanding. NASPE estimated that up to 30,000 patients in the United States would receive ICD devices in 1995. Sudden cardiac death, typically due to ventricular tachyarrhythmia, is a leading cause of death in the United States affecting up to 400,000 persons annually. Many of these persons might have been candidates for an ICD device, had it been possible to stratify risk. Appreciation that drugs are not ideal preventive therapy,[12,13] improved risk stratification, and increased availability of reliable ICD systems (including ones with antitachycardia and back-up bradycardia pacing) have made ICD therapy more attractive as preventive therapy. As a result, the number of individuals with ICD devices will likely increase substantially over the next decade. By the end of 1991, there was a worldwide experience of 25,000 implants with one manufacturer's device (AICD™, Cardiac Pacemakers, Inc. [CPI], St. Paul, MN).[30] Since then, other ICD devices have been approved (Pacer-Cardioverter-Defibrillator [PCD™, Transvene PCD™], Medtronic, Minneapolis, MN; Ventak™/Endotak™ System, CPI; Cadence™, Ventritex, Sunnyvale, CA; and others), so that possibly more than 80,000 persons had received some type of ICD device in the United States by 1995. However, because of underlying cardiovascular and other systemic disease, many are not alive today.

Anesthesia and critical care practitioners in larger referral centers are more likely to encounter patients with pacing or ICD devices than their colleagues elsewhere. Apart from significant cardiovascular and systemic disease, the chief concern with pacing and ICD devices is the potential for malfunction stemming from electromagnetic or mechanical interference in surgical and critical care environments (see Chapter 8).

CONCURRENT DISEASE

As mentioned earlier, the most common indication for pacemaker implantation is symptomatic bradycardia, whether from AV heart block or sinus node dysfunction. Both of these conditions are commonly the result of advancing age, coronary artery disease, or other myocardial degenerative processes. Consequently, these patients often have severely impaired cardiac function, along with other major systemic (central nervous system, endocrine, pulmonary, renal disease). Further, they may be receiving multiple-drug therapy that increases their potential for adverse effects and interactions in perioperative and critical care environments. Patients with ICD devices usually have the most severe cardiac functional impairment and associated systemic disease, especially if the device has been implanted for prevention of sudden death from ventricular tacharrhythmias complicating chronic MI or end-stage cardiomyopathy.

TEMPORARY PACING

Much imbalance that causes or aggravates serious cardiac rhythm disturbances in critical care and perioperative settings is transient. Transient imbalance can often be attributed to the untoward effects of drugs and drug interactions, or to inappropriate therapeutic and corrective interventions. If so, it makes little sense to compound such imbalance by the addition of still more drugs, especially if the rhythm disturbance is prevented or treated by temporary cardiac pacing. Some tachyarrhythmias, however, must first be treated by electroversion, without attempts at pacing: (1) DC cardioversion for tachycardia with life-threatening circulatory compromise; and (2) DC defibrillation for ventricular fibrillation or tachycardia when R(S) waves cannot be distinguished from T waves. Pacing may then be provided for prevention of recurrences, especially if bradycardia predisposes to tachycardia. Nevertheless, distinct limitations to more widespread use of temporary pacing have been that reliable methods (transvenous or epicardial pacing) are too invasive, and noninvasive methods (transesophageal or transcutaneous pacing) are limited to single chamber pacing (see Chapter 7). However, expected developments in transesophageal pacing may remove these limitations (see Chapter 7).

Approach to Management

In contrast to arrhythmias managed by cardiologists, an arrhythmia in the perioperative or critical care setting is rarely the patient's central problem. It may become the central problem or a significant annoyance because of the imposed imbalance occasioned by the circumstances of the perioperative or critical care environment. If so, provided the cardiac rhythm disturbance is not life-threatening, the immediate management goal is more to remove or correct the underlying imbalance and institute measures to prevent recurrences, rather than to provide definitive antiarrhythmic treatment.

CORRECT DIAGNOSIS

The importance of correct diagnosis for cardiac rhythm disturbances can never be stressed enough, given the possible dangers with improper or overly aggressive treatment discussed above. This is especially true when diagnosing wide QRS complex tachycardias. Just because the QRS complex is widened or bizarre and there is hemodynamic compromise (Fig. 1–3), does not mean one should administer a syringe of lidocaine. Not only would lidocaine be ineffective for the disturbance shown in Figure 1–3, but it might also increase the ventricular rate.

HEMODYNAMIC IMPACT

What is the hemodynamic impact of the rhythm disturbance? Do not treat unless there is reason to; rather, correct the cause. Again, given the potential dangers of drugs used to treat arrhythmias, one should withhold definitive treatment unless there is severe circulatory compromise. Even with some circulatory compromise, time taken to find and correct or remove inciting factors will reduce the need for specific antiarrhythmic treatment, or make subsequent specific treatment more effective.

FIRST CORRECT THE IMBALANCE

While this caveat has been repeatedly mentioned, it merits further amplification. The approach to management of a new or worsening cardiac rhythm disturbance, particularly in the perioperative or critical care setting, should be no different from that to other unexpected circulatory imbalances, such as hypotension or hypertension. The rhythm disturbance should first be viewed as a sign of some imposed imbalance: The rhythm disturbance was not there a minute ago, but now is. What happened; and why? Maybe the wrong drug was given, or too much or not enough drug. Or maybe the patient was hypokalemic and the respiratory alkalosis produced by mechanical ventilation worsened the hypokalemia. Or the patient was anesthetized too lightly, triggering a catecholamine surge, hypertension, sinus tachycardia, and perhaps atrial or ventricular tachyarrhythmia, depending on the underlying cardiac pathophysiology and other factors (Fig. 1-7). Initial treatment in this circumstance is not necessarily with antiarrhythmic drugs or a cardioverter. It does include deepening anesthesia and perhaps giving a short-acting beta-adrenergic blocker.

DEFINITIVE TREATMENT

Some arrhythmias do require more definitive initial treatment. However, such treatment is more likely to be effective if directed at the altered cardiac electrophysiology responsible for the arrhythmia or sustaining it (see Chapter 2). Treatment should never be haphazard, but rather carefully thought out and measured. For example, VT with acute myocardial infarction should respond to lidocaine, but that with chronic infarction might be more responsive to procainamide, sotolol or amiodarone (see Chapters 5 and 10). Similarly, for VT due to a catecholamine surge (Fig. 1-7), while lidocaine may be effective, a short-acting beta-blocker such as esmolol is more specific and sometimes more effective.

Summary

New or worsening cardiac arrhythmias within the context of anesthesia and critical care are often the result of transient physiologic imbalance, which may or may not be imposed on underlying structural heart disease (a "substrate") conducive to arrhythmias. This suggests that correction or removal of the imbalance may be sufficient treatment, which is important considering the risk of untoward effects with more specific treatment by drugs or ICD devices. The working definition for what constitutes a cardiac arrhythmia is more than just ECG appearance alone, since sinus bradycardia at 30 beats/min with severe circulatory compromise might not be considered an arrhythmia. In addition to appearance, the practitioner must also consider the functional consequences. For example, seemingly innocuous AV junctional rhythm in a patient with ischemic cardiomyopathy may be as dangerous as VT. Alternatively, sinus bradycardia in patients with

PERSPECTIVES ON ARRHYTHMIAS AND PACEMAKERS   **21**

```
                          LIGHT ANESTHESIA
                                 ↓
                      ┌─────────────────────┐
                      │ CATECHOLAMINE SURGE │
                      └─────────────────────┘
                                 ↓
                      ┌─────────────────────┐
                      │ Tachycardia, ↑ Wall Tension │
                      │   & Vascular Resistance     │
                      └─────────────────────┘
```

Normal Heart & no Systemic Disease	Coronary Disease (chronic & ischemia)	COPD, ↑ PVR, CHF by Hx, Cardiac Myopathies	WPW, AFIB-FLUT, any Non-sinus SVT
Sinus Tachycardia	Ventricular Extrasystoles	Atrial Extrasystoles	Reciprocating Tachycardia, Non-sinus SVT
(or)	(or)	(or)	(or)
Ventricular Arrhythmias with Sensitization	Ventricular Tachycardia/ Fibrillation	AFIB-FLUT AAT-MAT	Fast AFIB-FLUT
		(or)	(or)
		Ventricular Arrhythmias	Ventricular Fibrillation (WPW)

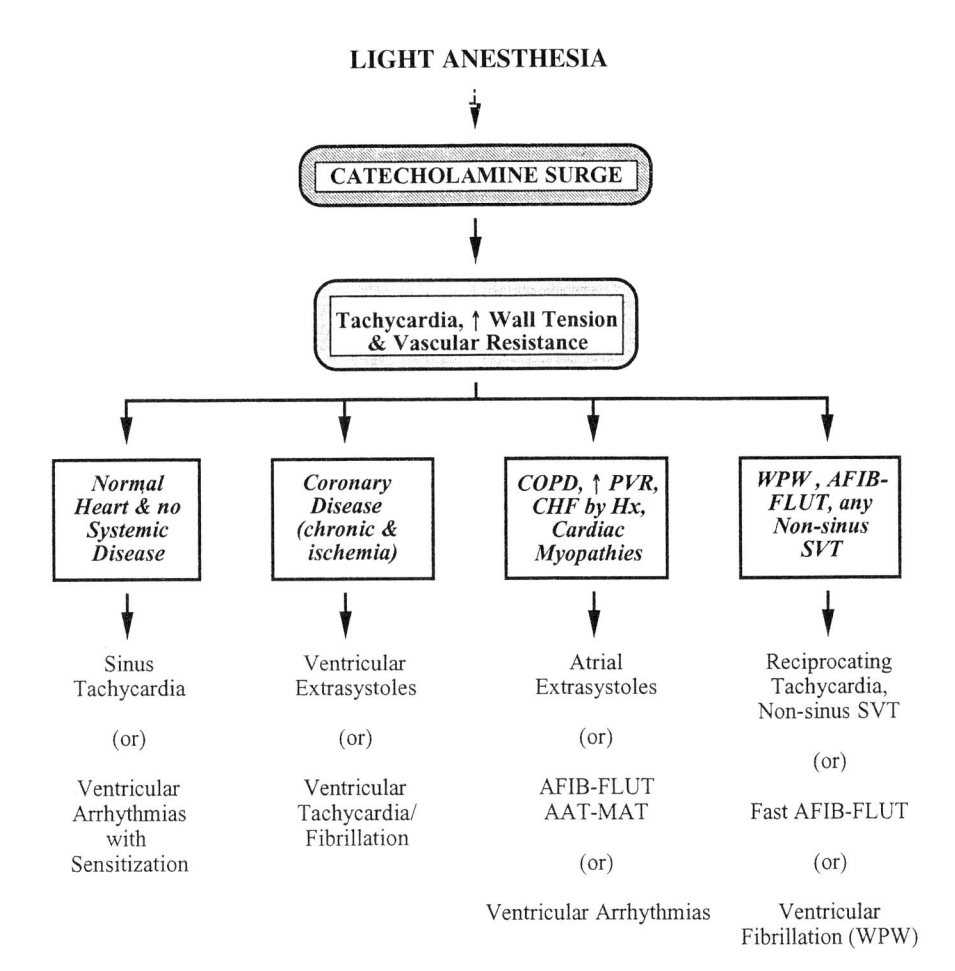

FIGURE 1-7 *A catecholamine surge produced by too light anesthesia can trigger a variety of atrial or ventricular arrhythmias depending on the circumstances. Common to all patients will be initial sinus tachycardia, increased ventricular wall tension, and increased systemic and pulmonary vascular resistance (PVR) due to the alpha- and beta-stimulating effects of catecholamines. Shown are the types of arrhythmias that might be facilitated by catecholamines in patients with normal hearts and no systemic disease or the specified conditions. COPD, chronic obstructive pulmonary disease; CHF by Hx, congestive heart failure by history; AFIB-FLUT, atrial flutter or fibrillation; AAT-MAT, automatic or multiform atrial tachycardia; SVT, supraventricular tachycardia.*

acquired Q–T interval prolongation may predispose to life-threatening torsades de pointes VT, or atrial flutter-fibrillation to ventricular fibrillation in patients with the WPW syndrome.

The incidence of cardiac arrhythmias depends on both the definition of the term (morphologic, functional, or both) and methods used for surveillance. With continuous ECG surveillance, incidence can exceed 80 percent in some surgical populations. With visual inspection only in a general population of surgical patients, it may be below 30 percent. Aside from medical conditions that predispose to arrhythmias, the incidence of arrhythmias in perioperative and critical care settings is increased with structural heart and major systemic disease, as well as patients having cardiothoracic, major vascular, and intracranial surgery. Cardiac arrhythmias within the context of anesthesia and critical care are an important public health problem in terms of patient morbidity and mortality, as well as increased costs of treatment and hospitalization. It can be estimated that 200 thousand or more patients in the United States each year will suffer adverse outcomes from arrhythmias, measured as the need for significant additional treatment or cardiopulmonary resuscitation, with or without full recovery or death. This definition does not include the added cost of treatment itself or that of complications.

Management of cardiac arrhythmias in anesthesia and critical care has usually been mostly with drugs, except for those post-cardiac surgical patients with epicardial pacing. This is not ideal, since drugs are often implicated as the cause of or a contributing factor to arrhythmias. There are other limitations to drugs as well, chief among which are their unpredictable onset and duration of action, and untoward side effects. Cardiac pacing and electroversion are much more attractive, since their onset of effect is immediate and they cause fewer adverse effects. Additionally, dose (i.e., paced pulses/min, current for shocks) is precisely and easily regulated. However, a distinct limitation to more widespread use of pacing has been the lack of reliable noninvasive methods. This will likely soon change with recent advances in noninvasive temporary cardiac pacing.

References

1. Atlee JL. Perioperative cardiac dysrhythmias in perspective. In Perioperative Cardiac Dysrhythmias. 2nd ed. Chicago: Year Book Medical Publishers, 1990: pp. 1–13.
2. Katz RL, Bigger JJ Jr. Cardiac arrhythmias during anesthesia and operation. Anesthesiology 1970;33:193–213.

3. Atlee JL, Bosnjak ZJ. Mechanisms for cardiac dysrhythmias during anesthesia. Anesthesiology 1990;72:347–374.
4. Forrest JB, Rehder K, Cahalan MK, Goldsmith CH. Multicenter Study of General Anesthesia. III. Predictors of severe perioperative adverse outcomes. Anesthesiology 1992;76:3–15.
5. Forrest JB, Cahalan MK, Rehder K, et al. Multicenter Study of General Anesthesia. II. Results. Anesthesiology 1990;72:262–268.
6. Lown B, Wolff M. Approaches to sudden death from coronary heart disease. Circulation 1971;44:130–142.
7. Myerburg RJ, Kessler KM, Luceri RM, et al. Classification of ventricular arrhythmias based on parallel hierarchies of frequency and form. Am J Cardiol 1984;54:1355–1358.
8. Surawicz B. Ventricular arrhythmias: Why is it so difficult to find a pharmacologic cure? J Am Coll Cardiol 1989;14:1401–1416.
9. Lowery N, De Marchena EJ, Castellanos A, et al. Interrelationship of variable coupling, multiformity and repetitive forms: Implications for classification of ventricular arrhythmias. Am Heart J 1990;119:301–307.
10. Zipes DP. Proarrhythmic events. Am J Cardiol 1988;61:70A–75A.
11. Creamer JE, Nathan AW, Camm AJ. The proarrhythmic effects of antiarrhythmic drugs. Am Heart J 1987;114:397–406.
12. The Cardiac Arrhythmia Suppression Trial (CAST) Investigators. Preliminary report: Effect of encainide and flecainide on mortality in a randomized trial of arrhythmia suppression after myocardial infarction. N Engl J Med 1989;321:406–412.
13. The Cardiac Arrhythmia Suppression Trial II Investigators. Effect of the antiarrhythmic agent moricizine on survival after myocardial infarction. N Engl J Med 1992;217:227–233.
14. Anderson JL. Reassessment of benefit–risk ratio and treatment alogorithms for antiarrhythmic drug therapy after the cardiac arrhythmia suppression trial. J Clin Pharmacol 1990;30:981–989.
15. Coumel P. Future trends in antiarrhythmic therapy. J Cardiovasc Pharmacol 1991;17:S95–S100.
16. Smith JJ, Kampine JP. Circulatory Physiology: The Essentials. 3rd ed. Baltimore: Williams & Wilkins, 1990: pp. 31–46.
17. Harvey W. Movement of the heart and blood in animals. An anatomical essay (translated by Franklin). Oxford, England: Blackwell Scientific, 1957: p. 34.
18. Gesell RA. Auricular systole and its relation to ventricular output. Am J Physiol 1911;29:32–63.
19. Gesell RA. Cardiodynamics in heart block as affected by auricular systole, auricular fibrillation and stimulation of the vagus nerve. Am J Physiol 1916;40:267–313.
20. Atlee JL 3d, Pattison CZ, Mathews EL, Hedman AG. Transesophageal atrial pacing for intraoperative sinus bradycardia or AV junctional rhythm: Feasibility as prophylaxis in 200 anesthetized adults and hemodynamic effects of treatment. J Cardiothorac Vasc Anesth 1993;7:436–441.

21. Packer M. Abnormalities of diastolic function as a potential cause of exercise intolerance in chronic heart failure. Circulation 1980;81 (Suppl. III):78–86.
22. Dean JW, Poole-Wilson PA. Therapeutic implications of diastolic dysfunction in heart failure. Postgrad Med J 1990;66:932–937.
23. Bonow RO. Regional left ventricular nonuniformity. Effects on left ventricular diastolic function in ischemic heart disease, hypertrophic myopathy, and the normal heart. Circulation 1990;81 (Suppl III):54–65.
24. Baig MW, Perrins EJ. The hemodynamics of cardiac pacing. Prog Cardiovasc Dis 1991;33:283–298.
25. Bosnjak ZJ, Warltier DC. New aspects of cardiac electrophysiology and function: Effects of inhalational anesthetics. In Conzen P, Peter K (eds): Inhalation Anaesthesia. Vol. 7. London: Bailliere-Tindall, 1993: pp. 937–960.
26. Schechter DC. Cardiac pacing in perspective. In Varriale P, Naclerio E (ed): Cardiac Pacing. Philadelphia: Lea & Febiger, 1979: pp. 1–12.
27. Platia EV, Watkins LJ, Mower MM, et al. Automatic implantable defibrillators. In Platia E (ed): Management of Cardiac Arrhythmias. Philadelphia: JB Lippincott, 1987: pp. 272–303.
28. Barold SS, Zipes DP. Cardiac pacemakers and antiarrhythmic devices. In Braunwald E (ed): Heart Disease. 4th ed. Philadelphia: WB Saunders, 1992: pp. 726–755.
29. Barold SS. ACC/AHA guidelines for implantation of cardiac pacemakers: How accurate are the definitions of atrioventricular and intraventricular conduction blocks? PACE 1993;16:1221–1226.
30. Holmes DJ. The implantable cardioverter defibrillator. In Furman S, Hayes DL, Holmes DJ (eds): A Practice of Cardiac Pacing. 3rd ed. Mt. Kisco, NY: Futura, 1993: pp. 465–508.

2

Overview of Mechanisms for Arrhythmias

Abbreviations Used in Chapter Two	
ATP	Adenosine tryphosphate
AP	Action potential
AV	Atrioventricular
DAD	Delayed afterdepolarization
DFR	Depressed fast response
EAD	Early afterdepolarization
ETP	Electrotonic potential
LMP	Loss of membrane potential
MDP	Maximum diastolic potential
MI	Myocardia infarction
RMP	Resting membrane potential
RRP	Relative refractory period
SA	Sinoatrial
SVT	Supraventricular tachycardia
TMP	Transmembrane potential

TP	Threshold potential
Vmax; phase 0	Maximum upstroke velocity
VT	Ventricular tachycardia
WPW	Wolff–Parkinson–White

The heart's primary function is to generate adequate cardiac output to meet changing body needs. To do this, atrial and ventricular contractions must be orderly and properly synchronized with each other. The function of the specialized cardiac conducting system is to generate and propagate the tiny electrical impulses required for excitation–contraction coupling in atrial and ventricular muscle. Autonomic modulation adapts this process to meet changing body needs.

SPECIALIZED CARDIAC CONDUCTING SYSTEM

The specialized cardiac conducting system includes automatic (pacemaker) and conducting fibers. Pacemaker fibers spontaneously depolarize to generate tiny electrical potentials (≤ 120 mV) termed *action potentials* (AP). Conducting fibers do not normally undergo spontaneous depolarization, and must be depolarized by propagating AP or external stimulation. AP generated by pacemaker fibers are propagated to the rest of the heart over preferential or specialized conducting pathways.

Normally, AP originate in the primary (dominant) pacemaker of the heart—the sinoatrial (SA) node. AP then propagate via preferential internodal conducting pathways to excite atrial tissue and the atrioventricular (AV) node (Fig. 2–1). While these internodal pathways are functionally discreet conducting pathways, they are not anatomically distinct (i.e., recognized on visual or histologic examination). At the AV node, the excitatory AP wavefront is delayed to provide adequate time for ventricular filling. It then propagates over anatomically distinct, specialized ventricular conducting pathways to both ventricles (Fig. 2-1). Any disruption in the rate, timing, or sequence of these processes for impulse generation and propagation constitutes some form of cardiac arrhythmia. Thus, cardiac arrhythmias can be viewed as primary disorders of impulse generation, impulse propagation, or both.

LATENT PACEMAKERS

If the SA node fails to generate AP for propagation to the rest of the heart, latent (or secondary, subsidiary) pacemaker fibers can assume

OVERVIEW OF MECHANISMS FOR ARRHYTHMIAS **27**

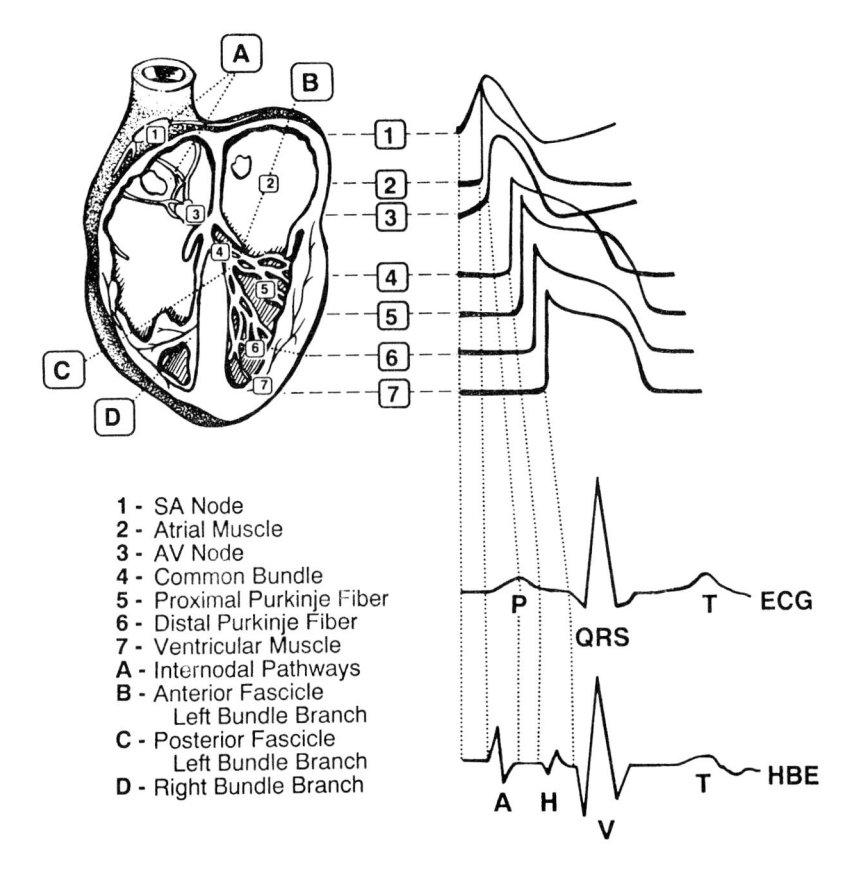

1 - SA Node
2 - Atrial Muscle
3 - AV Node
4 - Common Bundle
5 - Proximal Purkinje Fiber
6 - Distal Purkinje Fiber
7 - Ventricular Muscle
A - Internodal Pathways
B - Anterior Fascicle
    Left Bundle Branch
C - Posterior Fascicle
    Left Bundle Branch
D - Right Bundle Branch

FIGURE 2-1 *Depiction of the heart showing the approximate location of the primary pacemaker (SA node), atrial preferential (internodal) conducting pathways, AV node, bundle branches, left anterior and posterior fascicular branches, and the terminal Purkinje network. Representative AP from each of these locations are shown to the right. Note that the duration of AP from the fascicular branches (proximal Purkinje fibers) is longer than those of fibers from the terminal Purkinje network (distal Purkinje fibers). In turn, the timing of AP from the above locations is shown in relation to events of the surface electrocardiogram (ECG) and His bundle electrograms (HBE).*

pacemaker function. Latent pacemakers are found throughout the heart, and include (1) subsidiary atrial pacemakers along the sulcus terminalis from the classic SA node region to the inferior vena cava–atrial junction; (2) pacemaker fibers found in the AV valve leaflets, Bachmann's bundle, and coronary sinus; (3) junctional pacemakers at the upper and lower AV node margins; and (4) Purkinje fibers throughout the specialized ventricular conducting system.[1,2] Latent pacemakers probably do not exist within the AV node proper, hence the widespread preference for the term *AV junctional* versus *AV nodal* rhythm disturbances. The rate of automaticity of latent pacemakers is less than that of the SA node. Automaticity progressively decreases from the atria to ventricles, with intrinsic automaticity of subsidiary atrial, AV junctional, and Purkinje pacemaker fibers 80 to 85, 60 to 65, and 40 to 50 percent that of SA node fibers, respectively. SA node fibers are most affected by changes in autonomic tone, and Purkinje fibers least so. Finally, latent pacemakers are normally prevented from assuming control of the heart by overdrive suppression of automaticity by the SA node, as described later.

CARDIAC ELECTROPHYSIOLOGY

Basic cardiac electrophysiology is the study of normal and abnormal cellular mechanisms for the generation and propagation of cardiac AP. Studies in basic cardiac electrophysiology have contributed greatly to our current understanding of mechanisms for normal sinus rhythm and cardiac arrhythmias. Indeed, cellular mechanisms are fairly well established for most clinical arrhythmias. Consequently, contemporary therapy for arrhythmias, whether by drugs or devices, is targeted at interrupting one or more of the responsible electrophysiologic mechanisms. The following abbreviated account of normal and abnormal cardiac electrophysiology provides the basis for later discussion of the contributions of drugs and other imbalances to cardiac arrhythmias (see Chapter 3), and antiarrhythmic drug action (see Chapter 5). Postulated cellular electrophysiologic mechanisms for clinical arrhythmias are discussed at the end of this chapter.

Normal Cardiac Electrophysiology

Normal is distinguished from abnormal cardiac electrophysiology. Abnormal electrophysiologic phenomena result from the effects of disease, drugs, or other imbalances that change electrical properties of single or groups of cardiac cells. For example, cells that are not normally automatic might become so. Or, the propagating AP wavefront does not die out once all tissue in front of it has been excited, but instead continues to circulate as reentrant beats or rhythm. Triggered sustained rhythmic activity is yet another abnormal electrophysiologic phenomenon. Abnormal electrophysiologic properties will be discussed in more detail later.

CARDIAC CELL MEMBRANE

The cardiac cell membrane (sarcolemma) is a phospholipid bilayer, with a nonpolar hydrophobic core and a polar hydrophilic surface. The sarcolemma provides a high-resistance enclosure for the cell, one that is selectively permeable to biologic ionic species. Ions move across the sarcolemma through ion-specific, voltage-gated, protein channels that span the entire membrane.[3] In addition to membrane ion channels, other sarcolemmal protein complexes serve as receptors for hormones and neuro- and cellular transmitters, or as supplementary active or passive ion transport pumps.

TRANSMEMBRANE POTENTIAL AND TERMINOLOGY

The transmembrane potential (TMP) is recorded by inserting microelectrodes with tip diameters of approximately 0.5 μm into single cardiac cells. Two types of TMP are recorded: (1) *resting membrane potential* (RMP), the TMP recorded during electrical diastole (quiescence) in working atrial and ventricular, and nonautomatic Purkinje fibers; and (2) *action potential* (AP), the changes in the TMP after the cell is brought to threshold potential for regenerative depolarization. Quiescent fibers with stable RMP do not undergo spontaneous depolarization during diastole. They must rely on the propagating AP wavefront to bring them to threshold potential. In contrast, primary and latent pacemaker fibers do not have stable RMP. They slowly depolarize during diastole until they reach threshold potential or are depolarized first by propagating AP, a property termed *automaticity*. Therefore, for automatic fibers the term corresponding to RMP is *maximum diastolic potential* (MDP), the maximum TMP reached during diastole. AP for the principal cardiac fiber types are shown in Figure 2–1, with AP characteristics for these fiber types provided in Table 2–1.[4]

The terminology used to describe changes in the TMP is illustrated in Figure 2–2. Depolarization during the cardiac AP makes the TMP more positive (or less negative), and repolarization restores the TMP to its former, more negative (or less positive) potential. A "higher" level of TMP is more negative than the reference value. *Loss of membrane potential* (LMP) means that the RMP (MDP in automatic fibers) is less negative than the reference value. Finally, if the RMP becomes more negative than normal, it is said to be *hyperpolarized* (Fig. 2–2).

TABLE 2-1 *AP characteristics for different cardiac fiber types*

CHARAC-TERISTIC	SA NODE	ATRIA	AV NODE	PURKINJE	VENTRI-CLES
RMP or MDP (mV)	−50 to −60	−80 to −90	−60 to −70	−90 to −95	−80 to −90
Amplitude (mV)	60 to 70	110 to 120	70 to 80	120	110 to 120
Overshoot (mV)	1 to 10	30	5 to 15	30	30
Duration (msec)	100 to 300	100 to 300	100 to 300	300 to 500	200 to 300
Vmax, phase 0 (V/sec)	1 to 10	100 to 200	5 to 15	500 to 700	100 to 200
Conduction (m/sec)	< 0.05	0.3 to 0.4	0.1	2 to 3	0.3 to 0.4

Data from Sperelakis[4], Origin of the cardiac resting potential. In Berne R (ed): Handbook of Physiology. Section 2. The Cardiovascular System. Vol. 1: The Heart. Bethesda, MD: American Physiological Society, 1979, pp. 187–267.

CARDIAC ACTION POTENTIAL

The AP of a quiescent Purkinje fiber has five distinct phases (Fig. 2–2): (1) *phase 0*, upstroke or rapid depolarization; (2) *phase 1*, early rapid repolarization; (3) *phase 2*, the plateau phase; (4) *phase 3*, final rapid repolarization; and (5) *phase 4*, RMP in quiescent fibers, and diastolic potential in automatic fibers—not strictly part of the cardiac AP. That portion of the AP during phases 0 and 1 when membrane potential is positive to 0 mV is termed the *overshoot* (Fig. 2–2).

Ionic currents and exchange mechanisms responsible for the RMP and AP, ion concentrations during the RMP, and refractory periods are illustrated in Figure 2–3. The ionic basis for the cardiac RMP and AP, summarized below, is discussed in more detail elsewhere.[4-10]

BASIS FOR RESTING MEMBRANE POTENTIAL (PHASE 4)

During phase 4, the sarcolemma is quite permeable to potassium, relatively impermeable to other ions (e.g., sodium, calcium, and chloride), and virtually impermeable to large, intracellular, anionic protein species. As a direct result, and also because of the sodium–potassium exchange pump (Fig. 2–3), the intracellular sodium and

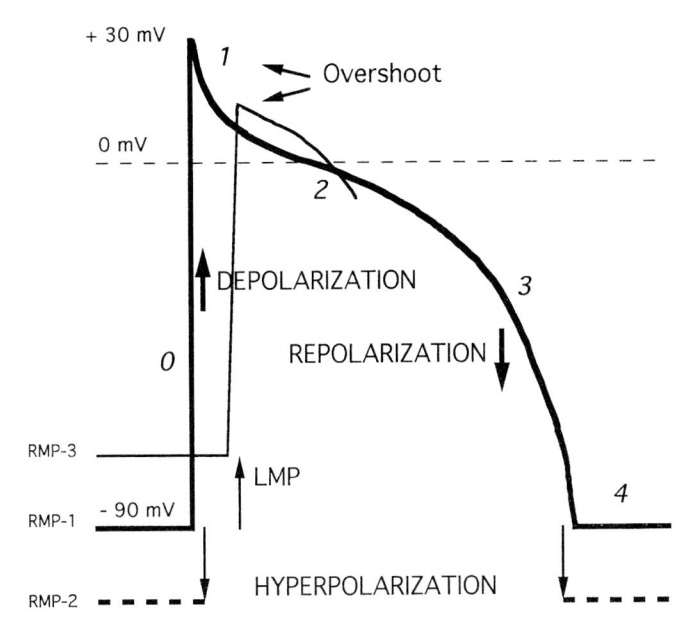

FIGURE 2-2 *Schematic of cardiac AP from a quiescent Purkinje fiber showing the five AP phases and terminology used to describe TMP changes.* With **depolarization, the TMP is more positive;** and with **repolarization, more negative.** With **hyperpolarization, the RMP is more negative than normal. If the RMP is reduced by the effects of disease, loss of membrane potential (LMP) has occurred. Overshoot describes that portion of the AP during phase 0 or 1 when the TMP is positive to 0 mV.**

potassium concentrations are low and high, respectively, with the inside of the cell negative with respect to the outside. The membrane-bound sodium–potassium exchange pump depends on energy supplied by hydrolysis of adenosine triphosphate (ATP), and transports three sodium ions out of the cell for two transported into the cell during phase 4. This pump is electrogenic because it generates net outward current. Also, depending on TMP and the sodium and calcium concentrations inside and outside the cell, a non-ATP-dependent sodium–calcium exchanger can run in the forward or reverse direction to move these ionic species inside or outside the cell (Fig. 2–3). Finally, in parallel with the sodium–calcium exchanger, an ATP-dependent calcium transport system also exists in the sarcolemmal membrane (Fig. 2–3).

32 OVERVIEW OF MECHANISMS FOR ARRHYTHMIAS

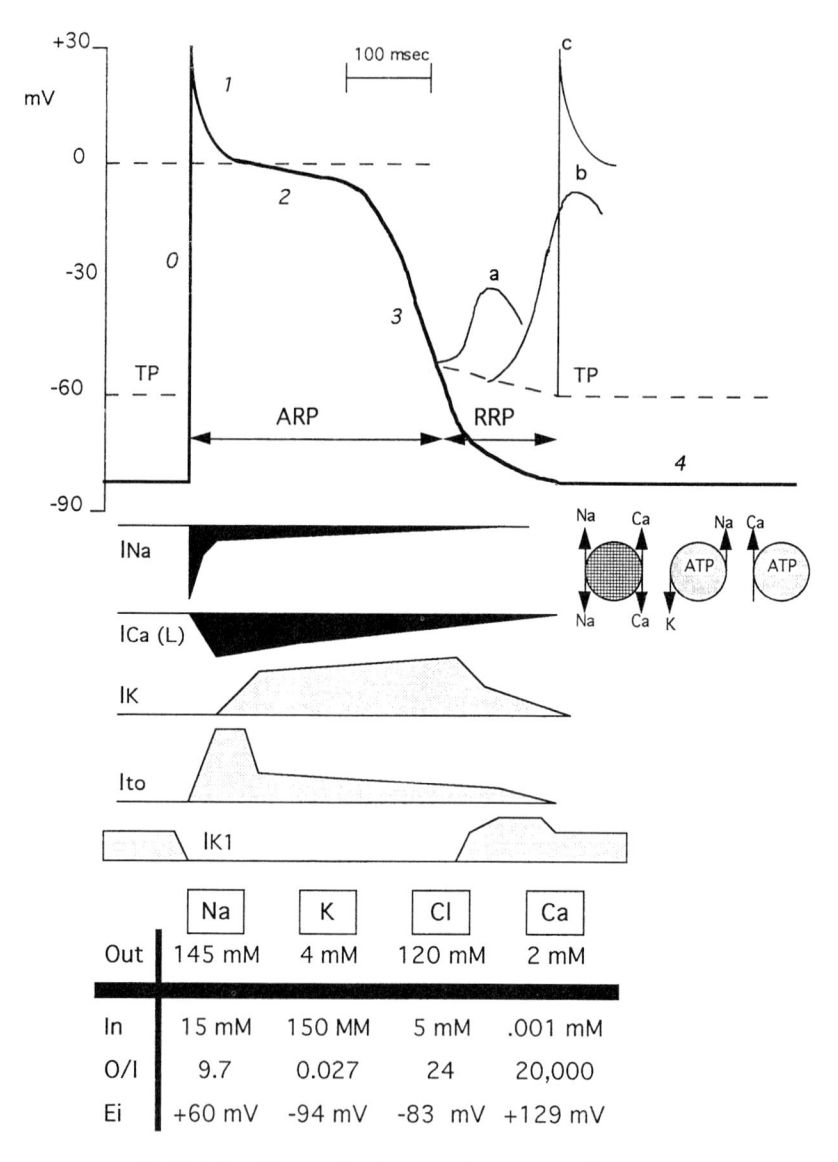

	Na	K	Cl	Ca
Out	145 mM	4 mM	120 mM	2 mM
In	15 mM	150 MM	5 mM	.001 mM
O/I	9.7	0.027	24	20,000
Ei	+60 mV	-94 mV	-83 mV	+129 mV

FIGURE 2-3   *See legend on opposite page*

BASIS FOR THE ACTION POTENTIAL
Phase 0 (Upstroke)

The depolarizing stimulus, usually the propagating AP, must be of sufficient strength to reduce membrane potential to the threshold potential (TP) for a regenerative ("all-or-none") depolarization. The TP is about − 60 mV in Purkinje fibers. Once the TP has been reached, regenerative depolarization produces an AP that can be propagated to adjacent fibers. Small depolarizing stimuli, which do not bring the cell to the TP, result in nonpropagated AP, termed *electrotonic potentials* (Fig. 2–3). These are important because they can affect the conduction of subsequent propagating AP through electrotonic interactions. Phase 0 depolarization in *fast-response fibers* (atrial and ventricular muscle, Purkinje fibers) is largely dependent on the fast inward current (I_{Na}, Fig. 2–3) carried mainly by sodium through ion-specific membrane protein channels. Fast-response fibers have rapid maximum upstroke velocities, and high RMP, amplitudes and overshoots (Table 2–1). In contrast, in *slow-response fibers* (SA and AV node fibers), depolarization during phase 0 is largely dependent on the slow inward current (I_{Ca}, Fig. 2–3), carried mainly by calcium through ion-selective membrane protein channels.

FIGURE 2-3 *Representation of the five AP phases of a quiescent Purkinje fiber, along with the major ionic currents (I_{Na}, $I_{Ca(L)}$, I_K, I_{to}, I_{K1}) responsible for AP depolarization and repolarization. Inward currents are shown in black, and outward ones in gray, with the relative timing and magnitude of each shown only as rough approximations. The five AP phases are the result of selective membrane permeability to individual ions, changes in intracellular ion concentrations during inscription of the AP, and active or passive ion-exchange mechanisms that restore intracellular concentrations of ions during phase 4. Individual ion concentrations outside (Out) and inside (In) the cell during phase 4 are shown below, along with their respective outside/inside ratios (O/I) during phase 4 and ionic equilibrium potentials (Ei). Finally, during the absolute refractory period (ARP), the fiber is inexcitable. During the relative refractory period (RRP), only small electrotonic potentials ("a" and "b") that cannot be propagated occur. At the end of the RRP, a normal AP ("c") capable of propagation occurs. Note that the TP is more positive during the RRP.*

Two types of inward calcium current exist in cardiac fibers: (1) the *long-lasting, large or "L-type,"* a slowly inactivating, high-threshold, dihydropyridine-sensitive current ($I_{Ca(L)}$); and (2) the *transient, tiny or "T-type,"* a rapidly inactivating, low-threshold, dihydropyridine-insensitive current ($I_{Ca(T)}$). The L-type calcium channel is the major type in cardiac fibers, and the calcium current carried by it also contributes to the excitation–contraction process. Both sodium and calcium channels in cardiac fibers exhibit time- and voltage-dependent gating characteristics. However, the calcium channel has slower activation and inactivation gating kinetics than does the sodium channel. Consequently, current moving through the calcium channel also contributes to the AP plateau (phase 2).

Phases 1 to 3 (Repolarization and Plateau)

Several different potassium repolarizing currents, the sodium "window" current, and the calcium current contribute to early rapid AP repolarization (phase 1), the AP plateau (phase 2), and final rapid AP repolarization (phase 3), as shown in Figure 2–3. A transient outward current (I_{to}), carried mainly by potassium, in conjunction with the rapid inactivation of the fast inward current and the slow inactivation of the L-type calcium current are responsible for phase 1. Inward movement of chloride through a chloride channel may also contribute to phase 1. Membrane conductance for all ions is reduced during phase 2. Several currents are believed to contribute to maintaining the membrane potential at or just below 0 mV during phase 2 (Fig. 2–3): (1) the sodium "window" current, possibly due to different populations of sodium channels with different activation–inactivation kinetics; (2) the slowly inactivating inward Ca current during phase 2; (3) the delayed-rectifier potassium current (I_K); and (4) the transient outward, mainly potassium current (long-lasting component), which inactivates as membrane potential is restored. The chloride current and electrogenic sodium–potassium and sodium–calcium exchange are also believed to contribute to phase 2. Both the inward (I_{K1}) and delayed-rectifier potassium currents are responsible for phase 3. Other potassium currents that may be involved in AP repolarization under special circumstances are listed in Table 2–2. Concerning potassium repolarization currents, as the membrane potential becomes more negative during repolarization, potassium conductance increases as a result of rectification. Most potassium channels of the heart rectify, in that they tend to show lower conductance with depolarization. Rectification enhances outward movement of potassium during repolarization, thereby accelerating repolarization by further increasing potassium conductance. This regenerative increase in potassium

TABLE 2-2 **Potassium repolarization currents under special circumstances**

Ca-activated	Accelerates repolarization in calcium-overloaded myocardium
Na-activated	Promotes repolarization in sodium-overloaded myocardium
ATP-sensitive	Promotes repolarization with depletion of ATP (e.g., ischemia)
ACh-activated	Activates with cholinergic stimulation to hyperpolarize RMP
AA-activated	Activated by arachidonic acid and other fatty acids at low pH

conductance partly explains "all-or-none" repolarization. As a result, a large repolarizing current toward the end of phase 2 will result in full repolarization to the former RMP, or MDP in automatic fibers. With subthreshold repolarizing current, however, the membrane potential returns to its former plateau level.

REFRACTORINESS

One characteristic of cardiac fibers as opposed to nerve tissue is prolonged refractoriness.[8] During phase 2 of the AP, fibers cannot be reexcited, regardless of stimulus strength. They are said to be *absolutely refractory* (Fig. 2–3). The reason for this is that the inward sodium and calcium current channels are both inactivated during the plateau, and repolarization must occur before they can reopen. In fast-response fibers, restoration of the normal RMP is usually sufficient for full recovery of excitability. This marks the end of the *relative refractory period* (RRP) (Fig. 2–3). During the RRP, the stimulus required to elicit an AP is larger than normal, and the resulting AP may be too small to propagate (i.e., an ETP), or it propagates quite slowly. In slow-response fibers (SA node, AV node), or depressed fast-response fibers with reduced TMP (described below), the RRP may extend several hundred milliseconds beyond full repolarization.

AUTOMATICITY

Automatic (pacemaker) fibers do not have a stable level of TMP during phase 4. Instead, after reaching some MDP during phase 3, they immediately begin to depolarize during phase 4 toward the TP. Under the right circumstances, pacemaker fibers will depolarize to the TP for

36 OVERVIEW OF MECHANISMS FOR ARRHYTHMIAS

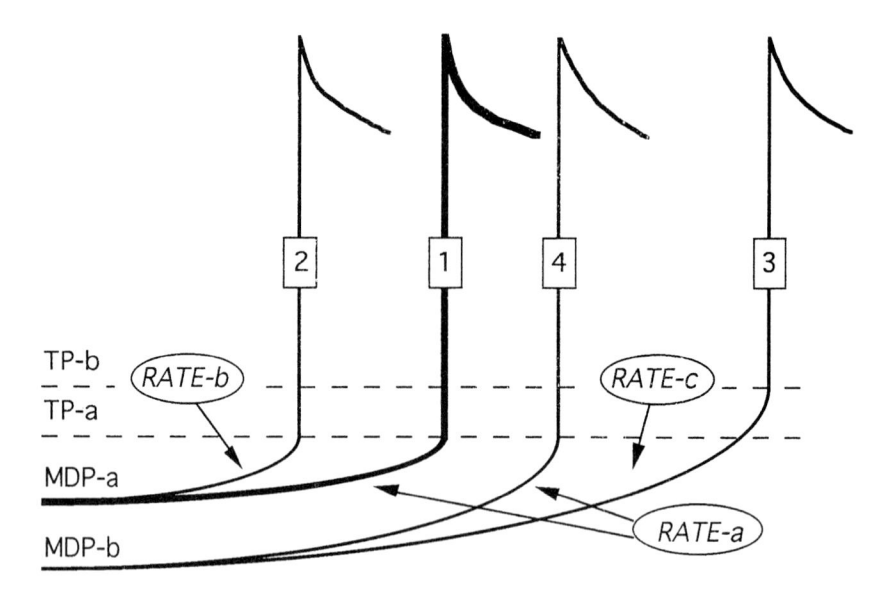

FIGURE 2-4 *Schematic of mechanisms whereby the rate of pacemaker discharge in an automatic Purkinje fiber may be altered. TP, threshold potential; MDP, maximum diastolic potential; Rate, rate of diastolic (phase 4) depolarization. 1, Normal automaticity (MDP-a; TP-a; Rate-a). 2, The rate of automaticity is increased (Rate-b) following catecholamines. Since MDP and TP are unchanged, TP is reached sooner. 3, The rate of automaticity has been decreased (Rate-c) by exposure to acetylcholine. Also, MDP is hyperpolarized (MDP-b), and TP reduced (TP-b). Automaticity is slowed since it takes longer to achieve TP. 4, With simultaneous cholinergic and sympathetic stimulation, MDP remains hyperpolarized (MDP-b), but TP and the rate of phase 4 depolarization are restored to normal. Automaticity is faster than in 3, but slower than in 1 because MDP-b is further from TP-a than MDP-a.*

regenerative AP, AP that can propagate successfully. Occasionally, however, the pacemaker fiber will depolarize only to some lower, but stable, level of membrane potential. The rate of automaticity is affected by changes in the rate of spontaneous phase 4 depolarization, the MDP, and the TP (Fig. 2-4).

Ionic Basis for Automaticity

Automaticity results from a net reduction in the outward movement of positive charges during phase 4.[5,6,8-10] This causes the interior of an automatic fiber to become progressively less negative with respect to the outside. Although the ionic mechanism is not fully resolved, and probably varies among fiber types depending on the MDP, there seems to be agreement on several points: (1) In SA node fibers, the excitatory inward current is subserved by L-type calcium channels, but T-type current may be activated during the latter of phase 4 depolarization. (2) In Purkinje fibers, the pacemaker current (I_f) is likely to be an inward current carried mainly by sodium and calcium that is inactivated by membrane potential less negative than − 50 mV. (3) Most SA node cells also have the pacemaker current, which passes through the same membrane protein channels as in Purkinje fibers. (4) Sodium–potassium and sodium–calcium ion-exchange pumps are not required for automaticity, but probably help to modify the rate of phase 4 depolarization. (5) The inward rectifier current is small or absent in SA node fibers, increasing the instability of the TMP during electrical diastole. Therefore, automaticity involves the interaction of several currents, which differ for SA node and automatic Purkinje fibers.

SA NODE. Automaticity results from an imbalance between slowly decaying delayed-rectifier and slowly recovering inward calcium currents. The pacemaker current is involved only when the membrane potential is more negative than about − 50 mV. Also, while the inward Na–Ca exchange current may contribute to a small extent immediately after repolarization to the MDP, it declines as the intracellular calcium concentration is reduced by calcium buffering and sodium–calcium exchange. The contribution of current from sodium–potassium exchange is small and time-invariant.

PURKINJE FIBERS. Automaticity has three phases: (1) initial depolarization during phase 4, which depends upon deactivation of delayed-rectifier current; (2) a middle phase, dominated by slowly rising pacemaker current, combined with little or no rise in outward potassium current because the inward potassium channel shows inward rectification; and (3) a final phase of accelerating depolarization due to partial activation of the fast inward current, and possibly also the calcium current through the T-type calcium channels.

AUTOMATICITY IN OTHER LATENT PACEMAKERS. As noted earlier, latent pacemakers include subsidiary atrial and AV junctional pacemakers. Importantly, these pacemakers have MDP intermediate between those of automatic Purkinje fibers and those of the SA node. While specific ionic mechanisms for automaticity have not been identified for these fibers, they should be similar to those for SA node or Purkinje fibers, with differences depending most on the MDP reached in individual fibers. Thus, in fibers with MDP higher than -70 mV, the mechanism possibly involves the pacemaker current, similar to the middle phase of automaticity in Purkinje fibers. For fibers with MDP more positive than -70 mV (more similar to SA node), the mechanism should involve slowly decaying delayed-rectifier and excitatory inward calcium currents.

OVERDRIVE SUPPRESSION OF AUTOMATICITY. Dominant pacemaker fibers of the SA node have a faster rate of automaticity than latent pacemakers elsewhere in the heart. The SA node maintains dominance over latent pacemakers by overdrive suppression of automaticity. SA node automaticity can also be suppressed following a period of rapid overdrive pacing. Overdrive suppression of automaticity is believed to result from the intracellular accumulation of sodium in suppressed pacemaker fibers.[6,11] Elevated intracellular sodium increases the turnover rate of the sodium–potassium exchange pump. Because this pump normally exchanges three intracellular sodium ions for two extracellular potassium ions, there is a small net gain in intracellular negative charges. As a result, the MDP becomes more negative, increasing the time needed for phase 4 depolarization to bring the fiber to threshold for regenerative depolarization. The spontaneous rate of the suppressed fiber will remain slow until the intracellular sodium concentration returns to its previous level. Purkinje fibers, with AP upstrokes more dependent on sodium influx, are more easily overdrive-suppressed SA node fibers.

ACTION POTENTIAL PROPAGATION

Membrane factors that determine the success of AP propagation are the active membrane generator and passive membrane properties.[8] The "generator" or current source is the inward sodium or calcium current during AP phase 0. The passive cell membrane absorbs energy introduced from the current source, and therefore is the "sink." The interaction of the source with the sink determines the characteristics of conduction.

Current Source

Experimental studies of cardiac conduction have dealt more with properties of the source. Therefore, while properties of the source such as Vmax, phase 0 (Table 2–1) may be considered determinants of conduction velocity, this is only an approximation, one that is most applicable to conduction in single Purkinje fiber strands.[8] At branching sites, or in atrial and ventricular muscle, there is less correlation between Vmax, phase 0 and conduction velocity. In slow-response or depressed fast-response fibers (see following), there is little correlation between Vmax, phase 0, and conduction velocity.

Current Sink

Cable analysis has often been used to describe properties of the sink.[8] A biologic cable (e.g., free-running strands of Purkinje fibers) consists of a low-resistance intracellular core surrounded by the relatively high-resistance cell membrane, with the latter surrounded by low-resistance extracellular fluid. As a result, the coordination of AP propagation, AP conduction itself, and aspects of normal and abnormal excitability are influenced by the cable properties of the fiber strand. This can be so because current communicated from one cell to the next depends on characteristics of the cell membrane, myoplasm, and intercellular connections. However, there are limitations to cable analysis of cardiac conduction. Varying structural complexities of cardiac cells, especially the presence of low-resistance gap junctions[12] and variations in fiber geometry,[13] play an important role in determining the speed of conduction. For example, cable analysis would not predict a dependence of the speed of conduction on the direction of conduction, which has been shown by several investigators.[14-16] Because the degree of intercellular coupling through low-resistance gap junctions varies with the specific geometry of cellular connections and fiber orientation (described by the term *effective axial resistivity*),[16] conduction in the longitudinal direction is several times faster than that in the transverse direction. A number of factors can lead to cell-to-cell uncoupling, thereby increasing resistance to current flow and lowering conduction velocity. Among these are myocardial ischemia, hypoxia, acidosis, calcium overload, and anesthetics.[17]

Safety Factor of Conduction

The relationship between the current source and the sink will determine whether AP propagation is successful, or only local or electrotonic effects will occur (Fig. 2–3). The *safety factor of conduction* is simply the excess of source current over the sink. This is large for highly polarized fast-response fibers, and small or marginal for slow and depressed fast-response fibers. For example, conduction is expected to be successful in Purkinje fibers with high RMP, Vmax, phase 0, AP amplitudes, and overshoots (Table 2–1). In contrast, conduction is much slower in slow-response fibers (SA and AV nodes) with lower RMP, Vmax, phase 0, AP amplitudes, and overshoots (Table 2–1). In depressed fast-response fibers, depending on the amount of depolarization, AP propagation may fail altogether, only electrotonic effects will occur, or minimal to pronounced reduction in conduction velocity will continue.

AUTONOMIC INNERVATION

There is substantial autonomic innervation of the atrial portions of the specialized AV conducting system, especially the SA and AV node regions. There is some "sidedness" to this innervation, with right-sided sympathetic dominance at the SA node, but more even distribution at the AV node. Therefore, stimulation of the right versus the left sympathetic ganglia has more effect on SA node rate, while stimulation of either has nearly the same effect on AV nodal conduction. Stimulation of the preganglionic parasympathetic fibers has a pronounced effect on the SA node rate and AV nodal conduction, and is even capable of beat-to-beat modulation of these parameters.[17] However, there is relatively less parasympathetic than sympathetic innervation of the ventricles. Nonetheless, enhanced parasympathetic and sympathetic and efferent activity produce highly localized changes in ventricular refractoriness that may significantly influence arrhythmogenesis.[17]

Abnormal Cardiac Electrophysiology

One or more abnormal cardiac electrophysiologic processes may underlie the genesis of individual cardiac arrhythmias, including impaired conduction and uneven refractoriness with the depressed fast response, abnormal automaticity, early or delayed afterdepolarizations and triggered activity, and reentry of excitation. These abnormal processes may result from underlying myocardial disease, or they may be initiated in normal or diseased hearts by effects of physiologic imbalance (Table 2–3).

TABLE 2-3 *Imbalances that might initiate abnormal electrophysiologic phenomena*

Temperature extremes	Hypoxia or ischemia	Hypercarbia/hypocarbia
Acidosis/alkalosis	Hyper- or hypokalemia	Magnesium deficiency
Hyper- or hypocalcemia	Adverse drug interactions	Toxicity with drugs
Malnutrition, cachexia	Autonomic imbalance	Stress, catecholamines

LOSS OF MEMBRANE POTENTIAL AND DEPRESSED FAST RESPONSE

Many abnormal electrophysiologic processes in the heart result from or are associated with partial depolarization (i.e., loss of membrane potential [LMP]) of fast-response fibers. Recall that the latter are fibers with AP upstrokes mostly dependent on inward Na current (i.e., atrial and ventricular muscle, and Purkinje fibers). Fast-response fibers with LMP are referred to as *depressed fast-response* (DFR) *fibers.* Cellular depolarization responsible for LMP and the DFR can have a number of causes, including ischemic injury, reperfusion of ischemic myocardium, and hyperkalemia.[6] Partial membrane depolarization in DFR fibers alters the depolarization and repolarization phases of the AP, so that DFR AP contours (Fig. 2–5) more closely resemble those of slow-response fibers (i.e., the SA and AV node, Figure 2-1). Reduced upstroke velocity following LMP (Fig. 2–5) is explained by incomplete recovery from inactivation of the sodium channel. This reduces the number of available Na channels for reactivation, and therefore the magnitude of current flowing during phase 0. Membrane depolariza-

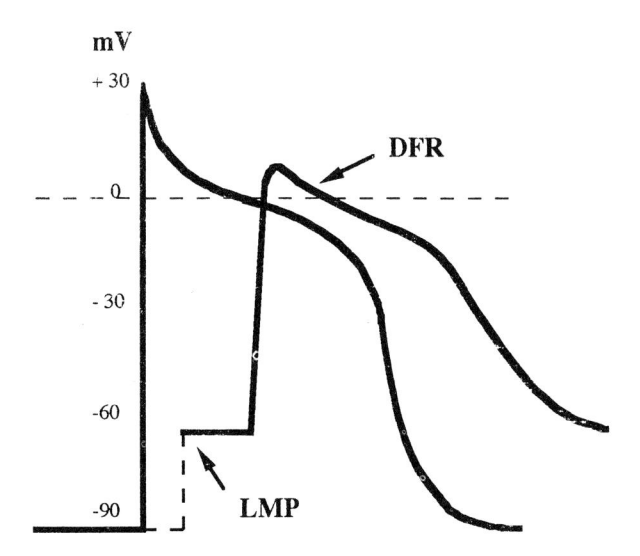

FIGURE 2-5 *Loss of membrane potential (LMP) in a Purkinje fiber with normally high RMP (– 90 mV) and overshoot (+ 30 mV). This produces a depressed fast response (DFR) AP with reduced RMP (– 65 mV), upstroke velocity, and overshoot. The AP contours of fibers with moderate to severe LMP more closely resemble those of slow-response fibers (SA or AV node, Fig. 2–1).*

tion to − 70 to − 60 mV may inactivate half the sodium channels, while that to − 50 mV or less may inactivate all the sodium channels.[6,18] At membrane potentials positive to − 50 mV, the slow inward calcium current may be activated to generate the AP upstroke.

The AP changes in DFR fibers are likely to be heterogeneous, with varying degrees of sodium-channel inactivation. This may lead to minimal conduction impairment in some areas and complete conduction block in others. Also, in DFR fibers, refractoriness may outlast full restoration of the RMP, similar to what is observed in slow-response fibers (see preceding). These changes in conduction and refractoriness in DFR fibers are favorable for reentry of excitation,[18] and also contribute to abnormal automaticity and afterdepolarizations with triggered activity.[11,19]

ALTERED NORMAL AND ABNORMAL AUTOMATICITY

Altered normal and abnormal automaticity are not the same. By *altered normal automaticity* is meant that the ionic mechanisms responsible for spontaneous phase 4 depolarization in dominant or latent pacemaker fibers remain unchanged, although the kinetics or magnitude of currents responsible for depolarization have changed.[6,11] Thus, the rate of pacemaker discharge may increase or decrease, but is still within the expected range for the type of pacemaker tissue (Table 2–4). With abnormal automaticity, the ionic mechanism for phase 4 depolarization is substantially different from that for normal automaticity in the same fiber type, or it occurs in fibers that do not normally exhibit automaticity. Because partial depolarization of atrial or ventricular muscle, or nonautomatic Pukinje fibers, can induce automaticity in previously quiescent fibers, the term *depolarization-induced automaticity* is sometimes used instead of abnormal automaticity. Abnormal automaticity is commonly associated with myocardial ischemia and reperfusion injury. The ionic mechanisms have not been established, and probably vary depending on the fiber type, MDP, and the

TABLE 2-4 *Expected rates for pacemakers*

SA node	50–220 beats/min
Subsidiary atrial	50–180 beats/min
AV junctional	45–110 beats/min
Purkinje fibers*	30–60 beats/min

*Normal (nondepolarized) fibers only.

condition that produced abnormal automaticity. That the slow inward (calcium) current may be involved is suggested by suppression of automaticity in partially depolarized Purkinje fibers by verapamil but not lidocaine.[20]

AFTERDEPOLARIZATIONS AND TRIGGERED ACTIVITY

Afterdepolarizations are small depolarizations in the TMP that occur after (delayed afterdepolarizations, (DAD) or before (early afterdepolarizations EAD) full restoration of the TMP following the AP (Fig. 2–6).[5,6,19,21] Afterdepolarizations can occur at virtually any level of TMP, and may or may not trigger sustained rhythmic activity. Triggered rhythmic activity is not the same as spontaneous automaticity, since it cannot arise de novo. Triggered activity is always consequent to a preceding beat or series of beats; otherwise, there is electrical quiescence.

Delayed Afterdepolarizations

Delayed afterdepolarizations and triggered rhythmic activity usually occur under circumstances where there is intracellular calcium excess, termed *calcium overload.* This may occur with excessive adrenergic stimulation along with high extracellular calcium,[6] or digitalis excess with sodium–potassium exchange pump inhibition. Myocardial ischemia and reperfusion injury are also causes for DAD and triggered rhythms.[8,19] DAD are believed to result from "transient inward current" caused by oscillatory calcium-induced calcium release from an overloaded sarcoplasmic reticulum.[22,23] This current, carried mainly by Na, may result from activation of a nonselective cation channel or be due to inward current generated by electrogenic sodium–calcium exchange.[6,8,19] DAD and triggered activity have been observed experimentally in all types of fast-response fibers. Drugs that reduce inward calcium current and overload (calcium-channel and beta-adrenergic blockers), inhibit calcium release from the sarcoplasmic reticulum (caffeine, ryanodine), or reduce inward sodium current and intracellular sodium concentration (tetrodotoxin, lidocaine, phenytoin), can inhibit DAD.[6] Finally, DAD increase in amplitude and the likelihood that they will trigger sustained rhythmic activity with faster spontaneous or paced rates, or increased prematurity of prior impulses.

Early Afterdepolarizations

Early afterdepolarizations are oscillations of the TMP that occur during the plateau or repolarization phases of AP arising from a high

44 OVERVIEW OF MECHANISMS FOR ARRHYTHMIAS

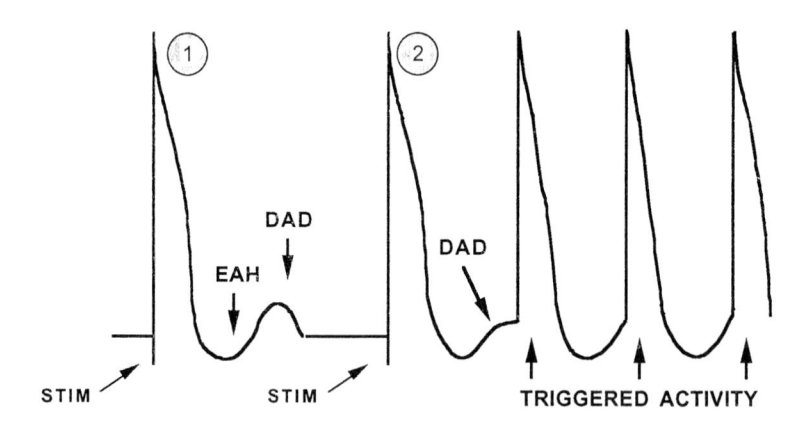

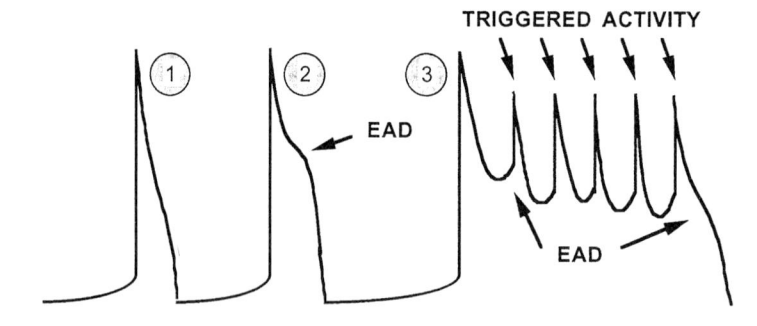

FIGURE 2-6 Schematic depiction of delayed or early afterdepolarizations (DAD, EAD), and triggered activity in Purkinje fibers. Top, Both the first and second AP are stimulated (STIM) beats, and are followed by early afterhyperpolarizations (EAH). The DAD following the first stimulated AP fails to trigger AP, but that following the second AP does trigger three AP (i.e., triggered activity). Bottom, AP from an automatic Purkinje fiber. The first AP is normal, but the second is associated with a subthreshold EAD (arrow). The third AP is associated with a threshold EAD, which then initiates a series of five triggered AP (i.e., triggered activity). The fifth triggered AP is followed by a subthreshold EAD and return to normal MDP.

TABLE 2-5 *Experimental interventions associated with EAD and triggered activity*

Quinidine*	Cesium chloride†	Aconitine‡	Veratridine‡
Alpha stimulation¶	Hypoxia	Hypercarbia	Acidosis
BAY K8644§	Toxic bupivacaine	Electrotonic effects	Low or absent potassium

* Also, any drugs that prolong AP duration.
† Inhibits the outward potassium current.
‡ Reduces TMP by increasing sodium permeability.
¶ Adrenergic.
§ Experimental calcium agonist.

level of TMP (− 75 to − 90 mV).[8,19] Under certain conditions EAD may trigger a second AP, which may self-perpetuate as triggered sustained rhythmic activity, also at a reduced level of TMP (Fig. 2–6). EAD-triggered rhythmic activity may continue for a variable number of beats, but terminates when repolarization of the initiating AP returns the TMP to its normal high level. EAD and triggered rhythmic activity can be produced by a variety of experimental interventions (Table 2–5). Potassium-channel activators (pinacidil, chromakalim), magnesium, alpha-adrenergic blockade, antiarrhythmics that shorten AP duration (e.g., lidocaine), tetrodotoxin, and nitrendipine all may oppose EAD and triggered activity, depending on the conditions that produced them.[6,19,24] EAD likely result from abnormalities involving the AP plateau or repolarization currents. Normally, net outward membrane current shifts the TMP progressively in a more negative direction, culminating in final rapid repolarization. An EAD might occur if there was a shift in the current–voltage relationship, resulting in a region of net inward current during the plateau range of TMP. This would retard or prevent repolarization, perhaps leading to secondary depolarizations or AP if a regenerative inward current was activated. The ionic current activated would depend on the level of TMP at which the EAD-triggered AP occurred. If during the plateau phase or early phase 3 repolarization, when most sodium channels are still inactivated, the upstroke would be more dependent on the slow inward calcium current. At higher TMP, with increasing recovery from inactivation by the sodium channels, the inward sodium current should contribute. Finally, in contrast to DAD, EAD increase in amplitude and the likelihood that they will trigger rhythmic activity as spontaneous heart rate slows.

REENTRANT EXCITATION

Normally, the propagating impulse dies out after sequential activation of the atria and ventricles because it becomes surrounded by refractory tissue or encounters the inexcitable annulus fibrosus.[18] On occasion, however, the impulse may persist to reexcite no longer refractory atrial or ventricular myocardium. This phenomenon is termed *reentry of excitation.* Extrasystoles due to reentry are called *echo* or *reciprocal beats,* and tachycardia due to reeentry is called *circus movement* or *reciprocating tachycardia.*

The criteria for ascribing arrhythmias to reentry were formulated by Mines more than 80 years ago.[25,26] These can be summarized as follows: (1) An area of unidirectional conduction block must be shown. (2) The reentry circuit must be defined; that is, the excitatory wavefront should be observed to progress through the pathway, return to its point of origin, and then again follow the same pathway. (3) Reentry can be terminated by interrupting the circuit at some point. If impulses continue to arise after interruption of the supposed circuit, this argues for an automatic or triggered origin.[18]

One of the essential requirements for initiation of reentry is unidirectional conduction block. Also, slowed conduction in an alternate conduction pathway facilitates reentry by allowing tissue proximal to a site of conduction block time to recover from refractoriness. Causes for unidirectional conduction block and slowed conduction are explored in more detail below, followed by discussion of the different types of reentry and myocardial sites for reentry.

Unidirectional Conduction Block

Unidirectional conduction block may be caused by regional differences in recovery of excitability, occur at connecting sites between adjacent fibers, or result from geometric factors (e.g., fiber branching or orientation).[18]

RECOVERY OF EXCITABILITY. Usually as impulses propagate through tissue with nonuniform refractoriness, propagation fails in tissue with the longest refractory periods. These tissues will be available for reexcitation if impulses can propagate through an alternate pathway with shorter refractoriness and return to the site of former block before arrival of the next normal impulse. In the normal heart there is substantial diastolic time during which excitability is normal, so that uneven refractoriness is usually present only during the propagation of rapid or premature spontaneous or stimulated beats. Reentry is facilitated because refractory periods shorten with such beats, so that the pathways over which potential reentrant impulses must circulate are also shortened. The degree of nonuniformity in refractory periods is smaller for atrial compared to ventricular reentry. Interventions that increase refractory period disparity in the ventricles (e.g., local temperature differences, carbachol) are required to show ventricular reentry in normal heart. Variable depression of fibers by ischemia, however, will produce uneven refractoriness conducive to ventricular reentry.

CELLULAR CONNECTIONS. Sites where the cross-sectional area of interconnected cells suddenly increases may be sites for unidirectional block. One such site is the Purkinje fiber–ventricular muscle junction, where Purkinje fibers overlay ventricular muscle. Activation of ventricular muscle from the Purkinje fiber layer occurs only at specific junctional sites; otherwise, a considerable resistive barrier exists between adjacent cell layers. However, retrograde propagation from ventricular muscle to the Purkinje fiber layer can occur at sites where conduction in the opposite (anterograde) direction is not possible. Explanations for such unidirectional block include (1) differences in excitability between the two layers; (2) greater thickness of the muscle compared to Purkinje fiber layer, so that the former presents a larger "load" for the latter than vice versa; and (3) increased coupling resistance at sites with unidirectional block. A similar situation may exist in patients with concealed accessory AV conducting pathways (see Chapter 9). During sinus rhythm, there is no evidence for ventricular preexcitation because conduction is over the AV node (normal) pathways, so that the accessory pathway is "concealed." However, a premature ventricular beat that encounters the AV node while it is still refractory may initiate reentrant tachycardia if it is conducted back to the atria over the concealed accessory pathway.

GEOMETRIC FACTORS. Unidirectional conduction block required for reentry is the result of several geometric factors: (1) Branching sites or junctions of separate bundles of muscle fibers form areas with a low safety factor of conduction. (2) Conduction velocity in the longitudinal versus transverse fiber direction is about three times that in the transverse direction, explained by comparative differences in intra- and extracellular resistance. (3) In fibers with reduced excitability or anisotropic tissue (i.e., with uneven conduction and refractoriness), transverse conduction may be faster. (4) There is no consistent relationship between fiber orientation and conduction velocity in ischemic myocardium.

Slowed Conduction

As already mentioned, reentry is facilitated by slowed conduction, which provides time for tissue proximal to a site of unidirectional block to recover its excitability. The SA and AV nodes with slow conduction are potential sites for reentry, and reentry may occur during slow propagation of rapid or premature impulses in tissue with uneven refractoriness. Reentry facilitated by slow conduction also occurs in partially depolarized (depressed) fast-response fibers. Variable depression of conduction in these fibers can lead to slowed conduction in some areas with conduction block in more severely depressed ones. The chance for reentry with premature stimulation is even greater in DFR tissue. When all sodium channels are inactivated, AP propagation is dependent on the slow inward calcium current. Such slow-response AP propagate very slowly and likely underlie the occurrence of some reentrant arrhythmias.

TYPES OF REENTRY

The simplest form of reentry requires an *anatomically defined circuit.* In such a circuit, the duration of the refractory period and conduction velocity determine whether or not reentrant excitation can occur. How an atrial or ventricular reentrant tachycardia might be initiated by a premature beat is illustrated in Figure 2–7. Such premature beats may result from external stimulation, triggered AP, or foci of automaticity that somehow escape overdrive suppression from the dominant pacemaker (e.g., parasystole). An important feature of this model is the presence of an *excitable gap,* which implies that impulses arising outside the reentrant circuit may penetrate it and reset or terminate tachycardia (Fig. 2–8). Anisotropy or areas of depressed conduction can reduce the size of the anatomic obstacle necessary to sustain reentry.[18] *Leading circle reentry* does not require an anatomic obstacle. The premature impulse initiating tachycardia or tachycardia wavefront propagates toward tissue with shorter refractoriness, but blocks in the direction of longer refractoriness (Fig. 2–9). Other types of reentry include *anisotropic reentry* and *reflection,* which are discussed elsewhere.[6,18] Finally, distinction has been made between *ordered* and *random reentry.*[27] Ordered reentry occurs over a relatively fixed pathway and results in a regular rhythm (e.g., AV node reentry tachycardia; atrial flutter). In contrast, with random reentry, the reentry pathways are continuously changing their size and shape with time, so that the resulting rhythm is irregular (e.g., atrial and ventricular fibrillation).

NSR PB TACH

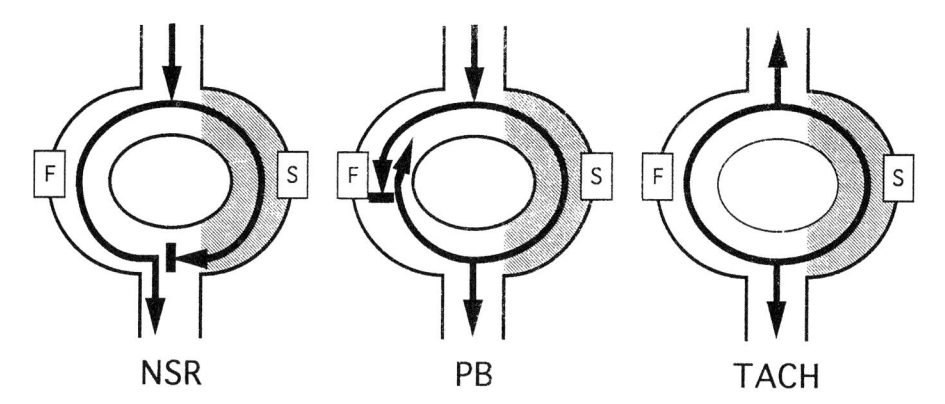

FIGURE 2-7 *Initiation of reentrant tachycardia with an anatomical obstacle. Left, During normal sinus rhythm (NSR), activation of myocardium distal to the reentry circuit is through a fast-conducting pathway (F). While the impulse also travels through the slow-conducting pathway (S), it blocks near the cricuit exit point when it encounters refractory tissue behind the impulse from F. Middle, A premature beat (PB) enters the circuit after a normal beat (not shown). PB blocks in F with longer refractoriness, but conducts through S with shorter refractoriness. PB also returns through F in the opposite (retrograde) direction to reexcite nonrefractory proximal myocardium. Right, If PB reaches nonrefractory myocardium in S before the next normal impulse from above, then a period of reentrant tachycardia may ensue.*

SITES FOR REENTRY

Because of normal areas of slow conduction, anatomic obstacles, anisotropic conduction, nonuniform refractoriness, or pathologic changes, most myocardial tissue is at least a potential site for reentry (Table 2–6). This potential is briefly discussed below, based on evidence reviewed elsewhere.[18]

SA Node

While clinical studies suggest that 5 to 10 percent of reentrant (paroxysmal) supraventricular tachycardia (SVT) may be due to SA node reentry,[28] it is difficult to experimentally produce sustained circus movement in the normal heart. Echo beats, however, are relatively easy to produce by premature stimulation. They are possibly the result of functional longitudinal dissociation between SA node fibers during propagation of the premature impulse (Fig. 2–10).[6,18,29]

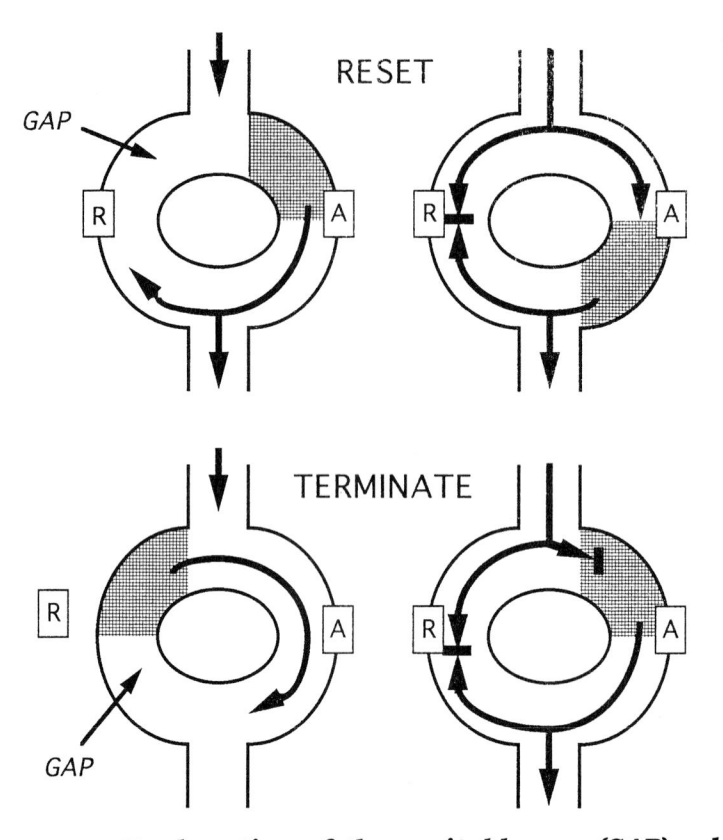

FIGURE 2-8 *Explanation of the excitable gap (GAP), whereby reentrant tachycardia with an anatomic obstacle is affected by external impulses. All panels: R, retrograde pathway; A, anterograde pathway. Also, a zone of relative refractoriness (hatched) trails the circulating wavefront of tachycardia, but tissue within the wavefront is absolutely refractory. Top left, An external impulse (short arrow) enters the reentry circuit within the excitable gap (GAP) of nonrefractory tissue between the receding and advancing wavefronts of tachycardia. Top right, It penetrates the reentry circuit in both directions, blocking in the retrograde pathway, where it encounters the advancing wavefront of tachycardia. However, it advances in the anterograde, resetting the phase of tachycardia (RESET). Bottom left, Another external impulse (short arrow) arrives sooner. Bottom right, It blocks in the zone of relative refractoriness trailing the wavefront of tachycardia. It conducts for a short distance in the retrograde pathway, but then blocks when it encounters the advancing wavefront of tachycardia. Thus, reentrant tachycardia is terminated by a single premature impulse (TERMINATE).*

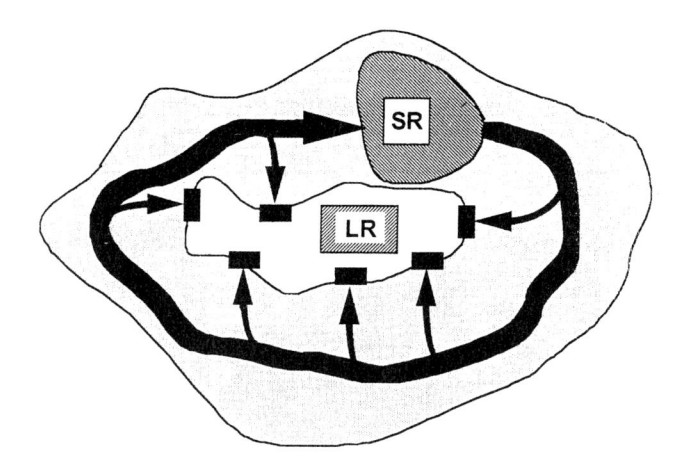

FIGURE 2-9 *Concept of leading circle reentry. The circulating wavefront of tachycardia (bold arrow) propagates in the direction of tissue with shorter refractoriness (SR), the relatively refractory tail of the propagating wavefront. However, it blocks in tissue with longer refractoriness (LR), the absolutely refractory core. Note the absence of a gap of fully excitable tissue between the head and tail of the circulating impulse or wavefront.*

TABLE 2-6 *Potential tissue sites for reentry*

SA or AV node	His–Purkinje system
Atrial myocardium	Ischemic ventricle
Accessory pathways	Infarcted ventricle

In contrast, in diseased SA node tissue or with altered conduction and refractoriness (e.g., due to autonomic imbalance or drugs) the chances for sustained SA node reentry are increased.

Atrial Myocardium

While it is widely believed that *atrial flutter* is caused by circus movement around a large anatomic obstacle (the caval orifices), evidence also points to leading circle reentry as a cause. The presence of an excitable gap and the ability to terminate slow atrial flutter (see Chapter 9) with single premature stimuli favor anatomic reentry. The absence of an excitable gap with fast atrial flutter (see Chapter 9)

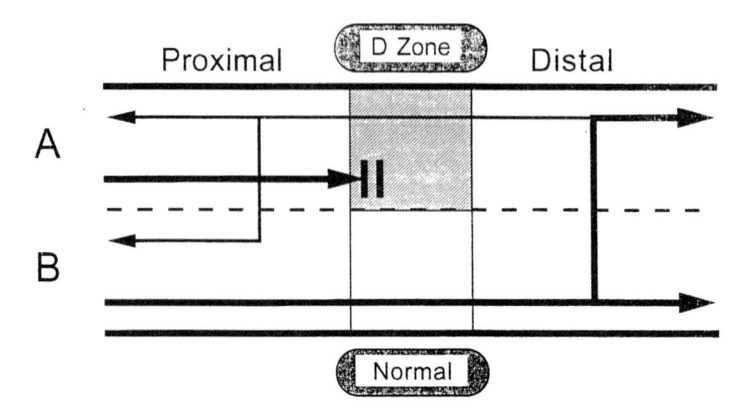

FIGURE 2-10 *Concept of functional longitudinal dissociation (linear reentry). Depicted is a linear bundle of fibers with a zone of depressed conduction (D ZONE, fiber A) and unidirectional block. A similar model (turtle heart) was first proposed by Schmitt and Erlanger.[29] The propagating impulse moves from proximal to distal through the nondepressed zone (NORMAL) in fiber B, but blocks in fiber A. In distal fiber B, the impulse crosses over to fiber A via lateral connections, then conducts back through D ZONE (now sufficiently recovered for slow conduction) to reexcite proximal fibers A and B.*

is consistent with leading circle reentry. The multiple-wavelet hypothesis best explains reentry with *atrial fibrillation*. Multiple, independent, propagating wavelets of excitation, some as small as several millimeters and some much wider, have been mapped in experimental atrial fibrillation. Individual wavelets may persist for several hundred milliseconds before extinction, either by fusion, collision, reaching the atrial borders, or encountering refractory tissue.

Accessory Pathways

Fast-conducting, muscular bundles of tissue connecting the atria and ventricles (accessory AV connections or pathways) are the cause for ventricular preexcitation in patients with the Wolff–Parkinson–White (WPW) syndrome (see Chapter 10). They also participate with the atrium, AV node, His–Purkinje system, and ventricular myocardium in a type of circus movement tachycardia known as *AV reciprocating tachycardia*. Of all the clinical tachyarrhythmias ascribed to reentry, AV reciprocating tachycardia most completely satisfies Mines' criteria for reentry. Namely, AV reciprocation is easily terminated by surgical transection or catheter ablation of the accessory pathway.

AV Node

The basis for AV node reentry could be functional longitudinal dissociation within the node into slow (alpha) and fast (beta) conducting pathways, more the result of electrophysiologic than anatomic differences between the two pathways. While such pathways have been demonstrated in isolated rabbit heart, they have not in human heart. However, the human AV node has two atrial inputs, one via the crista terminalis and the other via the interatrial septum, which could serve as the alpha and beta pathways. Another possibility is that reentry is produced by functional dissociation based on tissue anistropy (e.g., different coupling resistances depending on the direction of conduction and complex branching). While it is difficult to induce AV node reentry by premature stimulation in normal hearts, it is possible to do so in patients with paroxysmal (reentrant) SVT, or when conduction through the AV node is impaired by disease or drugs.

His-Purkinje System

Both macroreentry and microreentry are possible. When differences in refractory periods exist between the right and left bundle branches, an atrial, AV junctional, or His bundle premature impulse may be blocked in one of the branches and conducted in the other. If the branch where block occurred is invaded by a retrograde impulse from the other side of the interventricular septum, and reexcitation of tissue proximal to the site of block occurs, reentry as echo beats or tachycardia might occur. Premature stimulation of the ventricles may induce another type of reentry involving the bundle branches. Because refractory periods of the bundle branches are longer than those of ventricular myocardium, a premature impulse originating on the right side of the septum may fail to propagate retrogradely in the right bundle branch. However, it would conduct through septal myocardium to activate the left bundle branch, then back to the right bundle branch after retrograde His bundle activation. Finally, the combination of very slow conduction and very short refractory periods can lead to microreentry involving distal Purkinje fibers and ventricular myocardium. Such microreentry is promoted by acutely locally elevated extracellular potassium and increased catecholamines with myocardial ischemia.

Ischemic Myocardium

Within a few minutes of coronary occlusion, conduction velocity in ischemic myocardium decreases, and epimyocardial activation becomes delayed.[18,30] Such delayed activation coincides with the spontaneous occurrence of ventricular tachycardia and fibrillation. This, and the demonstration of continuous fragmented electrical activity during diastole with experimental mapping, has been interpreted as evidence for reentry as the mechanism for ventricular tachycardia and fibrillation in ischemic myocardium. Certainly, shortened refractoriness, slowed conduction, and increased dispersion of refractory periods with acute ischemia are all conducive to reentry. Ischemic ventricular tachycardia is likely caused by intramural reentry, while multiple independent wavelets are responsible for ventricular fibrillation. These could block in refractory tissue or collide with each other, but summation of wavefronts could also occur. Finally, it is possible that one or more rapidly discharging foci coexist with reentrant excitation during ventricular fibrillation.

Infarcted Myocardium

Experiments in which recordings are made simultaneously from multiple sites have provided direct evidence for reentry in infarcted canine heart.[18,30] Essentially, two types of infarction are produced: (1) transmural infarction after complete coronary occlusion; or (2) mottled infarction after coronary occlusion with reperfusion. With the latter, more or less viable myocardium is interspersed with infarcted myocardium, depending on the duration of occlusion before reperfusion. Sustained tachycardia is more easily induced by premature stimulation in mottled infarctions, probably because surviving fiber bundles provide the pathways for reentry. However, it is uncertain whether surviving intramural or subendocardial fibers form the reentrant pathways. Reentry can also be easily induced in large superfused infarct preparations 24 to 72 hours following coronary occlusion. This is because Purkinje fibers overlying the infarct have abnormally prolonged AP and form the site of unidirectional block, whereas conduction is maintained in fibers with shorter AP. What role these fibers play later following infarction is uncertain. Evidence that chronic-phase ventricular arrhythmias in human infarction are caused by reentry includes the following: (1) Arrhythmias are reproducibly induced and terminated by premature stimulation, which suggests an excitable gap; (2) Continuous electrical activity is present during tachycardia in multiple-catheter recordings; (3) Mapping studies during surgery demonstrate the activation sequence of tachycardia; (4) Tachycardia can be interrupted by strategically placed incisions, tissue resection, and sometimes catheter ablation.

Postulated Mechanisms for Clinical Arrhythmias

As will be appreciated from preceding discussion, most information concerning mechanisms for cardiac arrhythmias has come from in vitro studies, and much of this from intracellular recording. Intracellular recording cannot be performed in the intact heart, since it is not possible to maintain microelectrode impalements in the beating heart. Even so, phenomena similar to EAD have been observed in monophasic AP recordings in patients with polymorphic VT and the long-Q–T interval syndrome.[6,19] Otherwise, except for some reentry tachycardia (above), there is no conclusive evidence that one or another cellular mechanism is *the responsible* mechanism for a

TABLE 2-7 *Postulated cellular electrophysiologic mechanisms for clinical arrhythmias*

MECHANISM	CLINICAL ARRHYTHMIAS
Altered Normal Automaticity	Sinus bradycardia and tachycardia; sinus arrhythmia; wandering atrial pacemaker; AV junctional rhythm; idioventricular escape rhythm
Abnormal Automaticity	Slow monomorphic VT (acute MI); some automatic atrial tachycardia; accelerated AV junctional and idioventricular rhythms with ischemia
Triggered Activity (DAD)	VT due to myocardial ischemia or reperfusion of ischemic myocardium; catecholamine-mediated VT in normal heart; arrhythmias with digitalis toxicity
Triggered Activity (EAD)	Torsades de pointes with Q–T-interval prolongation (along with reentry?); ventricular arrhythmias with bupivacaine toxicity
Macroreentry	Atrial flutter; AV reciprocating tachycardia with manifest (WPW syndrome) or concealed* accessory AV pathways; paroxysmal SVT; VT with chronic MI
Microreentry	Mechanism that sustains atrial and ventricular fibrillation, but fibrillation likely triggered by other mechanisms

*Concealed because accessory pathways conduct only from ventricles to atria during tachycardia, but not from atria to ventricles to manifest as preexcitation (see Chapter 9).

particular clinical rhythm disturbance. Criteria used by clinical cardiac electrophysiologists to assign mechanisms for clinical arrhythmias are beyond the scope of this work, but are discussed elsewhere.[6,11,18,19,28,31,32] In essence, presumptive evidence exists when, during electrophysiologic study, behavior of the rhythm disturbance is consistent with that of the postulated cellular mechanism under in vitro conditions. With these reservations, postulated electrophysiologic mechanisms for clinical cardiac arrhythmias are given in Table 2-7.

References

1. Randall W, Talano J, Kaye M, et al. Cardiac pacemakers in absence of the SA node: responses to exercise and autonomic blockade. Am J Physiol 1978;234:H465–470.
2. Randall WC, Rinkema LE, Jones SB, et al. Functional characterization of atrial pacemaker activity. Am J Physiol 1982;242:H98–106.
3. Katz A. Cardiac ion channels. N Engl J Med 1993;328:1244–1251.
4. Sperelakis N. Origin of the cardiac resting potential. In Berne R (ed): Handbook of Physiology. Section 2. The Cardiovascular System. Vol. 1: The Heart. Bethesda, MD: American Physiological Society, 1979: pp. 187–267.
5. Atlee JL III, Bosnjak Z. Mechanisms for cardiac dysrhythmias during anesthesia. Anesthesiology 1990;72:347–374.
6. Zipes D. Genesis of cardiac arrhythmias: Electrophysiological considerations. In Braunwald E (ed): Heart Disease. 4th ed. Philadelphia: WB Saunders, 1992: pp. 588–627.
7. Gintant G, Cohen I, Datyner N, Kline R. Time-dependent outward currents in the heart. In Fozzard H, Haber E, Jennings R, et al (eds): The Heart and Cardiovascular System. 2nd ed. New York: Raven Press, 1992: pp. 1121–1169.
8. Fozzard H, Arnsdorf M. Cardiac electrophysiology. In Fozzard H, Haber E, Jennings R, Katz A, Morgan H (eds): The Heart and Cardiovascular System. 2nd ed. New York: Raven Press, 1992: pp. 63–98.
9. Baumgarten C, Fozzard H. Cardiac resting and pacemaker potentials. In Fozzard H, Haber E, Jennings R, et al (eds): The Heart and Cardiovascular System. 2nd ed. New York: Raven Press, 1992: pp. 963–1001.
10. Atlee JL, Bosnjak Z. The origin of the heart beat. In Brown BJ, Prys-Robers C (eds): General Anaesthesia. 6th ed. London: Butterworth-Heinemann, 1995:(in press).
11. Gilmour RJ, Zipes D. Abnormal automaticity and related phenomena. In Fozzard H, Haber E, Jennings R, et al (eds): The Heart and

Cardiovascular System. New York: Raven Press, 1986: pp. 1239–1257.
12. Gros D, Jongsma H. The cardiac connection. News Physiol Sci 1991;6:34–40.
13. Goldstein S, Rall W. Changes in action potential shape and velocity for changing core conductor geometry. Biophysical J 1974;14:731–757.
14. Sano T, Takayama N, Shimamoto T. Differential difference of conduction velocity in cardiac ventricular syncytium studied by microelectrodes. Circ Res 1959;7:262–267.
15. Spach M, Miller W, Geselowitz D, et al. The discontinuous nature of propagation in normal canine cardiac muscle. Evidence for recurrent discontinuities of intracellular resistance that affect membrane currents. Circ Res 1981;48:262–267.
16. Spach M, Miller W, Dolber P, et al. The functional role of structural complexities in the propagation of depolarization in the atrium of the dog. Cardiac conduction disturbances due to discontinuities of effective axial resistivity. Circ Res 1982;50:175–191.
17. Turner L, Bosnjak Z. Autonomic and anesthetic modulation of cardiac conduction and arrhythmias. In Lynch CI (ed): Clinical Cardiac Electrophysiology. Philadelphia: JB Lippincott, 1994: pp. 53–84.
18. Janse M. Reentrant arrhythmias. In Fozzard H, Haber E, Jennings R, et al (eds): The Heart and Cardiovascular System. 2nd ed. New York: Raven Press, 1992: pp. 2055–2094.
19. Wit A, Rosen M. Afterdepolarizations and triggered activity: Distinction from automaticity as an arrhythmogenic mechanism. In Fozzard H, Haber E, Jennings R, et al (eds): The Heart and Cardiovascular System. 2nd ed. New York: Raven Press, 1992: pp. 2113–2163.
20. Elharrar V, Zipes D. Voltage modulation of automaticity in cardiac Purkinje fibers. In Zipes D, Bailey J, Elharrar V (eds): The Slow Inward Current and Cardiac Arrhythmias. The Hague: Martinus-Nijhoff, 1980: pp. 357–373.
21. Cranefield P. Action potentials, afterpotentials, and arrhythmias. Circ Res 1977;41:415–423.
22. Tsien R, Kass R, Weingart R. Cellular and subcellular mechanisms of cardiac pacemaker oscillations. J Exper Biol 1979;81:205–215.
23. Fabiato A. Calcium-induced release of calcium from the cardiac sarcoplasmic reticulum. Am J Physiol 1983;245:C1–C14.
24. Fisch F, Prakash C, Roden D. Suppression of repolarization-related arrhythmias in vitro and in vivo by low-dose potassium channel activators. Circulation 1990;82:1362–1369.
25. Mines G. On dynamic equilibrium in the heart. J Physiol (Lond) 1913;46:349–382.
26. Mines G. On circulating excitations in heart muscles and their relation to tachycardia and fibrillation. Trans R Soc Can Sect IV 1914;43–52.

27. Hoffman B, Rosen M. Cellular mechanisms for cardiac arrhythmias. Circ Res 1981;49:1–15.
28. Zipes D. Specific arrhythmias: diagnosis and treatment. In Braunwald E (ed): Heart Disease. 4th ed. Philadelphia: WB Saunders, 1992: pp. 667–725.
29. Schmitt F, Erlanger J. Directional differences in the conduction of the impulse through heart muscle and their possible relation to extrasystolic and fibrillary contractions. Am J Physiol 1928;87:326–347.
30. Janse M, Wit A. Electrophysiological mechanisms of ventricular arrhythmias resulting from myocardial ischemia and infarction. Physiol Rev 1989;69:1049–1169.
31. Kastor JA. Arrhythmias. Philadelphia: WB Saunders, 1994.
32. Josephson ME. Clinical Cardiac Electrophysiology. 2nd ed. Philadelphia, Lea & Febiger, 1993.

3

Arrhythmia Causes and Associations

Abbreviations Used in Chapter 3	
A/C-LQTS	Acquired/congenital Long-QT-interval syndrome
AV	Atrioventricular
CNS	Central nervous system
ECG	Electrocardiogram, electrocardiography
MAC	Minimum alveolar concentration
MVPS	Mitral valve prolapse syndrome
NDMR	Nondepolarizing muscle relaxant
OCR	Oculocardiac reflex
SA	Sinoatrial
SVT	Supraventricular tachycardia
VES	Ventricular extrasystoles
VPB	Ventricular premature beats
VT	Ventricular tachycardia
WPW	Wolff–Parkinson–White (syndrome)

In this chapter, the concepts of physiologic imbalance and arrhythmia substrate are explained before discussion of specific causes and associations for cardiac arrhythmias. These concepts have particular relevance to prevention and management of arrhythmias in anesthetized or critically ill patients, in whom arrhythmias are usually due to interactions between imbalance and arrhythmia substrates, as opposed to those in patients with acquired or congenital structural heart disease. In these patients, cardiac arrhythmias are more likely the direct result of the disease process ("substrate") itself. References include several recent reviews or monographs,[1-6] and other listed sources.

Imposed or Physiologic Imbalance

In contrast to patients with heart disease, in whom cardiac arrhythmias are usually a consequence of that disease, arrhythmias in anesthetized or critical care patients are often triggered by adverse drug effects or interactions, altered states, and complications related to diagnostic or therapeutic interventions. Collectively, these may be referred to as *imposed or physiologic imbalance.* Some more common causes for such physiologic imbalance in perioperative settings are listed in Table 3-1. These may occur in patients with normal hearts, major systemic disease, structural heart disease, or major systemic and structural heart disease.

Major systemic disease predisposes to arrhythmias with imposed or physiologic imbalance. Structural heart disease, on the other hand, not only predisposes to arrhythmias with such imbalance, but also provides a "substrate" for arrhythmias (discussed further later), which

TABLE 3-1 *Causes for acute physiologic imbalance in perioperative settings*

Autonomic imbalance	Electrolyte imbalance	Temperature extremes
Acid–base imbalance	Hypoxia or ischemia	Hypercarbia; hypocarbia
Pain; anxiety	Light anesthesia	Anesthetic overdose
Inappropriate drugs	Drug toxicity	Drug interactions
Airway manipulation	Surgical manipulation	Traction reflexes
Metabolic imbalance	Endocrine imbalance	↑ Intracranial pressure
Central vascular access	Device malfunction	Microshock
Acute heart failure	Malnutrition; cachexia	Myocardial injury

could be a focus of altered normal, abnormal, or triggered automatic activity, and/or potential reentry circuits. Therefore, the combination of imposed physiologic imbalance with major systemic disease and/or structural heart disease is far more likely to trigger significant cardiac arrhythmias than imposed imbalance alone in patients with normal hearts and no systemic disease.

Because new or worsening arrhythmias in perioperative settings are often triggered by imposed or physiologic imbalance (Table 3–1), prevention and treatment are not necessarily with antiarrhythmic drugs or devices, as they are prone to be in patients with rhythm disturbances due to primary heart disease. Indeed, antiarrhythmic drugs or devices have recognized potential to compound imbalance and worsen arrhythmias. Therefore, indicated remedial or preventive measures for any identifiable imbalance are often the *only* required treatment.

Arrhythmia Substrates

Anesthetized, recovering, or critically ill patients with certain conditions (Table 3–2) appear at increased risk for new or exacerbated forms of arrhythmias from altered states because of imposed or physiologic imbalance. It is suggested that these conditions somehow provide a "substrate" for arrhythmias, perhaps by causing myocardial changes conducive to reentry, or by increasing susceptibility to triggered or abnormal automaticity. For example, patients with the Wolff–Parkinson–White (WPW) syndrome are prone to a special type of reentrant supraventricular tachycardia (SVT) called atrioventricular (AV) reciprocating tachycardia. However, without an altered state produced by some imposed or physiologic imbalance (Fig. 3–1),

TABLE 3-2 *Conditions or substrates that increase risk of arrhythmias with altered states*

Coronary artery disease	Hypertension	Hypertrophic myopathy
Dilated myopathy	Congestive heart failure	Sick sinus syndrome
Morbid obesity	Chronic lung disease	CNS pathology
Autonomic dysfunction	Endocrinopathies	Renal failure
Advanced age	Malnutrition; cachexia	Mitral valve prolapse

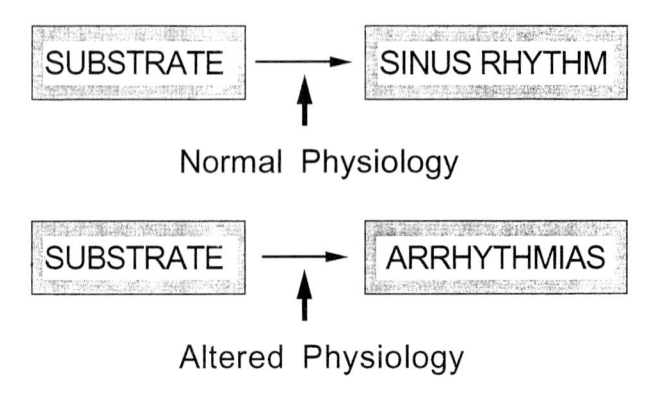

```
  SUBSTRATE  ──▶  SINUS RHYTHM
                ▲
         Normal Physiology

  SUBSTRATE  ──▶   ARRHYTHMIAS
                ▲
         Altered Physiology

(Autonomic, electrolyte, metabolic, acid-base,
 temperature imbalance; medical intervention)
```

FIGURE 3-1 *Concept of how arrhythmias are triggered by altered states in patients with substrates for arrhythmias (Table 3-2), but who do not necessarily have arrhythmias. With no imbalance from an altered state (Normal Physiology), the patient has sinus rhythm or relatively innocuous rhythm disturbances. With imbalance (Altered Physiology), more ominous arrhythmias can occur.*

reciprocating SVT may manifest not at all or only as extrasystoles. Stable coronary artery disease, another condition that provides an altered substrate for arrhythmias, requires no further explanation. Other conditions or substrates listed in Table 3-2 do require additional explanation.

HYPERTENSION, CARDIOMYOPATHY, AND CONGESTIVE HEART FAILURE

Hypertension acutely increases myocardial wall tension, as does hypertrophic cardiomyopathy with chronic hypertension, and aortic or pulmonary valvular stenosis or outflow-tract obstruction. Increased wall tension can produce subendocardial ischemia, particularly during tachycardia. Subendocardial ischemia, in turn, facilitates reentrant ventricular arrhythmias (see Chapter 2). Dilated cardiomyopathy and congestive heart failure also reduce subendocardial perfusion, and patients with dilated or hypertrophic cardiomyopathy may have cellular changes affecting conduction and refractoriness that are conducive to reentry.

SICK SINUS SYNDROME

Sick sinus syndrome sinus node dysfunction results from degenerative changes in the sinoatrial (SA) node or its atrial margins, autonomic dysfunction, or combinations of both. These changes are the basis for a variety of rhythm disturbances, including bradycardia, escape rhythms, and tachyarrhythmias (see Chapter 9). Anesthetic drugs or adjunct treatment that increase vagal tone, reduce sympathetic tone, or depress SA node automaticity may unmask or aggravate sinus node dysfunction with the sick sinus syndrome.

MORBID OBESITY

Morbid obesity and chronic pulmonary disease, both associated with pulmonary hypertension and right heart failure, increase the risk for atrial tachycardia, flutter, or fibrillation, presumably by causing SA changes (stretch, ischemia, fibrosis) conducive to reentry or ectopic (automatic, triggered) rhythm disturbances. Stress during anesthesia, surgery, emergence, or the immediate postoperative period may exacerbate pulmonary hypertension, heart failure, and arrhythmias.

OTHER CONDITIONS

Central nervous system (CNS) pathology, autonomic dysfunction, and endocrinopathies may produce sympathetic or parasympathetic dominance, and other physiologic derangements as well. For example, dysautonomia might increase disparity of ventricular refractoriness or prolong repolarization, both of which are conducive to reentrant or triggered ventricular tachyarrhythmias (see Chapter 10). Renal failure, cachexic states, and advanced age, aside from underlying cardiovascular disease, also promote arrhythmias due to metabolic or electrolyte derangements affecting myocardial electrophysiology. Finally, many of the conditions associated with arrhythmias may also provide arrhythmia substrates.

Drugs and Imbalance as Causes for Arrhythmias

AUTONOMIC IMBALANCE

No one can contest the ubiquitous involvement of autonomic—or "reflex-caused"—imbalance in the genesis of cardiac rhythm disturbances in perioperative and critical care settings. This, perhaps more than any single other factor, distinguishes the origin of arrhythmias in these settings from those in patients with primary heart disease. Among the factors contributing to autonomic imbalance are anxiety, stress, inadequate anesthesia, awareness, and pain. Tachycardia, bradycardia, and hyper- and hypotension are the usual manifestations, but with conditions or substrates that increase risk for arrhythmias (Table 3–2), supraventricular or ventricular arrhythmias are possible. Causes for autonomic imbalance during anesthesia and surgery are listed in Table 3–3, along with the anticipated predominant autonomic (vagal or sympathetic) mediation of the cardiovascular response. In postanesthetic care units, emergence delirium from general anesthesia, disorientation, and acute perception of pain are important causes for sympathetic predominance, along with an overly distended bladder. While bladder distension may be experienced as pain or discomfort in conscious patients, it may not be in patients with residual block from spinal or epidural anesthesia. Depending on the sensory level of anesthesia, there could be exaggerated hypertension with reflex bradycardia, much as with autonomic dysfunction in paraplegics and quadriplegics. In critical care units, inability to communicate and sensory deprivation are additional causes for sympathetic predominance.

TEMPERATURE IMBALANCE

Sinus bradycardia, AV junctional rhythm, and QT-interval prolongation are early manifestations of *hypothermia*. With more severe

TABLE 3-3 *Causes for autonomic imbalance during anesthesia and surgery with anticipated vagal (V) or sympathetic (S) mediation of the cardiovascular response*

Laryngoscopy (V, S)*	Tracheal intubation (S)
Oculocardiac reflex (V)	Pharyngeal stimulation (V, S)*
Traction on hilum of lung (V, S)*	Pericardial stimulation (S, V†)
Aortic dissection (S, V†)	Intra-abdominal traction (V, S)*
Anorectal dilation (V, S)*	Peritoneal stimulation (S)
Periosteal stimulation (V, S)*	Brainstem traction (V)
Carotid sinus stimulation (V)	Electroconvulsive therapy (V, S‡)

*Predominant component listed first.
†Secondary to hypertension.
‡Bradycardia first followed by hypertension and tachycardia.

hypothermia, conduction becomes depressed throughout the specialized conduction system. With extreme hypothermia, depressed intraventricular conduction is characterized by prominent notching of the terminal QRS complex with ST-segment elevation, the so-called Osborn or J wave (Fig. 3-2). The threshold for ventricular fibrillation is reduced by hypothermia, with fibrillation likely at temperatures below 28°C. Without adequate rewarming, treatment of ventricular fibrillation is difficult, and pharmacologic therapy is largely ineffective.[3]

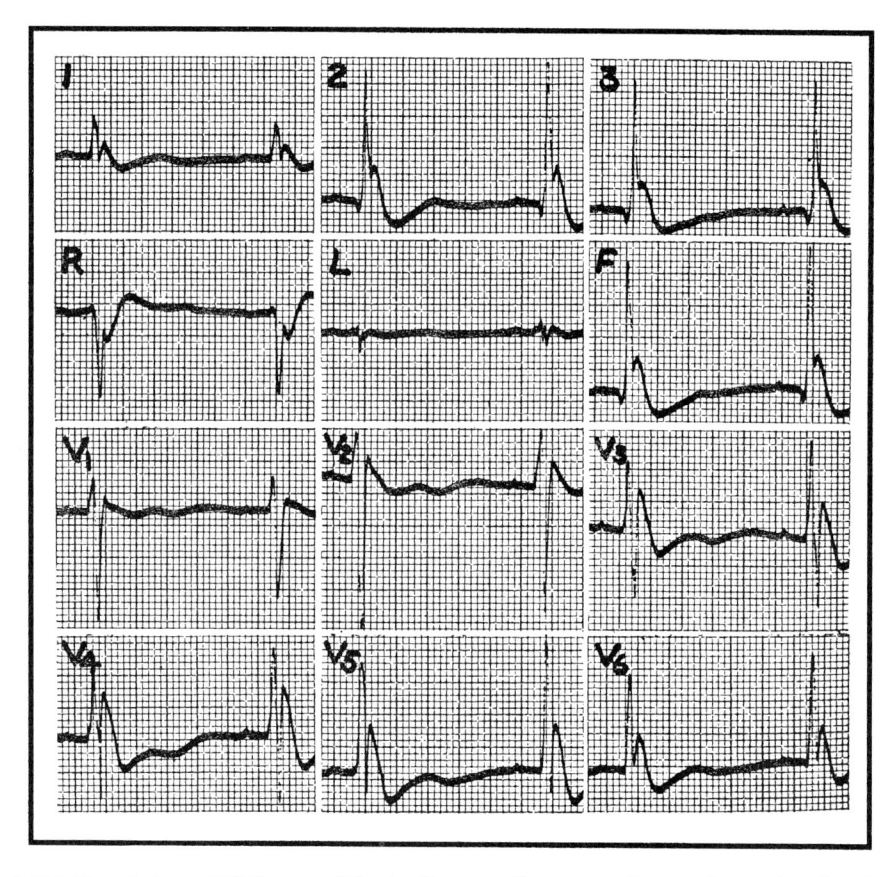

FIGURE 3-2 ECG manifestations of severe hypothermia (body temperature = 33°C). Note sinus bradycardia (50 beats/min), Q–T interval prolongation, and the characteristic Osborn or J waves; namely, notching of the terminal QRS complex with S–T segment elevation. (From Wagner GS: Mariotts Practical Electrocardiography. 9th ed. Baltimore, MD: Williams and Wilkins, 1994: p. 178, with permission.)

Indeed, class I antiarrhythmic drugs such as lidocaine or procainamide may actually increase the temperature required for defibrillation.[3] Sinus tachycardia is the most common rhythm disturbance with *hyperthermia*. Malignant ventricular arrhythmias can occur with extreme hyperthermia in association with hypoxia and metabolic acidosis (i.e., malignant hyperpyrexia).

MEDICAL INTERVENTION

Inappropriate or overly aggressive treatment with drugs probably heads the list of medical interventions that may contribute to or cause arrhythmias in anesthesia or critical care settings. Anesthetic overdose is cause for bradycardia and escape rhythms. Mechanical and electrical interference is more likely to trigger arrhythmias in patients with acute physiologic imbalance (Table 3–1) or conditions or substrates that increase the risk of arrhythmias (Table 3–2). Ventricular arrhythmias might be triggered in patients with pulmonary artery or transvenous pacing catheters during mechanical ventilation. Also, patients with central access catheters have a low-resistance pathway directly to the heart, and are at increased risk for microshock-caused arrhythmias.

DRUG TOXICITIES AND INTERACTIONS

It is not possible to mention all possibilities for arrhythmias due to drug toxicities or interactions. Only drug toxicities or interactions with certain arrhythmic potential are discussed here.[1,7–12] In general, concerning arrhythmic potential, drugs that reduce SA node automaticity or prolong AV conduction time may worsen bradycardia and escape rhythms in patients with sinus node dysfunction or impaired AV conduction. Drugs that cause hypotension by means of vasodilation may be associated with reflex tachycardia. Those that depress myocardial contractility are also likely to depress sinus node function and AV nodal conduction, but not necessarily ventricular conduction. Drugs that impair myocardial perfusion through direct vasoconstriction or vasodilation with coronary steal may provoke ischemic arrhythmias. Finally, electrophysiologic safety can be predicted for older anesthetics (especially, halothane) with more complete electrophysiologic profiles,[1,2] but not for newer drugs such as propofol, etomidate, midazolam, desflurane, and sevoflurane, which have not been investigated. This is far from ideal, since these newer drugs are commonly used in patients with heart disease or conditions conducive to arrhythmias, but with no knowledge of the potential for adverse cardiac electrophysiologic effects.

Anesthetics and Catecholamines

Anesthetic facilitation of catecholamine arrhythmias *(sensitization)* is the classic example of an adverse drug interaction. Sensitization with older anesthetics has been reviewed by Katz and Bigger,[13] and more recently by Atlee and Bosnjak[2]. Halothane is the most sensitizing contemporary anesthetic, with enflurane intermediate and isoflurane least sensitizing. Based on human and dog (similar to human) studies, the estimated median dose for ventricular arrhythmias with halothane is 2.0 µg/kg, enflurane > 4.0 µg/kg, and isoflurane > 6.0 µg/kg, although other drugs or factors can alter these doses. Desflurane and sevoflurane appear as sensitizing as isoflurane.[14-16] In dogs, thiopental halves the mean epinephrine dose for ventricular extrasystoles (VES) and tachycardia with halothane, enflurane, or isoflurane.[17,18] Thiamylal, aminophylline, ketamine, propofol, and cocaine facilitate halothane–epinephrine arrhythmias,[1,19] but etomidate and midazolam have no effect.[15,20] Factors that increase the dose of epinephrine for ventricular arrhythmias with anesthetics are listed in Table 3-4.[1]

Adrenergic Blockers and Agonists

ALPHA-ADRENERGIC BLOCKERS. While alpha-1 blockers are sometimes used as vasodilators, the beta-adrenergic effects of sympathetic stimulation are not blocked. Hence, direct or reflex sympathetic stimulation of heart rate is not inhibited, and there can be tachycardia during anesthesia with drugs or techniques that preserve or increase sympathetic tone.

CENTRAL ALPHA-2 AGONISTS. Clonidine, dexmedetomidine, and other central alpha-2 agonists may be used in perioperative and critical care settings for their sedative, anxiolytic, and analgesic properties, as well as their ability to promote hemodynamic stability. However, these drugs can produce disadvantageous bradycardia, and should be used with extreme caution in patients with SA node dysfunction or AV heart block, or with drugs that slow heart rate. The

TABLE 3-4 *Drugs or factors that increase epinephrine dose for arrhythmias*

Lidocaine, bupivacaine, etidocaine	Beta-adrenergic blockers
Alpha-adrenergic blockers	Central alpha-2 adrenergic agonists
Verapamil and diltiazem	Infants and children (halothane)

potential for interactions with anesthetic drugs that slow heart rate has not been adequately studied.

BETA-ADRENERGIC DRUGS. *Beta-blockers* such as esmolol and propranolol slow sinus rate and prolong AV node conduction time. These drugs have additive effects to those of potent volatile anesthetics or opiates, and will produce exaggerated effects in patients with SA or AV node dysfunction. *Beta-1 or -2 agonists* in sufficient dose may be associated with pronounced sinus tachycardia, but not necessarily ventricular arrhythmias. For example, isoproterenol (4 µg/kg) did not induce ventricular arrhythmias with halothane in dogs.[21] Also, the author is aware of an instance where 200 µg of isoproterenol was inadvertently administered to a healthy adult asthmatic patient instead of thiopental. The patient developed maximum sinus tachycardia (220 to 230 beats/min) and ST-segment depression, and a small increase in systolic arterial pressure (~ 160 mmHg), but there were no ventricular arrhythmias or subsequent evidence of myocardial injury. Therefore, if ventricular arrhythmias do occur with beta-adrenergic stimulation, they appear more likely the result of subendocardial ischemia with tachycardia.

Calcium-Channel Blockers

All calcium-channel blockers inhibit calcium entry into the cell or affect its mobilization from intracellular stores. Electrophysiologic effects are most evident in slow-response or depressed fast-response fibers, since action potentials of these fibers are more dependent on the inward calcium current (see Chapter 2). The magnitude of calcium-channel blockers effect on sinus rate or AV nodal conduction time depends on whether the drug delays recovery of the calcium channel. Verapamil more than diltiazem delays calcium-channel recovery, but nifedipine, nicardipine, and other dihydropyridines do not. Therefore, verapamil and diltiazem, but not the dihydropyridines, may slow sinus rate and increase AV nodal conduction time. In fact, depending on the magnitude of underlying sympathetic tone and hypotension, there may be a modest to moderate reflex increase in heart rate with dihydropyridines secondary to vasodilation. Heart block, severe sinus bradycardia, sinus pause or arrest, and escape rhythms have been reported with verapamil or diltiazem, and halothane, enflurane, or isoflurane.[1] There were no available reports of such interaction with desflurane or isoflurane in 1994. The potential for sinus bradycardia or arrest, or heart block, appears greater with intravenous (IV) verapamil and any of the anesthetics, and greater with IV verapamil or diltiazem and halothane or enflurane compared to isoflurane.[22] It should be appreciated that at least in dogs, volatile anesthetics increase plasma calcium-channel blocker concentrations following IV but not oral dosing.[1] If the preceding is applicable to humans, caution is advised when administering IV diltiazem or verapamil to patients anesthetized with potent volatile anesthetics. Finally, it may be worth noting that "apparent" complete heart block with volatile anesthetics and IV diltiazem or verapamil in dogs was due to SA, not AV heart block, since there was 1:1 AV conduction during atrial pacing (Fig. 3-3).[22] If so, some cases of "apparent" heart block with calcium-channel blockers and anesthetics might be treated by temporary atrial pacing (see Chapter 7).

Methylxanthines

Several reports implicate theophylline as a cause for arrhythmias with halothane and pancuronium.[1] In dogs, acute (not chronic) theophylline interacts with halothane (not isoflurane) to facilitate epinephrine–anesthetic arrhythmias. Down-regulation of the beta-adrenergic receptors following chronic theophylline may explain this finding.

Drugs Affecting Catecholamine Turnover

TRICYCLIC ANTIDEPRESSANTS. Electrocardiographic (ECG) changes with tricyclic antidepressant toxicity include T-wave flattening or inversion and prolongation of conduction time throughout the AV conduction system. With QT-interval prolongation and QRS duration > 0.16 sec, there is some danger of ventricular arrhythmias. Older studies (1970s) indicate that patients receiving tricyclic antidepressants are at risk for arrhythmias related to stress, including anesthesia and surgery.[1] Finally, short- but not long-term administration of tricyclic antidepressants enhances halothane–epinephrine arrhythmias in dogs.

MONOAMINE OXIDASE INHIBITORS. Monoamine oxidase inhibitors block the oxidative deamination of naturally occurring monoamines, thereby increasing tissue catecholamine levels. As a result, exaggerated tachycardia, hypertension, and arrhythmias may occur with indirect-acting sympathomimetics. In contrast, direct-acting sympathomimetics are more likely to produce tachycardia, hypertension, or arrhythmias with tricyclic antidepressants.

Digitalis

Cardiotoxicity with digitalis manifests as almost any cardiac rhythm disturbance. The probability and severity of rhythm distur-

70   ARRHYTHMIA CAUSES AND ASSOCIATIONS

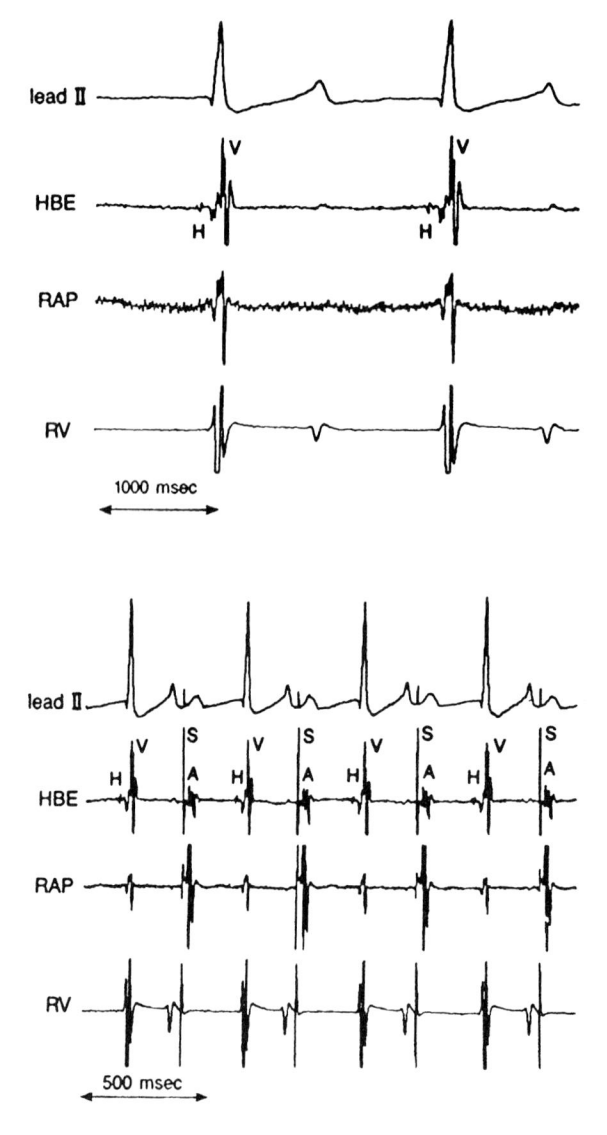

FIGURE 3-3   *See legend on opposite page*

bance is directly related to the presence or absence of heart disease.[23] After ingestion of large, but nonlethal quantities of digitalis, sinus bradycardia and AV heart block are the usual findings in patients with normal hearts. With structural heart disease or sinus node dysfunction, characteristic arrhythmias include paroxysmal (sudden-onset) and nonparoxysmal (gradual-onset) SVT, accelerated AV junctional rhythm, VES (especially, group beating), and ventricular tachycardia or fibrillation. Cardiotoxicity results both from direct and indirect actions of digitalis.[23] Direct effects result from an advanced stage of sodium–potassium pump inhibition and intracellular calcium overload. Indirect effects are due to central autonomic stimulation and increased cardiac sensitivity to adrenergic or cholinergic transmitters. Concurrent medication and other factors increase the risk of digitalis cardiotoxicity (Table 3–5). Most contemporary anesthetic agents or adjuncts have been experimentally shown either to oppose or to not affect digitalis arrhythmias.[1] However, under no circumstance should any anesthetic be relied upon to reverse clinical digitalis arrhythmias, even though it might have been shown in vitro to oppose the responsible cellular mechanisms. Older reports suggesting that succinylcholine or neostigmine worsened digitalis arrhythmias are suspect because no information was supplied about the status of digitalization.[1] Advice for management of digitalized patients or administration of digitalis in perioperative settings is provided in Table 3–6.

FIGURE 3-3   (Top) *Apparent complete AV heart block with AV junctional escape rhythm at 32 beats/min in a dog with 1.2 MAC halothane and verapamil. Simultaneous tracings of surface ECG lead II (lead II), His bundle (HBE), right atrial appendage (RAP), and right ventricular (RV) electrograms. In HBE, H and V denote His bundle and ventricular depolarization, respectively. Except for the RAP electrode there is no evidence of atrial depolarization in any lead (atrial quiescence).* (Bottom) *Same dog, test conditions, and lead designations as above during high right atrial pacing at 120 beats/min. Note that all paced beats are conducted, although with PR-interval prolongation. Therefore, the mechanism for apparent heart block must have been sinus arrest or SA block, since AV conduction was intact. A similar result was obtained for each of 13 additional occurrences of apparent complete heart block and AV junctional or idioventricular escape rhythms involving halothane, enflurane, or isoflurane with diltiazem or verapamil. (From Atlee et al.,[22] Anesthesiology 1990;72:889–01 with permission.)*

72 ARRHYTHMIA CAUSES AND ASSOCIATIONS

TABLE 3-5 *Drugs and factors that increase the likelihood of digitalis toxicity*

Catecholamines, stress	Potassium imbalance	Alkalosis and acidosis
Hyperthyroidism	Hypoxia, ischemia	Hypomagnesemia
Hypercalcemia	Quinidine, quinine*	Amiodarone*
Propafenone*	Diltiazem, verapamil†	Renal failure

*Elevates serum digitalis concentrations.
†Elevates serum digitalis concentrations plus additive effects on sinus automaticity and AV nodal conduction.

TABLE 3-6 *Advice for management of digitalized patients or administration of digitalis*

1. Without clinical evidence of toxicity or toxic serum levels (digoxin > 2.0 ng/ml), digitalis is unlikely to cause serious arrhythmias without other imbalance.
2. If rapid, acute rate reduction is required wth atrial flutter–fibrillation, edrophonium, esmolol, or calcium-channel blockers* are more reliable and safe compared to pushing digoxin.
3. Do not rely on anesthetics† or adjunct drugs to oppose presumed triggered rhythms with digitalis. Rather, correct imbalance and/or treat with digitalis-specific antibodies.

*The calcium-channel blockers diltiazem and verapamil may increase the ventricular rate in patients with WPW syndrome.
†See text.

Antiarrhythmic Drugs

USE DEPENDENCE. Some antiarrhythmic drugs show greater inhibitory effects on conduction with faster heart rates or following prolonged stimulation,[24] termed *use dependence.* Use dependence is thought to result from preferential interaction of the drug with open or inactive sodium or calcium channels compared to resting channels. With slower rates, more channels become free from drug and available for reexcitation.

CLASS 1 ANTIARRHYTHMICS. Class 1 drugs are sodium-channel blockers. Sodium-channel blockade is discussed in more detail under local anesthetics, below. Class 1 drugs show varying potential for use-dependent block, and are subclassified depending on the kinetics of sodium-channel block. Class 1B drugs (lidocaine-like) have fast onset–offset kinetics, and show little use dependence at normal heart rates. Class 1A (quinidine-like) drugs have intermediate kinetics, and class 1C (encainide-like) drugs slow kinetics. Class 1C drugs can show use-dependent block, even at physiologic heart rates. Increased potential for use-dependent block in part explains the greater proarrhythmic potential of 1C drugs. By *proarrhythmia* is meant the ability of some antiarrhythmics (notably, class 1A, 1C, and 3 drugs) to cause new arrhythmias or aggravate existing ones. Proarrhythmia is discussed in more detail in Chapter 6. Among the risk factors for ventricular proarrhythmia with antiarrhythmics are poor left ventricular function, prior QT-interval prolongation, and treatment with digitalis and diuretics.[24]

OTHER ANTIARRHYTHMICS. Volatile anesthetics, opiates and alpha-2 adrenergic agonists (e.g., clonidine) have potential to cause severe bradycardia or heart block with class 2 (beta-blockers) and some class 3 antiarrhythmics (amiodarone, sotolol). Bretylium, also a class 3 antiarrhythmic, may exacerbate ventricular arrhythmias due to initial release of catecholamines, depending on the available pool of catecholamines. AV heart block and junctional rhythm disturbances have been reported in anesthetized cardiac surgical patients receiving oral amiodarone. Since intravenous amiodarone may be available by the time this book appears, caution is advised for use in anesthetized patients until more data are available. Oral amiodarone has been associated with about a 2 percent incidence of ventricular proarrhythmia.[25] Recent evidence suggests that both proarrhythmia and pulmonary toxicity with amiodarone are dose related, and that smaller doses may be just as effective. Finally, among the class 4 antiarrhythmics (diltiazem, verapamil), the potential for bradycardia and escape rhythms appears least with diltiazem and isoflurane compared to with halothane or enflurane.[2,22]

Cocaine

Cocaine differs from other local anesthetics in that it also blocks the reuptake of norepinephrine at adrenergic nerve terminals. Therefore, cocaine also produces central and peripheral sympathomimetic effects. Myocardial ischemia or infarction related to cocaine abuse are documented, and possibly due to coronary spasm, intimal proliferation, or acceleration of arteriosclerosis.[26] Myocarditis, dilated cardiomyopathy, and congestive heart failure can also occur with chronic cocaine abuse. Sudden death and ventricular tachyarrhythmias may complicate acute cocaine intoxication. Cocaine prolongs ventricular conduction time and the QT interval. Type 1 antiarrhythmics may exacerbate ventricular arrhythmias in patients with a cocaine-prolonged QT interval or intracardiac conduction, and should be used

74 ARRHYTHMIA CAUSES AND ASSOCIATIONS

with caution.[26,27] Also, while beta-blockers may be used to reverse sympathetic hyperactivity with cocaine, there is potential for coronary spasm due to unopposed alpha-adrenergic stimulation. Finally, with cocaine for topical anesthesia or hemostasis in recommended doses, and no other significant imbalance, serious arrhythmias or coronary spasm appear unlikely.

Miscellaneous Drugs

Drugs with arrhythmic potential that might be used in perioperative settings, but that do not fit into the above categories, are mentioned here.[1,28,29]

BACLOFEN. Baclofen (Baclofen™, Lioresal™), a derivative of the inhibitory neurotransmitter gamma-aminobutyric acid, is commonly prescribed for treatment of spasticity following spinal cord injury or transection. It has produced severe hypotension and bradycardia (< 20 beats/min) in anesthetized patients (fentanyl, etomidate, isoflurane, atracurium). Bradycardia does respond to chronotropic drugs.

HISTAMINE. Histamine is the most important primary mediator released during anaphylaxis or anaphylactoid reactions (discussed later). Arrhythmic effects of histamine include H_1-mediated slowing of AV nodal conduction and H_2-mediated enhanced automaticity (SA node, ventricles). Since H_1 and H_2 actions are enhanced by volatile anesthetics and epinephrine, respectively, epinephrine to treat histamine-mediated reactions with some anesthetics, especially halothane, might provoke ventricular arrhythmias.

CIMETIDINE AND RANITIDINE. Histamine-increased sinus rate is opposed by H_2-blockade with cimetidine or ranitidine, and presumably also the newer H_2-blockers (famotidine, nizatidine). Sinus bradycardia, sinus arrest, and severe ventricular arrhythmias have been reported following IV cimetidine during anesthesia. Ranitidine has also been associated with profound bradycardia. The mechanism for these effects is not certain, but may involve unopposed H_1-stimulation (slowed conduction) with reduced SA node and latent pacemaker automaticity consequent to H_2-receptor blockade.

LITHIUM. Lithium is widely used for the treatment of affective disorders. In therapeutic doses (0.6 to 1.5 mEq/L), it may be associated with T-wave changes and QRS widening. With moderate

(1.6 to 2.5 mEq/L) to severe toxicity (≥ 2.6 mEq/L), ECG changes and arrhythmias resemble those with hypokalemia, including ST–T changes, SA block, bradyarrhythmias, AV block, intraventricular conduction and QT prolongation, and ventricular arrhythmias.[1,3,27] These occur because lithium enters the cell during depolarization, but it is not easily extruded. Thus, lithium accumulates within the cell and reduces resting membrane potential. It also interferes with adenyl cyclase and the cardiac effects of catecholamines. Extreme toxicity (≥ 4.0 mEq/L) may cause cardiovascular collapse. Paroxysmal bundle branch block and increased myocardial irritability have also been reported during anesthesia in patients receiving lithium.

METHYL METHACRYLATE. Methyl methacrylate is a space-filling substance used to facilitate fixation of prosthetic devices to bone. Insertion of the cement may produce sudden hypotension, postulated mechanisms for which are listed in Table 3–7. The magnitude of hypotension often depends on the volume status of the patient. If the venous capacitance is constricted, for whatever reason, hypotension is likely to be more severe. There has been one report of transient second-degree AV heart block with methyl methacrylate, and sinus bradycardia is also possible. As a rule, serious arrhythmias are not expected without compromised coronary perfusion.

METOCLOPRAMIDE. Metoclopramide acts peripherally to enhance the muscarinic actions of acetylcholine, and centrally to antagonize those of dopamine. Thus, the drug increases lower-esophageal sphincter tone, enhances gastric emptying time, and has antiemetic effects. Paroxysmal SVT has been reported with metoclopramide, but the mechanism was nonapparent and there was no history of SVT. While metoclopramide is structurally similar to procainamide, it lacks significant antiarrhythmic actions.

TABLE 3-7 *Mechanisms for hypotension with methyl methacrylate*

1. Vasodilation by absorbed methyl methacrylate monomer.
2. Systemic fat or marrow embolization with injection of cement.
3. Heating of bone marrow with release of vasoactive mediators.
4. Hydrolysis of methyl methacrylate to methacrylic acid.
5. Reflex circulatory changes with major pulmonary embolization.

ANESTHETIC DRUGS

Anesthetic drugs include inhalation and intravenous agents, local anesthetics, neuromuscular blockers, opioids, sedative–hypnotic–anxiolytics, and adjunct drugs. No contemporary anesthetic drug should be considered arrhythmic in the absence of causes (Table 3–1) or conditions (Table 3–2) that increase the likelihood of arrhythmias.[1-3,5,6,30] Unfortunately, knowledge of the pro- or antiarrhythmic potential of anesthetic drugs is sparse in comparison to that of cardiovascular drugs.

Direct and Indirect Effects

Both direct and indirect (reflex-caused) actions of anesthetic drugs will determine their net effect on cardiac arrhythmogenesis. Anesthetic drugs could alter properties of normal or abnormal myocardium in ways that might be conducive to or oppose the genesis of arrhythmias, depending on the nature of physiologic imbalance (Table 3–1) and the type of substrate (Table 3–2). Further, concurrent medication will influence the effects of anesthetic drugs on cardiac electrophysiologic properties. All of these considerations must be taken into account when projecting anesthetic arrhythmic potential in a particular patient.

Contemporary Inhalation Anesthetics

Contemporary volatile anesthetics include desflurane, enflurane, halothane, isoflurane, and sevoflurane. Rarely or no longer used agents (chloroform, cyclopropane, diethyl ether, fluroxene, methoxyflurane, trichlorethylene) are not discussed here, but are elsewhere.[1,13]

Desflurane, Sevoflurane, Nitrous Oxide

At this writing, there were no published reports of the direct electrophysiologic actions of the newer volatile anesthetics on normal or abnormal heart. Desflurane, however, is now well known to increase sinus rate through increased efferent sympathetic tone, particularly with high inspired concentrations. Neither were there no reports of the cardiac electrophysiologic effects of nitrous oxide, despite its widespread use as a supplement to volatile anesthetics or as part of balanced anesthetic techniques. A single report suggests that the addition of nitrous oxide to opioid-based or inhalation (enflurane, halothane, isoflurane) anesthesia can provoke AV junctional rhythm.[31] Aside from possible increased sympathetic tone with nitrous oxide, the authors offered no plausible explanation for this finding.

Normal Electrophysiology: Halothane, Enflurane, Isoflurane

It is generally known that direct depressant actions of halothane, enflurane, or isoflurane on normal or abnormal cardiac electrophysiologic properties are influenced by indirect effects, particularly the agent's ability to depress baroreceptor (halothane > enflurane > isoflurane) and other compensatory cardiovascular reflexes.

SA NODE AND LATENT PACEMAKERS. All agents produce equal direct depression of SA node rate. However, in patients with normal SA node function, there is little net effect of any agent to reduce heart rate, and isoflurane often increases rate. Wandering atrial pacemaker, ectopic atrial rhythm, and AV junctional rhythm (Fig. 3–4) are common in patients anesthetized with halothane, enflurane, or isoflurane, especially in patients with high resting vagal tone or sinus node dysfunction. It is postulated that (1) compared to secondary pacemaker automaticity, the SA node is more suppressed by direct anesthetic effects; (2) secondary pacemakers are less restrained by the vagus; (3) circulating catecholamines or increased sympathetic traffic produce a relative greater increase in automaticity of secondary pacemakers compared to the SA node; (4) accentuated antagonism[32], whereby vagal modulation of adrenergic effects on the heart is more pronounced with high sympathetic tone, enhances direct or indirect (i.e., opioids) vagal effects on the SA node; (5) enflurane, halothane, and isoflurane produce a small increase in automaticity of normal Purkinje fibers exposed to catecholamines or increased adrenergic tone; and (6) enflurane enhances recovery of latent pacemakers from overdrive suppression of automaticity by the SA node.[1,2,6] Additionally, available evidence suggests that none of the contemporary volatile anesthetics should suppress escape rhythms in patients with AV heart block or sinus node dysfunction.

AV CONDUCTION TIME. AV conduction time is subdivided into atrial, AV node, His–Purkinje and ventricular conduction times (see Fig. 2–1). As might be expected, since potent volatile anesthetics are calcium-channel blockers of sorts, but have little effect on sodium channels at clinical concentrations, these drugs cause more depression of AV node compared to atrial or ventricular specialized conduc-

78 ARRHYTHMIA CAUSES AND ASSOCIATIONS

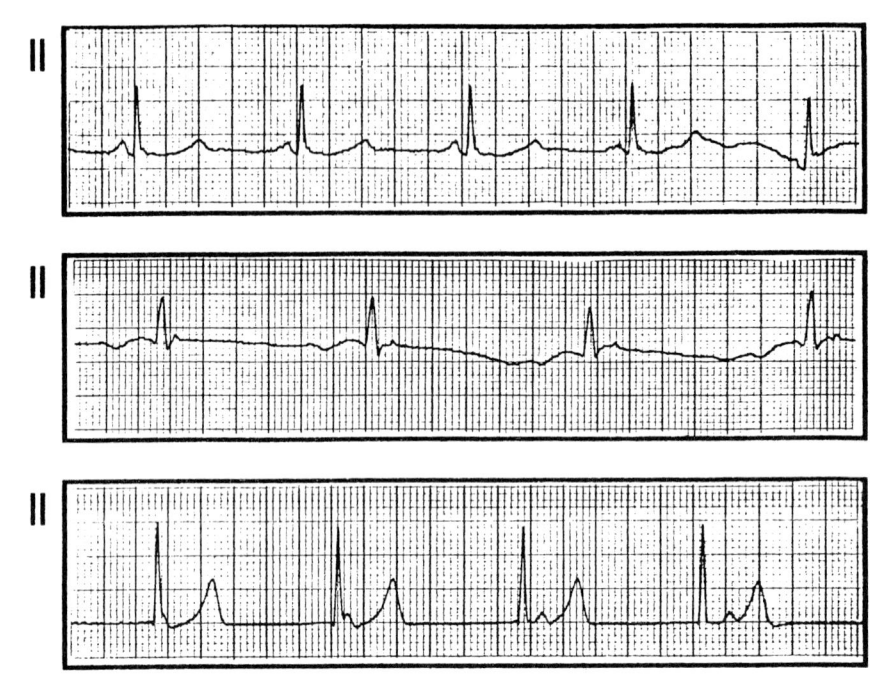

FIGURE 3-4 *Ectopic rhythm disturbances during anesthesia, presumably due to enhanced automaticity of secondary pacemakers. All tracings are surface ECG lead II (II). All patients received isoflurane–oxygen–fentanyl–midazolam–vecuronium (balanced) anesthesia. (Top) Wandering atrial pacemaker with dilated cardiomyopathy. Note tented, biphasic, and isoelectric P waves. (Middle) Ectopic atrial rhythm (bradycardia = 47 beats/min) with sinus node dysfunction. Note inverted P waves in lead II. (Bottom) AV junctional rhythm with isorhythmic AV dissociation in healthy young adult. Note upright P waves marching through QRS complex.*

tion. This depression is mediated by both direct and indirect effects (Fig. 3–5), since impairment of conduction is more pronounced by enflurane and halothane in the absence of autonomic blockade[33]. Enflurane, halothane, and isoflurane produce comparable prolongation of His–Purkinje or ventricular conduction time, both with and without autonomic blockade.[33] Prolongation of specialized AV conduction times by anesthetics is small in the absence of calcium-channel or beta-adrenergic blockers,[2,6,22] so these drugs should pose little risk of AV heart block without other cause for conduction impairment.

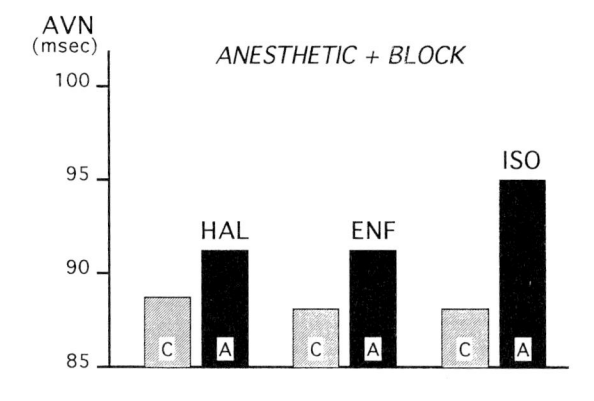

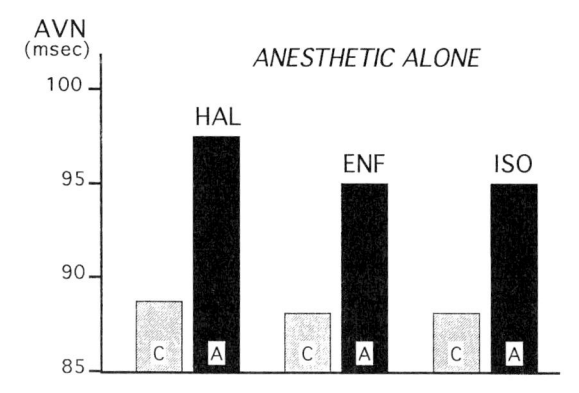

FIGURE 3-5 *Depression of AV nodal conduction time (AVN) by halothane (HAL), enflurane (ENF), or isoflurane (ISO) in dogs with pharmacologic autonomic blockade (ANESTHETIC + BLOCK) or without such blockade (ANESTHETIC ALONE). Values for AVN in conscious dogs (C) are compared to those for 1.7 MAC anesthesia (A). Note that for both HAL and ENF, conduction is somewhat more prolonged without autonomic blockade, suggesting that indirect effects (removal of sympathetic tone) are more important than with ISO. Based on data of Atlee et al.*[33]

AV REFRACTORY PERIODS. Enflurane, halothane, and isoflurane increase atrial and AV nodal refractoriness, with the latter effect additive to that of calcium-channel blockers.[2,6,22] Similar to anesthetic effects on specialized AV conduction times, these effects are both direct and indirect. Increased supraventricular refractoriness, particularly AV nodal refractoriness, should oppose paroxysmal SVT due to reentry. That this is so is suggested by the rare occurrence (author's impression and lack of published reports) of paroxysmal forms of SVT in patients with a history of paroxysmal SVT and anesthetized with halothane, enflurane, or isoflurane. Finally, all three inhalation anesthetics shorten ventricular refractoriness in normal heart.

Abnormal Cardiac Electrophysiology: Halothane, Enflurane, Isoflurane

Enflurane, halothane, and isoflurane have both anti- and proarrhythmic actions on abnormal cardiac electrophysiologic properties (see Chapter 2). These have been most tested in animal models of myocardial ischemia, infarction, or reperfusion injury. Arrhythmias originating in surviving, partially depolarized fibers following acute infarction or reperfusion injury may be caused by any abnormal phenomena (see Chapter 2), while those with healed infarction are most likely due to reentry.[34]

ACUTE INFARCTION AND ISCHEMIA. Halothane and isoflurane increase disparity of refractoriness in ischemic Purkinje fibers, as well as increase the conduction time of premature stimulated impulses into the zone of infarction (halothane more so than isoflurane).[1,5] While changes with both anesthetics should promote ventricular reentry, halothane is more conducive than isoflurane in this regard. In contrast, enflurane and halothane, but not isoflurane, oppose triggered activity from delayed afterdepolarizations in isolated infarcted heart.[5,6] However, no agent has discernible effects on abnormal automaticity in isolated infarcted heart.

CHRONIC INFARCTION. In contrast to reentry with acute infarction, halothane and enflurane more so than isoflurane oppose ventricular reentry with chronic infarction.[35] In part, this finding may be explained by greater prolongation of refractory periods by enflurane and halothane compared to isoflurane in both normal and infarcted tissue.[35] The fact that anesthetics oppose reentry in chronic but not acute infarcts may in part reflect the normalization of abnormal action potential characteristics several days following infarction.[34] Also, the substrate that supports reentry in chronic infarction may be more dependent on fiber geometry than abnormal electrophysiologic properties associated with partially depressed fibers.[34] In support of this idea, recent evidence suggests that reentry with chronic infarction may be of the leading circle type (see Fig. 2-9) in fibers with marked directional differences of conduction velocity and cell-to-cell coupling.[36]

TABLE 3-8 *Increased intracellular calcium with reperfusion injury*

1. Increased sacrolemmal membrane permeability to calcium.
2. Enhanced release of calcium from sarcoplasmic reticulum.
3. Less capacity of sarcoplasmic reticulum for binding calcium.
4. Impaired sodium–calcium exchange across the cell membrane.

REPERFUSION INJURY. Mechanisms underlying myocardial cell injury after reperfusion of ischemic myocardium are incompletely understood, although excessive calcium influx and intracellular accumulation of calcium appear important for development of arrhythmias (Table 3–8). Regardless of the mechanism, increased intracellular calcium can facilitate arrhythmias due to abnormal automaticity or triggered activity. Anesthetic effects against these mechanisms following reperfusion injury have not been examined, but should be similar to those with acute infarction (mentioned earlier). Finally, halothane, enflurane, and isoflurane oppose reperfusion ventricular fibrillation.[37]

Effects of Halothane, Enflurane, or Isoflurane on Clinical Arrhythmias

The following speculation is based on evidence summarized above. Enflurane, halothane (most), and isoflurane (least) should promote bradycardia in patients receiving negative chronotropes (beta- or calcium-channel blockers) or with sinus node dysfunction. In hyperadrenergic patients, with enhanced vagal tone or intrinsic sinus node dysfunction, they should facilitate ectopic atrial, AV junctional, or ventricular escape beats and rhythms. No anesthetic should promote paroxysmal SVT due to SA or AV node reentry; in fact, all should oppose it. Effects of enflurane, halothane, or isoflurane on reentry involving accessory AV pathways in patients with the WPW syndrome, or the ventricular rate response with atrial flutter or fibrillation in WPW syndrome patients, are not known and *cannot* be predicted based on available reports. Accelerated AV junctional or idioventricular rhythms due to abnormal automaticity in patients with ischemic heart disease should not be affected by enflurane, halothane, or isoflurane, but triggered VT with acute myocardial infarction or reperfusion injury might be slowed or terminated. Reentrant VT with ischemia or acute infarction might be unaffected, but that with chronic infarction should be slowed or terminated by volatile anesthetics.

Intravenous Anesthetics

Commonly used intravenous anesthetics include barbiturates, benzodiazepines, etomidate, ketamine, opiates, propofol, and droperidol. Very little is known of the cardiac electrophysiologic effects of any of these drugs. None is arrhythmic in normal heart.

BARBITURATES. Changes in action potentials of normal ventricular fibers suggest that thiopental reduces both inward calcium and repolarization potassium currents. Effects of thiopental and other short-acting barbiturates in other normal cardiac fiber types, or abnormal electrophysiologic properties, are unknown. Under experimental conditions, thiopental, thiamylal, and methohexital produce aftercontractions, possibly the result of delayed afterdepolarizations.[1] Finally, while atrial and ventricular arrhythmias often occur following anesthetic induction with short-acting barbiturates, especially during airway manipulation, these are unlikely due to the drugs. Rather, redistribution of the drugs, resultant light anesthesia, and increased sympathetic tone appear more responsible.

BENZODIAZEPINES. Parenteral benzodiazepines (diazepam, lorazepam, midazolam) do not cause arrhythmias by themselves. None appreciably alters heart rate, except that it may be decreased when benzodiazepines are used in combination with moderate to high doses of fentanyl-like opiates. The effects of diazepam or lorazepam on anesthetic–epinephrine arrhythmias or cardiac electrophysiologic properties are not known. Midazolam does not affect halothane-epinephrine arrhythmias.[38] With fentanyl, it appears to have no effects on cardiac refractoriness or arrhythmia inducibility in patients undergoing electrophysiologic testing.[39]

ETOMIDATE. Etomidate is not known to cause arrhythmias, nor does it affect epinephrine arrhythmias with halothane. One older report indicates that etomidate has no effects on atrial rate or action potential characteristics in atrial, Purkinje, or ventricular muscle fibers.[40] Effects on other electrophysiologic properties are not known, despite many practitioners' preference for this drug in patients with significant heart disease.

KETAMINE. Ketamine has a central sympathomimetic action that leads to increased heart rate, but not to catecholamine-mediated atrial or ventricular arrhythmias. Ketamine facilitates epinephrine arrhythmias with halothane in dogs.[1,2] While ketamine is not known to be proarrhythmic, there are no reports of its electrophysiologic actions, either in normal or abnormal heart.

OPIATES.   Except for meperidine, which increases heart rate, synthetic and natural opiates either have no effect on heart rate or reduce it. Opiate-related bradycardia can be marked in patients receiving beta-adrenergic or nondihydropyridine calcium-channel blockers. Also, opioids in association with benzodiazepines or potent anesthetics for general anesthesia can produce exaggerated bradycardia. The opiates are not known to be arrhythmic, and their cardiac electrophysiologic actions in the absence of other drugs are not known. The mechanism for bradycardia with opiates is thought to involve central vagal stimulation in conjunction with suppression of opiate-sensitive adrenergic mechanisms that regulate cardiovascular function.

PROPOFOL.   While propofol appears as sensitizing as halothane in dogs,[19] its effect on epinephrine arrhythmias in humans is not known. Whether propofol reduces epinephrine requirements for ventricular arrhythmias with volatile anesthetics, as thiopental does with enflurane, halothane, or isoflurane,[17,18] also is unknown. Similar to volatile anesthetics, propofol shortens action potential duration in ventricular muscle (guinea pig), but has no significant effects on other action potential characteristics.[41] Propofol is not known to facilitate arrhythmias in patients with preexisting arrhythmias.

DROPERIDOL.   Droperidol alone has no effect on heart rate. With fentanyl and other opioids, it may reduce heart rate. Droperidol's in vitro electrophysiologic properties are similar to those of quinidine and procainamide (see Chapter 5).[1,2] In cats, it prevents ventricular arrhythmias with halothane–epinephrine and following coronary ligation. Droperidol or fentanyl with droperidol (Innovar™) converts ouabain-induced ventricular arrhythmias to sinus or AV junctional rhythm in dogs. Droperidol alone or with fentanyl increases antegrade and retrograde refractoriness of accessory pathways in patients with the WPW syndrome, which may prevent, slow, or terminate reciprocating SVT.

Local Anesthetics

The cardiotoxic effects of local anesthetics appear most related to use-dependent cardiac sodium-channel blockade and autonomic effects. Class 1A and 1C antiarrhythmic drugs, which are also sodium-channel blockers, have potential cardiotoxicity similar to that with bupivacaine, etidocaine, or large IV doses of lidocaine. Therefore, what follows also applies to class 1A and 1C antiarrhythmics, although these drugs were briefly discussed above and in more detail in Chapter 5.

TABLE 3-9 **Modulated receptor hypothesis and possible sodium-channel states**

STATE	CORRESPONDING ACTION POTENTIAL PHASE	CONSEQUENCE
Open	Upstroke—phase 0	Cell depolarizes due to rapid influx of sodium ions
Inactivated	Plateau—phase 2	Cell is totally unavailable for depolarization
Resting	Repolarization—phase 3, diastolic—phase 4	Cell becomes or is available for depolarization

SODIUM-CHANNEL BLOCKADE. Toxic doses of sodium-channel blockers produce varying use-dependent block in ventricular specialized conducting tissue. This prolongs conduction and refractoriness, causing AV heart block or areas of functional conduction block. The latter are conducive to reentrant ventricular tachycardia. The prevailing explanation for use-dependent sodium-channel blockade with local anesthetics is the modulated receptor hypothesis, whereby the sodium channel is believed to exist in three states (Table 3–9).[42] Sodium-channel blockers interact with binding sites within the sodium-channel pore, so that when these sites are occupied (bound state), the channel can no longer conduct sodium ions. The sodium channel remains in the bound state until the drug leaves the binding site (unbound state). Although in high concentrations, sodium-channel blockers may bind to receptor sites in any state, clinical concentrations preferentially block open and/or inactivated sodium channels. In addition to drug concentration and binding affinity, the amount of block that develops depends on the duration and frequency of sodium-channel opening. If the diastolic interval is too short for dissociation of drug from its binding site (fast heart rates), block accumulates until a new steady-state level of blockade is reached. Conversely, if the diastolic interval is too long, drug will dissociate from its binding site so that less block can develop. Some characteristics of the interaction between sodium-channel blockers and the sodium channel are summarized in Table 3–10. Based on these, the potential for reentrant ventricular arrhythmias appears greatest with bupivacaine and class 1C antiarrhythmics. While the likelihood of this occurring is extremely small in normal heart without excessive drug concentrations (i.e., following inadvertent IV bupivacaine), it appears much greater in depressed (ischemic, hypoxic) myocardial tissue,[43,44] and possibly also with general anesthetics that

TABLE 3-10 *Interaction of sodium-channel blockers with the sodium-channel*

Lidocaine	Blocks I > O, little or no R; binds loosely; less use-dependent block; fast onset–offset kinetics
Bupivacaine	Blocks mainly I; binds avidly; more use-dependent block; slow onset–offset kinetics
Class 1A*	Blocks O and I, little R; intermediate binding; use-dependent block prominent; intermediate onset–offset kinetics
Class 1B*	Block I > O; time constant of unbinding slowed in depolarized cells; fast onset–offset kinetics
Class 1C*	Blocks O and I, also R > IA or IB; time constant of unbinding prolonged; slow onset-offset kinetics

*Antiarrhythmic drugs. O, I, R, open, inactivated, or resting sodium channels.

interact with cardiac sodium channels in less specific ways to prolong ventricular conduction time and refractoriness.[5]

AUTONOMIC EFFECTS. Early studies of bupivacaine cardiotoxicity implicated autonomic involvement along with cardiac sodium-channel blockade,[1,2] although no therapeutic strategies resulted from this. More recently, it was reported that the combination of dobutamine and clonidine reversed bupivacaine cardiotoxicity in dogs, including impaired ventricular conduction and hemodynamic changes.[45] Concerning clonidine's effect to reverse conduction defects, more recent work by the same group suggests that stimulation of ganglionic (nicotinic) receptors rather than central alpha-2 receptors is the mechanism.[46] However, clonidine should not be used alone to reverse ventricular conduction disturbances with bupivacaine, since it might worsen bradycardia and/or produce SA or AV nodal conduction block.[45]

Neuromuscular Blocking Drugs

No contemporary muscle relaxant alone is proarrhythmic. Succinylcholine, however, may cause exaggerated potassium release and arrhythmias in susceptible patients. Tachycardia or arrhythmias following tracheal intubation are more likely due to light anesthesia caused redistribution of IV anesthetics.

SUCCINYLCHOLINE. There have been reports of cardiac arrest after succinylcholine in seemingly healthy children or adolescents[47]

TABLE 3-11 *Potassium release following succinylcholine*

Extensive third-degree burns	Massive muscle injury
Ruptured cerebral aneurysm	Closed head injuries; stroke
Severe abdominal infections	Tetanus
Neuromuscular disease	Spinal cord injury

with skeletal myopathies. Rhabdomyolysis with acute hyperkalemia is the probable mechanism for cardiac arrest. The manufacturer advised that succinylcholine not be administered for elective intubation in children considered at risk for myopathies. Nevertheless, succinylcholine might be indicated when the airway must be secured immediately, although newer nondepolarizing relaxants (rocuronium, mivacurium) can provide intubating conditions within 60 to 90 sec. Finally, many reports have shown that succinylcholine can produce life-threatening conduction disturbances and ventricular arrhythmias through exaggerated potassium release in susceptible patients of all ages (Table 3-11).[1,2] While attempts have been made to identify the period of risk for exaggerated potassium release (i.e., 6 months following spinal cord injury), and methods are touted to reduce the risk of such release (e.g., self-taming dose of succinylcholine),[1,2] prudence teaches that there really are no fail-safe time constraints or techniques.

NONDEPOLARIZING MUSCLE RELAXANTS. None of the nondepolarizing muscle relaxants (NDMR) are considered arrhythmogenic. However, they may be associated with hypotension or tachycardia, and may potentiate bradycardia with opioids. Tachycardia and/or hypotension may cause myocardial ischemia in patients with coronary artery disease, and possibly ventricular arrhythmias consequent to myocardial ischemia. NDMR are competitive antagonists at the postjunctional (nicotinic) cholinergic receptors on the motor end plate, and also have prejunctional effects or cause histamine release. The latter along with ganglionic or muscarinic blockade explain most adverse cardiovascular side effects (Fig. 3-6). Doxacurium, pipecuronium, rocuronium, and vecuronium are essentially devoid of histamine release or significant side effects due to ganglionic or muscarinic blockade.

Anesthetic Adjuncts

Estimation of the arrhythmic potential of adjunct drugs used during anesthesia is based on available reviews and monographs.[1,2,10–12,28,29]

```
            ┌─────────────────────────┐      Histamine release
            │ Tubocurare > Metocurine >│  →   • Hypotension
            │ Atracurium > Mivacurium  │      • Reflex tachycardia
            └─────────────────────────┘      • Myocardial ischemia
                                              • Ventricular arrhythmias

                                              Muscarinic blockade
            ┌─────────────────────────┐      • Tachycardia
            │  Gallamine > Pancuronium │  →   • Myocardial ischemia
            └─────────────────────────┘      • Ventricular arrhythmias

                                              Ganglionic blockade
            ┌─────────────────────────┐      • Hypotension
            │  Tubocurare > Metocurine │  →   • Myocardial ischemia
            └─────────────────────────┘      • Ventricular arrhythmias
```

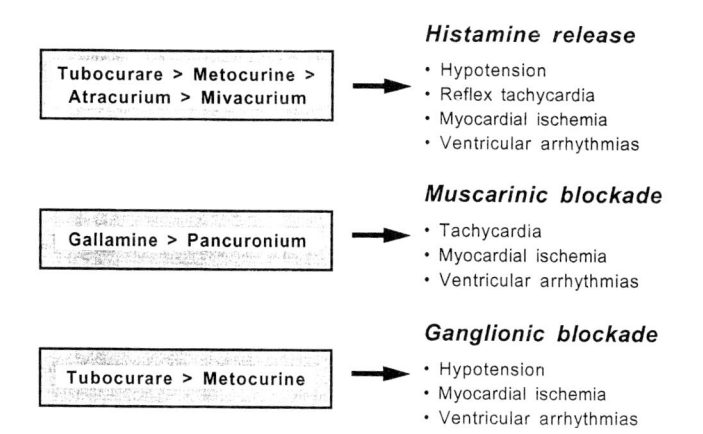

FIGURE 3-6 *Mechanisms for hemodynamic changes and consequent arrhythmias due to histamine release, muscarinic blockade, or ganglionic blockade with nondepolarizing muscle relaxants.*

ANTICHOLINESTERASE DRUGS. Edrophonium and neostigmine are used to reverse nondepolarizing neuromuscular blockade. Their cardiovascular actions are complex and sometimes unpredictable because of ganglionic (nicotinic), postganglionic (muscarinic), and central effects (medullary) of accumulated acetylcholine. Acetylcholine can have excitatory or inhibitory ganglionic effects, with the latter prevailing at higher concentrations. Central and muscarinic effects of acetylcholine are general inhibitory. In the absence of muscarinic blockade, the inhibitory effects of accumulated acetylcholine can produce severe bradycardia, asystole, or AV heart block.

ANTICHOLINERGICS. Atropine or glycopyrrolate are used to reverse the muscarinic effects of anticholinesterase agents, and less commonly as antisialogogues. Scopolamine is often used in cardiac surgical patients for its sedative–hypnotic–amnestic properties. These drugs have little effect at nicotinic receptors in usual doses. There may be transient bradycardia due to initial block of postganglionic vagal fibers preventing inhibition of terminal transmitter release. In patients with intrinsic sinus node dysfunction, antimuscarinics can have no discernible effect on heart rate or stimulate ectopic atrial junctional, or ventricular arrhythmias.

ANALEPTIC, OPIOID, ANTAGONIST, AND AROUSAL AGENTS. *Doxapram* increases minute ventilation, facilitating elimination of volatile anesthetics. Continuous infusion for a sustained effect on ventilation

TABLE 3-12 *Drugs with anticholinergic CNS effects*

Scopolamine; atropine*	Droperidol
Volatile anesthetics	Benzodiazepines
Antihistamines	Ketamine
Tricyclic antidepressants	Major tranquilizers

*And also glycopyrrolate, but only with high doses.

has produced subconvulsive CNS stimulation and arrhythmias. Otherwise, arrhythmias with doxapram are likely due to rapid reversal of anesthesia. Fulminant pulmonary edema and tachyarrhythmias have been reported in patients receiving large bolus doses of *naloxone* (0.4 mg IV). This is easily prevented by using smaller increments of naloxone (40 µg) for reversal. Finally, *physostigmine*, a tertiary anticholinesterase, is used to reverse central agitation and other CNS side effects with a variety of drugs that produce central anticholinergic effects (Table 3–12). Too high doses may cause bradycardia.

ELECTROLYTE IMBALANCE

There is still considerable controversy with regard to the arrhythmic potential of electrolyte imbalance, especially hypo- or hyperkalemia. While a number of studies have addressed this issue, many fall short because they fail to address the two most important issues: (1) How acute is the imbalance? and (2) What are the confounding effects of associated imbalance or pathophysiologic states? It is hoped that the discussion below provides a proper perspective on the problem.

Potassium

While the ECG is often used to monitor changes in serum potassium, it does not predict arrhythmic potential. Also, while there is good correlation between serum potassium and the surface ECG with *acute* potassium imbalance, this is not necessarily the case with *chronic* imbalance. Some effects of changes in serum potassium on the surface ECG are shown in Table 3–13. Not considered in Table 3–13 is the influence of other ion imbalance or drugs. Concerning arrhythmias with potassium imbalance, keep in mind that they are not caused by changes in serum K per se, but rather by the ratio between intracellular and extracellular potassium. This ratio is the most important determinant of cell membrane potential, which affects both normal and abnormal electrophysiologic properties (see Chapter 2). For example, only extremes of extracellular potassium (< 2.7 or >10 mEq/L)

TABLE 3-13 *Serum potassium (K) and the ECG with hypo- or hyperkalemia*

ECG	K ≤ 3.0 mEq/L	K > 4.0 mEq/L	K > 6.0 mEq/L	K > 8.0 mEq/L
P wave	Normal	↓ Amplitude	↓ Amplitude	Nonapparent
PR	Normal	Prolongation	Prolongation	Nonapparent
QRS	↑ Amplitude	Normal	Normal	Widening
T wave	Flat; inverted	Normal	Peaked; tented	Peaked; tented
QT	Normal	Normal	Decreased (±)	Decreased (±)
U wave	Present	Absent	Absent	Absent

significantly depolarize transmembrane potential in Purkinje or ventricular fibers.[48] Between these values, membrane potential increases toward more normal values. Finally, electrophysiologic changes with potassium balance are likely to be heterogeneous, so that some cells or tissues may be more affected than others.

Therefore, an isolated value for serum potassium of 3.0 mEq/L is quite meaningless. First, it must be confirmed. Second, it must be determined whether this value represents an acute change for the patient. Then, assuming the value is real and does represent an acute change, it must be considered within the context of the patient's overall medical condition, underlying cardiac disease, concurrent physiologic imbalance, and medication, as well as anticipated diagnostic, medical, or surgical intervention. Concerning acuteness of the condition, a decrease in potassium from 4.0 mEq/L to 3.0 mEq/L over minutes or hours compared to weeks or months is more likely to increase cellular electrophysiologic instability and risk of arrhythmias. This is due to insufficient time for compensatory changes to restore normal cell membrane potential. Even an apparently normal serum potassium may be associated with hypokalemic ECG changes and arrhythmias in patients with chronic hyperkalemia secondary to renal failure (Fig. 3–7). Issues such as these must be considered when determining the arrhythmic potential of serum potassium values in surgical or critical care patients.

HYPOKALEMIA.   Hypokalemia is far more likely than hyperkalemia to cause clinically important arrhythmias. It often results from dialysis, thiazide or loop diuretics, mechanical hyperventilation, or treatment with insulin or beta-adrenergic agonists. Repolarization abnormalities and loss of membrane potential with hypokalemia affect

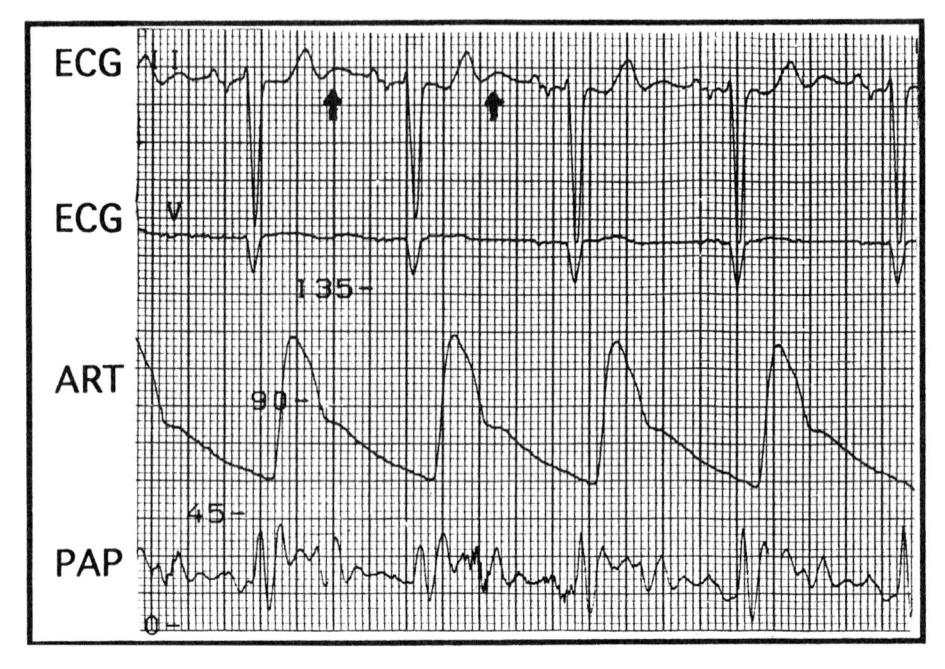

FIGURE 3-7 *U waves (arrows, lead II) suggestive of hypokalemia in a cardiac surgical patient with chronic renal failure. Initial and repeat serum potassium values at this time were 4.5 and 4.7 mEq/L, respectively. The patient's "normal" serum potassium was >5.5 mEq/L. Except for atrial extrasystoles (not shown), there were no arrhythmias. ART, radial arterial pressure; PAP, pulmonary arterial pressure. [ECG - 1.0 cm = 2.0 mV.]*

conduction and refractoriness, and are conducive to reentry and disturbed automaticity or triggered activity. Arrhythmias with severe hypokalemia include atrial and ventricular extrasystoles, automatic atrial tachycardia, reentrant SVT, and AV conduction disturbances. Torsades de pointes ventricular tachycardia (VT), polymorphic VT, and ventricular fibrillation are all possible with extreme hypokalemia. Accordingly, arrhythmias related to hypokalemia resemble those with digitalis toxicity. There is no generally accepted serum level of potassium below which there is increased risk of arrhythmias. While Vitez and colleagues found no evidence for increased risk of intraoperative arrhythmias with chronic hypokalemia (potassium values of 2.6 to 3.4 mEq/L),[49] there are several limitations to this study which must be considered before making recommendations for clinical practice (Table 3–14).[50,51] Based on the foregoing and evidence

TABLE 3-14 *Limitations to Vitez' study of chronic hypokalemia and arrhythmias*

1. Serum potassium determinations were not confirmed (single determination only).
2. Impossible to ascertain whether hypokalemia was an acute or chronic.
3. Most patients were at low risk for arrhythmias (no digitalis or heart disease).
4. Operations in hypokalemic group not usually associated with arrhythmias.
5. Power too small to detect differences between hypo/normokalemic patients.
6. Not addressed: increased incidence of adverse outcomes with heart disease?
7. Factors that increase the risk of arrhythmias with hypokalemia not identified.

reviewed elsewhere,[1] and with full realization that the required outcome studies are still lacking, it seems reasonable to suggest the following. Confirmed serum potassium values ≤ 2.5 mEq/L justify postponement of elective or nonemergent surgery because of possible increased likelihood of complications and in order to determine the cause and significance of potassium imbalance. Confirmed values between 2.6 and 3.0 mEq/L, especially with other factors that increase the risk of arrhythmias (Table 3–2), also justify postponement of elective surgery. Between 3.0 and 3.5 mEq/L, provided there has not been an acute decrease in potassium ≥ 1.5 mEq/L, there should be little risk of significant arrhythmias without overt digitalis toxicity, catecholamine excess, acute myocardial infarction, or significant other heart disease.

HYPERKALEMIA. The contribution of hyperkalemia (potassium ≥ 5.5 mEq/L) to cardiac arrhythmias in surgical or critical care settings is not known. Patients with chronic moderate hyperkalemia (serum potassium ≤ 7.5 mEq/L) are rarely reported to have atrial or ventricular ectopy or cardiac conduction disturbances.[1] This "antiarrhythmic" action of increased potassium might be due to reduced automaticity of ectopic pacemakers, termination of reentry because of altered conduction or refractoriness, or abolition of supernormal conduction and excitability. Arrhythmias or conduction disturbances caused by hyperkalemia usually occur following too rapid IV replacement or inadvertent central administration of potassium. Slow-response or depressed fast-response fibers (see Chapter 2) are more resistant to the effects of hyperkalemia than normal fast-response fibers. With severe hyperkalemia (potassium > 7.5 mEq/L), progressive slowing of AV conduction and decreased excitability terminate in cardiac arrest when potassium depolarizes ventricular fibers to the point of inexcitability. However, ventricular fibrillation can also occur with extreme hyperkalemia.

Magnesium

There are no specific ECG changes with hypo- or hypermagnesemia, although rapid administration of magnesium may shorten the QT interval. Rhythm disturbances with *hypomagnesemia* are similar to those with hypokalemia, and the two conditions often occur in association. Because magnesium is the second most abundant intracellular cation and essential for the sodium–potassium exchange pump, it helps to maintain resting membrane potential. Consequently, cardiac arrhythmias with hypomagnesemia likely result from loss of membrane potential and are similar to those with hypokalemia or digitalis toxicity. In patients with magnesium deficiency (Table 3-15), arrhythmias may occur even though serum levels are within the normal range. This can be so because only 5 percent of the available pool of magnesium is extracellular. Finally, *hypermagnesemia* has effects similar to those of hyperkalemia. Both AV and intraventricular conduction may be prolonged, although magnesium serum levels required for impaired conduction appear higher than those for respiratory arrest.[1]

Calcium and Sodium

ST-segment and QT-interval prolongation with *hypocalcemia* likely reflect increased action potential duration (consequent to increased plateau phase) in ventricular myocardium.[27,52,53] Hypocalcemia also increases ventricular irritability. If there is also hypokalemia with flattened T and U waves, there may be the impression of a

TABLE 3-15 *Conditions associated with magnesium deficiency*

Diuretic-induced hypokalemia	Critically ill adults and children
Acute myocardial infarction	After cardiopulmonary bypass
Cachexia of malignancy	Following chemotherapy
Malnutrition, starvation	Chronic ethanolism
Diarrhea; following dialysis	Type I diabetes

markedly prolonged QT interval due to TU fusion. In contrast, *hypercalcemia* shortens the ST segment and QT interval, and may also cause ST-segment depression with T-wave inversion. Hypercalcemia without associated ion imbalance should not be proarrhythmic. Hypo- and hypercalcemia augment and oppose, respectively, the effects of hyperkalemia. *Hyponatremia* or *hypernatremia* with hyperkalemia parallel the effects of changes in serum calcium. Otherwise, there are no independent effects of sodium imbalance on the ECG or arrhythmias.

Conditions Associated With Arrhythmias

Almost all systemic disease ultimately affects the heart and might be the cause for cardiac arrhythmias. Discussed below are medical conditions, interventions, and syndromes, or disease processes, with proven arrhythmic associations.[1,3,8,9,26,27] Cardiac rhythm disturbances with any of these might be aggravated by altered states in surgical or critical care settings.

ALCOHOL ABUSE

There are no adequately controlled studies that show a higher incidence of arrhythmias in anesthetized or critically ill patients with acute *ethanol* intoxication. Other abused drugs (e.g., central stimulants) along with ethanol or structural heart disease are the more likely cause for arrhythmias in such patients. Chronic ethanol abuse is commonly associated with hypomagnesemia and atrial flutter or fibrillation, but rarely VT in the absence of structural heart disease. *Ethylene glycol* or *methanol* intoxication is not associated with specific ECG changes or arrhythmias. *Isopropanol* toxicity may cause bradycardia, hypotension, and pulmonary edema.[27]

AMYLOIDOSIS

Cardiac arrhythmias and conduction disturbances are common in patients with systemic amyloidosis and myocardial involvement. Severe bradycardia and/or AV heart block in anesthetized patients with amyloidosis have been attributed to depressant effects of anesthetic drugs, dysautonomia, or exaggerated potassium release with succinylcholine. Although such disturbances may respond to chronotropic drugs, prophylactic temporary perioperative pacing in patients with amyloid heart disease and evidence of SA node dysfunction or AV conduction disturbances is strongly advised.

ANAPHYLAXIS AND ANAPHYLACTOID REACTIONS

Immunologic reactions, with IgE-mediated release of histamine and other primary mediators from mast cells or basophiles (Table 3-16), are termed *anaphylactic* as opposed to *anaphylactoid* reactions. The latter, caused by direct (non-IgE-mediated) release of histamine with certain drugs (Table 3-17), have clinical manifestations identical to those of anaphylaxis. Arrhythmic actions of histamine are discussed above under Drugs and Imbalance as Causes for Arrhythmias.

ARRHYTHMOGENIC RIGHT VENTRICULAR DYSPLASIA

The diagnosis of arrhythmogenic right ventricular dysplasia is based on the presence of ventricular arrhythmias along with motion or morphologic abnormalities involving the right ventricular free wall. VT with a left bundle branch block pattern is the most commonly observed arrhythmia.

TABLE 3-16 *Primary mediators of anaphylaxis and adverse physiologic effects*

PRIMARY MEDIATORS	EFFECTS THAT DIRECTLY OR INDIRECTLY CAUSE OR PROMOTE ARRHYTHMIAS
Histamine	Bronchospasm, hypoxia, hypercarbia; vasodilation with hypotension; coronary constriction; increased heart rate, inotropy, and oxygen demand; slowed conduction; enhanced automaticity of latent pacemakers
Platelet-activating factor	Bronchoconstriction; platelet activation-aggregation with coronary thrombosis and arrhythmias
Prostaglandins and leukotrienes	Bronchoconstriction; coronary constriction; increased vascular permeability causing airway edema, bronchial obstruction and hypoxia or hypercarbia
Adenosine	Bronchospasm, hypoxia and hypercarbia
Serotonin	Bronchoconstriction, hypoxia, hypercarbia; vasodilation; coronary vasoconstriction; increased heart rate, inotropy, and oxygen demand

TABLE 3-17 *Drugs that release histamine*

Morphine	Tubocurarine
Atracurium*	Protamine
Vancomycin	Thiopental
Radiographic contrast dyes	Salicylates; nonsteroidal anti-inflammatory drugs

*Dose ranges ≥ 0.4 mg/kg.

ATHLETE'S HEART SYNDROME

The heart adapts somewhat differently to exercise, depending on whether it produces pressure (isometric exercise) or volume overload (isotonic exercise). Free wall and septal thickness increase with chronic pressure overload. End-diastolic diameter increases to normalize stress with chronic volume overload. Whether such adaptations influence the incidence or type of arrhythmias is unknown, so no further distinction is made. Sinus bradycardia (resting rates < 30 beats/min have been reported), sinus arrhythmia, wandering atrial pacemaker and first-degree AV heart block are the most common rhythm disturbances in trained athletes. While all of these disturbances can be attributed to increased vagal tone, there may also be an intrinsic component (sinus node) as well. Regardless, exertion tends to reverse bradycardia or arrhythmias. Other rhythm disturbances in well-conditioned athletes include SA block, sinus pause, and type 1 (Wenckebach) second-degree AV heart block. Rare are type 2 (Mobitz) second-degree and complete AV block, atrial tachyarrhythmias during rest, and AV junctional or ventricular arrhythmias. While anesthesia is not known to affect arrhythmias with athlete's heart syndrome, hemodynamically significant bradycardia could occur in some patients, especially with bradycardic drugs.

CARDIOMYOPATHIES

Cardiomyopathies may be dilated, hypertrophic, or restrictive. Respectively, these are associated with ischemic heart disease or valvular regurgitation, obstruction to ventricular outflow and chronic hypertension, or cardiac tamponade and pericardial disease. Serious or lethal cardiac arrhythmias and conduction disturbances can occur with either dilated or hypertrophic cardiomyopathy. Restrictive cardiomyopathy has no special arrhythmic associations except for compensatory tachycardia. Nonsustained ventricular tachycardia in adults with cardiomyopathy during Holter monitoring is predictive of increased risk for sudden death. The absence of ventricular arrhythmias during Holter monitoring in children with cardiomyopathy does not necessarily predict reduced risk for sudden death. Whether cardiomyopathy is an independent risk factor for dangerous perioperative arrhythmias is not known.

CIRCADIAN VARIATION IN SUSCEPTIBILITY TO ARRHYTHMIAS

Several studies report an increased incidence of sudden death from arrhythmias in the early morning hours. Perhaps this reflects a precipitous increase in sympathetic tone with awakening in patients with significant occlusive coronary artery disease. Whether such circadian variation in cardiac susceptibility occurs in surgical or critical care patients is unknown.

CORONARY ARTERY DISEASE

Myocardial ischemia, infarction, or reperfusion injury can be associated with life-threatening ventricular arrhythmias due to a variety of electrophysiologic mechanisms (see Chapter 2). Lesser ventricular arrhythmias are also commonplace, but it is increasingly appreciated by cardiologists that Lown–Wolf grade premature ventricular extrasystoles (Table 3–18) are not necessarily predictive of increased risk for lethal arrhythmias, except with acute myocardial infarction (<48 – 72 hours).[54] Therefore, the usual practice of treating "R on T" or other high-grade ventricular premature beats (VPB) in the absence of myocardial ischemia or acute infarction, ECG rates equivalent to tachycardia, or significant hemodynamic compromise, must be questioned (see Chapter 10).

TABLE 3-18 *Lown–Wolf grading system for VES*

Grade 0	No VES
Grade 1	Occasional VES (< 30/hr)
Grade 2	Frequent VES (≥ 30/hr)
Grade 3	Multiform VES regardless of frequency
Grade 4A	Two consecutive VES (a couplet)
Grade 4B	Three or more consecutive VES (nonsustained VT if < 30 sec)
Grade 5	Extremely early ("R on T") VPB

DISORDERS WITH AUTONOMIC DYSFUNCTION

Arrhythmias due to autonomic dysfunction may occur with several disorders. *Sympathetic hypofunction* is seen in patients with Gill familial dysautonomia, and the Shy–Drager, Riley–Day, and Lesch–Nyhan syndromes. Arrhythmias in these patients may result from reduced coronary perfusion secondary to loss of autonomic compensatory mechanisms or exaggerated responses to direct-acting adrenergic drugs. Arrhythmias due to *sympathetic hyperfunction* occur with pheochromocytoma, neurofibromatosis, tetanus, thyrotoxicosis, and some types of chemodectomas. Characteristic ECG changes and arrhythmias with *subarachnoid hemorrhage* and autonomic dysfunction are listed in Table 3–19. Finally, after high thoracic (above T7) or cervical spinal cord injury, bradycardia and hypotension are more severe with complete compared to partial transection. The incidence of bradycardia declines after four days, with complete resolution by 2 to 6 weeks.

ELECTROCONVULSIVE THERAPY

Characteristic cardiovascular changes following electroconvulsive therapy result from initial vagal stimulation (tonic phase) followed by combined sympathetic vagal stimulation (clonic phase). The vagal component is secondary to hypertension. This sequence of events is not consistent because of varying autonomic competence among patients and concurrent drug therapy. Arrhythmias with vagal stimulation include sinus bradycardia, sinus pause, AV junctional or ventricular escape beats and rhythms, and SA or AV heart block. While atropine is sometimes used as prophylaxis for bradycardic arrhythmias, it may facilitate tachycardia or ventricular arrhythmias during the clonic phase. Since bradyarrhythmias with the tonic phase are

TABLE 3-19 *ECG changes and arrhythmias with subarachnoid hemorrhage*

ECG CHANGES	ARRHYTHMIAS
QT-interval prolongation	VPB
Peaked P waves	Nonsustained VT
ST-segment depression or elevation	Paroxysmal SVT or atrial fibrillation
Prominent upright or inverted T waves	SA block and sinus pause or arrest
Prominent U waves	Lethal ventricular tachyarrhythmias

transient (< 30 seconds), but those during the clonic phase more persistent, the author prefers not to pretreat with atropine. Instead, esmolol (0.25 to 0.5-mg/kg bolus), possibly along with short-acting nicardipine (1.0 to 2.0-mg bolus), is given during induction of anesthesia to obtund the cardiovascular effects of sympathetic stimulation.

EXTRACORPOREAL SHOCK WAVE LITHOTRIPSY

Supraventricular and ventricular arrhythmias have been observed in patients undergoing extracorporeal shock wave lithotripsy. Arrhythmias are likely triggered by improperly synchronized (to R-wave of ECG) therapeutic shocks in patients with atrial or ventricular vulnerability. Vulnerability might be conferred by myocardial chamber enlargement, cardiomyopathies, acute electrolyte imbalance, excessive catecholamines, myocardial ischemia, hypoxia, or digitalis and other drug toxicity.

LEFT VENTRICULAR HYPERTROPHY

The Framingham Heart Study showed a strong positive association between *echocardiographic evidence* of left ventricular hypertrophy and malignant ventricular arrhythmias. However, *ECG evidence* of left ventricular hypertrophy failed to predict such an association, possibly because the ECG does not assess left ventricular mass as well as the echocardiogram.

LONG QT INTERVAL SYNDROME

QT-interval prolongation may be congenital or acquired. Congenital long QT interval syndrome (C-LQTS) is a familial disorder that is (Jervell and Lange–Nielsen syndrome) or is not associated with deafness (Romano–Ward syndrome). Acquired QT interval syndrome (A-LQTS) is caused by a variety of drugs and conditions (Table 3–20). Torsades de pointes VT occurs with acquired or congenital LQTS (see Chapter 10). While left-sided sympathetic predominance may facilitate ventricular arrhythmias with C-LQTS, it is now believed that early afterdepolarizations with triggering are responsible for torsades de pointes VT. Early afterdepolarizations and triggering may be caused by defective potassium channels and altered ventricular repolarization. By way of speculation, it could be that patients with C-LQTS have genetic defects affecting the potassium channels, and those with A-LQTS a defect that confers increased susceptibility to drugs or factors that inhibit potassium channels. For management of A-LQTS

TABLE 3-20 *Drugs and conditions associated with QT-interval prolongation*

Amiodarone	Hypokalemia	Neck surgery
Anorexia nervosa	Hypomagnesemia	Organophosphates
Bepridil	Hypothermia	Phenothiazines
Cardiomyopathies	Hypothyroidism	Procainamide
Class 1C anti-arrhythmics	Hyperalimentation	Quinidine
Coronary artery disease	Lithium toxicity	Sotolol
CNS/autonomic disorders	Liquid protein diets	Thioridazine
Disopyramide	Malnutrition	Tricyclic antidepressants
Hypocalcemia	Mitral valve prolapse	Volatile anesthetics*

*Small effect and unlikely cause for ventricular arrhythmias without other causes for QT-interval prolongation or arrhythmias.

patients, inciting drugs or factors should be removed, electrolyte (potassium, magnesium) imbalance corrected, and atrial or AV sequential pacing instituted for bradycardia. Isoproterenol may also be useful, but atropine is considered unreliable. With C-LQTS patients, beta-adrenergic blockers, often at maximally tolerated doses, are required. Alpha-adrenergic blockers may be added as well. Dual-chamber pacing for bradycardia is recommended, because atrial pacing may be unreliable because of AV heart block. All contemporary anesthetic drugs appear safe in patients with C-LQTS, except that ketamine and high concentrations (>1.5 MAC) of volatile agents are probably best avoided, since the former is sympathomimetic and the latter is among drugs known to prolong the QT interval (Table 3–20).

MITRAL VALVE PROLAPSE SYNDROME

Mitral valve prolapse syndrome (MVPS) results from congenital and acquired conditions affecting the mitral valve apparatus.[1,55,56] Palpitations, diminished cardiac reserve and atypical chest pain are common symptoms, but many patients are asymptomatic. The positive association between MVPS and QT interval prolongation possibly contributes to ventricular arrhythmias in some patients. Characteristic ECG changes in symptomatic MVPS patients include inverted or biphasic T waves and nonspecific ST segment changes (inferior leads). Arrhythmias are listed in Table 3–21. Paroxysmal SVT is the most

TABLE 3-21 *Arrhythmias with the mitral valve prolapse syndrome*

> Atrial and ventricular premature beats
> Paroxysmal SVT
> Ventricular tachyarrhythmias (with long QT interval)
> Bradycardia due to sinus node dysfunction
> Various degrees of AV heart block

common sustained tachyarrhythmia, possibly because of the high incidence of left-sided AV bypass pathways in this condition.

MYOTONIC AND MUSCULAR DYSTROPHY

With myotonic dystrophy, cardiac involvement includes degeneration of the specialized AV conducting system. As a result, arrhythmias include those with the sick sinus syndrome (see Chapter 9), AV heart block, and bundle branch or fascicular heart block. Frequent PVB or VT have also been reported. Muscular dystrophy has no special arrhythmic associations. However, patients with the condition are susceptible to malignant hyperpyrexia and consequent ventricular tachyarrhythmias with an episode of triggering.

OCULOCARDIAC REFLEX

The oculocardiac reflex (OCR) can result from traction on the extrinsic eye muscles, acute glaucoma, stretching of the eyelid, sudden increased intraocular pressure, enucleation, ocular trauma, and intraorbital injections or hematomas. The OCR is trigeminal–vagal (afferent–efferent). Expected arrhythmias with stimulation of the OCR include severe sinus bradycardia, sinus pause and arrest, SA block, AV heart block, and junctional or ventricular escape rhythms. It is no longer believed that traction on the medial rectus muscle is necessarily more reflexogenic than that on the other extrinsic eye muscles. However, it is appreciated that gentle, nonsustained traction is less reflexogenic than strong, sustained traction. The routine use of anticholinergics to treat bradycardia with the OCR is discouraged: (1) Arrhythmias are usually self-limited, and either terminate or fatigue with removal of or repeated stimulation, respectively; (2) Anticholinergics often increase the instability of AV junctional and ventricular escape rhythms with the OCR. However, preoperative anticholinergics may reduce the severity of bradycardia and escape rhythms with OCR in children.

References

1. Atlee J. Causes for perioperative dysrhythmias. In Perioperative Cardiac Dysrhythmias. 2nd ed. Chicago: Year Book Medical, 1990: pp. 187–273.
2. Atlee J, Bosnjak Z. Mechanisms for cardiac dysrhythmias during anesthesia. Anesthesiology 1990;72:347–374.
3. Davis R. Etiology and treatment of perioperative cardiac arrhythmias. In Kaplan J (ed): Cardiac Anesthesia. 3rd ed. Philadelphia: WB Saunders, 1993: pp. 170–205.
4. Kastor J. Arrhythmias. Philadelphia: WB Saunders, 1994.
5. Turner L, Bosnjak Z. Autonomic and anesthetic modulation of cardiac conduction and arrhythmias. In Lynch C (ed): Clinical Cardiac Electrophysiology. Philadelphia: JB Lippincott, 1994: pp. 53–84.
6. Atlee J, Bosnjak Z. The origin of the heart beat. In Brown BJ, Prys-Roberts C (eds): International Practice of Anaesthesia. London: Butterworth-Heinemann, 1995: in press.
7. Becker R, Gore J. Cardiac rhythm disturbances: Recognition and treatment. In Rippe J, Invin J, Alpert J, Finck M (eds): Intensive Care Medicine. 2nd ed. Boston: Little, Brown, 1991: pp. 217–228.
8. Buxton A, Hurwitz J. Disorders of cardiac rhythm and conduction in the medical intensive care unit. In Carlson R, Gehab M (eds): Medical Intensive Care. Philadelphia: WB Saunders, 1993: pp. 1049–1078.
9. Rowlands D, Brownlee W. The cardiac dysrhythmias. In Zapol W, Tinker J (eds): Care of the Critically Ill Patient. New York: Springer-Verlag, 1992: pp. 217–241.
10. Tatro D (ed). Drug Interaction Facts. 4th ed. St. Louis: Facts and Comparisons, 1994.
11. AMA Drug Evaluations. Annual 1994. Chicago: American Medical Association, 1994.
12. Stockley I. Drug Interactions. 2nd ed. Oxford: Blackwell Scientific, 1991.
13. Katz R, Bigger J. Cardiac arrhythmias during anesthesia and operation. Anesthesiology 1970;33:193–213.
14. Hayashi Y, Sumikawa K, Tashiro C, et al. Arrhythmogenic threshold of epinephrine during sevoflurane, enflurane, and isoflurane anesthesia in dogs [letter]. Anesthesiology 1988;69:145–147.
15. Moore M, Weiskopf R, Eger E, Wilson C. Arrhythmogenic doses of epinephrine are similar during desflurane or isoflurane anesthesia in humans. Anesthesiology 1993;79:943–947.

16. Navarro R, Weiskopf R, Moore M, et al. Humans anesthetized with sevoflurane or isoflurane have similar arrhythmic response to epinephrine. Anesthesiology 1994;80:545–549.
17. Atlee J, Malkinson C. Potentiation by thiopental of halothane–epinephrine induced arrhythmias in dogs. Anesthesiology 1982;57:285–288.
18. Atlee J, Roberts F. Thiopental and epinephrine-induced dysrhythmias in dogs anesthetized with enflurane or isoflurane. Anesth Analg 1986;65:437–443.
19. Kamibayashi T, Hayashi Y, Sumikawa K, et al. Enhancement by propofol of epinephrine-induced arrhythmias in dogs. Anesthesiology 1991;75:1035–1040.
20. Metz S, Maze M. Halothane concentration does not alter the threshold for epinephrine-induced arrhythmias in dogs. Anesthesiology 1985;62:470–474.
21. Hayashi Y, Sumikawa K, Tashiro C, Yoshiya I. Synergistic interaction of alpha-1 and beta-1 adrenoceptor agonists on induction of arrhythmias during halothane anesthesia in dogs. Anesthesiology 1988;68:902–907.
22. Atlee J, Bosnjak Z, Yeager T. Effects of diltiazem, verapamil, and inhalation anesthetics on electrophysiologic properties affecting reentrant supraventricular tachycardia in chronically instrumented dogs. Anesthesiology 1990;72:889–901.
23. Hoffman B, Bigger J. Digitalis and the allied cardiac glycosides. In Gilman A, Rall T, Nies A, Taylor P (eds): The Pharmacological Basis of Therapeutics. 8th ed. New York: Pergamon Press, 1990: pp. 814–839.
24. Zipes D. Management of cardiac arrhythmias: Pharmacological, electrical, and surgical techniques. In Braunwald E (ed): Heart Disease. 4th ed. Philadelphia: WB Saunders, 1992: pp. 628–666.
25. Atlee J. Methods for treatment of cardiac dysrhythmias. In Perioperative Cardiac Dysrhythmias. 2nd ed. Chicago: Year Book Medical, 1990: pp. 274–372.
26. Mehta P, Kloner R. Metabolic and toxic effects on the cardiovascular system. In Carlson R, Geheb M (eds): Medical Intensive Care. Philadelphia: WB Saunders, 1993: pp. 1039–1049.
27. Rutledge D, Geheb M, Cronin S, Peppers M. Pharmacologic agents and poisoning. In Carlson R, Geheb M (eds): Medical Intensive Care. Philadelphia: WB Saunders, 1993: pp. 1686–1714.
28. Barash P, Cullen B, Stoelting R. Clinical Anesthesia. 2nd ed. Philadelphia: JB Lippincott, 1992.
29. Goodman A, Rall T, Nies A, Taylor P. The Pharmacological Basis of Therapeutics. 8th ed. New York: Pergammon Press, 1990.
30. Bosnjak Z, Warltier D. New aspects of cardiac electrophysiology and function. In Conzen P, Peter K (eds): Baillière's Clinical Anaesthesiology. Vol. 7. Inhalation Anaesthesia. London: Bailliere-Tindall, 1993: pp. 937–960.

31. Roizen M, Plummer G, Lichtor J. Nitrous oxide and dysrhythmias. Anesthesiology 1987;66:427–431.
32. Levy M, Martin P. Neural control of the heart. In Berne R (eds): Handbook of Physiology. Section 2. The Cardiovascular System. Vol 1. Bethesda, MD: American Physiological Society, 1979: pp. 581–620.
33. Atlee J, Brownlee S, Burstrom R. Conscious-state comparisons of the effects of inhalation anesthetics on specialized atrioventricular conduction times in dogs. Anesthesiology 1986;64:703–710.
34. Janse M, Wit A. Electrophysiological mechanisms of ventricular arrhythmias resulting from myocardial ischemia and infarction. Physiol Rev 1989;69:1049–1169.
35. Deutsch N, Hantler C, Tait A, et al. Suppression of ventricular arrhythmias by volatile anesthetics in a canine model of chronic myocardial infarction. Anesthesiology 1990;72:1012–1021.
36. Weiss J, Nademanee K, Stevenson W, Singh B. Ventricular arrhythmias in ischemic heart disease. Ann Int Med 1991;114:784–797.
37. Kroll D, Knight P. Antifibrillatory effects of volatile anesthetics in acute reperfusion arrhythmias. Anesthesiology 1984;61:657–661.
38. Court M, Dodman N, Greenblatt D, et al. Effect of midazolam infusion and flumazenil administration on epinephrine arrhythmogenicity in dogs anesthetized with halothane. Anesthesiology 1993;78:155–162.
39. Lau W, Kovoor P, Ross D. Cardiac electrophysiologic effects of midazolam combined with fentanyl. Am J Cardiol 1993;72:177–182.
40. Xhonneux R, Carmeliet E, Reneman R. The electrophysiological effects of etomidate (R-26490), a new, short-acting hypnotic, in various cardiac tissues. In Arias A, et al (eds): Recent Progress in Anaesthesiology and Resuscitation. Amsterdam: Excerpta Medica, 1975: pp. 157–161.
41. Azuma M, Matsumura C, Kemmotsu O. Inotropic and electrophysiologic effects of propofol and thiamylal in isolated papillary muscles of the guinea pig and the rat. Anesth Analg 1993;77:557–563.
42. Barber M. Class I antiarrhythmic agents. In Lynch C (ed): Clinical Cardiac Electrophysiology. Philadelphia: JB Lippincott, 1994: pp. 85–111.
43. The Cardiac Arrhythmia Suppression Trial (CAST) Investigators. Preliminary report: Effect of encainide and flecainide on mortality in a randomized trial of arrhythmia suppression after myocardial infarction. N Engl J Med 1989;321:406–412.
44. The Cardiac Arrhythmia Suppression Trial II Investigators. Effect of the antiarrhythmic agent moricizine on survival after myocardial infarction. N Engl J Med 1992;327:227–233.
45. de La Coussaye J, Bassoul B, Brugada J, et al. Reversal of electrophysiologic and hemodynamic effects induced by high dose of bupivacaine by the combination of clonidine and dobutamine in anesthetized dogs. Anesth Analg 1992;74:703–711.

46. de La Coussayc J, Eledjam J-J, Bassoul B, et al. Receptor mechanisms for clonidine reversal of bupivacaine-induced impairment of ventricular conduction in pentobarbital-anesthetized dogs. Anesth Analg 1994;78:624–637.
47. Kent R (Burroughs Wellcome Communication). Revised product labeling for succinylchoine. Research Triangle Park, NC: Burroughs Wellcome, 1993.
48. Atlee J. Normal electrical activity of the heart. In Perioperative Cardiac Dysrhythmias. 2nd ed. Chicago: Year Book Medical, 1990: pp. 14–56.
49. Vitez T, Soper L, Wong K, Soper P. Chronic hypokalemia and intraoperative dysrhythmias. Anesthesiology 1985;63:130–133.
50. McGovern B. Hypokalemia and cardiac arrhythmias. Anesthesiology 1985;63:127–129.
51. Glaser R. Chronic hypokalemia and intraoperative dysrhythmias (letter). Anesthesiology 1986;64:408–409.
52. Atlee J. Abnormal electrical activity of the heart. In Perioperative Cardiac Dysrhythmias. 2nd ed. Chicago: Year Book Medical, 1990: pp. 57–118.
53. Atlee J. Clinical electrocardiography and electrophysiology. In Perioperative Cardiac Dysrhythmias. 2nd ed. Chicago: Year Book Medical, 1990: pp. 119–186.
54. Lown B, Wolf M. Approaches to sudden death from coronary heart disease. Circulation 1971;44:130–142.
55. Braunwald E. Valvular heart disease. In Braunwald E (ed): Heart Disease. 4th ed. Philadelphia: WB Saunders, 1992: pp. 1007–1077.
56. Zipes D. Specific arrhythmias: Diagnosis and treatment. In Braunwald E (ed): Heart Disease. 4th ed. Philadelphia: WB Saunders, 1992: pp. 667–725.

4

Electrocardiographic Diagnosis of Cardiac Arrhythmias

Abbreviations Used in Chapter Four

AV(VA)	Atrioventricular (ventriculoatrial)
ECG	Electrocardiogram (-graphic, -graphy)
LA(P)FB	Left anterior (posterior) fascicular block
L(R)BBB	Left (right) bundle branch block
MCL	Modified bipolar chest lead
SA	Sinoatrial
VES	Ventricular extrasystole
VT	Ventricular tachycardia
WPW	Wolff–Parkinson–White (syndrome)

This chapter concerns use of the electrocardiogram (ECG) for detection and diagnosis of cardiac rhythm disturbances and conduction defects. Only passing mention is made of the ECG for diagnosis of myocardial ischemia and infarction, or other cardiac afflictions. More extensive discussion of the latter aspects of ECG diagnosis is found elsewhere.[1-7] While this chapter emphasizes only the more practical aspects of ECG arrhythmia diagnosis, sufficient information is provided for practitioners to recognize and diagnose most clinical rhythm and conduction disturbances.

Limitations of Electrocardiography

The surface ECG records constantly changing potentials from an electrical field generated by all myocardial cells, not just discreet electrical activity from specific regions of the heart, even though a given lead "views" the heart from one perspective. In fact, the surface ECG records only about 10 to 15 percent of the electrical potential generated by the heart.[2] To record discreet cardiac electrical activity requires that electrodes be applied to the heart's surface (epicardial) or within its chambers (endocardial). Therefore, depending on the electrode place-

TABLE 4-1 *Diagnostic and monitoring applications of the ECG*

CARDIAC RHYTHM	PATHOPHYSIOLOGY	IMBALANCE
Rate, regularity, rhythm	Coronary artery disease	Myocardial ischemia
Conduction disorders	Cardiomyopathies	Metabolic imbalance
Repolarization defects	Pericardial disease	Physiologic imbalance*
Specific ECG patterns	Chamber enlargement	Drug effects or toxicity
AMBULATORY ECG	INTRAOPERATIVE ECG	POSTOPERATIVE ECG
Suspected sinus node dysfunction	Heart rate; arrhythmias	Heart rate; arrhythmias
Cause for syncope†	Myocardial ischemia	Ischemia/infarction
Myocardial ischemia	Physiologic imbalance*	Physiologic imbalance*
Pacemaker (mal)function	Pacemaker (mal)function	Pacemaker (mal)function

*Electrolyte disorders; autonomic and temperature effects.
†Establish tachyarrhythmia, bradycardia, or vasomotor syncope as cause.

ment and leads selected, surface ECG may fail to detect localized cardiac pathology. For localized pathology to be detected, a lead must be selected that is oriented directly toward or away from (reciprocal changes) the affected region of the heart. Despite these limitations, ECG monitoring can be extremely useful for cardiac diagnosis and monitoring before, during, and after anesthesia and surgery, and in critical care units (Table 4–1). The technique is most sensitive for detecting pathophysiology involving the entire heart, such as cardiac rhythm disturbances. Indeed, ECG is the most sensitive and specific technique available for diagnosis of cardiac rhythm disturbances and conduction disorders, although other techniques (e.g., echocardiography, nuclear imaging, angiography, cardiac catheterization) are more sensitive or specific for detection and diagnosis of coronary artery or valvular heart disease. Finally, it is important to appreciate that ECG machines and monitors in current use have evolved considerably from units used as recently as 10 to 15 years ago. This is due to the incorporation of digital signal processing and microprocessors.[4]

Surface Electrocardiography: Basic Considerations

ELECTROCARDIOGRAPHIC WAVEFORMS AND INTERVALS

Nomenclature and Standards

While surface ECG recordings represent the sum total of electrical activity from all myocardial cells, such activity can be "seen" from a number of different perspectives. Normally, the 12 standard (bipolar) limb, augmented (unipolar) limb, and unipolar precordial leads comprise the conventional surface ECG, although most available ECG monitors display up to four simultaneous leads. The characteristic ECG waveforms (Fig. 4–1) result from changes in electrical potential produced by depolarization and repolarization of atrial and ventricular myocardium. Depolarization and repolarization of the sinus node and specialized atrioventricular (AV) conducting tissue is not recognized in surface ECG recordings, but may be in intracardiac or signal-averaged ECG.[1] By convention, a negative deflection at the onset of the QRS complex is the Q wave; a positive deflection following it the R wave; and a negative deflection following the R wave the S wave. Also by convention, positive or negative ECG deflections > 5 mm are Q, R, or S waves, and ones < 5 mm q, r, or s waves, respectively. Standard ECG amplification is 1 mV = 10 mm. Relatively isoelectric intervals (e.g., the

108 ELECTROCARDIOGRAPHIC DIAGNOSIS OF CARDIAC ARRHYTHMIAS

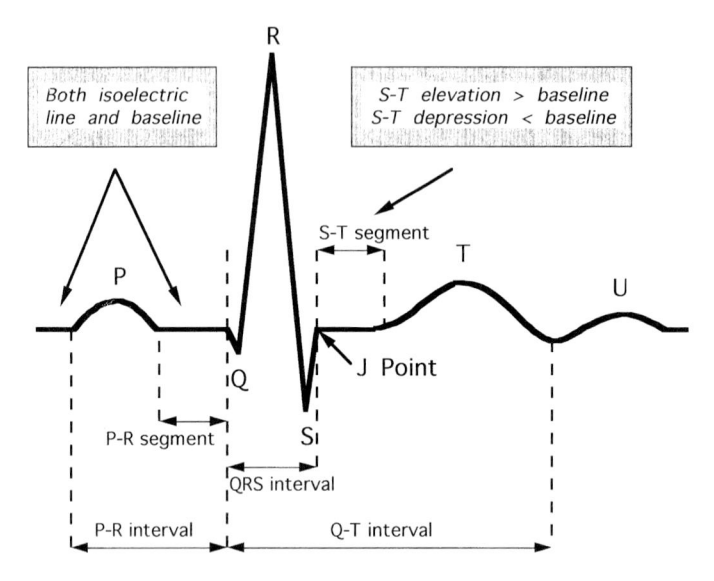

FIGURE 4-1 *Depiction of ECG waveforms, segments, and intervals. The junction of the QRS complex with the ST segment is called the J point. Especially with hypokalemia, T waves may be followed by U waves, which are probably due to delayed repolarization in some areas of the ventricle. The PR and TP intervals are at the same level of potential, and form the isoelectric line. This is also baseline for measuring amplitudes of the various waveforms. Upward and downward deviations of the ST segment from baseline are termed* **ST-segment elevation** *and* **depression,** *respectively.*

baseline) between the ECG waveforms (Fig. 4-1) occur because atrial and ventricular myocardium has recovered from excitation and is electrically silent.

Depolarization (R and S Waves)

Rapid ventricular depolarization (phase 0 of the action potential; see Figs. 2-2 and 2-3) produces a relatively high-frequency waveform, which is positive (R wave) or negative (S wave) depending on the lead selected and the mean QRS vector. With the normal, more vertical heart orientation, mean ventricular depolarization proceeds toward the positive terminal of inferior bipolar or augmented limb leads (e.g., II, aVF, and III), producing R waves in these leads (Fig. 4-2). Since the same ventricular depolarization proceeds away from the superior limb leads (e.g., I, aVL, and aVR), S waves are produced in these leads. Atrial depolarization is represented by the P wave. It too proceeds inferiorly with normal sinus rhythm and a more vertical heart orientation, so that P waves are negative, isoelectric, or biphasic in the superior limb leads, and positive in the inferior ones (Fig. 4–2). As depolarization persists during the action potential plateau (phase 2; see Figs. 2–2 and 2–3), the ECG returns to baseline as the ST segment. Late depolarization of the base of the heart is oriented superiorly, and may produce S(s) and R(r) waves in the inferior and superior limb leads, respectively. Early ventricular septal depolarization may produce q or r waves in some leads.

Repolarization (T and U Waves)

Repolarization of ventricular myocardium (phase 3 of the action potential; see Figs. 2–2 and 2–3) is much slower, and therefore produces a low-frequency waveform (the T wave in Fig. 4–1). The U wave, which may be seen in some ECG tracings, particularly with hypokalemia, follows the T wave and precedes the P wave. There is no general agreement as to the cause for U waves. They may represent delayed repolarization of ventricular endocardium or the Purkinje network.[6,7] Atrial repolarization is not seen in the surface ECG, probably because it has extremely small potential and occurs mostly during ventricular depolarization.

MONITORING LEADS

Although one can monitor any of the standard surface ECG leads or simultaneous multiple-lead combinations, depending on the monitor use and access to proper electrode positions, it is still common practice to use modified bipolar chest leads (MCL) in critical care units and for patient transport. The positive electrode is usually placed in the V_1 or V_5 precordial positions (Fig. 4–3), depending on whether one is more interested in detecting P waves for arrhythmia diagnosis (V_1 for MCL_1) or ST–T changes for diagnosis of myocardial ischemia or other imbalance (V_5 for MCL_5). For both MCL_1 and MCL_5, the negative electrode is placed near the left shoulder and a third (ground) electrode on the right shoulder or under the right clavicle.

NORMAL VALUES FOR ELECTROCARDIOGRAPHIC INTERVALS

Normal values for the PR, QRS, and QTc intervals are provided in Table 4–2. Table 4–2 assumes proper electrode placement and ECG stan-

110 ELECTROCARDIOGRAPHIC DIAGNOSIS OF CARDIAC ARRHYTHMIAS

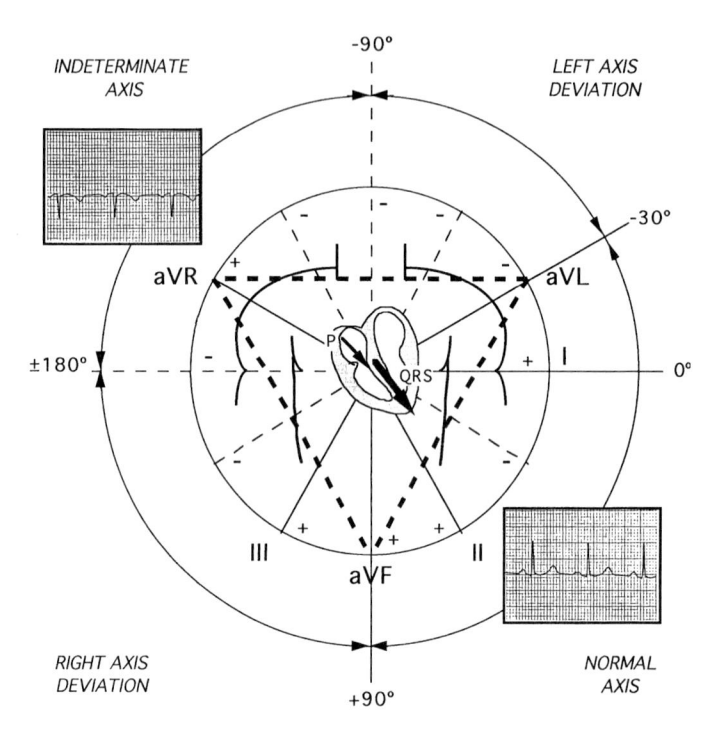

FIGURE 4-2 *Appearance of QRS complex and P waves with a normal (vertical) heart position and rotation (right ventricular chamber anterior). Shown is the hexaxial reference system, with the location of the positive and negative poles of each unipolar (aVR, aVL, and aVF) and bipolar limb lead (I, II, and III) shown. The axes of all leads intersect near the center of the heart, and each lead is designated at its respective positive pole. The solid or dashed portions of each axis indicate the positive and negative poles, respectively. Einthoven's triangle (dashed triangle) is formed by lines connecting the positive poles of aVR, aVL, and aVF, with its sides parallel to the axes of leads I, II, and III. These leads form a triaxial reference system. Mean vectors for the P wave and QRS are indicated by bold arrows. Note that P waves and QRS complexes are positive in lead II, but negative in aVR. Finally, normal mean QRS vector (axis) is between +90 and -30 degrees. Left axis deviation is +30 to -90 degrees, right axis deviation +90 to ±180 degrees, and indeterminate axis -90 to ±180 degrees. See text for further discussion.*

ELECTROCARDIOGRAPHIC DIAGNOSIS OF CARDIAC ARRHYTHMIAS **111**

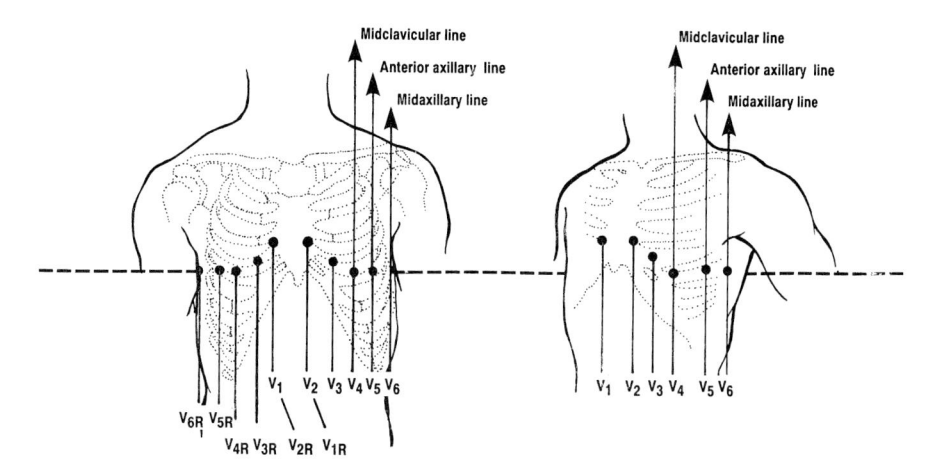

FIGURE 4–3 *Correct placement of the left (V_1 to V_6) and right precordial or chest leads (V_{1R} to V_{6R}). V_1 (V_{2R}) and V_2 (V_{1R}) are in the fourth intercostal space just to the right or left of the sternum, and V_4 (V_{4R}) in the fifth intercostal space in the midclavicular line. V_3 (V_{3R}) is halfway on a straight line between V_2 and V_4 (V_{2R} to V_{4R}), and V_5 (V_{5R}) and V_6 (V_{6R}) directly lateral to V_4 (V_{4R}) in the anterior axillary and midaxillary lines, respectively.*

TABLE 4-2 *Range of values for ECG intervals in adults, children, and adolescents*

INTERVAL (SEC)	ADULTS	CHILDREN	ADOLESCENTS
PR	0.12–0.22	0.10–0.12	0.11–0.16
QRS*	0.08–0.11	0.07–0.09	0.07–0.10
QTc†	0.37–0.46 (50–80)	0.31–0.38 (80–120)	0.31–0.36 (70–100)

*Values for limb and right precordial leads are about 0.01 to 0.015 sec shorter.
†Corrected QT interval for heart rates in parentheses (see text for discussion).

dardization (25 mm/sec; 1 mV = 10 mm). Proper electrode placement may not be practical or feasible in some circumstances, and this must be taken in to account when interpreting ECG. *PR Interval:* The PR interval includes atrial, AV node, and His–Purkinje conduction times, with AV node conduction delay accounting for most of the PR interval. The PR interval is influenced by heart rate, increasing with increased heart rate to the point of second-degree AV block of some beats within the AV node (i.e., the Wenckebach point). The Wenckebach point changes with age. It may exceed 240 beats/min in infants and children, but decrease to 130 beats/min or lower with advanced age, or if the patient is receiving beta- or calcium-channel blockers. However, when increased heart rate results from beta-adrenergic stimulation (e.g., stress, exercise, catecholamines, hyperthermia) as opposed to other causes (supraventricular tachycardia; atrial pacing), then the PR interval may increase little or even shorten somewhat despite substantial increases in rate. *QRS Interval (Complex):* The QRS complex may be slightly longer (~ 0.01 second) in males than females, and also longer by a similar amount in the left lateral precordial leads because of the larger mass of underlying ventricular myocardium. The QRS complex is lengthened by intraventricular conduction delay or ventricular hypertrophy. *QT Interval:* The QT interval measures the duration of ventricular activation and recovery. It varies inversely with heart rate, and should be corrected for heart rate (QTc interval) for reporting purposes. A simplified formula for QTc is QTc (msec) = QT (msec) + 1.75 (ventricular rate − 60).[9] The QTc interval is slightly longer in females, and tends to increase with age. There is commonly a variation in the QTc interval among the various leads, so that the longest value in multiple leads is generally reported.

LEAD SELECTION FOR SURFACE ELECTROCARDIOGRAPHIC MONITORING

The full 12-lead surface ECG is the standard for detection of myocardial ischemia and physiologic imbalance. Multiple leads are also useful for arrhythmia diagnosis, particularly with complex arrhythmias. "Complex arrhythmias" include those with varying sinoatrial (SA) or AV heart block, nonapparent P waves, and beats with ventricular aberration (i.e., widened or bizarre QRS complexes) present in one or more leads. While multiple-lead recording may become standard with future generations of ECG monitors designed for use in operating rooms and critical care units,[4] it is not at present. Therefore, most ECG diagnoses in operating and recovery rooms or critical care units are made from ECG monitors that usually display two, and sometimes up to four, simultaneous leads. Selection of multiple-lead displays, however, usually requires deselection of pressure waveforms.

Myocardial Ischemia

ST-segment depression is a common manifestation of subendocardial ischemia, and is almost always present in at least one of the anterolateral precordial leads (V_4 to V_6).[4] However, ST-segment depression fails to localize the responsible coronary lesion very well, and bears little relation to underlying segmental asynergy. In contrast, ST-segment elevation correlates well with segmental asynergy and localizes the coronary lesion relatively well.[4] Reciprocal ST-segment depression is often present in one or more of the other 12 leads. In patients with angiographically demonstrated single-vessel disease, ST-segment elevation or Q waves and inverted T waves in leads I, aVL, or V_1 to V_4 correlates closely with left anterior descending disease, and similar changes in I, III, and aVF with left circumflex or right coronary disease. The latter two cannot be distinguished by surface ECG criteria. Single-lead sensitivity for detection of intraoperative myocardial ischemia (ST-segment elevation or depression) based on continuous 12-lead ECG monitoring in 105 anesthetized surgical patients with known or suspected coronary artery disease is shown in Figure 4–4.[8] While multiple leads have increased sensitivity over single leads, note that leads II and V_5 are only 80 percent sensitive (Table 4–3).[8]

Arrhythmias

For correct arrhythmia diagnosis, it is essential to ascertain the relation of atrial to ventricular depolarization and the cause for aberration with widened or bizarre QRS complexes, both of which are discussed in more detail later. Importantly, not all beats associated with QRS aberration are of ventricular origin. In fact, with ventricular aberration, aberration may be difficult to detect in some leads (Fig. 4–5). Finally, while depolarization of the ventricles is apparent in most conventional surface ECG leads, atrial depolarization is best seen in the inferior limb leads II, III, and aVF, or the right precordial lead V_1 (Fig. 4–6).

STRIP-CHART RECORDINGS

It may be difficult to make the correct diagnoses of some arrhythmias from the monitor screen. A strip-chart recording may be required. Strip-chart recordings are also needed for the patient's chart to provide documentation of rhythm disturbances and their response to drugs and other interventions. Therefore, a strip-chart recorder should be an integral part of the monitoring system, or at least remotely connected to it. Strip-chart tracings should use standard electrode placement, leads, and calibrations (1 mV = 10 mm; 25 mm = 1 second), so that tracings may be compared to other ECG recordings in the patient's chart. The lead(s) recorded should be noted on the paper recording.

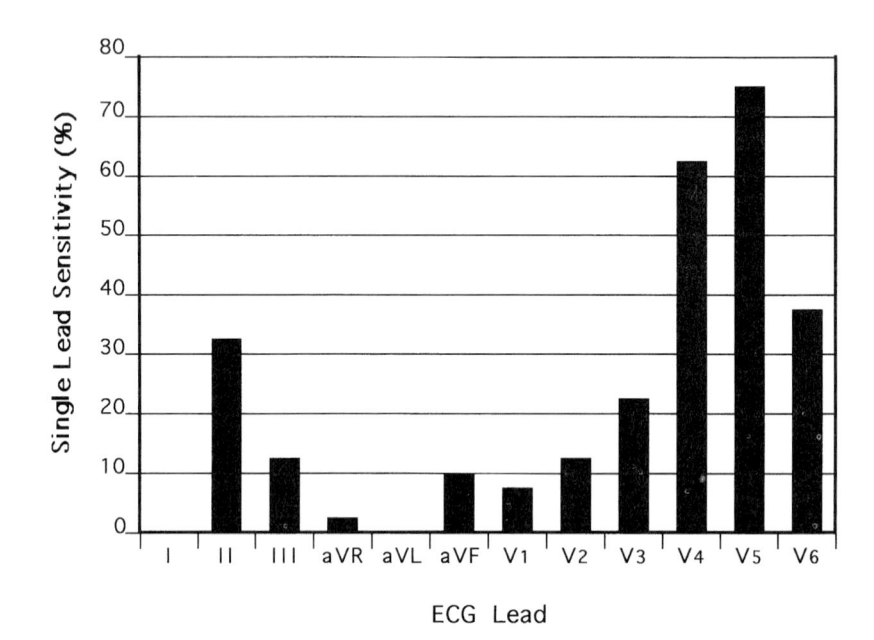

114 ELECTROCARDIOGRAPHIC DIAGNOSIS OF CARDIAC ARRHYTHMIAS

FIGURE 4-4 *Single-lead sensitivity for intraoperative detection of myocardial ischemia based on 51 episodes of ischemia detected in 25 of 105 patients with known or suspected coronary artery disease and having noncardiac surgery. (Redrawn from London et al.,[8] Anesthesiology 1988;69:232-241, with permission.)*

TABLE 4-3 *Different lead combinations for ischemia detection*

COMBINATION	LEAD(S)	% SENSITIVITY
One lead	II	33
	V_4	61
	V_5	75
Two leads	II/V_5	80
	II/V_4	82
	V_4/V_5	90
Three leads	$V_3/V_4/V_5$	94
	$II/V_4/V_5$	96
Four leads	II/V_3–V_5	100

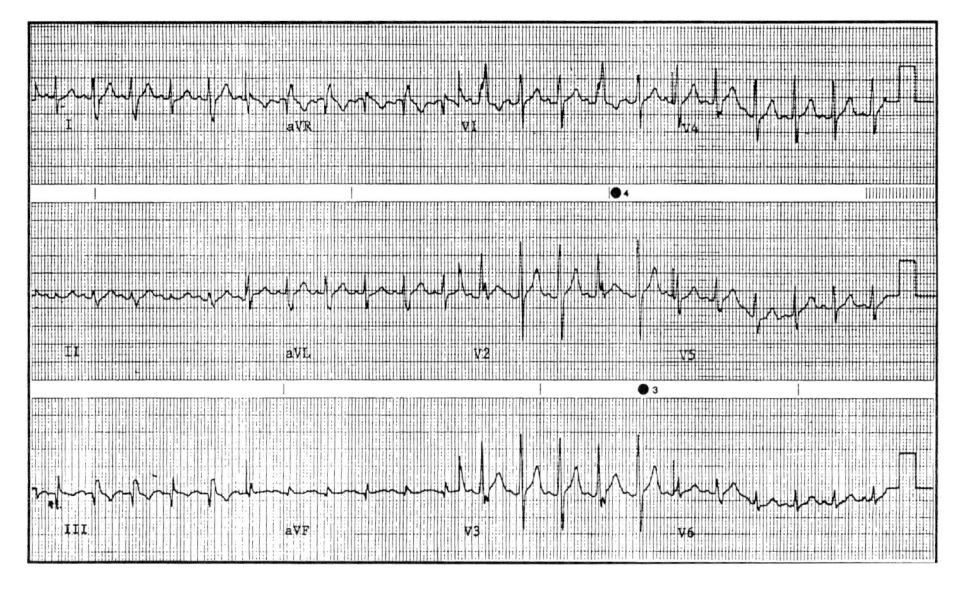

FIGURE 4-5 *Sinus tachycardia with intermittent right bundle branch block (RBBB) pattern aberration. Aberration is apparent in all leads, but least evident in leads I, aVL, aVF, and V_4 to V_6.*

LEAD PLACEMENT AND ELECTRODE APPLICATION

Lead Placement

Accurate ECG interpretation is possible only when individual electrodes for the ECG leads are correctly placed at their proper positions.[5] Under ideal circumstances in resting or immobile subjects, which may sometimes be impractical or not feasible in perioperative circumstances, the three frontal plane electrodes (left arm, left leg, and right arm) should be placed at the mid- or distal limb positions on the designated extremity. However, these positions will produce more artifact with limb movements. If more proximal positions are used, particularly with the left arm electrode, marked distortion of the QRS complex may occur.[9] A common error with application of frontal plane electrodes is reversal or switching of the limb or grounding electrodes.[5] For example, if the left and right arm electrodes are reversed, lead I will appear inverted, and leads II to III and aVR to aVL reversed. Lead aVF will not be affected. If the grounding (right leg) electrode is switched with the right or left arm electrodes, the amplitude of waveforms in lead II or III, respectively, will be extremely low. It is also possible for several of the precordial lead electrode positions to be reversed, which will

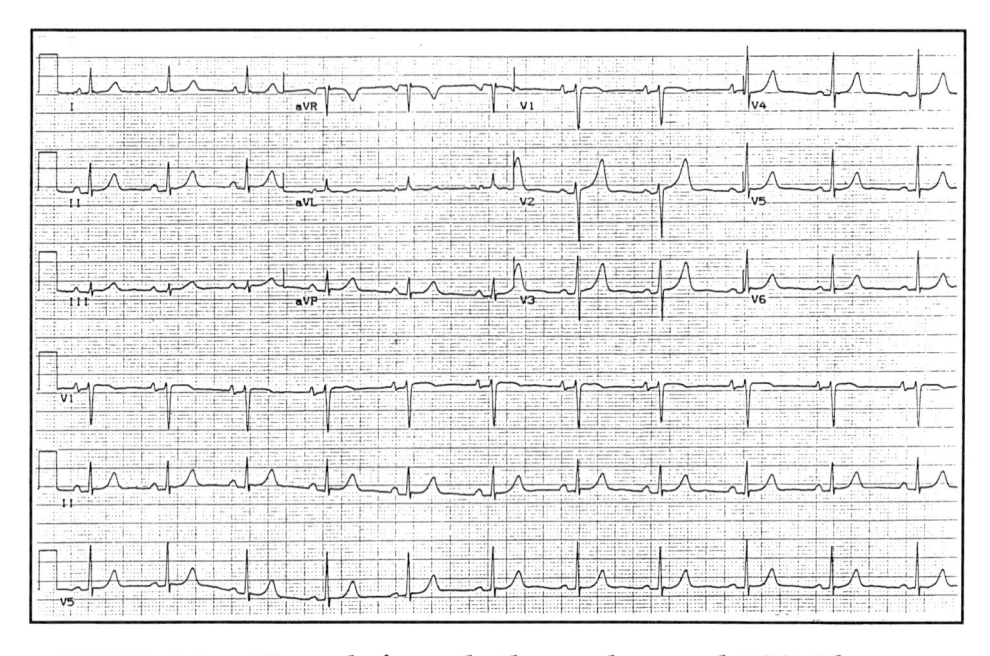

FIGURE 4-6 *Normal sinus rhythm and normal ECG. The ventricular rate is 66 beats/min, P-R interval 0.16 sec, QRS duration 0.08 sec, and the QTc interval 0.42 sec. The P-, R-, and T-wave axes are normal and +55, +30 and +60 degrees, respectively. Note that P waves are best seen in the inferior limb leads II, III, and aVF, and right precordial lead V_1.*

affect normal progression of the R- and S-wave amplitudes across the precordium.[5] However, a more common mistake with the placement of the precordial electrodes is to incorrectly position individual electrodes, which can significantly alter the appearance of ECG waveforms. Especially for serial ECG recordings, precise precordial electrode placement is critical for the correct interpretation of possible changes.

Electrode Application

Electrodes should be selected for maximum adhesiveness and minimum skin–electrode impedance based on standards published by the American Heart Association Council on Clinical Cardiology.[10] Electrode should not be used if they appear dried out or oxidized (e.g., greenish discoloration). Adequate contact gel should be present. To further reduce skin–electrode impedance, the skin should be cleansed with alcohol-moistened gauze to remove dry skin or oils that could increase impedance or reduce adhesiveness. If electrodes are in close proximity to a surgical field, they should be covered by a transparent adhesive dressing to prevent electrodes from becoming wet and detached during surgical field preparation.

INTERPRETATION OF THE ELECTROCARDIOGRAM

As with most medical diagnoses, a systematic approach to ECG interpretation will improve the practitioner's ability to detect abnormalities. Features of the ECG that should always be examined are listed in Table 4-4.[5] However, the emphasis on one or more of these will depend somewhat on whether one has a full 12-lead ECG report with rhythm strips, or only strip-chart recordings from one or two monitored leads. Therefore, to accurately assess cardiac rhythm requires examination not only of rate and regularity, but also each of the ECG waveforms and intervals listed in Table 4-4.

Rate

When the atrial and ventricular rates are the same, rate can be determined by measuring the RR or PP intervals. Otherwise, atrial and ventricular rates are determined separately. Each large (0.5 cm^2) grid on standard ECG recording paper is divided into 25 smaller grids by vertical and horizontal grid lines spaced 1 mm apart (Fig. 4-7). By convention, horizontal spacing is 0.04 sec/mm and vertical spacing 0.10 mV/mm. Therefore, each 0.5-cm grid is 200 msec "wide" × 0.5 mV "high." Rate in beats/min is calculated by dividing 60,000 (msec/min) by the RR or PP interval (msec/beats). Corresponding heart rates for RR intervals (in msec) are shown in Table 4-5. Another way to estimate rate is to count the number of cardiac cycles (i.e., beat-to-beat intervals) in 6 sec (30 large grids) and multiply by 10.

Regularity

Cardiac rhythm, even normal sinus rhythm, is never precisely regular. In part this is due to beat-to-beat autonomic and intrinsic

TABLE 4-4 *Systematic examination of ECG features*

1. Rate	6. ST segment
2. Regularity	7. T waves
3. P waves	8. U waves
4. PR interval	9. QTc interval
5. QRS complex	10. Rhythm

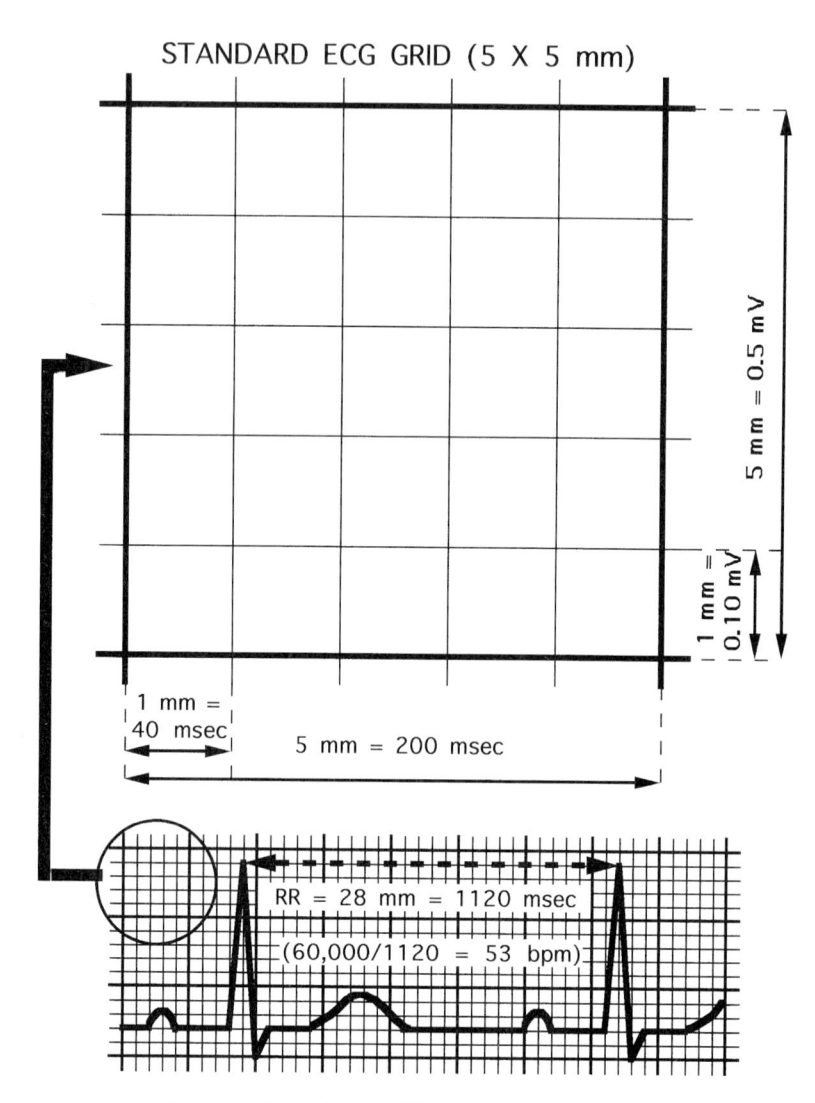

118   ELECTROCARDIOGRAPHIC DIAGNOSIS OF CARDIAC ARRHYTHMIAS

FIGURE 4-7   *Determination of heart rate from ECG grid lines. Each large grid has 25 1-mm squares within it, with each square corresponding to 40 msec "wide" × 0.1 mV "high." Heart rate in beats/min is 60,000 msec/min ÷ the R-R interval in msec/beats. In this example, the RR interval is 28 mm × 40 msec = 1,120 msec. Therefore, heart rate is 53 beats/min.*

TABLE 4-5 *Corresponding heart rates for RR intervals*

RR INTERVAL (MSEC)	RATE (BEATS/MIN)
200	300
240	250
300	200
400	150
500	120
600	100
800	75
1,000	60

modulation, which affects pacemaker rate and AV node conduction time. Also, the regularity of cardiac rhythm can provide valuable clues for diagnosis when P waves wave are nonapparent in monitored leads.

P Waves

Normally, atrial activation spreads to the left and inferiorly from the region of the sinus node (see Fig. 2–1). Because of this, the P wave is upright in leads with a leftward and inferior orientation (I, II, aVF, and V_4 to V_6), negative in aVR, and variable in the other standard limb or precordial leads except V_1 (Fig. 4–6). In V_1, the P wave is biphasic (Fig. 4–6) because it "sees" earlier right atrial depolarization as positive (coming toward V_1), and subsequent left atrial depolarization as negative (going away from V_1). This is the usual pattern, but anesthetized or sedated healthy young patients without arrhythmias commonly have inverted, biphasic, or nearly isoelectric P waves (Figs. 4–8 and 4–9). Such "wandering" or "shifting atrial pacemakers" are in fact ectopic atrial rhythms, and likely the result of a downward shift in pacemaker location from the SA node to inferior sites of subsidiary atrial pacemakers along the sulcus terminalis.[11-15] However, it is also possible that these ectopic atrial rhythms originate in secondary atrial pacemakers located in Bachman's bundle, the coronary sinus ostia, or the tricuspid valve ring. Because depolarization from inferior right atrial pacemakers would spread upward and to the left, this would produce the P-wave changes noted in Figures 4–8 and 4–9, but with little effect on the PR interval.

PR Interval

As noted earlier, the PR interval measures the time for the propagating impulse to depolarize the atrium, AV node, and specialized

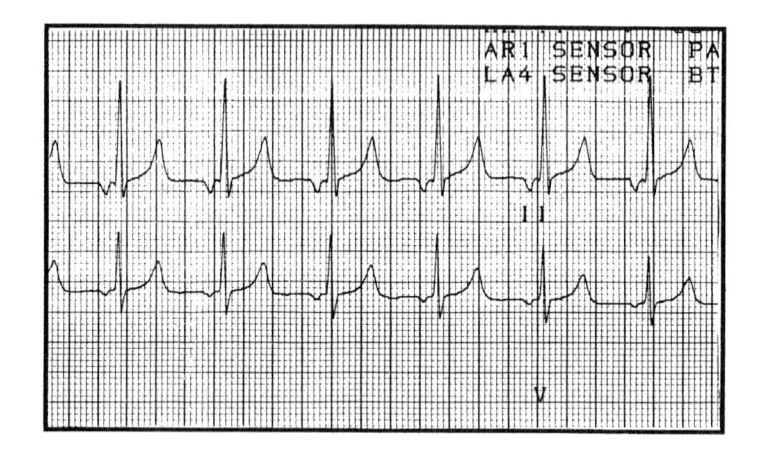

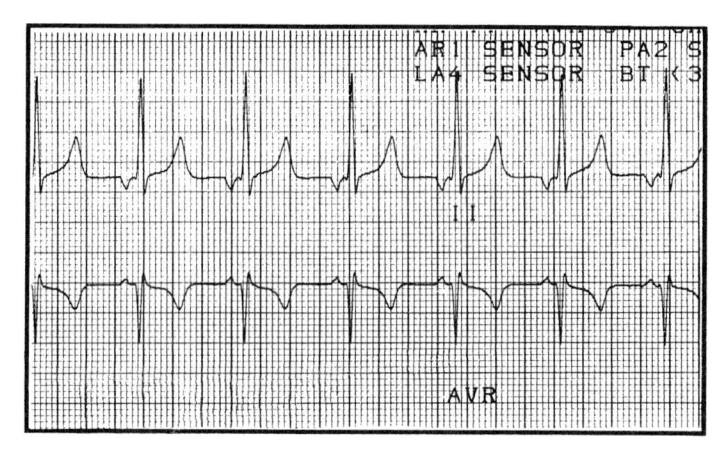

FIGURE 4–8 *P-wave changes with an ectopic atrial rhythm in healthy, young adult male under general anesthesia (propofol, fentanyl, desflurane, vecuronium). (Top) Shortly after induction of anesthesia, the P waves became inverted in monitored leads II and V$_5$. While a preanesthesia recording was not made, the P waves had been noted to be upright. (Bottom) Note that the P waves in aVR are positive with this ectopic atrial rhythm, suggesting that the rhythm originates in subsidiary atrial pacemakers located inferiorly along the sulcus terminalis toward the right atrial–inferior vena cava junction (see text).*

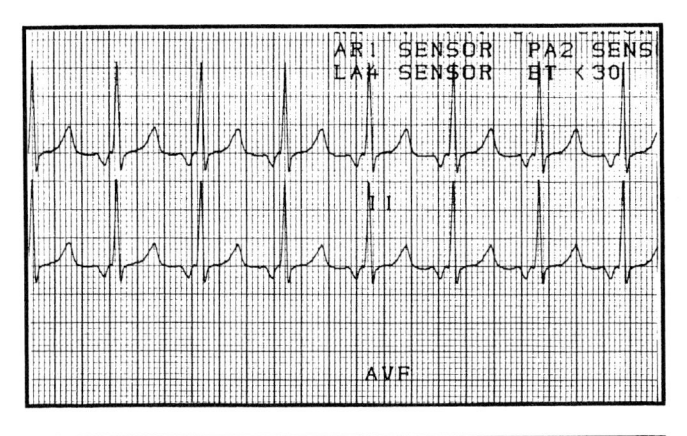

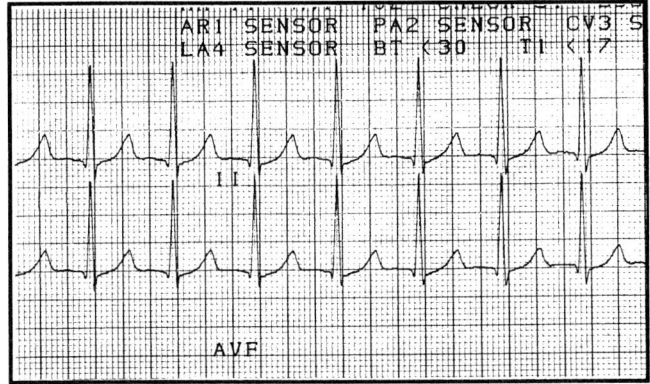

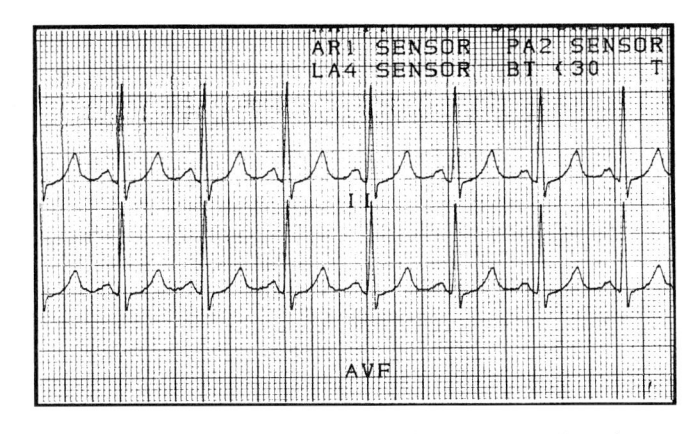

FIGURE 4-9 Same patient as in Figure 4-8. (Top) The patient remained in ectopic atrial rhythm for the duration of anesthesia. The P waves are also inverted in aVF, as would be expected. (Middle) Shortly after reversal of muscle relaxation, the P waves became nearly isoelectric in leads II and aVF, suggesting that the atrial pacemaker has migrated upward along the sulcus terminalis toward the sinus node region. (Bottom) As the patient awakened, there was return to normal sinus rhythm, with expected upright P waves in leads II and aVF.

ventricular conducting system. A shortened PR interval (≤0.10 msec) immediately suggests one of two possibilities: either the pacemaker is located at or in close proximity to the AV junction (it is uncertain whether pacemakers exist within the AV node proper), or AV impulse propagation has bypassed ("short-circuited") the AV node itself. The latter possibility is discussed later under Accessory Pathways and Ventricular Preexcitation (see Chapter 10).

QRS Complex

The QRS complex results from ventricular depolarization. The appearance of its component waveforms (Q, R, and S) will depend on the perspective of the selected surface ECG lead, as well as the ventricular activation sequence and underlying structural heart disease. The normal sequence of ventricular activation and evolution of the QRS complex, as might be seen in lead II, is depicted schematically in Figure 4–10. *Q Waves:* The presence of Q waves in leads V_1 to V_3 is considered abnormal, but Q waves in V_4 to V_6 are normal. In all other leads, except III and aVR, Q waves—if present—should be quite small. Ventricular septal hypertrophy or chamber dilatation can increase the size of Q waves. *R Waves:* The R wave normally increases in amplitude and duration from V_1 to V_4 or V_5. Right or left ventricular hypertrophy and chamber enlargement can produce larger R waves in leads V_1 to V_2 or V_5 to V_6, respectively. Loss of normal R-wave progression occurs with infarction of left ventricular myocardium. *S Waves:* S waves should be large in V_1 and largest in V_2, then progressively decrease in size in leads V_3 to V_6. Alteration in this sequence is produced by right or left ventricular enlargement or hypertrophy.

ST Segment

This represents the time during which ventricular myocardium remains depolarized following activation. The ST segment begins at the J point, where it forms close to a right angle with the QRS complex. It extends horizontally, perhaps with slight up- or down-sloping, or even horizontal depression (≤ 1 mm), until it gently curves into the T wave. The length of the ST segment is influenced by factors that alter ventricular activation, and points along this segment are designated by their distance from the J point (J + 60 msec, J + 80 msec, etc.). Normally, the first portion of the ST segment is at baseline voltage (i.e., at same voltage as the PR or TP intervals). In some individuals, particularly young black males, early ventricular repolarization may produce J-point elevation of several millimeters in the left precordial leads (V_1 to V_3).

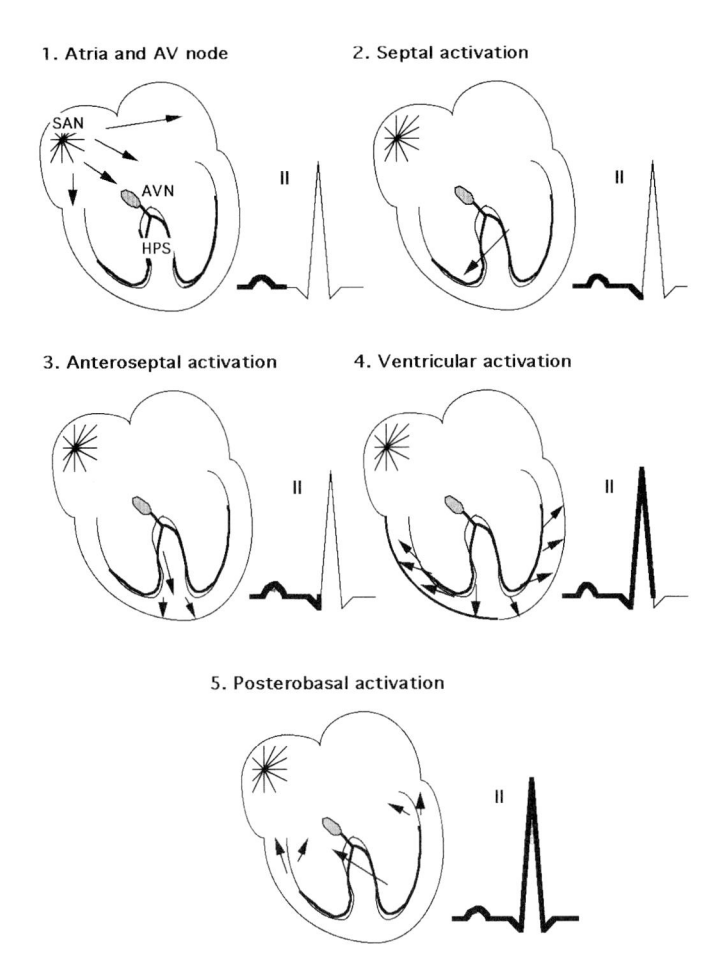

ELECTROCARDIOGRAPHIC DIAGNOSIS OF CARDIAC ARRHYTHMIAS   **123**

FIGURE 4–10 *Inscription of the P wave and evolution of the QRS complex in surface ECG lead II. (1) Atrial activation proceeds inferiorly and to the left, with the left atrium activated last. Conduction through the AV node is electrically silent. (2) Septal activation is downward and from left to right. (3) Activation of the distal interventricular septum is downward and then anteriorly. (4) Activation of the bulk of ventricular myocardium proceeds from the endocardial to epicardial surface. (5) Posterobasal ventricular and uppermost interventricular septal activation proceeds posteriorly and superiorly. SAN, sinoatrial node; AVN, AV node; HPS, His–Purkinje system.*

T Waves

Typically, the initial deflection of the T wave is longer than the terminal deflection, producing a slightly asymmetrical shape. The amplitude of the T wave tends to be larger in males compared to females, and diminishes with age. Normally, amplitude does not exceed 5 mm in any of the frontal plane (limb) leads or 10 mm in the precordial leads. The direction of the T wave (upward or downward) should be similar to the QRS complex; therefore, positive in the inferior limb leads and chest leads V_3 to V_6. The T wave is negative or biphasic in leads aVR, aVL, and V_1 to V_2. It is possible with fast heart rates that the T and P waves will merge, making the two waveforms difficult to distinguish from each other (Fig. 4–11).

U Waves

The U wave may be present or absent as a small wave following the T wave, and usually has a similar direction (Fig. 4–1). When present, the U wave is said to be most prominent in leads V_2 to V_3.[7] The U wave is larger at slower heart rates, and becomes smaller or merges with the following P wave at faster heart rates. Finally, there may be fusion of the T and U waves, making it difficult to measure the QTc interval.

QTc Interval

Measurement of the QTc interval was discussed earlier, and normal values are provided in Table 4–2. The diagnostic value of the QTc interval is limited by the difficulty in identifying the end of ventricular recovery (T wave), and its occasional mergence with T or P waves.

Rhythm

Certain irregularities of rate, regularity, P-wave morphology, or the PR interval may, in themselves, indicate the presence of cardiac rhythm abnormalities.[5] However, abnormalities involving the PR and QTc intervals, and QRS complex and T waves, may indicate only the potential for development of rhythm abnormalities.

RATE. The normal sinus rate is between 60 and 100 beats/min. Slower or faster rates in adults are termed *sinus bradycardia* or *tachycardia*, respectively. However, these are arbitrary upper and lower rate limits. What constitutes bradycardia or tachycardia must be considered for each patient and circumstance. For example, while resting sinus bradycardia of 40 beats/min in a conditioned athlete is normal, the same rate in an elderly patient signifies intrinsic or

Sinus rate 107 beats /min

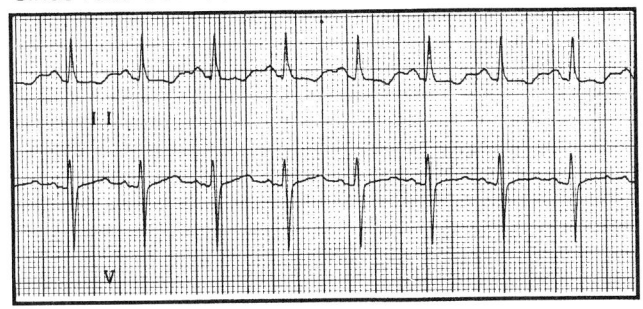

Sinus rate 118 beats/min

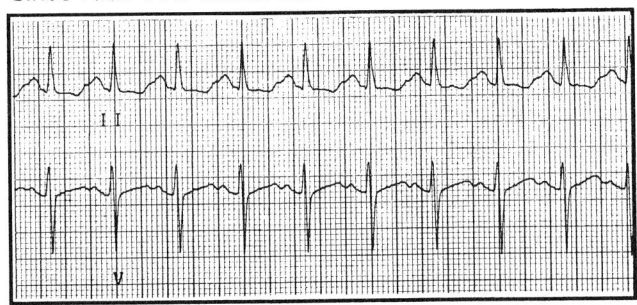

Sinus rate 133 beats/min

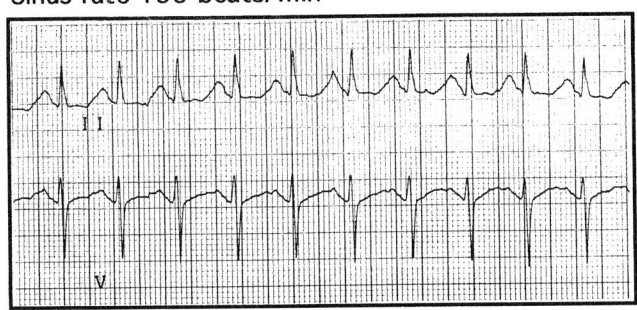

FIGURE 4-11   Merging of T and P waves with increased heart rate. When the sinus rate is 107 beats/min, the T and P waves are separate and distinct. When the rate increases to 118 beats/min, the T and P waves merge in lead II. When the rate is 133 beats/min, the T and P waves are merged in both leads II and V_5. Biphasic T waves (lead II) may be in part due to large doses of tricyclic antidepressants this patient was receiving. Also, the patient was anemic.

extrinsic sinus node dysfunction. Similarly, in adults, a sinus rate of 100 beats/min during sleep or with vigorous exercise would be abnormal.

REGULARITY. As noted earlier, sinus rhythm is not precisely regular because of the variation in autonomic tone and intrinsic modulation. As a result, sinus rate tends to accelerate with inspiration and slow with expiration, termed *respiratory sinus arrhythmia* when maximum–minimum cycle length variation exceeds 10 percent of the shortest cycle length (Fig. 4–12). Respiratory variation in sinus cycle length decreases with age, and is considered pathologic (i.e., a manifestation of sinus node dysfunction) in patients over 60 years of age. Pulse rate variability with sinus arrhythmia in some patients may sometimes be so pronounced as to suggest important arrhythmias.

P WAVES. Normally, the P-wave axis is between + 30 and + 75 degrees. When the P-wave axis is outside these limits, the rhythm must have originated in an ectopic atrial or AV junctional site.

PR INTERVAL. Ectopic P waves are sometimes associated with shortened PR intervals. However, a normal P wave with a short PR interval suggests the presence of an AV bypass pathway or an abnormally fast conducting pathway within the AV node. When the PR interval cannot be determined because of the absence of visible P waves in any lead, there is an obvious abnormality of cardiac rhythm.

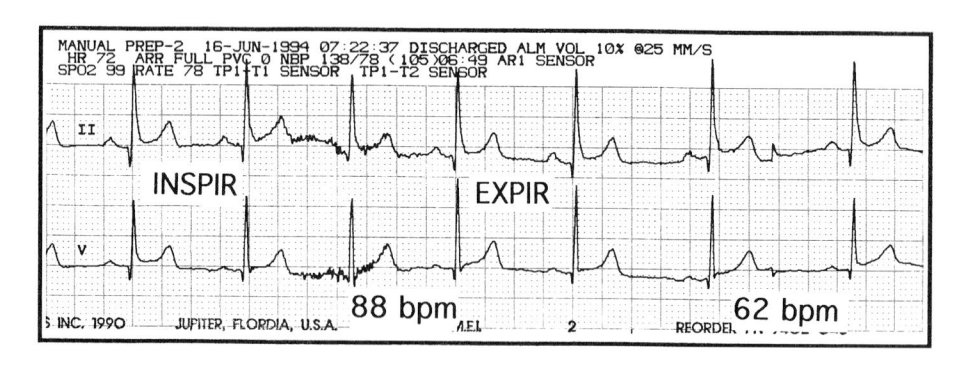

FIGURE 4–12 *Respiratory sinus arrhythmia in a conscious, healthy young adult. Note cyclical variation in sinus rate with inspiration (INSPIR) and expiration (EXPIR). The maximum cycle length (960 msec = 62 beats/min) exceeds the minimum cycle length (680 msec = 88 beats/min) by more than 10 percent.*

QRS MORPHOLOGY. A normal P-wave axis with shortened PR interval will be associated with a normal QRS complex if an AV bypass pathway inserts into the common (His) bundle or there is a fast pathway within the AV node (Fig. 4–13A). If the AV bypass pathway inserts beyond the bifurcation of the common bundle or directly into ventricular myocardium, there will be evidence of ventricular preexcitation (delta wave), as seen in patients with the Wolff–Parkinson–White (WPW) syndrome (Fig. 4–13B). The P wave and PR interval may be normal, but intraventricular conduction impaired to produce a

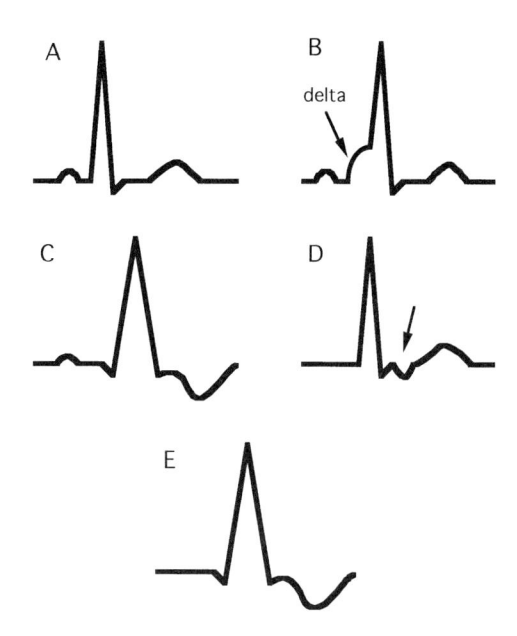

FIGURE 4–13 *QRS complex morphology and arrhythmias. (A) A normal P wave, shortened P-R interval, and normal QRS suggest an AV bypass pathway or fast pathway within the AV node. (B) A normal P wave and shortened P-R interval with evidence of ventricular preexcitation (delta wave) are observed in patients with the WPW syndrome. (C) A normal P wave and PR interval, but abnormal QRS morphology, are seen in patients with disturbed intraventricular conduction. (D) Retrograde P waves (arrow) with normal QRS morphology are consistent with AV junctional rhythm. (E) Absent or retrograde P waves with abnormal QRS morphology are consistent with ventricular origin beats, AV junctional beats conducted with ventricular aberration, or antidromic AV reciprocating tachycardia (see Chapter 10).*

rolonged QRS with abnormal morphology (Fig. 4–13C). Absent P waves or inverted (retrograde) P waves following normal QRS complexes (Fig. 4–13D) indicate an AV junctional origin for the rhythm disturbance. Finally, absent or retrograde P waves with abnormal QRS morphology usually indicate that the impulse originated somewhere in the ventricles distal to the His bundle (Fig. 4–13E). However, such beats could also be AV junctional with ventricular aberration or associated with antidromic AV reciprocating tachycardia (see Chapter 10).

ST SEGMENT, T WAVES, U WAVES AND QTC INTERVAL. ST segment changes, abnormal T waves, the appearance of new U waves or an increase in their amplitude, and a prolonged QTc interval indicate the presence of underlying cardiac pathology with the potential for development of significant ventricular arrhythmias.

ARRHYTHMIA DIAGNOSIS FROM MONITORED LEADS

It is essential that ECG leads be selected convey the ECG information of most interest. Since this is the information needed to make the diagnosis of myocardial ischemia or arrhythmias, leads II and V_5 (or V_4) are usually monitored. Either of these lead combinations (II to V_5, II to V_4) show about 80 percent sensitivity for detection of myocardial ischemia (Table 4–3). For diagnosis of arrhythmias, it is essential to detect P waves if present. For detection of P waves, V_1 is at least as good as or better than lead II, and certainly better than V_5. The problem is that available five-lead monitoring leads allow recording from only one precordial position, so that V_5 and V_1 cannot be monitored simultaneously. Therefore, leads V_1 or II and aVR or aVL are recommended for diagnosis of arrhythmias. Leads aVR or aVL will aid with diagnosis of ectopic atrial rhythms, since P waves may be nonapparent in II or V_1. However, the best leads for detection of P waves are intravascular or esophageal leads (below), since these greatly amplify atrial depolarization. When esophageal leads become more widely used for perioperative and critical care ECG monitoring, ECG lead selectors will be provided by manufacturers to allow easy switching between surface and esophageal ECG.

Computer Electrocardiographic Analysis

Microprocessor-based (computer) ECG analysis for detection of myocardial ischemia (i.e., ST-segment trending) is now the standard for most operating room and critical care units.[4] However, there has been less success with automated arrhythmia detection and diagnosis, at least in operating rooms and critical care units. The major problem has been differentiating between arrhythmias and artifact produced by electrical noise, patient movement, and other interference in these highly "contaminated" environments. As a result, little reliance has been placed on computer-aided arrhythmia detection and diagnosis by anesthesia or critical care practitioners. It is possible that this will change with expected advances in ECG signal processing and esophageal ECG.

Intracavitary Electrocardiography

Intracavitary ECG employs epicardial, intravascular, or esophageal leads. When available, epicardial or intravascular leads are extremely useful for arrhythmia diagnosis. Atrial depolarization is greatly amplified in these leads compared to that in surface ECG leads, provided the lead is situated within or on the atrium. With esophageal ECG, electrodes are also much closer to the atrium than with surface ECG, thereby greatly increasing (improving) the signal-to-noise ratio for detection of atrial depolarization.

UNIPOLAR EPICARDIAL AND ENDOCARDIAL LEADS

Unipolar epicardial and transvenous endocardial leads record electrical potentials from underlying myocardium without being influenced by potentials from an indifferent electrode. However, it should be understood that these unipolar leads do not just record the electrical potential from a small area of underlying myocardium, but rather all of the electrical events of the entire cardiac cycle as viewed from the particular lead location. Unipolar epicardial or endocardial leads are taken by connecting the respective lead to the V lead position and selecting the V lead position on the ECG monitor. To avoid direct microshock, latex gloves should be worn when handling endocardial or epicardial leads. Also, ECG monitoring equipment used with these leads should be isolated from ≤ 10 µA leakage current by isolation amplifiers (see AAMI standards: Safe Current Limits for Electromedical Apparatus—American Association for the Advancement of Medical Instrumentation). This is because currents as low as 10 µA can induce ventricular fibrillation in patients with increased susceptibility.

Epicardial Leads

Temporary atrial epicardial pacing wires can be used to record the right atrial electrogram. The proximal connector pin of one of the bipolar leads can be placed under the positive surface ECG electrode pad (V_1) of MCL_1. Alternatively, one of the bipolar leads can be connected to the V lead input of a five-lead monitoring system, and the V position selected to record a unipolar atrial ECG.

Intravascular Leads

Intracardiac electrode catheters, depending on the type, number, and position of electrode elements, can be used to record unipolar or bipolar right atrial or ventricular ECG. For unipolar ECG, the recording electrode is connected to the V lead input of the ECG monitor and the V position selected. For bipolar ECG, electrode pins are connected to the right and left arm ECG inputs, and lead I selected. Bipolar ECG, however, produces less baseline drift and artifact related to spontaneous or mechanical respiration. Pacing Swan–Ganz catheters (see Chapter 7) can also be used to record intracavitary ECG, as can saline-filled central venous access catheters. However, the nonconductive plastic hub of the central venous catheter must be modified with a conductive ECG adapter (e.g., RAECG adapter, Arrow International, Reading, PA). Changes in morphology of the P waves and QRS complexes identify the position of the electrode(s) in the right atrium or ventricle (Fig. 4–14).

UNIPOLAR AND BIPOLAR ESOPHAGEAL LEADS

A *unipolar esophageal lead* can be constructed from a vascular J-wire and a disposable esophageal stethoscope.[1] The J-wire is insulated (e.g., 8-Fr red Robinson catheter), and taped to the stethoscope barrel with its tip exposed at the level of the stethoscope diaphragm. This arrangement permits simultaneous auscultation and temperature monitoring while recording highly amplified P waves. The proximal J-wire is attached with an alligator clip lead to the V lead input of the ECG monitor, and the V position selected on the ECG monitor. However, unipolar esophageal ECG is subject to the same respiratory baseline drift-artifact as with unipolar intravascular ECG. Better and more convenient for recording esophageal ECG are commercially available, disposable, esophageal stethoscopes with closely spaced bipolar electrodes (Arzco Medical Systems, Inc., Tampa, FL). These can be used to record *bipolar atrial* or *ventricular esophageal ECG* (Figs. 4–15 and 4–16), and are a significant improvement over previously available esophageal ECG-recording stethoscopes with 10-cm interelectrode spacing. This is because the newer probes record fairly

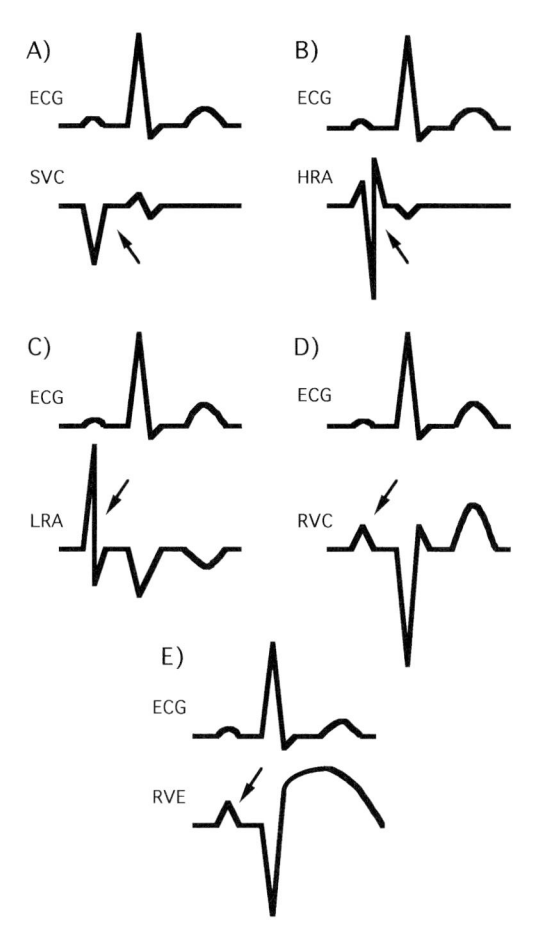

ELECTROCARDIOGRAPHIC DIAGNOSIS OF CARDIAC ARRHYTHMIAS **131**

FIGURE 4–14 *Depiction of unipolar catheter electrograms recorded from the superior vena cava (SVC—panel A), high right atrium (HRA—panel B), low right atrium (LRA—panel C), right ventricular cavity (RVC—panel D), and right ventricular endocardium (RVE—panel E). Catheter electrograms are shown with simultaneous surface ECG (ECG) to indicate timing of waveforms. Note especially the transition in amplitude and polarity of P waves with catheter ECG (arrows) as the electrode is advanced from the right atrium to ventricle. Finally, note the right ventricular injury potential (elevated ST segment) when the electrode contacts right ventricular endocardium (panel E).*

132 ELECTROCARDIOGRAPHIC DIAGNOSIS OF CARDIAC ARRHYTHMIAS

Pmax-1

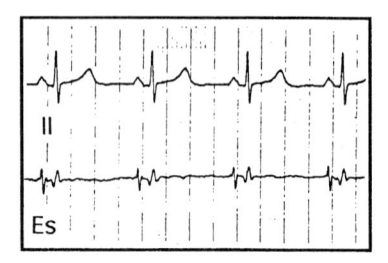

Pmax

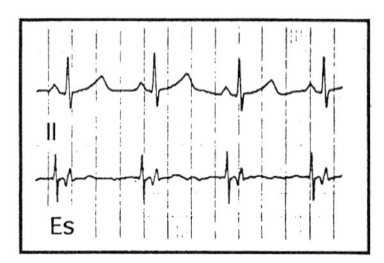

Pmax+1

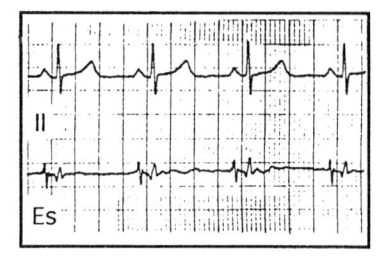

FIGURE 4–15 *Bipolar atrial esophageal ECG. Esophageal ECG recordings (Es) are shown with surface ECG lead II (II) at the point of a maximum amplitude P wave (Pmax), as well as points 1 cm proximal (Pmax − 1) and distal (Pmax + 1) to Pmax. Note that the amplitude of esophageal P waves is substantially reduced at Pmax − 1 and Pmax + 1.*

discreet atrial or ventricular ECG signals as opposed to global ECG. To record bipolar esophageal ECG, the proximal electrode pins are connected directly to the right arm and left arm surface ECG electrode inputs, and lead I selected on the ECG monitor. Alternatively, one of the bipolar stethoscope leads can be selected to record unipolar esophageal ECG (above).

ELECTROCARDIOGRAPHIC DIAGNOSIS OF CARDIAC ARRHYTHMIAS **133**

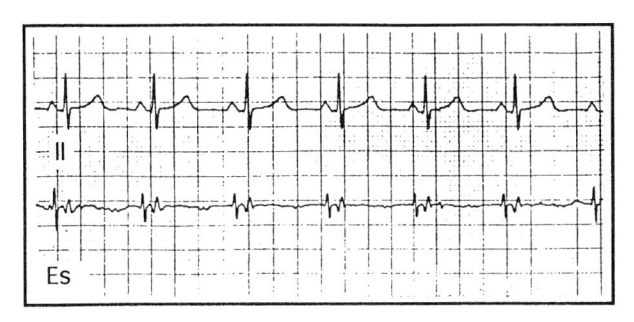

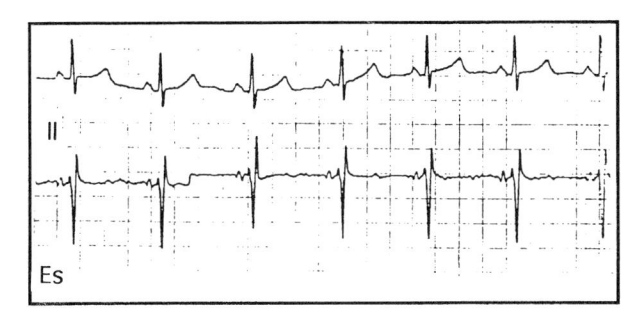

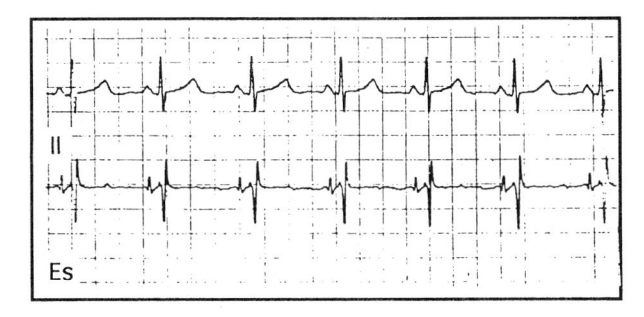

FIGURE 4–16 *Bipolar ventricular esophageal ECG. Esophageal ECG recordings (Es) are shown with surface ECG lead II (II) at the point of a maximum amplitude QRS complex (Vmax), as well as points 1 cm proximal (Vmax − 1) and distal (Vmax + 1) to Vmax. Note that the amplitude of esophageal V waves is substantially reduced at Vmax − 1 and somewhat so at Vmax + 1.*

Miscellaneous Topics Related to Electrocardiographic Arrhythmia Diagnosis

There are several topics that require further discussion to enable practitioners to detect and correctly diagnose cardiac rhythm disturbances. Discussed are patterns of beating, accessory pathways and preexcitation, QRS aberration, interference between pacemakers, AV dissociation, fusion and capture beats, retrograde and concealed conduction, exit and entrance block, parasystole, and ECG artifacts.

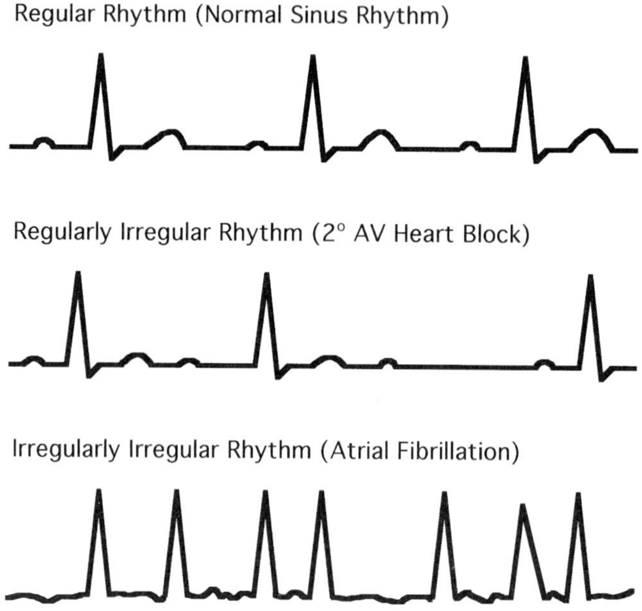

FIGURE 4–17 *Depiction of patterns of beating. (Top) If beat-to-beat intervals show no or minimal cycle length variation, the rhythm is regular (e.g., sinus rhythm). (Middle) If beat-to-beat intervals show a recurring pattern of cycle length variation, the rhythm is regularly irregular (e.g., second-degree AV heart block). (Bottom) If beat-to-beat intervals show no recurring pattern of cycle length variation, the rhythm is irregularly irregular (e.g., atrial fibrillation). Simulated ventricular aberration with the next to last beat (bottom) is due to the Ashman phenomenon, discussed later in the text under QRS Aberration.*

PATTERNS OF BEATING

While all beats on the ECG monitoring screen or rhythm strip may have similar morphology, beat-to-beat cycle lengths may be nearly the same (regular rhythm), or show recurring or nonrecurring cycle length variation. Cycle length is the time interval between successive beats. Rhythms with recurring cycle length variation are "regularly" irregular (also termed *group beating*), while those with nonrecurring cycle length variation are "irregularly" irregular (Fig. 4–17). Even when there is QRS aberration (below), a regularly irregular rhythm suggests a primary supraventricular mechanism for the rhythm disturbance, although perhaps associated with grouped extrasystoles (e.g., bigeminal, trigeminal, or quadrigeminal pattern) or second-degree AV heart block. A pattern of increasing PR-interval prolongation prior to dropped beats with second-degree AV heart block (Fig. 4–17) indicates presence of the *Wenckebach* phenomenon (also pattern, periodicity). While Wenckebach block can occur anywhere within the specialized AV conducting system, it is most commonly recognized at the AV node. The Wenckebach pattern is recognized whenever the first cycle (RR interval) of a group of beats is longer than the second, and the longest cycle between beats is less than twice the shortest.[5]

ACCESSORY PATHWAYS AND PREEXCITATION

Normally, ventricular myocardium is activated by impulses traveling over the common pathway: SA node, atria, AV node, common (His) bundle, bundle and fascicular branches, and Purkinje network to ventricular endocardium. This common pathway constitutes the *specialized AV conducting system*. However, in some individuals, a portion of the ventricular specialized conducting system or myocardium may receive earlier than expected excitation *(preexcitation)* from above via accessory or AV bypass pathways. Accessory pathways (Fig. 4–18) or connections are small, discreet bundles of cardiac (usually atrial) muscle fibers with electrophysiologic properties typical of fast-response fibers (see Chapter 2). Note that accessory pathways can affect the ECG in one or two ways (Fig. 4–18): (1) shorten the P–R interval if all or part of AV impulse propagation bypasses the AV node; (2) cause a fusion QRS complex if part of the ventricle is preexcited. As shall be seen in Chapters 9 and 10, accessory pathways form part of the reentry circuit with AV reciprocating tachycardia.

QRS ABERRATION

The term *QRS (ventricular) aberration* is reserved for a supraventricular impulse with abnormal ventricular. This gives rise to a widened,

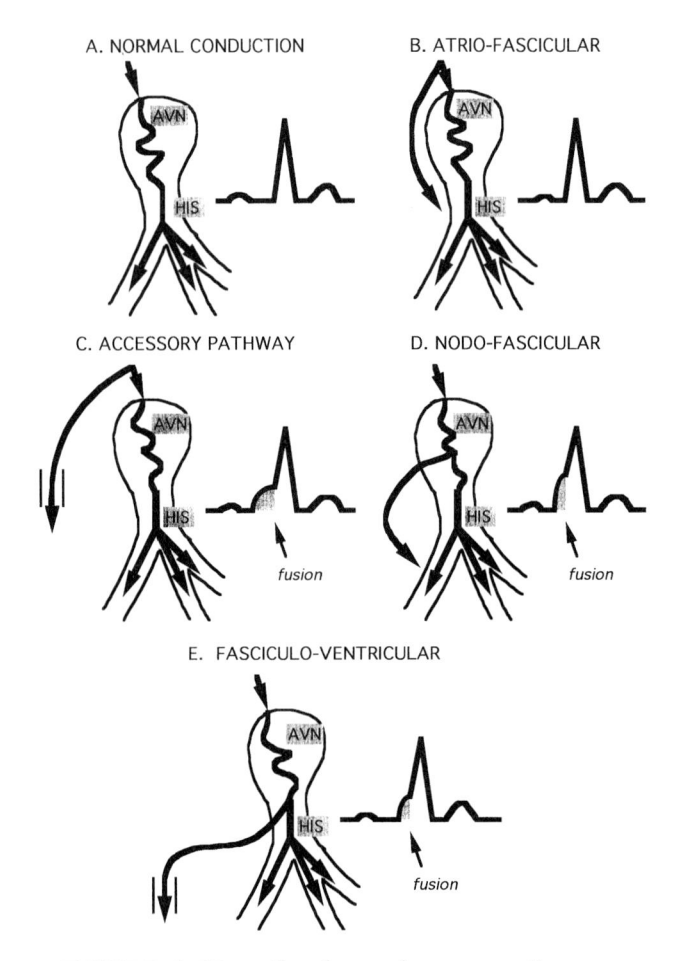

136 ELECTROCARDIOGRAPHIC DIAGNOSIS OF CARDIAC ARRHYTHMIAS

FIGURE 4–18 *See legend on opposite page*

sometimes bizarre, QRS complex compared to that with normal beats. The clinical significance of aberrant beats is that they are easily mistaken for ventricular beats and mistreated as such. Most commonly (80 to 85 percent of instances),[5] QRS aberration occurs with a right bundle branch block (RBBB) pattern (Fig. 4–19; Table 10–5). However, in patients with significant heart disease, left bundle branch (LBBB) pattern aberration (Figs. 4–20 and 4–21; Table 10–5) may account for up to one-third of QRS aberration.[5] Causes for ventricular aberration are summarized in Table 4–6. The ECG manifestations of QRS aberration are related to nonuniform changes in parameters affecting normal ventricular conduction (see Chapter 2). The term *aberration* does not include fixed ventricular conduction defects, such as bundle branch or fascicular heart block. However, as just noted above, aberrant beats are usually conducted with the pattern of RBBB or LBBB (Table 10–5), or left anterior or posterior fascicular block (LBBB, LPFB; see Table 10–11). RBBB and LBBB pattern aberration often occur in association (Figs. 4–20 and 4–21). Causes for ventricular aberration (Table 4–6) are further discussed.

FIGURE 4–18   *PR-interval and QRS morphology with accessory or AV bypass pathways. (A) Normal conduction through the AV node, His bundle, and bundle branches with normal PR interval and QRS complex. (B) An atriofascicular pathway bypasses the slower-conducting AV node and inserts into the His bundle, producing a shortened PR interval. Because the bundle branches, Purkinje network, and ventricular myocardium are activated from the His bundle, the QRS is normal. (C) An accessory AV pathway bypasses the AV node and inserts into the ventricular free wall, causing earlier than expected activation (preexcitation) of a portion of the ventricle. This produces both a short P–R interval and ventricular fusion (gray zone), since the QRS complex results both from preexcitation and activation via normal pathways. (D) A nodofascicular pathway from the AV node to a bundle branch also causes earlier than expected activation of a portion of the ventricle and a fusion beat. Nonetheless, even though the PR interval is shortened, most ventricular activation is via normal pathways, and the fusion wave is less pronounced. (E) A fasciculoventricular pathway causes preexcitation of an even smaller portion of the ventricle, explaining the smaller fusion wave. Most ventricular activation is via the normal pathways, and the P–R interval is not shortened because the AV node is not bypassed.*

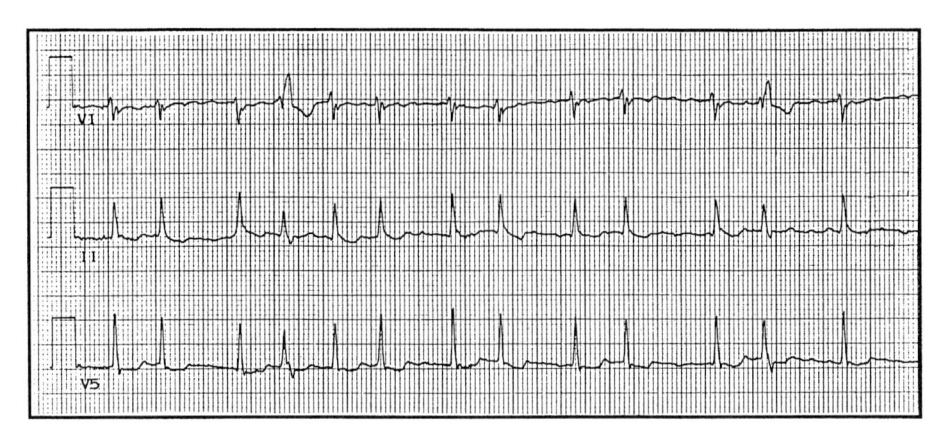

138 ELECTROCARDIOGRAPHIC DIAGNOSIS OF CARDIAC ARRHYTHMIAS

FIGURE 4–19 *RBBB pattern ventricular aberration with atrial fibrillation. Note that aberrant beats follow beats with a long preceding R–R interval (i.e., the Ashman phenomena; see text).*

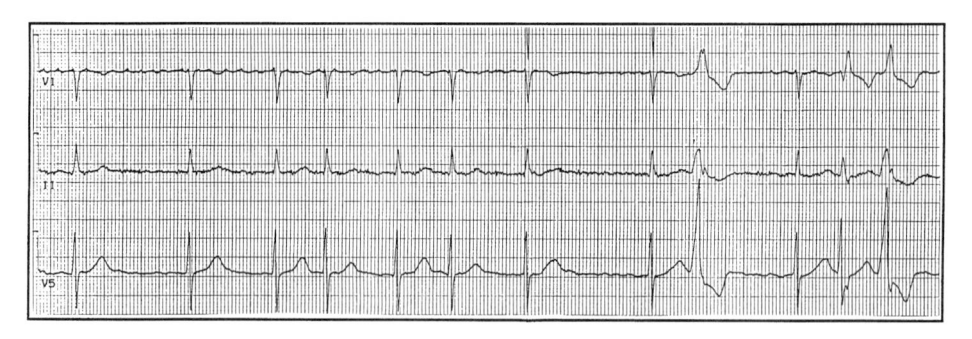

FIGURE 4–20 *Mainly LBBB pattern ventricular aberration in patient with atrial fibrillation. The second aberrant beat is more consistent with right bundle branch pattern aberration. The first and second aberrant QRS complexes are probably due to the Ashman phenomenon (text).*

Premature Beats

Conduction of premature beats can be delayed as a result of relative refractoriness of the ventricular specialized conducting system or myocardium. This is more likely with slower heart rates, since refractoriness tends to increase with slow heart rates. Also, because refractoriness is longer in the RBBB compared to LBBB, this explains why premature beats are more likely to be conducted with RBBB pattern aberration.

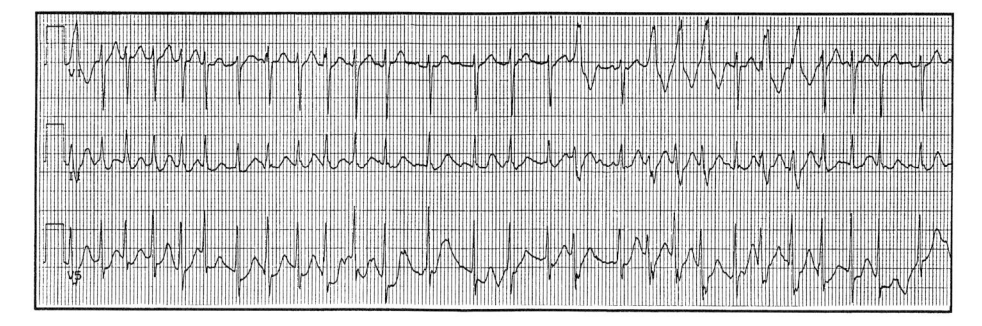

FIGURE 4–21 *Atrial fibrillation with a rapid ventricular response and beats conducted with LBBB pattern aberration, except for the final two aberrant beats.*

TABLE 4-6 *Causes for ventricular aberration*

1. Abrupt change in heart rate; prematurity
2. Change in electrophysiologic properties
3. Anomalous conduction within ventricles
4. Drugs; metabolic or electrolyte disorders

Ashman Phenomenon

Prolonged refractoriness following long cycle length beats can give rise to aberrant conduction of one or more successive beats because of the Ashman phenomenon (Figs. 4–17 and 4–19). The Ashman phenomenon is common with atrial fibrillation, and QRS aberration due to this phenomenon almost always has a RBBB pattern.

Acceleration-Dependent Aberration

Acceleration-dependent aberration results from impaired ventricular conduction at critical heart rates. In contrast to the Ashman phenomenon, it is not dependent on the cycle length of the preceding beat, and usually has a LBBB pattern. Acceleration-dependent aberration is almost always due to underlying (organic) heart disease.

Deceleration-Dependent Aberration

Deceleration-dependent aberration differs from the acceleration-dependent form in that slowing of heart rate (longer cycle lengths) is associated with QRS aberration, while increased rate (shorter cycle lengths) normalizes the QRS complex. Deceleration-dependent aberration also occurs with a predominantly LBBB pattern, and in patients with significant underlying heart disease.

Diffuse Myocardial Depression

Finally, diffuse myocardial depression from drugs, electrolyte disorders, hypoxia, ischemia or metabolic disturbances may produce ventricular aberration. This type of aberration is distinguished from bundle branch or fascicular block pattern aberration in that there is distortion of both the initial and terminal portions of the QRS complex. Additionally, QRS aberration due to this cause is often rate dependent.

INTERFERENCE AND ATRIOVENTRICULAR DISSOCIATION

Interference

Interference is due to refractoriness in cardiac tissue, usually the AV node. Therefore, in contrast to ventricular aberration, it is often a normal ECG phenomenon. For example, interference might be produced by nearly simultaneous discharge of two pacemakers, one in the SA node and the other in the AV junctional tissues. Physiologic refractoriness within the AV node produced by AV junctional pace-

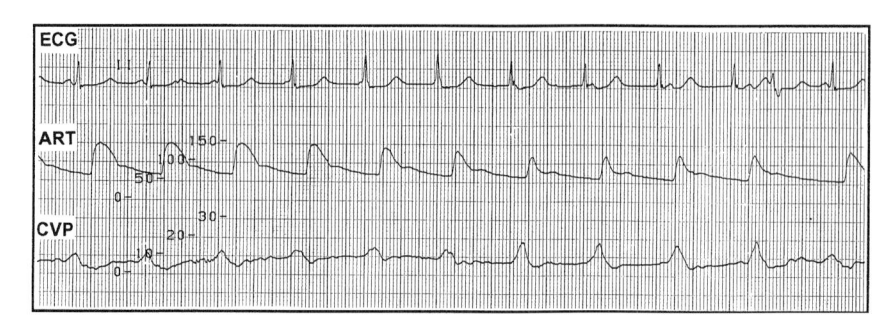

FIGURE 4–22 *Interference between SA node and AV junctional pacemakers produces AV dissociation in an anesthetized patient with heart disease. The atria are controlled by the SA node, and ventricles by an AV junctional pacemaker. Note that P waves appear to "march in and out of the QRS complex," a phenomenon (not a primary rhythm disturbance) often termed* **isorhythmic AV dissociation.** *Note the cannon A waves (CVP) and reduction in blood pressure ($\geq$ 40 mmHg decrease) when P waves occur at the end of or just after the QRS complex. The next to last beat may be a junctional premature beat with a retrograde (inverted) P wave.*

maker discharge will prevent conduction of the impulse from above, so that the AV junctional pacemaker can control the ventricles (Fig. 4–22). However, since the atria are still controlled by the SA node, the P waves remain upright and appear to "march in and out" of the QRS complex (Fig. 4–22). This *phenomenon* is often referred to as *isorhythmic AV dissociation,* since pacemakers controlling the atria and ventricles have similar rates.

Atrioventricular Dissociation

With AV dissociation, the atria and ventricles are controlled by different pacemakers, producing independent beating of the atria and ventricles. *AV dissociation is never a primary rhythm disturbance.* One cannot make a diagnosis of AV dissociation. The primary disturbance is always the rhythm (junctional or ventricular) that controls the ventricles. Alternatively, it could be AV heart block and idioventricular escape rhythm with AV dissociation. The primary causes for AV dissociation are listed in Table 4–7.

FUSION AND CAPTURE BEATS

Fusion

A fusion QRS complex results when the ventricles are simultaneously excited by impulses originating in two different pacemakers, commonly the atria and ventricles. A fusion complex during wide-QRS tachycardia confirms the diagnosis of ventricular tachycardia (Fig. 4–23). The fusion QRS complex by definition must differ from a normal (supraventricular) complex, but the amount of aberration can vary from subtle to considerable. Multiple ECG leads may be required to ascertain fusion beats.

Capture Beats

Capture beats are produced if the ventricles are occasionally activated by atrial beats in the presence of third-degree AV heart block,

TABLE 4-7 *Primary causes for AV dissociation*

Default	Slowing of the primary pacemaker permits latent pacemaker escape
Usurpation	Latent pacemaker rate increases so that it can control the rhythm
Heart block	Primary pacemaker impulse fails with escape rhythm or asystole

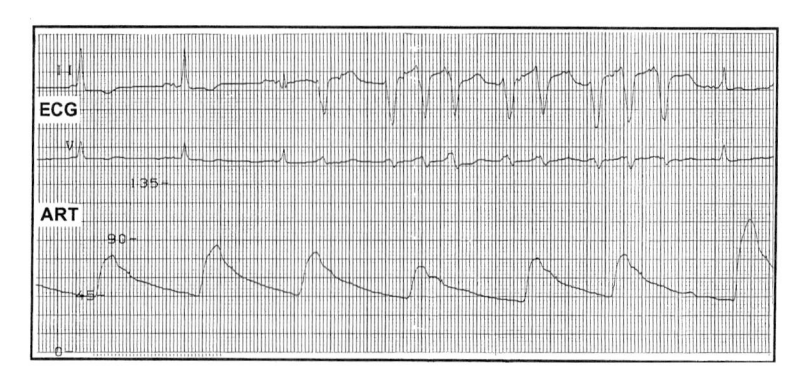

FIGURE 4–23 *Fusion beats with nonsustained ventricular tachycardia (beats 4 to 9). Ventricular conduction with the first two beats (AV junctional and SA nodal origin) is nearly normal except for a small amount of intraventricular conduction delay related to previous myocardial infarction. Beats 3 and 10 are fusion beats, with QRS aberration intermediate between that of normal beats and those during VT.*

and AV junctional or ventricular rhythms. Capture beats may produce normal QRS complexes or beats with QRS aberration. The latter also qualify as fusion beats if the ventricles are simultaneously activated by a ventricular and supraventricular focus. The presence of capture beats during wide-QRS tachycardia (Fig. 4–24) provides strong evidence for ventricular tachycardia (VT).

RETROGRADE AND CONCEALED CONDUCTION

Ventriculoatrial (Retrograde) Conduction

Ventriculoatrial (VA) (retrograde) conduction may be seen with AV junctional or ventricular rhythms (Fig. 4–25). One-to-one VA conduction during VT makes it nearly impossible to distinguish VT from ectopic atrial tachycardia with aberrant conduction or antidromic AV reciprocating tachycardia (see Chapter 10). Regardless, it is prudent to assume a ventricular origin for wide-QRS tachycardia with retrograde P waves, since VT is much more likely than the other disturbances.

Concealed Conduction

Concealed conduction occurs when an atrial or ventricular impulse penetrates specialized conduction tissue (e.g., AV node),

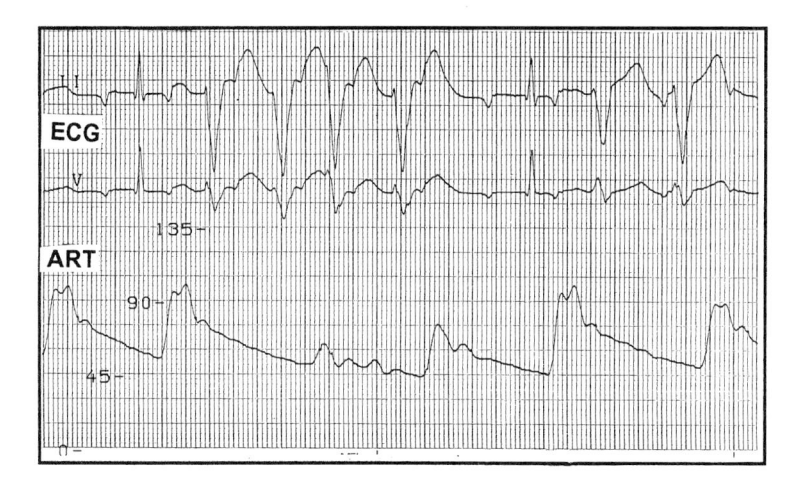

ELECTROCARDIOGRAPHIC DIAGNOSIS OF CARDIAC ARRHYTHMIAS

FIGURE 4-24 *Ventricular capture beats from an AV junctional pacemaker during consecutive runs of nonsustained VT. The basic rhythm is AV junctional escape rhythm with advanced second- or third-degree AV heart block, and an ectopic pacemaker controlling the atria.*

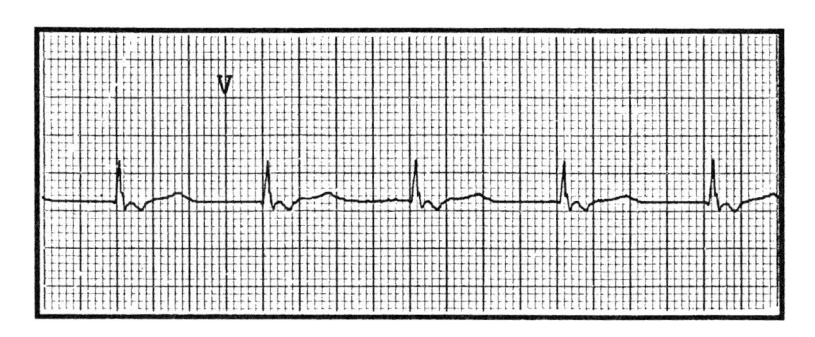

FIGURE 4-25 *Retrograde conduction. AV junctional rhythm with inverted P waves following each QRS complex. Inverted P waves are the result of VA (retrograde) conduction. Only lead V_5 was recorded.*

without emerging. Propagation of this impulse is electrically silent on the surface ECG, and therefore "concealed." However, such concealed conduction may affect transmission of ensuing impulses. For example, retrograde penetration of the AV node by a ventricular extrasystole may block conduction of the next sinus beat producing a fully compensa-

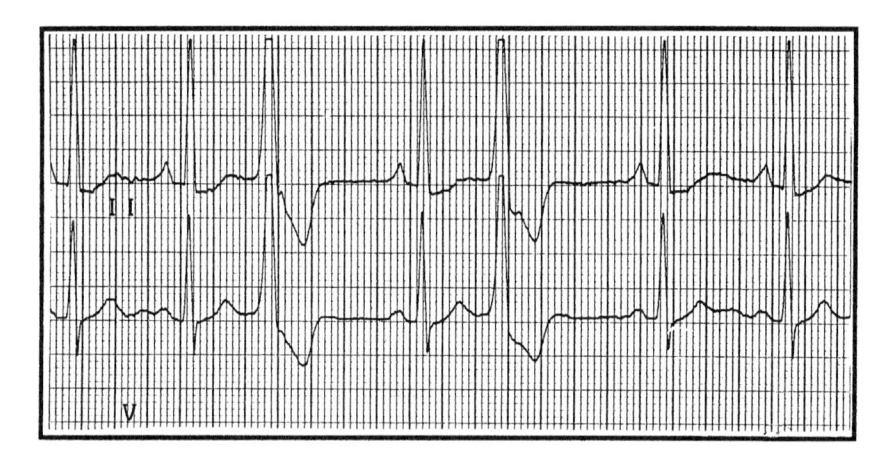

144 ELECTROCARDIOGRAPHIC DIAGNOSIS OF CARDIAC ARRHYTHMIAS

FIGURE 4-26 *Concealed conduction. Sinus rhythm with fully compensated premature ventricular extrasystoles (VES). RR intervals interrupted by VES are almost exactly twice those between successive normal sinus beats (i.e., the first and last pairs of normal beats). This is because VES conduct back to and penetrate the AV node, blocking anterograde conduction of the normal sinus beat. Since the next sinus beat occurs at the expected time and is conducted without delay, the pause between sinus beats is fully compensatory (twice the normal PP interval).*

tory pause (Fig. 4-26). However, if the extrasystole is interpolated (see Chapter 10), concealed conduction may delay AV node conduction, causing PR interval prolongation with the next sinus beat.

EXIT AND ENTRANCE BLOCK

The response of cardiac tissue to primary or secondary pacemaker discharge depends not only on pacemaker rate, but also on conductivity of tissue immediately surrounding the pacemaker. Impulses can propagate into or out of the pacemaker focus, provided surrounding tissue is not refractory. If the pacemaker is no longer refractory from previous discharge, impulses entering it can reset its rate of automaticity to cause a noncompensatory pause (see Chapter 10). However, if surrounding tissue is relatively or absolutely refractory, impulse propagation away from the pacemaker will be delayed or blocked. *Exit block* is a delay or failure of impulse propagation away from a primary or secondary pacemaker, with the result that myocardial activation does not occur at the expected time

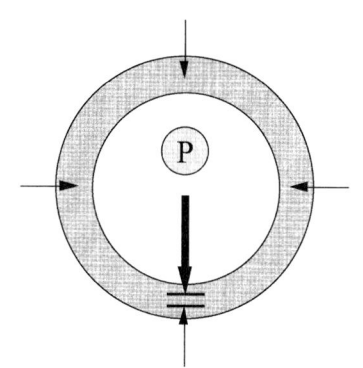

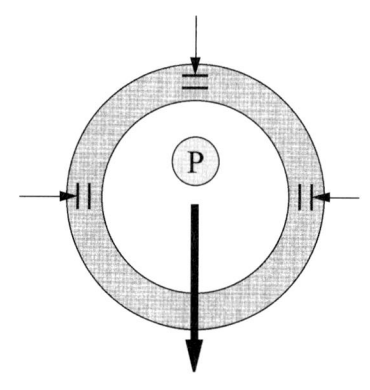

FIGURE 4-27 *Exit and entrance block.* (Top) *Exit block. Propagation of the an impulse (bold arrow) from a pacemaker (P) is prevented by refractoriness of tissue immediately surrounding the pacemaker (gray zone). Such refractoriness may be caused by impulses from adjacent myocardium (small arrows) penetrating tissues around the pacemaker, or it may be due to persistent refractoriness created by previous pacemaker discharge.* (Bottom) *Entrance block. The pacemaker is now "protected" from premature discharge by surrounding impulses (small arrows) by persistent refractoriness in its immediate vicinity caused by previous pacemaker discharge. However, subsequent impulses from the pacemaker (bold arrow) can propagate to depolarize adjacent myocardium if the surrounding tissues have recovered from refractoriness.*

(Fig. 4–27). *Entrance block* is the failure of impulses from adjacent myocardium to penetrate and discharge or reset a pacemaker (Fig. 4–27). Entrance block protects an ectopic pacemaker from premature discharge by impulse from above, so that ectopic beats or rhythms can become manifest.

PARASYSTOLE

Parasystole is a rhythm disturbance in which a single heart chamber is activated by two pacemakers, the dominant and a latent (ectopic) pacemaker. The latter is protected by entrance block (Fig. 4–27). Parasystole is characterized by a varying coupling interval between ectopic pacemaker beats and those of the dominant (usually sinus) rhythm. Also, intervals between ectopic beats are the same or near multiples of each other (Fig. 4–28), and there may be fusion beats. Presumably, parasystolic foci can exist anywhere in the heart.

ARTIFACTS

ECG artifacts often occur as a result of poor contact between electrodes and skin, or between the lead pins and ECG cable. Proper lead application is essential to reduce artifact and resulting misdiagnosis. A few extra moments to properly prepare the skin before electrode application, especially when electrode sites will be inaccessible during surgery, will save later annoyance if artifacts confuse ECG interpretation. Common causes for ECG artifact aside from poor electrode application are listed in Table 4–8, with examples provided in Figures 4–29 and 4–30.

Concerning the diagnosis of artifact, it is important to remember that artifact does not affect the underlying rhythm, although it does distort its ECG appearance. Observation of a normal pulse waveform or heart sounds may be required to rule out malignant tachyarrhythmias with large, continuous artifact produced by electromagnetic interference. ECG baseline artifact, for example, that produced by succinylcholine-induced fasciculations (Fig. 4–31), might easily be misdiagnosed as atrial fibrillation except that the RR intervals are regular or nearly so. Similarly, that produced by bumping leads might be misdiagnosed as nonsustained ectopic atrial or ventricular tachycardia (Fig. 4–32). So, inspection of the pulse waveform, listening to heart sounds, and careful examination of the ECG baseline and pattern of QRS complexes can provide important clues for correct diagnosis of "arrhythmias" due to artifact.

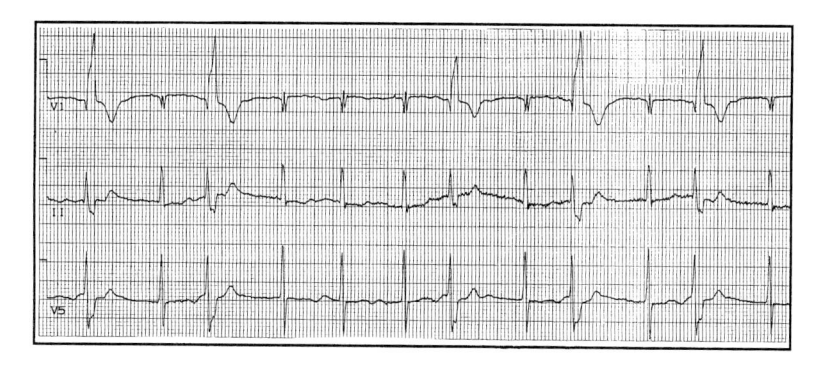

FIGURE 4-28 *Parasystole. The primary rhythm is atrial fibrillation. However, this is interrupted by wide QRS beats with RBBB pattern aberration. On close inspection, shorter RR intervals are separated by similar amounts (1,320 to 1,340 msec), and longer ones by twice this amount (2,640 msec). This behavior is consistent with discharge from a protected (i.e., parasystolic) ectopic ventricular focus.*

TABLE 4-8 *Common causes for ECG artifacts*

Patient movement	Respirations
Muscle tremors	Shivering
Fasciculations	Seizures
Electrocautery	Lead movement
Touching electrodes	Saws, drills, hammers
Infusion/roller pumps	Broken leads
Poor electrode contact	Poor standardization

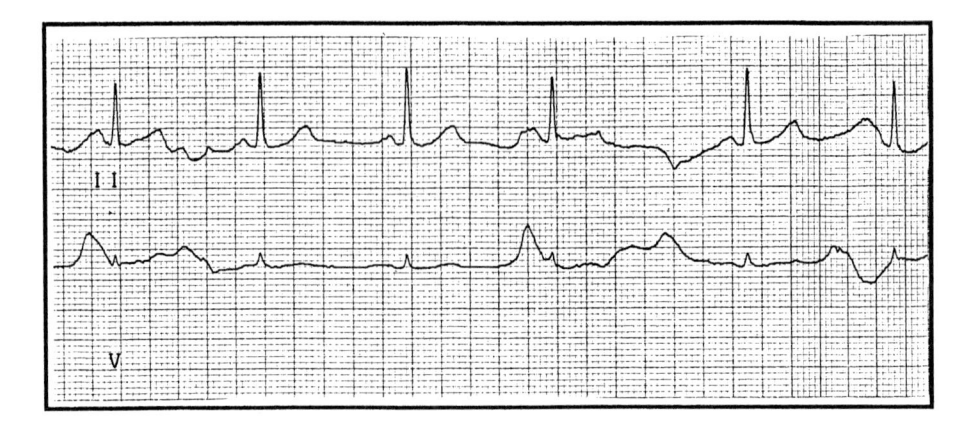

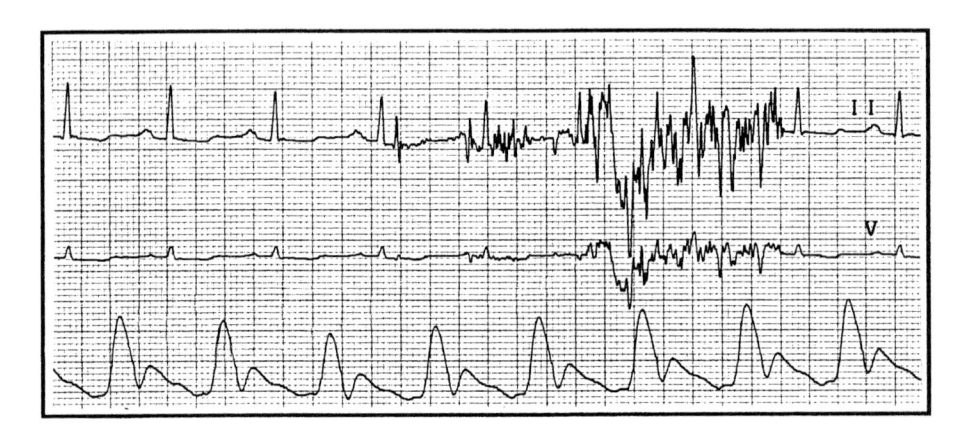

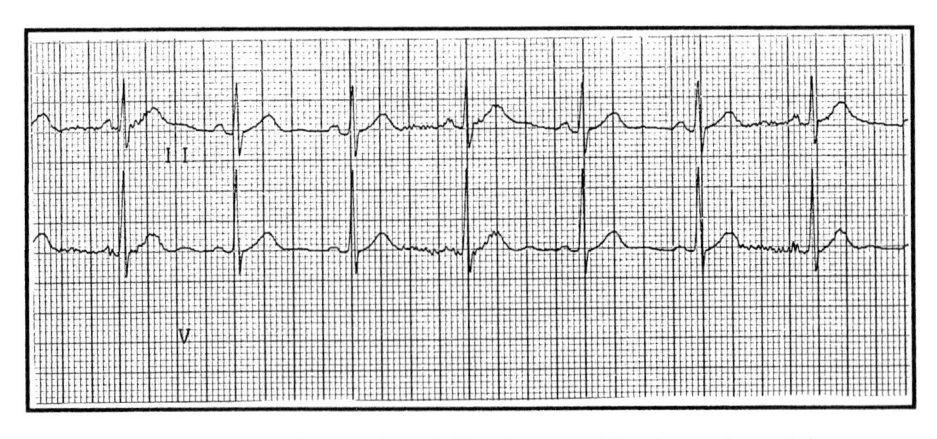

FIGURE 4-29 *Artifacts. (Top) Motion artifact produced by gagging. (Middle) Artifact with unipolar electrocautery. (Bottom) Shivering artifact.*

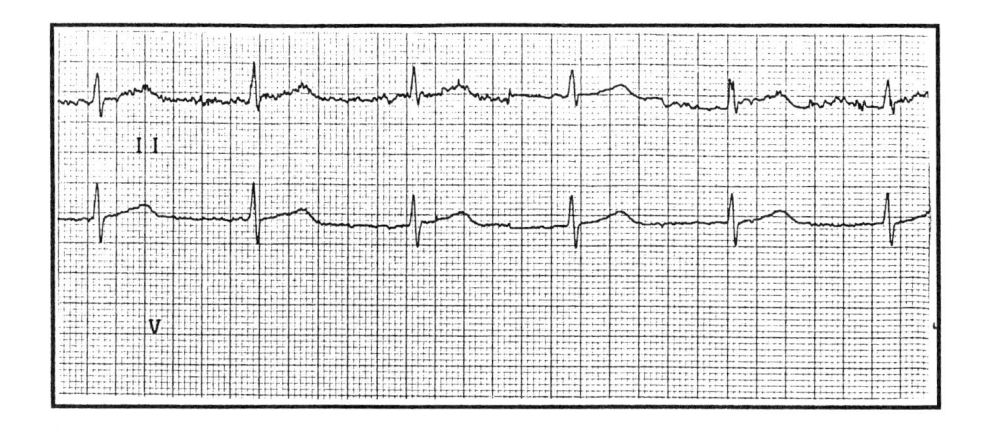

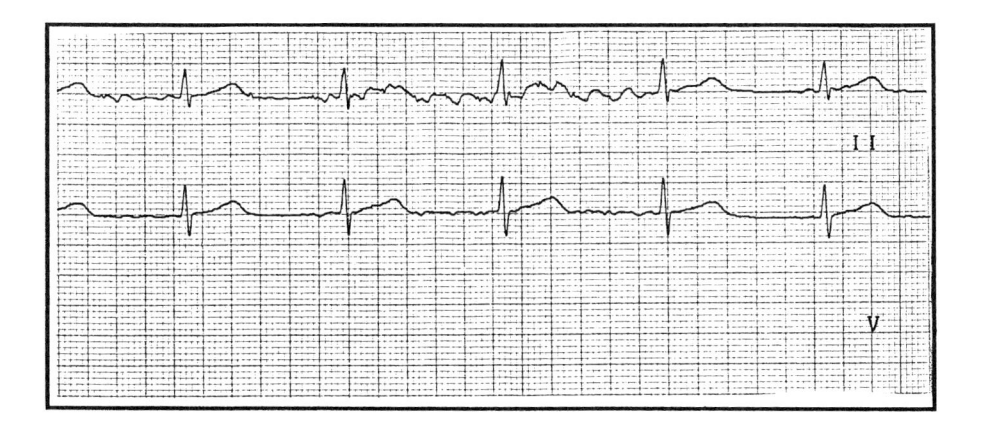

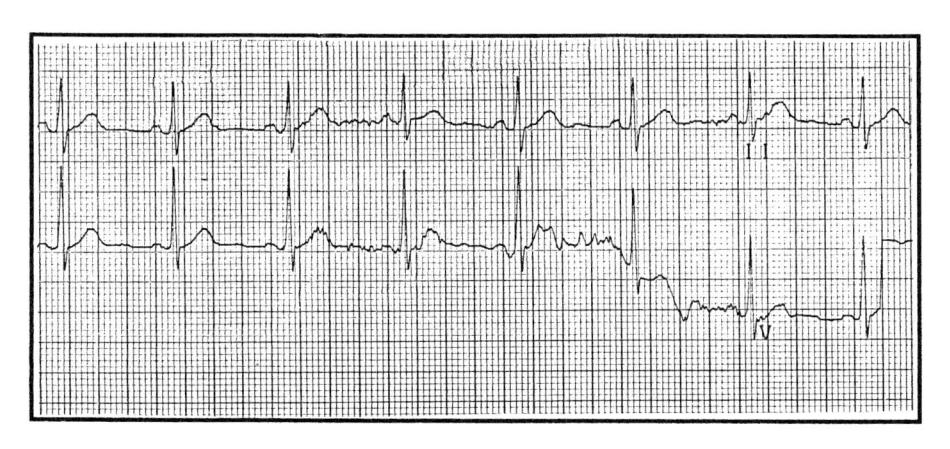

FIGURE 4-30 *Artifacts. (Top) Artifact produced by bipolar electrocautery. (Middle) Artifact produced from bone hammer. (Bottom) Artifact produced by bumping left arm electrode.*

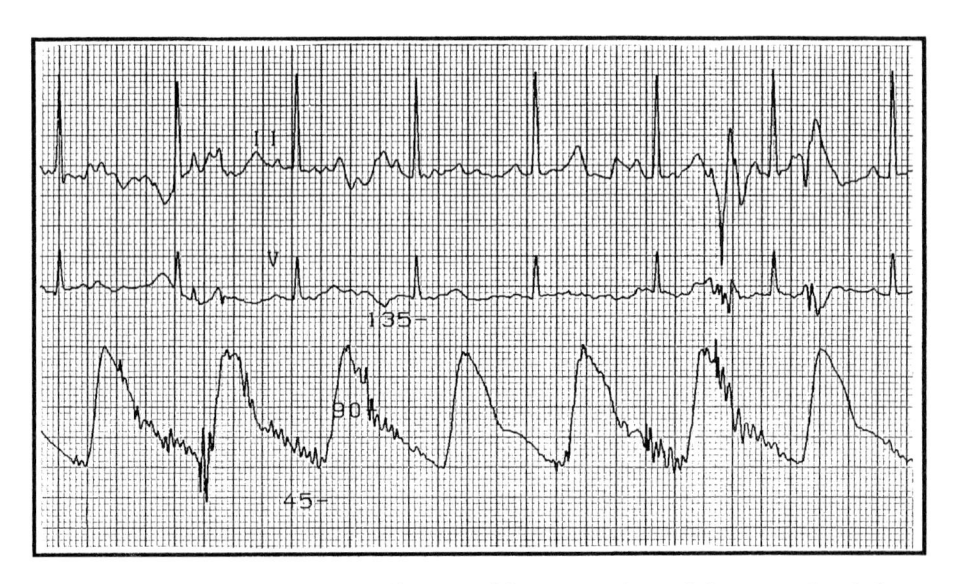

FIGURE 4–31 *ECG baseline artifact produced by succinylcholine-induced fasciculations. Artifact might be misdiagnosed as coarse atrial fibrillation with interpolated ventricular extrasystoles between the last three beats. However, note that artifact also affects the arterial pressure waveform, there are normal P waves before many QRS complexes (leads II or V_5), and the RR intervals are regular. The latter are consistent with the diagnosis of atrial fibrillation.*

ELECTROCARDIOGRAPHIC DIAGNOSIS OF CARDIAC ARRHYTHMIAS **151**

ECTOPIC VENTRICULAR RHYTHM OR ARTIFACT?

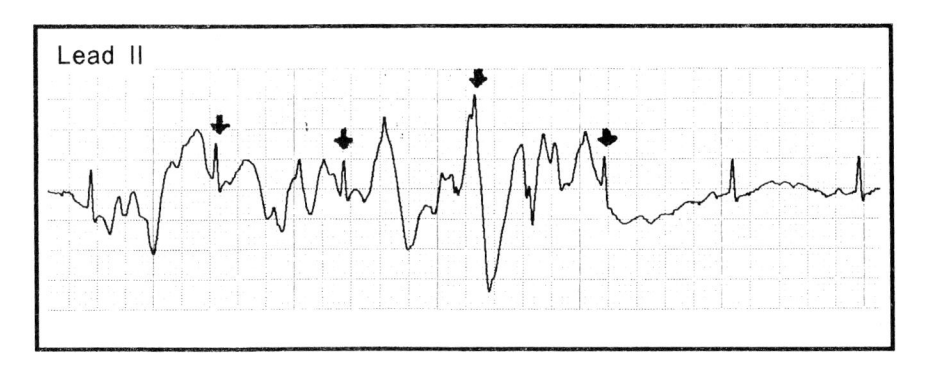

Lead II

ECTOPIC ATRIAL RHYTHM OR ARTIFACT?

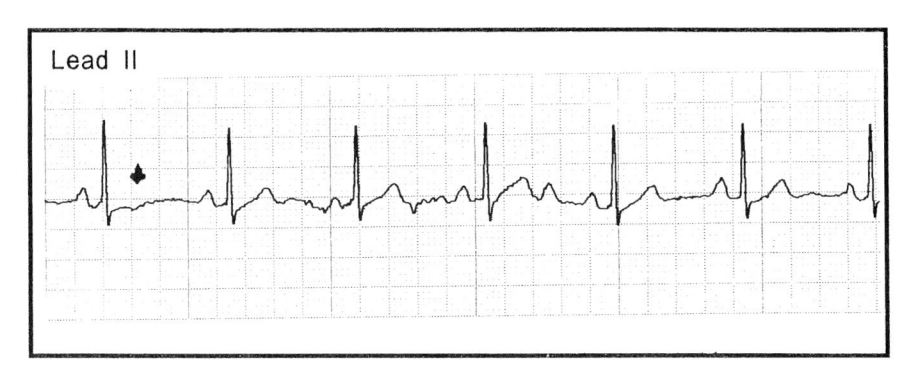

Lead II

FIGURE 4-32   *ECG artifact produced by bumping leads may simulate ectopic rhythms, especially on casual inspection of the ECG monitoring screen. (Top) Marked baseline artifact could be misdiagnosed as nonsustained polymorphic VT or ventricular fibrillation. On closer inspection, regularly recurring QRS complexes (arrows) can be recognized. (Bottom) Baseline artifact with normal P and T waves could create the initial impression of nonsustained atrial flutter, coarse atrial fibrillation, or ectopic atrial tachycardia with 2:1 AV heart block. The T wave with the first beat (arrow) is probably also distorted by artifact.*

References

1. Atlee J. Perioperative Cardiac Dysrhythmias. 2nd ed. Chicago: Year Book Medical Publishers, 1990.
2. Fisch C. Electrocardiography and vectorcardiography. In Braunwald E (ed): Heart Disease. 4th ed. Philadelphia: WB Saunders, 1992: pp. 116–161.
3. Kaplan J, Thys D. Electrocardiography. In Miller R (ed): Anesthesia. 3rd ed. New York: Churchill Livingstone, 1990: pp. 1101–1127.
4. London M, Kaplan J. Advances in electrocardiographic monitoring. In Kaplan J (ed): Cardiac Anesthesia. 3rd ed. Philadelphia: WB Saunders, 1993: pp. 299–341.
5. Wagner G. Practical Electrocardiography. 9th ed. Baltimore: Williams & Wilkins, 1994.
6. Goldman M. Principles of Clinical Electrocardiography. 12th ed. Los Altos, CA: Lange Medical Publications, 1986.
7. Underwood D. Clinical Electrocardiography. Philadelphia: WB Saunders, 1993.
8. London M, Hollenberg M, Wong M, et al. Intraoperative myocardial ischemia: localization by continuous 12-lead electrocardiography. Anesthesiology 1988;69:232–241.
9. Pahlm O, Haisty W, Edenbrandt L, et al. Evaluation of changes in standard electrocardiographic QRS waveforms recorded from activity-compatible proximal limb lead positions. Am J Cardiol 1992;69:253–257.
10. A Report for Healthcare Professionals by a Task Force of the Council on Clinical Cardiology A. Instrumentation and practice standards for electrocardiographic monitoring in special care units. Circulation 1989;79:464–471.
11. Randall WC, Rinkema LE, Jones SB, et al. Functional characterization of atrial pacemaker activity. Am J Physiol 1982;242(1):H98–106.
12. Polic S, Atlee J, Laszlo A, et al. Anesthetics and automaticity in latent pacemaker fibers. II. Effects of halothane and epinephrine or norepinephrine on automaticity of dominant and subsidiary atrial pacemakers in the canine heart. Anesthesiology 1991;75:298–304.
13. Boban M, Atlee J, Vicenzi M, et al. Anesthetics and automaticity in latent pacemaker fibers. IV. Effects of isoflurane and epinephrine or norepinephrine on automaticity of dominant and subsidiary atrial pacemakers. Anesthesiology 1993;79:555–562.
14. Woehlck H, Vicenzi M, Bosnjak Z, Atlee J. Anesthetics and automaticity of dominant and latent pacemakers in chronically instrumented dogs. I. Methodology, conscious state and effects of halothane during exposure to epinephrine with and without muscarinic blockade. Anesthesiology 1993;79:1304–1315.

15. Vicenzi M, Woehlck H, Bosnjak Z, Atlee J. Anesthetics and automaticity of dominant and latent pacemakers in chronically instrumented dogs. II. Effects of enflurane and isoflurane during exposure to epinephrine with and without muscarinic blockade. Anesthesiology 1993;79:1316–1323.

5

Drug Treatment for Arrhythmias

Abbreviations Used in Chapter Five

APD	Action potential duration
AV	Atrioventricular
BB/CCB	Beta-/calcium-channel blocker
CNS	Central nervous system
ECG	Electrocardiogram
ERP	Effective refractory period
SA	Sinoatrial
SVT	Supraventricular tachycardia
VT-VF	Ventricular tachycardia–fibrillation
WPW	Wolff–Parkinson–White (syndrome)

Most available monographs on drug treatment for arrhythmias emphasize oral drugs. For obvious reasons, oral therapy is often not practical or feasible in perioperative or critical care settings. Therefore, discussion in this chapter emphasizes drugs available for parenteral use. However, enough surgical or critically ill patients receive concurrent oral antiarrhythmic therapy, so that oral drugs are also discussed.

Antiarrhythmic drugs are not a panacea.[1] Most antiarrhythmic drugs have a narrow therapeutic window, that is, there is a small margin between doses that are effective in controlling arrhythmias or preventing sudden death, and those that aggravate or worsen arrhythmias (proarrhythmia), produce bradyarrhythmias or atrioventricular (AV) heart block, cause cardiovascular depression and heart failure, or are associated with troublesome noncardiac side effects. Since arrhythmias in anesthesia and critical care settings are more often than not transient occurrences, precipitated by a potentially correctable physiologic or metabolic imbalance, and antiarrhythmic drugs may compound such an imbalance, it behooves the clinician to first identify, correct, or remove obvious imbalance before attempting more definitive drug treatment. Additionally, such remedial intervention usually improves success with subsequent drug treatment.

Antiarrhythmic Drug Action

Antiarrhythmic drug action depends on *direct* and *indirect* effects. The former are those that affect normal and abnormal cardiac electrophysiologic properties (see Chapter 2). Direct effects are mediated at the cellular level by block of one or more ion channels responsible for generation of the cardiac action potential. Indirect effects, in contrast, are mediated more at the tissue level by autonomic receptors.

DIRECT ANTIARRHYTHMIC ACTION

Specific antiarrhythmic drugs affect primarily the sodium, potassium, or calcium (ionic) currents involved in depolarization and repolarization phase of cardiac action potentials (see Fig. 2–3). Recall from Chapter 2 that defective or deficient ion currents caused by myocardial disease or physiologic imbalance are the basis for altered normal or abnormal forms of automaticity, reentry of excitation, and triggered arrhythmias. By affecting ionic currents responsible for these electrophysiologic phenomena, antiarrhythmic drugs may oppose one or more of the cellular mechanism(s) responsible for arrhythmias. Some examples of direct antiarrhythmic action are listed in Table 5–1. These

TABLE 5-1 *Examples of how antiarrhythmic drugs act directly to oppose arrhythmias*

ARRHYTHMIA	MECHANISM	DIRECT EFFECT
Sinus bradycardia	Altered normal automaticity	Increase rate of automaticity
Junctional rhythm	Abnormal automaticity	Alter pacemaker current
Paroxysmal SVT	AV node reentry	Increase AV node refractoriness
Reciprocating SVT	AP reentry	Increase AP refractoriness
Digitalis VT	Triggered activity	Decrease cellular calcium overload
VT after MI	Ventricular reentry	Reduce RP disparity; ↑ RP

MI, myocardial infarction; RP, refractory period; AP, accessory pathway.

involve altering the magnitude of normal pacemaker currents, resisting abnormal pacemaker currents, reducing intracellular calcium overload (delayed afterdepolarizations), affecting calcium plateau and potassium repolarization currents (early afterdepolarization), or producing changes in conduction and refractoriness that are nonconducive to reentry.

Antiarrhythmic Drugs and Reentry

How drugs affect reentry requires further elaboration. They can terminate, prevent, or promote reentry by effects on conduction and refractoriness.[2] Recall from Chapter 2 that reentry requires critical changes in conduction and refractoriness so that the circulating impulse can return to excite nonrefractory tissue before the arrival of the next normal impulse from above. Drugs that improve conduction or decrease refractoriness may eliminate an area of unidirectional conduction block. Or, they may cause the circulating impulse to return while fibers are still refractory. Drugs that delay conduction, on the other hand, may terminate or prevent reentry by converting an area of unidirectional conduction block to bidirectional conduction block. Conversely, a drug that slows conduction without causing conduction block may facilitate reentry. Finally, most antiarrhythmic drugs share the ability to prolong refractoriness relative to their effects on action potential duration, so that the ratio of the effective refractory period to action potential duration (ERP/APD) exceeds 1.0. This is an important measure of drug action against reentry arrhythmias, since if a drug produces sufficient prolongation of refractoriness, the reentry pathway may not regain excitability in time to be depolarized by the returning impulse.

INDIRECT ANTIARRHYTHMIC ACTION

Most indirect antiarrhythmic effects are ultimately mediated by stimulation or block of autonomic neuraxis or specific end-organ receptor types. Indirect effects are very important to antiarrhythmic drug action in perioperative settings, since autonomic imbalance is often a major cause or at least contributes to the genesis of arrhythmias. How drugs or interventions might oppose some arrhythmias by indirect actions is summarized in Table 5–2.

DRUG CLASSIFICATION

Vaughan Williams Classification

Given that at least 20 drugs are currently approved as antiarrhythmics, it is useful to have a classification that groups drugs with similar actions. Vaughan Williams proposed a classification that grouped drugs by cellular electrophysiologic actions (Table 5–3).[3] Harrison further subdivided class I drugs—sodium-channel blockers—into class 1A, 1B, or 1C based on their effects on ventricular conduction and APD (Table 5–4).[4] These effects are the result of differences in interaction of class 1 drugs with the sodium channel.[5] Class 1A antiarrhythmic drugs interact very slowly, having a binding constant on the order of 1 to 3 seconds, and a dissociation constant of 1 to 10 seconds. Because of this, block accumulates more at fast compared to slow heart rates, termed *use dependence*. Class 1B drugs interact very rapidly with the sodium channel, with binding constants of 0.1 to 1.0 seconds and dissociation constants of 0.1 to 0.8 seconds,

TABLE 5-2 *How drugs or interventions indirectly oppose arrhythmias*

ARRHYTHMIA	DRUG OR INTERVENTION	INDIRECT EFFECT
Sinus bradycardia	Atropine; local anesthetic	Block receptor or reflex arc
Junctional rhythm	Nitroglycerin; beta-blockers	Reduce myocardial ischemia
Paroxysmal SVT	Valsalva; carotid massage	↑ AV node refractoriness (vagus)
Sinus tachycardia	Opiates; anesthesia	Reduce pain or awareness
Ventricular ectopy	Vasodilators; beta-blockers	↓ wall stress and SE ischemia
VT with long QT	Beta-blockers; pacing	Shorten QT; ↓ RP disparity

SE, subendocardial ischemia; RP, refractory period.

TABLE 5-3 *Classification of antiarrhythmic drugs by electrophysiologic (EP) and other actions*

CLASS	DISSOCIATION*	CELLULAR EP ACTION	EFFECT ON ECG
1A. Quinidine group	Intermediate	↑APD, ERP; ↑ERP/APD	↑QTc; (±) ↑ QRS
1B. Lidocaine group	Fast	↓APD, ERP; ↑ERP/APD	Small ↓ QTc
1C. Flecainide group	Slow	↑ERP; ↑ERP/APD	↑PR; ↑QRS; ↑QT
1A&B. Moricizine†	Fast–intermediate	↓APD, ERP	↑PR; ↑QRS
2. Beta-blockers		↓APD, ERP; ↓ phase 4‡	↓ SA node rate; (±) ↑PR
3. Prolong repolarization		↑APD, ERP	↑QT
4. Calcium-channel blockers		↑ERP (AV node); ↓ phase 4‡	↓ SA node rate; (± ↑PR

*Speed of dissociation from sodium channels. †Moricizine has 1A and 1B actions. ‡Phase 4 automaticity.

TABLE 5-4 *The Harrison subdivision of class 1 drugs according to effect on EP properties*

SUBDIVISION	APD	CONDUCTION	INDIVIDUAL DRUGS
Class 1A	Prolong	Moderate ↓	Quinidine, *procainamide*, disopyramide
Class 1B	↓ or no effect	Little ↓	*Lidocaine, phenytoin*, mexiletine, tocainide, moricizine*
Class 1C	No effect	Marked ↓	Flecainide, encainide, lorcainide, propafenone

*Moricizine has both 1A and 1B activity (see Table 5-3). Italicized drugs are available for IV use.

and there is little use dependence except at very fast heart rates or in association with other drugs that affect the sodium channel. As a result, 1B drugs move on and off the sodium channel rapidly in *normal* heart. However, because 1B drugs bind preferentially to inactivated sodium channels, they are expected to exert greater effects in partially depolarized fibers (e.g., by ischemia).[5,6] Finally, class 1C antiarrhythmics interact very slowly with the sodium channel, with binding constants of 1 to 8 sec and dissociation constants exceeding 10 sec. Therefore, class 1C drugs are expected to affect resting sodium channels to a greater extent than the other two class 1 subclasses. This would result in slow accumulation and relief of block, both in normal and depressed fibers. Recall from Chapter 3 that the long-acting local anesthetics bupivacaine and etidocaine have kinetics of interaction with the cardiac sodium channels similar to those of class 1C antiarrhythmics.

Classification Limitations

Josephson[6] and others[2,7] point out deficiencies of the Vaughan Williams–Harrison classification (Tables 5–3 and 5–4). *First,* the classification is based on electrophysiologic actions of arbitrary drug concentrations on normal fibers of one animal species. Further, this may be only one type of fiber—Purkinje fibers. Aside from possible species differences, antiarrhythmic drugs commonly affect more than one cardiac tissue type (Fig. 5–1). *Second,* the classification does not

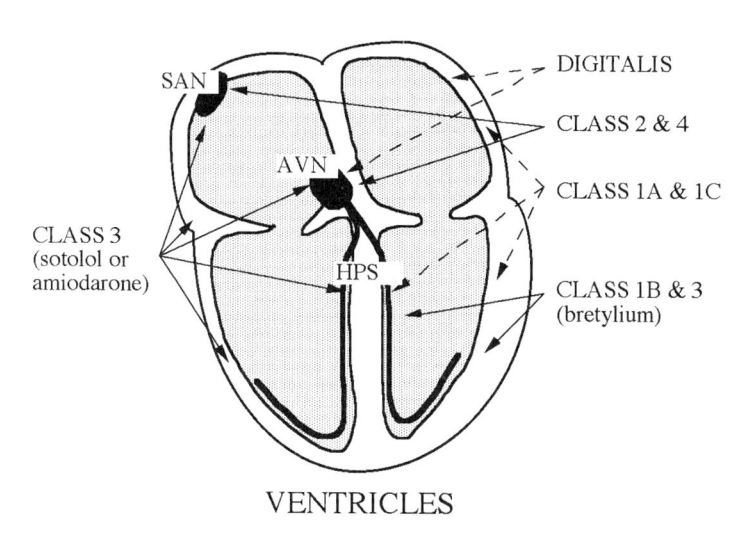

FIGURE 5–1 *Major cardiac sites of action for digitalis and antiarrhythmic drugs based on the Vaughan Williams classification. These are the atria, ventricles, sinoatrial node (SAN), atrioventricular node (AVN), and His–Purkinje system (HPS).*

TABLE 5-5 *Complex actions of representative antiarrhythmic drugs that contribute to antiarrhythmic or cardiovascular effects*

DRUG	CLASS	OTHER ACTIONS
Amiodarone	3	Sodium- and calcium-channel blockade; beta-adrenergic blockade
Beta-blockers	2	Sodium-channel blockade with high concentrations of some drugs
Procainamide	1A	Vagolytic; active metabolite (NAPA) with class 3 activity
Sotolol	3	Beta-adrenergic blockade; partial beta-1 agonist
Quinidine	1A	Vagolytic; alpha-adrenergic blockade

consider actions on abnormal fibers, especially depressed ones. Thus, it may provide misleading information concerning effectiveness against clinical arrhythmias due to structural heart disease. *Third,* many antiarrhythmic drugs have complex actions. They may block more than one ion channel, as well as have indirect effects, active metabolites, or hemodynamic actions that affect antiarrhythmic activity (Table 5-5). *Fourth,* some drugs exert greater effects at faster rates of stimulation or following prolonged stimulation (i.e., use dependence). Use dependence may lead one to entirely different conclusions about a particular drug's actions compared to those predicted based on observations in slowly beating myocardial fibers. *Fifth,* physiologic imbalance (electrolyte, drugs, metabolic, temperature, pH, autonomic, etc.) may greatly alter the actions of antiarrhythmic drugs. *Sixth,* little attention has been paid to the effect of antiarrhythmic drugs on passive membrane properties (e.g., gap junctional conductance, anisotropic tissue, etc.—see Chapter 2), which effects can differ substantially among drugs of the same class or subclass. Despite these limitations, the Vaughan Williams–Harrison classification is still the most widely used classification system for antiarrhythmic drugs, and will be commonly referred to throughout this book.

Pharmacokinetics

For an antiarrhythmic drug to produce its desired effect, it must be present in an appropriate concentration at its site of action. The term

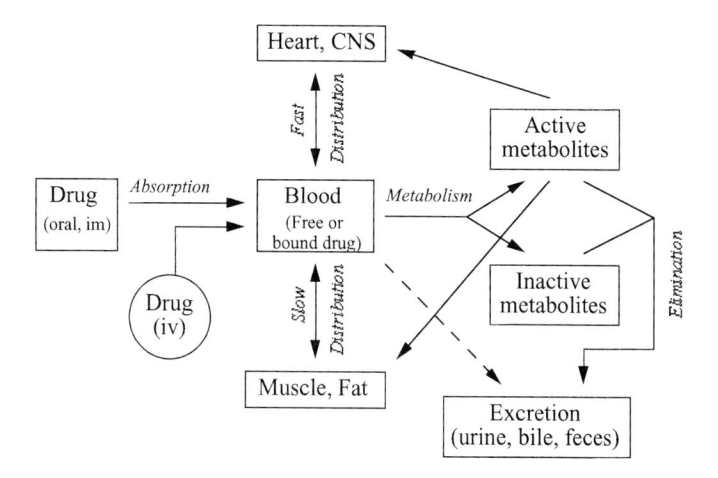

FIGURE 5-2 *Drug disposition in the body (pharmacokinetics), including the processes of absorption, distribution, metabolism, and elimination. See text for further discussion.*

pharmacokinetics describes drug disposition in the body over time, and includes the processes of absorption, distribution, metabolism, and excretion (Fig. 5-2).[2,7,8]

ABSORPTION

Absorption of oral antiarrhythmic drugs is affected by the preparation (vehicle, regular versus extended release), physicochemical properties of the drug and cell membrane, and gastric pH and emptying time (affected by many anesthetic and adjunct drugs). *Bioavailability* describes the amount of oral or intramuscular (IM) drug that reaches the systemic circulation compared to that following intravenous (IV) administration. After IV administration, bioavailability is 100 percent. Following oral or IM administration, it reflects the amount of drug absorbed as well as that removed by presystemic *(first-pass)* elimination or metabolism in the gut wall or liver. Drugs with significant first-pass metabolism may require much higher oral compared to IV dosing (e.g., verapamil, propranolol), or they may be unsuitable for oral use (e.g., lidocaine).

Disease and other factors affect the rate and completeness of absorption. Low cardiac output or shock states, by decreasing intestinal perfusion or causing mucosal edema, may impair drug absorption. Diarrhea, malabsorption syndromes, or drugs that alter gastrointestinal motility also affect absorption. Injection of drug into poorly perfused fat as opposed to better-perfused muscle may also cause incomplete absorption. Since most antiarrhythmic drugs are basic compounds, they are mostly ionized and poorly absorbed at normal gastric pH. Some may even decompose at this pH. Use of histamine (H_2) blockers or antacids that increase gastric pH may increase absorption and bioavailability of some antiarrhythmics (e.g., diltiazem following ranitidine or cimetidine),[9] which has relevance to the usual practice of continuing cardiac medications on the morning of surgery and routine use of antacids and H_2 blockers prior to anesthesia.

DISTRIBUTION

Two-Compartment Pharmacokinetic Model

Once a drug has entered the systemic circulation, its plasma concentration first declines rapidly, then slowly, because of tissue distribution and elimination, respectively. The distribution and elimination of most antiarrhythmic drugs follows a two-compartment pharmacokinetic model (Fig. 5–3). Following drug administration in this model, the curve of decline in plasma drug concentration has two phases: (1) The early *(alpha)* distribution phase is characterized by rapidly declining plasma concentrations. This early decline is caused by distribution of drug throughout the blood volume and to well-perfused tissues such as heart, brain, lung, gut, liver, and kidneys (i.e., the central compartment). (2) A second, slower decline in plasma concentration results mainly from drug elimination (see following), but also in part to redistribution of drug to less well-perfused peripheral tissues such as muscle, fat, skin, and bone (i.e., the peripheral compartment). The characteristic effects of a particular drug can result from accumulation in either or both compartments.

Bound and Unbound (Free) Drug

Drugs exist in plasma in both the free and protein- (mostly albumin) bound forms. In general, it is the free (unbound) drug in plasma that interacts at the site of action to produce desired or untoward effects. Commercial assays, however, routinely measure the total plasma concentration of drug, which includes both the free and bound (inactive) portions. However, while the fraction of bound drug varies greatly among antiarrhythmic drugs, it is fairly constant for individual drugs at clinically relevant plasma concentrations. How-

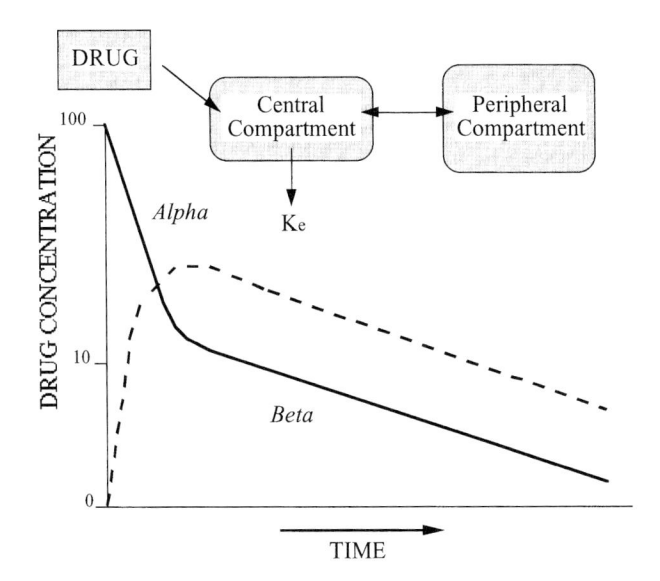

FIGURE 5-3 *Two-compartment pharmacokinetic model for drug distribution (Alpha) and elimination (Beta) phases from the central compartment (blood and well-perfused tissue). There is a dynamic equilibrium between the smaller central and larger peripheral (less perfused) tissue compartments, with elimination from the former described by the elimination rate constant (K_e). The semilogarithmic plot depicts drug concentrations in the central (bold line) and peripheral compartments (dashed line) over time. See text for further discussion.*

ever, phenytoin, lidocaine, propafenone, and disopyramide saturate tissue-binding sites at high therapeutic plasma concentrations, so that assays for free drug may be required to monitor therapy and avoid systemic toxicity. With drugs that saturate tissue-binding sites, doubling measured plasma concentrations may reflect a more than doubling of free drug. Finally, bound and free portions of drug may change without affecting total plasma concentration. For example, the protein binding of phenytoin decreases in renal failure, producing more free drug and potential toxicity.

Volume of Distribution

The *volume of distribution* of a drug is the apparent or theoretical volume into which it is distributed. It does not correlate with the volume of the central or peripheral compartments, and may exceed the total-body volume if there is extensive tissue binding. Under steady-state conditions provided by a constant drug infusion, the volume of distribution is the total amount of administered drug divided by the plasma concentration.

METABOLISM AND EXCRETION

Active Metabolites

Most antiarrhythmic drugs are metabolized to some extent in the body, usually in the liver. In many instances, physiologically active metabolites are produced (e.g., N-acetyl procainamide, NAPA) that may have similar electrophysiologic actions to the parent drug.

Kinetics of Elimination

With therapeutic plasma concentrations of most antiarrhythmic drugs (except phenytoin and propafenone), a constant *proportion* of drug is eliminated per unit time, the definition of a *first-order* or exponential elimination process. This can be so because plasma concentrations of drug do not approach those required to saturate the elimination process. If, however, the elimination process becomes saturated, only a constant *amount* of drug present can be eliminated per unit time, a *zero-order* elimination process. The elimination of phenytoin and propafenone are zero-order processes.

Time Course of Elimination

The time course of elimination is described by the elimination half-life, which is the time required for the plasma concentration of a drug to fall by one-half of its maximal value following IV bolus administration. Alternatively, this could also be after stopping a constant IV infusion or following absorption of an oral or IM dose. After one half-life, the plasma concentration is 50 percent of its initial value; after two half-lives 75 percent; and after four half-lives over 90 percent.

Time Course of Accumulation

The process of drug accumulation mirrors that of elimination. Therefore, plasma concentrations of drug rise to near steady-state levels after four or five half-lives. This should be kept in mind when increasing drug dosage to avoid drug toxicity. One should wait until four or more half-lives have passed or adjust the added dose downward depending on the number of half-lives since drug administration.

Altered Elimination

Elimination half-life is directly proportional to the volume of distribution and inversely proportional to clearance. Therefore, conditions that lower both the volume of distribution and clearance do not change the half-lives of drugs eliminated mainly by the liver (e.g., lidocaine with congestive heart failure). Conditions that reduce only clearance are expected to prolong the half-life (e.g., lidocaine with impaired hepatic perfusion; quinidine or procainamide with impaired renal perfusion).

Intravenous Drug Infusions

Drugs with a short half-life are convenient for IV infusion, but not long-term oral administration because of the requirement for frequent dosing. During an IV infusion, steady-state plasma concentration is directly proportional to dosage or infusion rate and inversely proportional to clearance. Doubling the infusion rate, or halving clearance, doubles the plasma concentration, but does not affect the time to reach steady state. To quickly achieve a therapeutic plasma concentration of drug may require one or two bolus (loading) doses followed by a continuous infusion. The volume of distribution alone determines the plasma concentration of drug following a single IV bolus dose.

Proarrhythmia

DEFINITION

While antiarrhythmic drugs are expected to terminate or suppress arrhythmias, on occasion they may exacerbate or worsen arrhythmias, an event termed *proarrhythmia*.[1,2,8] However, before calling an untoward drug result "proarrhythmia," one must determine whether the result was due to drug failure or spontaneous variability of the arrhythmia.[7] This requires some knowledge of the natural history of the progression of cardiac disease and arrhythmias in a given patient. Usually, the term *proarrhythmia* implies ventricular tachyarrhythmias (tachycardia or fibrillation), but it could also be applied to supraventricular tachyarrhythmias. New bradyarrhythmias can also occur, especially with toxic plasma concentrations of antiarrhythmic drugs.

CARDIAC ARRHYTHMIA SUPPRESSION TRIAL

It has long been known that nonsustained ventricular arrhythmias following acute myocardial infarction increase the risk of sudden cardiac death. Therefore, it was reasonable for the Cardiac Arrhythmia Suppression Trial (CAST) investigators to attempt chronic suppression of nonsustained ventricular arrhythmias with drugs, with the expectation of reducing the incidence of sudden cardiac death.[10,11] The CAST investigators found that patients with asymptomatic ventricular arrhythmias following acute myocardial infarction had a two- to three-fold higher incidence of late (1 to 2 years after infarction) sudden death when treated with encainide or flecainide compared to placebo.[10] This occurred despite suppression of ambient ventricular extrasystoles and nonsustained tachycardia by encainide or flecainide. Treatment with moricizine was also associated with increased late mortality due to arrhythmias.[11] While the CAST results do not directly apply to treatment of arrhythmias in anesthesia and critical care settings, the following caveats are proffered: (1) Do not presume that asymptomatic or nondisadvantageous, worrisome ventricular extrasystoles (e.g., frequent, complex, R-on-T, etc.) predispose to malignant ventricular tachyarrhythmias. (2) Intolerance of arrhythmias rather than appearance provides sufficient justification for prompt drug treatment. (3) Treatment of lesser arrhythmias with drugs does not necessarily afford protection against more ominous arrhythmias, and may produce other adverse circulatory effects. (4) Antiarrhythmic drugs may on occasion paradoxically precipitate malignant ventricular tachyarrhythmias. For these reasons, anesthesia and critical care practitioners are advised against overly aggressive therapy with antiarrhythmic drugs. However, it must also be noted that proarrhythmia is at present an undefined problem in perioperative and critical care settings.

PREDISPOSITION TO PROARRHYTHMIA

Certain conditions appear render patients more susceptible to proarrhythmia with antiarrhythmic drugs.[1,2,6,8] Patients with congestive heart failure or recurrent sustained ventricular arrhythmias (lasting > 30 seconds) are more likely to experience ventricular proarrhythmia during treatment with class 1A, 1C, or 3 (sotalol, amiodarone) antiarrhythmic drugs. Impaired left ventricular function, treatment with digitalis and diuretics, and prolonged QT intervals prior to treatment also favor ventricular proarrhythmia (below) with these drugs. Patients with intrinsic sinus node dysfunction or impaired conduction are at increased risk for disadvantageous bradycardia or AV heart block with therapeutic concentrations of most antiarrhythmic drugs. However, this is more likely with class 2, 3 (amiodarone, sotalol), and 4 antiarrhythmics.

VENTRICULAR PROARRHYTHMIA

Most proarrhythmic events occur within several days of beginning treatment or changing the dosage of drugs.[2,6,8] Incessant ventricular tachycardia (VT) or QT interval prolongation with torsades de pointes VT are the common types of ventricular proarrhythmia. *Incessant VT* is invariably produced by drugs that slow intraventricular conduction. Thus, it can occur with class 1A and 1C drugs, as well as amiodarone. VT with 1A drugs is said to be identical with that occurring spontaneously (before treatment) in the same patient.[6] VT with 1C drugs can be similar to that in patients receiving 1A drugs or more malignant, including a sine wave-like tachycardia or flutter.[6] The latter is likely to produce life-threatening hemodynamic instability. *Torsades de pointes VT* is a rapid, polymorphic VT associated with QT-interval prolongation (see Fig. 1–2). It is most commonly seen with class 1A and 3 antiarrhythmics (e.g., quinidine syncope), especially in association with hypokalemia, hypomagnesemia, liquid-protein diets, bradycardia, concomitant treatment with tricyclic antidepressants, or congenital QT-interval prolongation.

Antiarrhythmic Drugs

Discussion of individual drugs is subdivided into parenteral antiarrhythmic drugs, adjunct parenteral drugs, and oral antiarrhythmics. Most information is provided for parenteral drugs (many of which are also available for oral use), since these are the ones most likely to be administered by anesthesia or critical care practitioners.

PARENTERAL ANTIARRHYTHMIC DRUGS

Adenosine

Adenosine is a ubiquitous endogenous nucleoside with negative chronotropic and dromotropic effects at the sinoatrial (SA) and AV nodes, respectively.[2,8,12–15] It is used to terminate supraventricular tachycardia (SVT) and for differential diagnosis of wide or narrow QRS tachycardias with nonapparent P waves.

ACTIONS. Adenosine is not classified (Tables 5–3 and 5–4), but has actions and indications similar to those of class 4 drugs. *Electrophysiologic Actions:* Adenosine interacts with cardiac A_1 receptors to increase potassium current, similar to acetylcholine. This shortens action potential duration and hyperpolarizes resting or maximum diastolic membrane potential. Adenosine antagonizes catecholamine-stimulated adenylate cyclase to reduce cyclic AMP accumulation, inward calcium conductance, and the pacemaker current. These effects explain decreased SA node and latent pacemaker automaticity with adenosine, as well as increased AV node conduction time. The latter may produce transient first-, second-, or third-degree AV heart block. Initial sinus bradycardia with adenosine is followed by a transient, but longer-lasting, reflex sinus tachycardia.[16] Adenosine has little effect on conduction and refractoriness in normal atrial or ventricular myocardium, or the His–Purkinje system. It opposes catecholamine-stimulated triggered activity and ventricular automaticity.[8] *Hemodynamic Actions:* Adenosine is a direct coronary vasodilator. Bolus doses produce a biphasic blood pressure response, with an initial increase in systolic and diastolic blood pressure coincident with increased AV node conduction time, followed by a decrease coincident with secondary tachycardia. The initial blood pressure increase may be mediated by stimulation of aortic chemoreceptors.[16] In patients with autonomic incompetence, the initial increase in blood pressure is greatly attenuated and the delayed decrease accentuated.[14] Except for reduced pulmonary and systemic vascular resistance, adenosine has little effect on other hemodynamic variables at usual clinical doses. Adenosine's hemodynamic effects are short lived (< 1 minute).

PHARMACOKINETICS. Adenosine is rapidly cleared from the vascular compartment by enzymatic degradation to inosine, phosphorylation to adenosine monophosphate, or reuptake into cells. The elimination half-life is less than 10 seconds.

CLINICAL USE. Suggested use for adenosine for the diagnosis or treatment of *regular* tachycardias is presented in Table 5–6. Adenosine is not used for diagnosis or treatment of *irregular* narrow or wide QRS tachycardia. Irregular tachycardia suggests underlying atrial fibrillation, although polymorphic VT or torsades de pointes VT are also associated with irregular RR intervals. Adenosine may accelerate the ventricular rate in patients with accessory pathways and atrial fibrillation, and is ineffective for VT except for exercise-induced right ventricular outflow tract tachycardia in patients without structural heart disease.[14] Adenosine should not be used to treat tachycardia with (imminent) hemodynamic collapse, unless the mechanism for tachycardia is certain and responsive to adenosine. Concerning use of adenosine for treatment or differential diagnosis of wide QRS tachycardia, an algorithm is provided in Figure 5–4.[14,15] Illustration of the use of adenosine to produce transient AV block and

TABLE 5-6 *Adenosine for the diagnosis and treatment of regular tachycardias (tachy)*

DIAGNOSIS	TREATMENT
Differential diagnosis wide QRS tachy	Paroxysmal SVT (SA or AV node reentry)
Mechanism for narrow QRS tachy	Junctional tachycardia with poor left ventricular function
To unmask latent preexcitation*	Exercise/catecholamine-induced RVOT†

*See text. †Right ventricular outflow tract tachycardia, a relatively uncommon VT in patients without structural heart disease.

```
            Regular Wide QRS
               Tachycardia
             (Possibly SVT)
                    │
                    ▼
                ADENOSINE
       ┌────────────┼────────────┐
       ▼            ▼            ▼
   Terminate   Transient AV block  No effect on
   tachycardia  to unmask P waves  tachycardia
```

1. AVN reentry
2. AV reentry
3. SAN reentry
4. Ectopic atrial
5. RVOT tachy

1. Atrial flutter
2. Ectopic atrial
3. Intra-atrial reentry

1. Ventricular tachycardia with structural heart disease

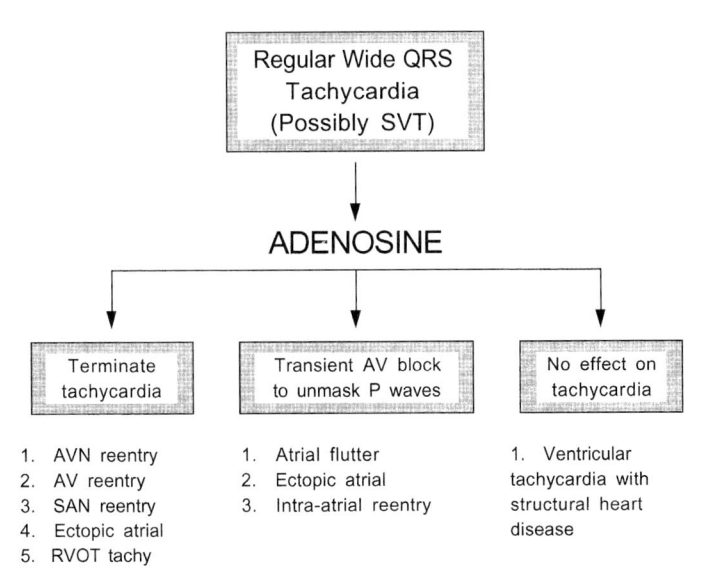

FIGURE 5-4 *Algorithm for use of adenosine in treatment or differential diagnosis of* regular wide-QRS *tachycardia. If, after careful analysis of the patient's history, surrounding circumstances and the 12-lead ECG (if practical), wide-QRS tachycardia could be SVT with ventricular aberration, or findings are still inconclusive for VT, then adenosine can be administered for differential diagnosis provided the tachycardia is reasonably well tolerated and there is no immediate danger of hemodynamic collapse. AV(N), atrioventricular (node); SAN, sinoatrial node; RVOT, right ventricular outflow tract; tachy, tachycardia.*

unmask atrial activity with regular wide QRS tachycardia is shown in Figure 5–5. Finally, adenosine may be of special diagnostic value in patients with suspected ("latent") ventricular preexcitation and SVT.[14] Adenosine may reveal preexcitation by blocking AV nodal conduction to expose the accessory AV pathway (Fig. 5–6). Patients with latent as opposed to intermittent preexcitation[17] are at risk for rapid ventricular rates if atrial fibrillation develops.

ADVERSE EFFECTS. Adenosine frequently causes flushing, dyspnea, or angina-like chest pain in conscious patients. These symptoms are usually mild and transient (< 1 min). Because dyspnea is likely due to bronchoconstriction, adenosine should be used with care in patients with reversible airways disease, and is best avoided in asthmatic patients. Adenosine can produce transient asystole in patients with sinus dysfunction or receiving beta-adrenergic blocking

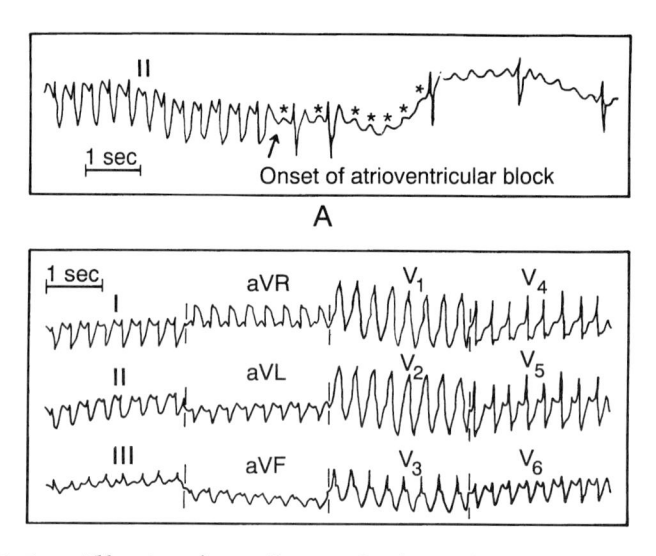

FIGURE 5–5 *Illustration of use of adenosine in the differential diagnosis of wide-QRS tachycardia. (A) Fifteen seconds after adenosine, the ventricular rate slowed to reveal flutter waves at a rate identical to the rate of wide-QRS tachycardia. Note that the QRS complexes are narrow with the slower ventricular rate, indicating that QRS aberration was probably rate related. (B) Note that the 12-lead ECG during wide-QRS tachycardia in the same patient is consistent with the diagnosis of VT. (From Camm and Garrat,[14] the New England Journal of Medicine. Vol 325, page 1626, 1991, with permission.)*

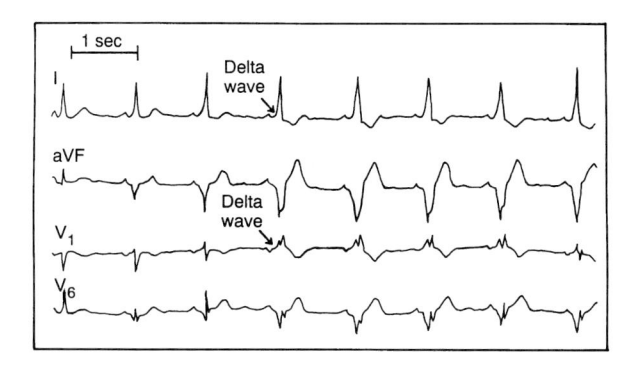

FIGURE 5-6 *Use of adenosine to slow AV nodal conduction and unmask latent ventricular preexcitation. See text for further discussion. (From Camm and Garrat,[14] the New England Journal of Medicine. Vol 325, page 1625, 1991, with permission.)*

drugs (beta-blockers, BB), diltiazem, or verapamil. Sinus bradycardia or AV nodal conduction block is not reversed by atropine. Dipyridamole potentiates adenosine's effects by inhibiting cellular uptake, and methylxanthines are competitive antagonists.

ADMINISTRATION. Because of its extremely short elimination half-life, adenosine should be administered through a central or large peripheral vein with a 10-mL saline flush. It is best administered by incremental dosing (1- to 2-minute intervals). In adults, the initial dose is 6 mg. This can be increased to 12 or 18 mg if required and tolerated. Alternatively, 0.05 mg/kg is the initial and incremental dose.

Amiodarone

While admiodarone was available only in oral form in late 1994, it was nearing approval for IV use; hence, discussion of the drug under antiarrhythmics available for parenteral use. Amiodarone, a benzofuran derivative, was developed in Europe as part of a systematic search for coronary vasodilators.[2,7,8]

ACTIONS. Amiodarone is not a "clean" class 3 antiarrhythmic drug. In addition to blocking potassium repolarization currents, it also blocks sodium and calcium channels, produces noncompetitive alpha- and beta-adrenergic blockade, and blocks conversion of thyroxine (T_4) to triiodothyronine (T_3). *Electrophysiologic Actions:* Amiodarone's electrophysiologic properties have been difficult to characterize because the drug is poorly soluble in water. Additionally, the vehicle for IV amiodarone (Tween 80) and amiodarone metabolites have electrophysiologic effects of their own. Important in vitro electrophysiologic effects include increased action potential duration and refractoriness in all cardiac tissues, but no effect on resting membrane potential. Amiodarone inhibits abnormal automaticity, and normal automaticity of the SA node and latent pacemakers. Amiodarone produces use-dependent sodium-channel block and increased conduction time in fast-response fibers. In patients, it prolongs the ERP of all cardiac tissues. These in vitro effects are responsible for increased QRS and QT intervals, T-wave changes, and U waves in the surface electrocardiogram (ECG), which ECG changes become more pronounced at fast heart rates. Sinus rate is slowed and AV nodal conduction time prolonged. Except for AV nodal conduction time, less increase in conduction time or refractoriness occurs after IV compared to oral amiodarone.[2] *Hemodynamic Actions:* Amiodarone is a peripheral and coronary vasodilator. When administered IV in doses between 2.5 and 10 mg/kg, it decreases heart rate, systemic vascular resistance, and left ventricular contractility.[2] Oral doses of amiodarone sufficient to control arrhythmias do not reduce left ventricular ejection fraction, even in patients with reduced ejection fractions.[2] However, IV amiodarone should be given cautiously to such patients.

PHARMACOKINETICS. Oral doses of amiodarone are poorly and slowly absorbed, with bioavailability ranging from 20 to 65 percent because of marked patient variability. Peak plasma concentrations occur 3 to 7 hours after a single oral dose. Amiodarone is highly protein bound, accumulates extensively in most body tissues, and is metabolized slowly in the liver. Concentrations in body tissue, including myocardium, can be 10 to 50 times those in plasma. The volume of distribution is large and variable ($\geq$ 60 liters/kg). The onset of action following IV administration is generally within several hours, but may be up to several weeks following oral administration. The half-life of elimination is biphasic, with an initial 50 percent reduction in plasma concentration 3 to 10 days after cessation of oral therapy, followed by a terminal half-life of 26 to 107 days (mean 53 days).[2] This difference probably reflects initial rapid clearance from well-perfused tissue, and greater accumulation in poorly perfused tissue. Therefore, to reach steady-state plasma concentrations in the therapeutic range (1.0 to 2.5 µg/ml), it can take many months.

CLINICAL USE. Amiodarone is effective for the treatment of ventricular (40 to 60 percent efficacy) and supraventricular tachyarrhythmias (60 to 80 percent efficacy), including SVT due to intra-atrial and AV nodal reentry, automatic atrial tachycardia, and atrial flutter–fibrillation with or without preexcitation. However, because of the potential for serious side effects, and the difficulty in starting another antiarrhythmic drug due to residual amiodarone effects, amiodarone is not used for treatment until other agents have been tried. If amiodarone is approved for IV use, it is hard to predict use in perioperative and critical care settings, even though its efficacy equals or exceeds that of all other antiarrhythmics. It is suggested that amiodarone will be found most useful for treatment or prophylaxis of arrhythmias following cardiac surgery.

PRECAUTIONS. The high incidence of adverse effects with amiodarone (up to 75 percent after 5 years) appears directly related both to dose and duration of treatment. Serious complications include pulmonary toxicity (10 to 15 percent), proarrhythmia (2 to 5 percent), worsening of heart failure (2 percent), and cirrhosis (uncommon). Amiodarone may interact with inhalation anesthetics and other negative inotropic, chronotropic, or dromotropic drugs to produce severe cardiovascular depression, bradycardia, or AV heart block.[18] Other adverse effects include development of hyper- or hypothyroidism, gastrointestinal and visual disturbances, neurologic dysfunction, increased pacing and defibrillation thresholds, and bluish skin discoloration. The dose of warfarin, digitalis, and other antiarrhythmics is reduced by up to one-half in patients receiving amiodarone.

ADMINISTRATION. The recommended *IV dose* for amiodarone is 5 to 10 mg/kg over 20 to 30 min, followed by 1 g/24 h for several days.[2] Additional boluses of 1 to 3 mg/kg may be given several hours after the first bolus if necessary. The drug should be administered (IV) with great caution to patients with depressed ejection fractions. An optimal *oral dosing* regimen has not been developed. One authority suggests 800 to 1600 mg daily for 1 to 3 weeks, 800 mg daily for next 2 to 4 weeks, 600 mg daily for next 4 to 8 weeks, and finally 400 mg or less daily.[2]

Bretylium

Bretylium is a quaternary ammonium compound approved for IV or IM use against life-threatening ventricular tachyarrhythmias. It was developed in the 1950s as an antihypertensive agent.[2,7,8]

ACTIONS. Bretylium is selectively concentrated in sympathetic ganglia and postganglionic adrenergic nerve terminals. Initially, it causes norepinephrine release. Subsequently, it prevents norepinephrine release by depressing sympathetic nerve terminal excitability. It does not deplete catecholamines, interfere with sympathetic neural or ganglionic transmission, or decrease responsiveness of adrenergic receptors. With more prolonged use, beta-adrenergic responsiveness to circulating catecholamines may be increased. *Electrophysiologic Actions:* Initial catecholamine release may aggravate ventricular arrhythmias with myocardial infarction or digitalis excess. Bretylium's principal action (class 3) is to increase the APD and ERP. The ERP/APD ratio does not change, nor does conduction velocity. APD prolongation is more pronounced in tissue with short APD, so that bretylium reduces APD disparity. This action is nonconducive to reentry, and the probable explanation for why bretylium increases ventricular fibrillation threshold. Concerning ECG effects, bretylium does not affect QRS duration but does prolong the QT interval. *Hemodynamic Actions:* Bretylium may produce a transient ($\leq$ 15 minutes) increase in heart rate, contractility, and blood pressure due to initial norepinephrine release. This is followed by a reduction in heart rate, systemic vascular resistance, and blood pressure. There may be severe postural hypotension in some patients. Bretylium does not affect myocardial contractility.

PHARMACOKINETICS. While bretylium can be administered orally or IM, its absorption by these routes is slow and unpredictable. Bioavailability is less than 50 percent, elimination is almost exclusively renal, and there is no significant metabolism or active metabolites. The half-life of elimination is 5 to 10 hours, with fairly wide variability. This may be longer than 13 hours in patients with renal insufficiency, and doses should be reduced in such patients. However, bretylium can be significantly removed by hemodialysis. Bretylium is almost universally administered IV. The onset of antiarrhythmic effect is within 10 to 20 minutes of IV bolus administration, but full effects may not be apparent for several hours.

CLINICAL USE. Bretylium is usually not effective for treating supraventricular tachyarrhythmias. The drug is currently recommended only for treatment of life-threatening ventricular tachyarrhythmias that have not responded to conventional therapy (i.e., correction of imbalance, lidocaine, procainamide). The response of ventricular fibrillation to bretylium has been impressive. Bretylium may even cause spontaneous conversion in some instances. Bretylium is generally reserved for use in closely monitored circumstances.

ADVERSE EFFECTS. Transient aggravation of arrhythmias (particularly those caused by digitalis), tachycardia, and hypertension due to initial catecholamine release can be troublesome. Subsequently, hypotension, typically orthostatic, is the most significant side effect, especially in patients with depressed left ventricular function or fluid depletion. Vasodilator drugs, hypovolemic states, sympathetic blockade (spinal or epidural anesthesia), and anesthetic or adjuvant drugs that are circulatory depressants can be expected to enhance the hypotensive effects of bretylium. Finally, rapid IV administration may be associated with nausea and vomiting in some patients.

ADMINISTRATION. The initial IV (or IM) dose for life-threatening arrhythmias is 5 to 10 mg/kg as a rapid bolus. This can be repeated in a dose of 5 to 10 mg/kg every 10 to 30 minutes until a maximum dose of 30 mg/kg has been reached. For treatment of VT with reasonable hemodynamic stability, and to reduce the incidence of nausea and vomiting, 5 to 10 mg/kg of bretylium is diluted in 50 to 100 ml of saline or 5 percent dextrose and water, and administered over 10 to 30 minutes. For maintenance, an IV infusion of 1 to 4 mg/min is used.

Diltiazem and Verapamil

Diltiazem and verapamil are benzothiazepine and phenylalkylamine calcium-channel blockers (CCB), respectively. In contrast to dihydropyridine-type CCB (nicardipine, nifedipine nimodipine), diltiazem and verapamil have class 4 antiarrhythmic efficacy at useful clinical concentrations in addition to their vasodilator properties.[2,7,8,12,19] Both drugs, hereafter referred to collectively as CCB, are approved for IV use and have similar actions, efficacy, indications, and adverse effects.

ACTIONS. CCB block L-type calcium channels that lead to generation of the slow-inward current in SA or AV node and partially depolarized fast-response fibers (atrial, ventricular and Purkinje fibers). The slow-inward current also contributes to the action potential plateau in fast-response fibers. *Electrophysiologic Actions:* In slow-response fibers, CCB produce use-dependent reduction in action potential upstroke velocity and conduction time. CCB also slow the rate of normal automaticity in the SA node and latent pacemakers, as well as abnormal automaticity in partially depolarized fast-response fibers. CCB increase AV nodal conduction time and refractoriness. In fast-response fibers, CCB may reduce action potential plateau amplitude and duration. In intact heart, CCB have no effect on QRS duration or the QT interval, but do prolong the PR interval. The above direct effects of CCB on the SA and AV nodes are countered to a variable extent by the reflex increase in sympathetic tone consequent to systemic vasodilation (more so with diltiazem than verapamil). CCB do not affect conduction or refractoriness in fast-response fibers or AV bypass (accessory) pathways. However, conduction in accessory pathways may be enhanced by increased sympathetic tone after CCB. *Hemodynamic Actions:* CCB relax vascular smooth muscle by blocking voltage-dependent calcium channels. This leads to a reduction in blood pressure and systemic vascular resistance, and increased coronary flow. However, there is little effect on venous capacitance beds. CCB are potent negative inotropes (verapamil more so than diltiazem), countered to some extent by reflex-increased sympathetic tone. Nevertheless, CCB may trigger heart failure in patients with poor ventricular function or receiving BB.

PHARMACOKINETICS. After IV *verapamil*, there is a slowing of AV nodal conduction within 1 to 2 minutes (30 minutes after an oral dose), which lasts 4 to 6 hours. Absorption is nearly complete after oral dosing, but bioavailability is reduced (20 to 35 percent) because of extensive first-pass, hepatic metabolism. Verapamil's major metabolite (norverapamil) contributes to its antiarrhythmic action. Verapamil's elimination half-life is 3 to 7 hours, and that of norverapamil 8 to 10 hours. *Diltiazem's* onset and duration of action following oral or IV administration are similar to those of verapamil, but bioavailability is greater (35 to 55 percent) and protein binding less.[19] While diltiazem is extensively metabolized in the liver, its metabolites are not known to be active.

CLINICAL USE. After vagal maneuvers, possibly along with adenosine or edrophonium, CCB may be used for termination of paroxysmal (reentrant) SVT, as well as AV reciprocating tachycardia in patients with the Wolff–Parkinson–White (WPW) syndrome. These drugs should be tried before attempts at termination with digitalis, vasopressors, pacing, or DC cardioversion, unless SVT produces serious hemodynamic compromise and requires immediate conversion. CCB are also used to slow the ventricular rate with atrial flutter–fibrillation, *except in patients with the WPW syndrome,* in whom it may cause dangerous acceleration of ventricular rate. While there are reports of success with CCB as treatment for VT,[2,18] unless tachycardia is known to be SVT with QRS aberration, it is generally best to use drugs other than CCB for initial treatment of new wide-QRS tachycardia.

ADVERSE EFFECTS. CCB can interact with negative chronotropes, inotropes, or dromotropes (BB, inhalation anesthetics, amiodarone, etc.) to produce severe bradycardia, heart block, hypotension, or sudden cardiac decompensation. CCB can cause severe bradycardia or asystole in patients with sinus node dysfunction. Calcium administration is effective for hemodynamic dysfunction secondary to CCB, and temporary pacing (Fig. 3–3) or positive chronotropes–dromotropes (isoproterenol, glucagon) for bradycardia. Atropine is only partially effective for reversing bradycardia with CCB.[2]

ADMINISTRATION. *Diltiazem:* The initial IV dose of diltiazem is 20 mg (0.25 mg/kg) in the average adult. If ineffective after 15 minutes, a second dose (25 mg or 0.35 mg/kg) may be tried. The maintenance infusion is 10 to 15 mg/hr. Oral diltiazem has no approved antiarrhythmic indications, although doses of 60 to 90 mg every 6 hours have been used for SVT prophylaxis.[7] *Verapamil:* The initial IV bolus dose is 5 to 10 mg over 1 to 3 minutes. This dose may be repeated after 30 minutes. To prevent recurrences of SVT or for continued rate control with atrial flutter–fibrillation, verapamil is infused at 0.005 mg/kg/min. The oral dose is 240 to 480 mg daily in divided doses.

Digitalis

The cardiac glycosides share a common action on the heart, so are collectively referred to here as "digitalis." While these drugs are primarily used for the treatment of congestive heart failure, they are also used in the management of supraventricular tachyarrhythmias.

ACTIONS. Digitalis has both direct and indirect (autonomic) actions that contribute to its cardiac effects.[8,20] Its direct action is due to sodium–potassium pump inhibition, which increases intracellular sodium and also calcium via enhanced sodium–calcium exchange. The latter, along with increased inward calcium current, contribute to the inotropic and chronotropic effects of digitalis. *Electrophysiologic actions:* Direct and indirect actions of therapeutic and toxic digitalis on the SA and AV nodes, and atrial, Purkinje, or ventricular fibers are summarized in Table 5–7. Note that digitalis–AV nodal effects, needed for ventricular rate reduction with atrial flutter–fibrillation, are actually a toxic manifestation of digitalis. Sympathetic excitation is more evident with toxic digitalis. In patients with ventricular preexcitation (WPW syndrome), digitalis can decrease refractoriness in the accessory conducting pathway. This may cause dangerous acceleration of ventricular rate with atrial flutter–fibrillation. Delayed afterdepolarizations and triggered activity are believed responsible for some tachyarrhythmias caused by digitalis toxicity. Digitalis ECG effects include PR-interval prolongation, QT-interval shortening, decrease in T-wave amplitude or inversion, and ST-segment depression. The QRS complex and duration are unaffected, even with toxic plasma concen-

TABLE 5-7 *Direct and indirect effects of digitalis on various myocardial fiber types*

	SA NODE	AV NODE	PURKINJE	A OR V MUSCLE
Therapeutic (direct)	None or minimal slowing	↑ conduction time (small)	↓ RMP; ↓ APUV; ↓ APD; ↑ rate automaticity	↓ APD; ↑ slope plateau; ↓ slope phase 3
Toxic (direct)	SA block; sinus pause/arrest	↑ conduction and ERP; AV block	DAD; ↓ gap junctional conductance	↓ APA and RMP, conduction and excitability; DAD
Vagal (V) or sympathetic (S) indirect	Potentiate (V) therapeutic/toxic direct effects	Potentiate (V) therapeutic/toxic direct effects	↑ automaticity and arrhythmias—toxic digitalis (S)	↓ Atrial ERP (V); little effect on ventricular muscle

A, V, atrial, ventricular; RMP, resting membrane potential; APUV, action potential upstroke velocity; DAD, delayed afterdepolarization.

trations. Following exercise, there can be J-point depression mimicking ischemia. *Hemodynamic Actions:* Digitalis increases arterial pressure, systemic vascular resistance, and venous tone in normal subjects, but has little effect on cardiac output and heart rate. In patients with heart failure, digitalis-increased contractility is associated with reduced efferent sympathetic activity, systemic resistance and venous tone. Therefore, heart rate decreases and cardiac output increases, with expected improvement in renal perfusion, and consequent diuresis and edema reduction.

PHARMACOKINETICS. Discussion centers on digoxin, the most widely used digitalis compound. Following oral administration, absorption is highly variable (40 to 90 percent) depending on the preparation.[20] The onset of action and time to maximal effect are also quite variable (1.5 to 6 and 4 to 6 hours, respectively). After an IV dose, these are 5 to 30 minutes and 1.5 to 4 hours, respectively. Digoxin has a fairly large volume of distribution because of high tissue uptake (~ 3 liters/kg in patients with normal cardiac and renal function). Heart failure slows the rate at which steady-state distribution is attained. Concentrations of digoxin in myocardial tissue following equilibration are 15 to 30 times those in plasma. The half-life for elimination of digoxin (1.5 days) is increased in patients with impaired renal function. Monitoring steady-state plasma concentrations during the distribution and equilibration phases is important for reducing digoxin toxicity. For treatment of congestive heart failure, the therapeutic range is 0.5 to 2.0 ng/ml. Ventricular rate control with atrial flutter–fibrillation may require somewhat higher plasma concentrations (≤ 2.5 ng/ml), but optimal dosing for this indication is better gauged by the ventricular rate response and toxic ECG manifestations (e.g., accelerated AV junctional rhythm, paroxysmal atrial tachycardia with block, ventricular arrhythmias).

CLINICAL USE. The principal antiarrhythmic use of digitalis today is to slow the ventricular rate in patients with atrial flutter–fibrillation and left ventricular systolic dysfunction who are poor candidates for treatment with CCB or BB. Since digitalis increases AV nodal conduction and refractoriness, it is sometimes used for treatment or prophylaxis of AV node reentry tachycardia. It is also used to slow the ventricular response in intra-atrial reentry and automatic (ectopic) atrial tachycardias. Since digitalis can accelerate accessory pathway conduction, it is contraindicated for ventricular rate reduction in patients with ventricular preexcitation, unless conduction over the accessory pathway is slow or absent.

ADVERSE EFFECTS. The incidence of adverse effects with digitalis has been reduced with better preparations and monitoring of plasma concentrations. Yet life-threatening cardiac toxicity still occurs in patients with overdose or renal failure. Cardiac toxicity can manifest as almost every conceivable type of rhythm disturbance, and noncardiac toxicity usually involves the gastrointestinal and central nervous systems (Table 5–8). Digitalis arrhythmias can occur in patients with *therapeutic* plasma concentrations, and are facilitated by acid–base imbalance, myocardial ischemia, hypoxia and hypercarbia with chronic pulmonary disease, catecholamines, hypokalemia, hypomagnesemia, hypercalcemia, hyperthyroidism, and potassium-wasting diuretics. Aside from correcting obvious imbalance, ventricular arrhythmias with digitalis may respond to phenytoin or lidocaine, and bradycardia to atropine or temporary cardiac pacing. With life-threatening arrhythmias, digoxin-specific antibodies effectively bind the drug and promote renal excretion.

ADMINISTRATION. For rapid digitalization with digoxin, the IV dose is 0.5 to 1.0 mg in divided doses over 12 to 24 hours. The oral dose is 0.75 to 1.5 mg. The usual maintenance dose is 0.25 to 0.5 mg/day, although children may require higher doses for control of atrial

TABLE 5-8 *Common cardiac and noncardiac toxicities with digitalis compounds*

CARDIAC TOXICITY	NONCARDIAC TOXICITY
Sinus bradycardia; AV heart block	Anorexia; nausea, vomiting (CTZ)
SA or intra-atrial block	Diarrhea; abdominal discomfort or pain
Paroxysmal, nonparoxysmal SVT	Headache; fatigue/drowsiness; malaise
Accelerated AV junctional rhythm*	General muscle weakness; neuralgias
Premature ventricular beats (bigeminy)	Disorientation, aphasia, delirium
Ventricular tachycardia-fibrillation	Visual disturbances; gynecomastia

CTZ, chemoreceptor trigger zone. *Recognized as normalization of ventricular rate response with atrial fibrillation.

TABLE 5-9 *Cardiac electrophysiologic actions of esmolol*

Slow sinus rate; ↑ SA conduction and refractoriness
↑ AV nodal conduction time and refractory periods
Oppose arrhythmias due to catecholamines or digitalis
↓ catecholamine-enhanced latent pacemaker automaticity

fibrillation. IM administration is not recommended because of pain and necrosis at the injection site, as well as unpredictable pharmacokinetics.

Esmolol

Of the BB currently approved for IV antiarrhythmic use (metoprolol, esmolol, propranolol), esmolol, because of its short duration of action, is the one most likely to be used for treatment of tachycardia and arrhythmias in anesthetized or critically ill patients.[2,7,8,12] Other BB are discussed later under Oral Antiarrhythmics.

ACTIONS. *Electrophysiologic Actions:* The cardiac electrophysiologic actions of esmolol are typical of other BB that interact selectively (i.e., cardioselective) with beta-1 adrenergic receptors. Cardioselective BB include acebutolol, atenolol, esmolol, and metoprolol. Esmolol's electrophysiologic actions (Table 5–9) are more obvious when tachycardia or arrhythmias are due to heightened adrenergic tone or digitalis. Also, if hypertension or myocardial ischemia provoke tachycardia and arrhythmias, and are relieved by esmolol, then esmolol may be of benefit against these disturbances as well. *Hemodynamic Actions:* Esmolol and other beta-1 selective blockers depress myocardial contractility and heart rate, leading to a reduction in cardiac output and blood pressure. There may be a compensatory increase in systemic vascular resistance, which can precipitate heart failure in patients with marginal left ventricular function.

PHARMACOKINETICS. The half-life for esmolol distribution to tissues is ~ 2 minutes. The ester bond of esmolol is hydrolyzed by red blood cell esterases. The half-life of elimination is about 9 minutes, and there are no active metabolites.

CLINICAL USE. In addition to approved antiarrhythmic indications for BB (Table 5–10), esmolol may slow the ventricular rate with or terminate ectopic atrial tachycardia. Also, esmolol may slow the rate of paroxysmal (reentrant) SVT, but not necessarily terminate the disturbance.[21,22] The role of esmolol and other IV BB for the prevention and treatment of malignant ventricular arrhythmias related to cardiac surgery requires further definition.

TABLE 5-10 *Beta-blockers approved for antiarrhythmic use*

DRUG	APPROVED INDICATION(S)
Acetbutolol (oral only)	Reduce the number and complexity of VPB, including group beating, multiform VPB, or "R-on-T" phenomenon
Esmolol (IV only)	Ventricular rate control with atrial flutter–fibrillation; noncompensatory ST; reflex tachycardia secondary to tracheal/surgical stimulation
Metoprolol (oral or IV)	To reduce morbidity and mortality from ventricular arrhythmias, including incidence of sudden death following MI
Propranolol (oral or IV)	Noncompensatory sinus tachycardia; SVT; VT caused by digitalis or catecholamines; to reduce incidence of symptomatic VPB
Timolol (oral only)	To reduce morbidity and mortality from ventricular arrhythmias, including incidence of sudden death following MI

VPB, ventricular premature beats; MI, myocardial infarction.

ADVERSE EFFECTS. Because esmolol lacks significant beta-2 blocking activity at clinical doses, it appears safe for use in patients with chronic obstructive pulmonary or reactive airways disease. Esmolol can aggravate heart failure, or cause bradycardia or AV heart block in patients with sinus node dysfunction. Esmolol may produce additive effects to those of catecholamine-depleting drugs. Esmolol does not alter warfarin plasma concentrations, but may increase plasma digoxin concentrations by 10 to 20 percent. Esmolol may prolong succinylcholine neuromuscular block, increase bradycardia with narcotics, or cause bradycardia due to sinus node dysfunction or AV heart block in patients receiving BB or CCB. Finally, esmolol has at least the potential to interact with inhalation anesthetics to cause bradycardia or AV heart block.

ADMINISTRATION. Esmolol is supplied in 10-ml ampules containing 2.5 g, which must be diluted to 10 mg/ml for infusion. It also comes prepared as 10 mg/ml for bolus administration. The single bolus dose is 0.25 to 1.0 mg/kg. For extended use, loading is by bolus or infusion (0.5 mg/kg for 1 minute every 5 minutes × 4). The maintenance dose ranges from 50 to 200 µg/kg/min. If continued treatment with BB beyond 24 to 48 hours is required, the patient should be transferred to a longer-acting beta-blocker or other indicated antiarrhythmic drugs.

Lidocaine and Phenytoin

Lidocaine and phenytoin, which have few adverse hemodynamic effects, are useful for the acute treatment of ventricular arrhythmias related to myocardial infarction, catecholamines, or digitalis excess. Phenytoin is especially effective against the latter.

ACTIONS. *Electrophysiologic Actions:* Lidocaine and other class 1B drugs (phenytoin, mexiletine, tocainide) have no appreciable effects on atrial myocardium, and produce only small changes in action potential upstroke velocity and resting membrane potential in *normal* Purkinje or ventricular muscle fibers. However, depressant effects of class 1B drugs on these parameters are greatly intensified in partially depolarized fibers or with fast rates of stimulation. Class 1B drugs hasten action potential repolarization in Purkinje and ventricular fibers, which effect is most apparent in fibers with the longest action potential duration. This reduces temporal and spatial dispersion of refractoriness. Class 1B drugs have little effect on normal His–Purkinje or ventricular conduction. With abnormal conduction, however, these drugs may decrease or increase His–Purkinje and ventricular conduction time.[7] In ischemic tissue, conduction time usually decreases substantially, whereas in tissue depolarized by stretch or low extracellular potassium, conduction time is prolonged. Thus, class 1B drugs might oppose ventricular reentry by one of two mechanisms: (1) by converting an area of unidirectional conduction block to bidirectional block; or (2) by improving conduction and removing an area of unidirectional conduction block. It is unusual for therapeutic concentrations of class 1B drugs to affect sinus node automaticity in the absence of intrinsic dysfunction. However, normal automaticity of Purkinje fibers and depolarization-induced (abnormal) automaticity may be suppressed. Both lidocaine and phenytoin are effective in abolishing triggered activity due to digitalis-induced delayed afterdepolarizations. Class 1B drugs may shorten the QT interval but have no other effects on the surface ECG. Except for phenytoin, class 1B drugs have little autonomic interaction. Phenytoin, however, owes most of its antiarrhythmic action to autonomic effects. It modulates central efferent vagal activity and reduces increased cardiac sympathetic nerve traffic with digitalis toxicity. Phenytoin has no peripheral anticholinergic or beta-adrenergic blocking activities. *Hemodynamic Actions:* In the absence of severe left ventricular dysfunction, class 1B antiarrhythmics in usual doses have little effect on hemodynamics. All 1B drugs may aggravate myocardial depression and hypotension in patients with heart failure.

PHARMACOKINETICS. Because of extensive first-pass hepatic metabolism following oral administration, which leads to unpredictable and/or low plasma concentrations and excessive toxic metabolites, *lidocaine* is only administered parenterally. Lidocaine kinetics follow a two-compartment model (Fig. 5–3), with a distribution (alpha phase) half-life of 8 minutes. Plasma concentrations correlate well with antiarrhythmic activity (therapeutic range 2.0 to 5.0 µg/ml). The elimination half-life (beta phase) is 1.5 to 2 hours. Steady-state plasma lidocaine concentrations are not reached until 8 to 10 hours after starting a maintenance infusion. The drug is extensively metabolized in the liver, and its clearance approaches the rate of hepatic blood flow (first-order kinetics). The two major metabolites of lidocaine have antiarrhythmic activity as well as central nervous system (CNS) toxicity, and are excreted by the kidneys. Clearance of lidocaine may be decreased during prolonged infusion, and maintenance infusions should be reduced by one-third to one-half in patients with a low cardiac output. *Phenytoin:* Phenytoin is slowly and unpredictably absorbed following oral administration. After IV administration, phenytoin is rapidly distributed to tissues. It is extensively protein bound and metabolized in the liver, the latter being a saturable process (zero-order kinetics). Metabolism is relatively slow and not greatly altered by changes in hepatic blood flow. Thus, during therapy, a small increase in dose can lead to a dramatic rise in plasma concentration. The elimination half-life ranges from 16 to 24 hours. Therapeutic plasma concentrations (bound and unbound forms) range from 10 to 20 µg/ml.

CLINICAL USE.   *Lidocaine:* The principal use of lidocaine is for suppression of ventricular arrhythmias that require rapid control. Lidocaine is not effective for treatment of supraventricular arrhythmias, and it may accelerate the ventricular rate in patients with ventricular preexcitation and atrial fibrillation. Lidocaine is efficacious against a variety of ventricular arrhythmias of diverse causes. While it may not be as effective as bretylium in preventing recurrences of ventricular fibrillation *during* resuscitation (controversial), it appears as effective as bretylium for preventing recurrences of ventricular tachyarrhythmias *after* successful resuscitation. Lidocaine prophylaxis in patients with acute myocardial infarction is also controversial, since it has not been clearly shown to reduce the risk of ventricular fibrillation or to improve survival.[2,8] Also, lidocaine-related side effects and the possible risk of developing asystole lead one to the conclusion that lidocaine is probably not indicated for all patients.[2] *Phenytoin:* Phenytoin is also not effective against supraventricular arrhythmias, unless due to digitalis toxicity. Phenytoin is as or more effective than lidocaine for treating ventricular arrhythmias with digitalis toxicity, but lidocaine is easier to administer. However, phenytoin is not as effective as lidocaine and other drugs against ventricular arrhythmias with myocardial infarction. Finally, phenytoin (or beta-blockers) is useful for treating ventricular arrhythmias associated with sympathetic predominance or imbalance (e.g., anesthesia and surgery, congenital long QT-interval syndrome).

ADVERSE EFFECTS.   *Lidocaine.* The most common toxicity with lidocaine is that of the CNS. Manifestations include dizziness, paresthesias, tinnitus, confusion, delirium, tremor, stupor, coma, and seizures. Nausea and vomiting are the most common gastrointestinal symptoms. Too rapid administration may cause transient hypotension due to negative inotropy and vasodilation, particularly with left ventricular dysfunction. Lidocaine may cause bradycardia or heart block in patients with sinus node dysfunction or impaired conduction. *Phenytoin:* As with all class 1B drugs, CNS toxicity (see lidocaine) is the most common adverse effect. Progression of symptoms correlates with increasing plasma concentrations of phenytoin. Nausea, epigastric pain, and anorexia are also relatively common. Other toxicity following chronic administration includes hyperglycemia, hypocalcemia, gingival hypertrophy, lymphoid hyperplasia, skin rashes, microcytic anemia, peripheral neuropathy, and drug-induced systemic lupus erythematosus.

ADMINISTRATION. *Lidocaine:* The total loading dose is 3 to 4 mg/kg over 30 minutes, with the initial dose 50 to 100 mg (~ 1.0 mg/kg). Maintenance infusions are 1 to 4 mg/min, but if the arrhythmia recurs, the plasma concentration of lidocaine should be measured (if feasible) and a 50-mg bolus administered. The lidocaine dose should be reduced by up to one-half in patients with hepatic insufficiency, taking drugs that reduce the clearance of lidocaine (norepinephrine, beta-blockers, cimetidine), or with heart failure. *Phenytoin:* Phenytoin should be administered slowly in a large peripheral or central vein to avoid pain, sclerosis, thrombosis, or phlebitis at the injection site. The initial dose (100 mg) is repeated every 5 minutes until the arrhythmia is controlled, side effects result, or 1.0 g has been given. This dose is reduced by at least one-half on subsequent days. Constant IV infusion is not recommended (because of pain, sclerosis, etc.). The oral dose is 1.0 g on the first day, 500 mg on the second and third days, and 400 mg daily thereafter. Cimetidine, isoniazid, sulfonamides, dicumarol, phenothiazines, disulfiram, carbamazepine, chloramphenicol, amiodarone, and barbiturates reduce the clearance of phenytoin.[2,8] Lidocaine, quinidine, disopyramide, theophylline, mexiletine, and thyroxin levels may decrease following phenytoin.[8]

Procainamide

Of the class 1A sodium-channel blockers, only procainamide is suitable for IV administration. Intravenous quinidine can cause severe hypotension due to reduced preload and afterload (alpha-adrenergic blockade), as well as impaired contractility with high doses. Disopyramide has even more potent negative inotropic and vasodilator effects, and may cause severe circulatory compromise in patients with left ventricular dysfunction.

ACTIONS. Procainamide, a structural analog of procaine, is useful for urgent and long-term treatment of ventricular and supraventricular arrhythmias.[2,5,7,8] *Electrophysiologic Actions:* Similar to quinidine and disopyramide, procainamide increases the ERP/APD ratio in fast-response fibers. When this exceeds 1.0, the earliest premature impulse that can be initiated during repolarization arises when cells have returned to their most negative potential. Such impulses will have higher action potential amplitudes and upstroke velocities, therefore conduct more rapidly, reducing the likelihood of sustained reentry. Compared to quinidine and disopyramide, procainamide exerts the least anticholinergic effects, but does produce more local anesthetic effects. Procainamide slows conduction in the AV node, accessory pathways, and ventricular muscle, manifest as PR-, QRS, and QT-interval prolongation. Procainamide does not normally affect SA node automaticity, but may slow automaticity in latent pacemakers, abnormal forms of automaticity, or triggered and catecholamine-induced automaticity. The drug's major metabolite (NAPA) has class 3 antiarrhythmic activity. NAPA prolongs action potential duration and refractoriness, but has little effect on resting membrane potential, or action potential amplitude and upstroke velocity. Toxic concentrations of NAPA can produce early afterdepolarizations, triggered activity, and ventricular tachyarrhythmias. *Hemodynamic Actions:* Procainamide has a small negative inotropic effect, which may be clinically significant with higher doses or too rapid administration. In addition, there can be hypotension and bradycardia consequent to mild ganglionic blockade and impairment of cardiovascular reflexes.

PHARMACOKINETICS. Procainamide is well absorbed following oral administration (80 to 90 percent bioavailability), and reaches peak plasma concentrations within 30 minutes to several hours. The elimination half-life is from 2 to 5 hours. Renal excretion accounts for 50 to 70 percent of the drug, while the remainder is metabolized in the liver to mainly NAPA (renal excretion with half-life of 6 to 12 hours). The enzyme that acetylates procainamide to NAPA is genetically determined. Roughly half the North American population are slow acetylators, and accumulate less NAPA than do rapid acetylators. Both procainamide and NAPA concentrations should be monitored in patients receiving chronic treatment with procainamide.

CLINICAL USE. The indications for procainamide with ventricular arrhythmias are similar to those for lidocaine, and it is likely the second drug of choice after lidocaine. Procainamide may convert recent-onset atrial fibrillation to sinus rhythm, but prior treatment with digitalis, BB, or CCB is required to prevent acceleration of the ventricular rate response if atrial fibrillation persists. Procainamide IV is the treatment of choice for patients with atrial fibrillation and preexcitation, a rapid ventricular response over the accessory conducting pathway, but not in immediate danger of circulatory collapse. It slows conduction over the accessory pathway, and may "chemically" convert atrial fibrillation to sinus rhythm.

TABLE 5-11 *Usual, noncardiac adverse effects with chronic procainamide*

Skin rashes; myalgias	Digital vasculitis	Vomiting; diarrhea
Arthralgias; fever*	Raynaud's phenomenon	Nausea; anorexia
Pericardial effusion*	Hallucinations; insomnia	Hepatomegally; hepatitis
Pleurocarditis*	Depression; psychosis	Agranulocytosis

*Manifestations of systemic lupus erythematosus-like syndrome in some patients.

ADVERSE EFFECTS. Noncardiac side effects limit use of procainamide for long-term treatment (Table 5–11). Cardiovascular side effects include depression of left ventricular function, especially with concurrent antiarrhythmic drug therapy. Torsades de pointes VT is less frequent than with quinidine, but other ventricular proarrhythmias occur in some patients. Finally, sinus node dysfunction, AV heart block, and intraventricular conduction disturbances are common with preexisting conduction system disease.

ADMINISTRATION. The ECG and blood pressure should be monitored closely during administration of IV procainamide. Twenty-five to 50 mg/min are given every 5 minutes until a total of 1.0 to 2.0 g is given, hypotension results, or the QRS complex is prolonged by more than 50 percent.[2] The maintenance infusion is 2 to 6 mg/min. Oral dosing is 2 to 6 g/day, but the initial loading dose may be somewhat higher.

ADJUNCT PARENTERAL DRUGS

Atropine, beta-1 adrenergic agonists, edrophonium, and magnesium sulfate are commonly used as adjunct drugs in the management of bradycardia and arrhythmias in anesthesia and critical care settings. Discussion for each focuses on mechanism of action, cardiovascular and side effects, suggested clinical use, and administration. It is cautioned that none of these drugs are approved antiarrhythmic drugs. Nonetheless, there is widespread clinical precedent for suggested use below.

Atropine

CARDIOVASCULAR EFFECTS. Atropine sulfate and similar drugs (atropine methyl nitrate, glycopyrrolate, hyoscyamine, scopolamine) increase sinus rate and prolong AV nodal conduction and refractoriness by blocking the cardiac muscarinic effects of acetylcholine.[18,23] Scopolamine's CNS side effects (drowsiness, confusion, delirium) limit its usefulness for this purpose. Atropine has minimal effects on His–Purkinje and ventricular conduction or refractoriness, and no direct cardiac electrophysiologic effects.

CLINICAL USE. Atropine is used to treat bradycardia due to sinus node dysfunction or AV heart block when *excessive vagal tone or reflex vagal stimulation* is suspected as the cause. Small doses of atropine (< 0.4 mg) may cause initial, transient (< 30 seconds) slowing of heart rate in some patients. While first-degree or type 1 second-degree (Wenckebach) AV heart block due to AV nodal conduction delay may be reversed by atropine, in some patients block may be worsened. Such paradoxical prolongation of conduction by atropine occurs because doses that have little effect on AV node conduction still increase sinus rate, which in turn facilitates use-dependent AV nodal conduction delay, which is not opposed by atropine.[23] Atropine is also sometimes used to treat symptomatic bradycardia in patients with ischemic heart disease or following cardiopulmonary bypass. However, in these circumstances, reduced vagal tone could lead to sympathetic predominance or hyperactivity, sinus tachycardia or other SVT, myocardial ischemia, and accelerated junctional rhythm or ventricular arrhythmias consequent to ischemia. For these reasons, temporary pacing or cautious use of beta-1 agonist drugs is preferred by the author to atropine for treating bradycardia in patients with ischemic heart disease. Finally, 2.0 mg or more of atropine may be required to block the cardiac effects of vagal stimulation in adults, depending on such factors as physical status, age, concurrent medication, and physical conditioning.

Beta- or Mixed Adrenergic Agonists

Beta- or mixed adrenergic agonists directly stimulate heart rate and conduction, and do not rely on removal of vagal tone for their effect. Because of this, beta-agonists are preferred to atropine or related drugs by the author for increasing heart rate and improving conduction (Table 5–12).

ISOPROTERENOL. Isoproterenol, which has beta-1 and beta-2 activity, is used to increase the rate of primary and secondary atrial pacemakers, and to decrease AV node conduction time with heart block.[18,24] Advantages of the drug compared to atropine are listed in Table 5–12. Positive chronotropic effects on junctional and His–Purkinje pacemakers are less pronounced, and isoproterenol has little

TABLE 5-12 *Beta-adrenergic agonists* **(B)** *versus atropine* **(A)**

1. Contribution of vagus to bradycardia or heart block variable.
2. A can cause sympathetic predominance and tachyarrhythmias.
3. Doses of A to produce effect are unpredictable and variable.
4. A may have no effect on bradycardia with sinus dysfunction.
5. B more easily titrated to effect; effects are more predictable.

---

effect on atrial, His–Purkinje, or ventricular conduction. The bolus and infusion doses are 1 to 5 µg and 1 to 5 µg/min, respectively.

EPHEDRINE. Ephedrine is a mixed agonist with predominant beta-1 effects. It is also used to increase heart rate and improve conduction, but is more reliable for increasing blood pressure than isoproterenol because of its alpha-1 effects. The initial dose of ephedrine is 5 to 10 mg, but larger doses may be required.

Edrophonium

PHARMACOLOGY. Edrophonium (and other anticholinesterase agents) are quite useful for diagnosis and initial management of SVT.[12,25-27] Edrophonium's effects are due to accumulation of acetylcholine at muscarinic and nicotinic sites.[28,29] Sufficient doses can produce the following effects: (1) stimulation of muscarinic receptors at all cholinergic sites; (2) stimulation then depression or paralysis of nicotinic receptors (autonomic ganglia; skeletal muscle); and (3) stimulation then depression of CNS cholinergic receptors. However, with doses used to reverse muscle relaxant drugs in anesthesia, edrophonium's muscarinic effects prevail.

CARDIOVASCULAR EFFECTS. Edrophonium slows the rate of all pacemakers under cholinergic control. Thus effects are most pronounced at the sinus node and subsidiary atrial pacemakers. The rate of accelerated AV junctional or ventricular rhythms is little changed. Atrial refractoriness is shortened, but ventricular refractoriness is unchanged. SA and AV nodal conduction time are increased by edrophonium, as is AV nodal refractoriness. In contrast to BB, CCB, or adenosine, edrophonium does not impair myocardial contractility or cause significant vasodilation in doses required for diagnosis or treatment of SVT.

NONCARDIAC SIDE EFFECTS. Bronchoconstriction and increased airway secretions are the most troublesome potential noncardiac effects of edrophonium and other anticholinesterase agents (Table 5-13) in doses used for the diagnosis and treatment of SVT. Edrophonium alone is best avoided in patients with asthma or chronic obstructive pulmonary disease. Beta-blockers and adenosine may also be problematic in these patients. Aside from these precautions, the suggested edrophonium doses for SVT (below) have not produced the effects listed in Table 5-13, at least in the author's experience.

SUGGESTED CLINICAL USE. Compared to BB or CCB for SVT, similarly effective doses of edrophonium do not produce cardiac depression, vasodilation, or hypotension. Also, recurrence of SVT is less likely than with adenosine. Ventricular rate reduction is much more prompt and reliable with edrophonium compared to digoxin, especially with atrial flutter. Edrophonium is ideal for establishing the benefit of rate reduction with noncompensatory sinus tachycardia, especially if the patient is hypotensive and has impaired ventricular function. If reduced diastolic time with tachycardia compared to ventricular dysfunction is more responsible for hypotension, then it is reasonable to continue treatment with BB or CCB. Finally, edrophonium, similar to adenosine, can be used for the differential diagnosis of regular, wide-QRS tachycardia (Fig. 5-4).

ADMINISTRATION. The initial dose of edrophonium is for diagnosis or treatment of SVT is 5 to 10 mg in the average adult. Up to a total of 25 to 30 mg may be given as divided doses every 5 minutes. For continuous ventricular rate reduction with atrial flutter–fibrillation, Frieden and colleagues used a loading dose of 5 to 10 mg followed by a continuous infusion of 0.25 mg/min.[27] The infusion was increased

TABLE 5-13 *Potentially troublesome noncardiac side effects of edrophonium and other anticholinesterase drugs*

PULMONARY	GASTRO-INTESTINAL	GENITO-URINARY	MISCEL-LANEOUS
Bronchoconstriction	Anorexia; nausea	↑ Ureteral peristalsis	Generalized weakness
↑ Airway secretions	Belching; diarrhea	Detrusor constriction	Reverse NMR drugs
Difficulty breathing	Intestinal cramps	↓ Bladder capacity	Confusion; ataxia
Laryngospasm	↑ Gastric secretion	↓ Sphincter tone	Impaired vision

NMR, neuromuscular relaxant.

by 0.25 mg/min amounts every 10 minutes until the desired effect occurred or 2.0 mg/min was infused.

Magnesium sulfate

MAGNESIUM AND ARRHYTHMIAS. Magnesium is the second most abundant intracellular cation.[30] It plays an important role in neurochemical transmission and muscular excitability, and is essential for the activity of many enzymes. Magnesium activates the sodium–potassium exchange pump. Recall that digitalis inhibits this pump. Therefore, it should not be surprising that arrhythmias with digitalis toxicity and magnesium deficiency (Table 5–14) are often the same, and may have similar cellular mechanisms. Indeed, it has been observed that adequate ventricular rate control with digoxin is difficult in patients with atrial fibrillation and magnesium deficiency.[31] Having said all this, it is necessary to point out that a cause-and-effect relationship between magnesium deficiency and cardiac arrhythmias has not been clearly established.[32,33] Further, practitioners should be aware that serum magnesium concentrations can be normal in patients with significant intracellular deficits, since only 5 percent of the available pool of magnesium is extracellular.[30]

SUGGESTED CLINICAL USE. While magnesium sulfate may be effective against a wide variety of ventricular and supraventricular arrhythmias (Table 5–15),[12,18,31,33–35] most authorities recommend reserving its use for those situations where magnesium deficiency causes or contributes to arrhythmias (Table 5–14), and more conventional treatment has failed. The one exception to this recommendation is that magnesium is the treatment of choice for torsades de pointes VT.[36] It should also be considered for any polymorphic VT associated with QT-interval prolongation.

ADVERSE EFFECTS. Magnesium depresses cardiac and vascular smooth muscle, which can cause significant hypotension. Too rapid

TABLE 5-14 *Magnesium deficiency: causes and common clinical associations*

Diets low in magnesium	Thiazide-loop diuretics	Diarrhea or steatorrhea
Chronic ethanolism	Hemodialysis	Diabetes mellitus
Renal tubular damage	Hyperaldosteronism	Starvation; malnutrition
Chemotherapy	Cirrhosis of the liver	Critically ill patients
Myocardial infarction	Open heart surgery	Cachexic states

TABLE 5-15 *Magnesium as ancillary or principal treatment for arrhythmias*

SUPRAVENTRICULAR	VENTRICULAR
Automatic (ectopic) atrial tachycardia	Torsades de pointes (with long QT)
Multiform (chaotic) atrial tachycardia	Arrhythmias due to digitalis toxicity
To ↓ rate with atrial flutter–fibrillation*	VT–VF refractory to usual drugs
Arrhythmias due to digitalis toxicity	Dilated ischemic cardiomyopathy

*To ↑ digitalis effect with magnesium deficiency.

administration or large doses can produce sinus bradycardia or arrest, or AV heart block.[30,36] Other toxicity with magnesium includes potentiation of muscle relaxants, or direct peripheral neuromuscular blockade and central respiratory paralysis with very high doses. Based on similar actions, there is potential for additive or synergistic cardiovascular depressant effects with any of the potent volatile anesthetics, and beta-adrenergic or calcium-channel blockers.

ADMINISTRATION. The effective dose of magnesium for treating cardiac arrhythmias has not been established. For torsades de pointes VT, the adult Advanced Cardiac Life Support Guidelines specify a 1- to 2-g loading dose mixed in 50 to 100 ml of 5 percent dextrose and water over 5 to 60 minutes.[36] The infusion is 0.5 to 1 g/hr for up to 24 hours. While this may not be the ideal dose for arrhythmias listed in Table 5–15, the author has found the same initial dose (adults) effective and tolerated for these arrhythmias as well. However, the dose of magnesium should be reduced in infants and children.

ORAL ANTIARRHYTHMICS

None of the antiarrhythmics discussed here are approved for parenteral administration. However, they may be among the concurrent medications in surgical or critically ill patients, so that their principal actions, indications, and adverse effects may be of interest to anesthesia and critical care practitioners.[2,7,8]

Quinidine (Class 1A)

ACTIONS. Quinidine is the prototype class 1A drug. Its antiarrhythmic actions and clinical use are the same as for procainamide (above). Quinidine has both antimuscarinic and alpha-adrenergic blocking properties. The latter explain significant vasodilation and hypotension following parenteral administration. The antimuscarinic action and reflex-increase in sympathetic tone with vasodilation facilitates AV nodal conduction. This counters direct depression of the AV node by quinidine to produce paradoxical acceleration of the ventricular rate with atrial flutter–fibrillation. Direct myocardial depression occurs only with excessive doses or following too rapid IV administration.

ADVERSE EFFECTS. Quinidine cardiotoxicity includes QT-interval prolongation (used to monitor therapy), proarrhythmia, and polymorphic or torsades de points VT. The latter are the cause for "quinidine syncope" and sudden death. Gastrointestinal distress and CNS toxicity with quinidine (i.e., cinchonism) are common. Symptoms of the latter include tinnitus, hearing loss, blurred vision, headache, diplopia, photophobia, altered color perception, confusion, and psychosis. Allergic reactions may manifest as fever, rash, or immune-mediated thrombocytopenia. Adverse effects preclude long-term administration of quinidine in one-third or more of patients. Of concern to anesthesia and critical care practitioners, quinidine potentiates depolarizing and nondepolarizing muscle relaxants. Also, cimetidine and propranolol reduce quinidine clearance.

ADMINISTRATION. The usual oral dose for quinidine is 300 to 600 mg four times daily. Although quinidine can be given IM, it causes pain at the injection site and a substantial increase in plasma creatine kinase activity. It is no longer administered IV because of the danger of severe cardiovascular depression.

Disopyramide (Class 1A)

ACTIONS. Disopyramide has similar antiarrhythmic action and use as quinidine and procainamide. In contrast to quinidine or procainamide, disopyramide produces significant, dose-dependent, negative inotropic effects when administered to patients with normal or impaired left ventricular function. Additionally, vasoconstrictor properties, which increase afterload and oxygen consumption, contribute to myocardial depression. Disopyramide also has antimuscarinic effects, which increase heart rate and reduce AV node conduction time. However, resting heart rate usually does not change due to direct depression of SA node automaticity.

ADVERSE EFFECTS. In addition to myocardial depression, which is additive to that produced by BB or CCB, disopyramide is associated with proarrhythmia, QT-interval prolongation, and torsades de pointes or polymorphic VT. Symptoms related to its parasympatholytic effects include urinary hesitancy or retention, constipation, blurred vision, closed-angle glaucoma, and dry mouth. Symptoms of gastrointestinal upset are less common than with quinidine.

ADMINISTRATION. Disopyramide is administered orally in doses of 100 to 300 mg four times daily. It is not administered IV because of its potent vasoconstrictor and negative inotropic actions, especially in patients with impaired left ventricular function.

Mexiletine and Tocainide (Class 1B)

MEXILETINE. Mexiletine has similar electrophysiologic and antiarrhythmic actions to lidocaine. It is used for the treatment of symptomatic ventricular arrhythmias. Mexiletine can produce severe bradycardia in patients with sinus node dysfunction. It increases His–Purkinje, but not AV nodal, conduction time or the QT interval. Ventricular proarrhythmia is rare. Oral mexiletine has minimal hemodynamic effects, even in patients with impaired myocardial function. The usual starting dose is 150 to 200 mg three times daily, which is increased to a maximum of 1200 mg daily. A third or more of patients require dose reduction or treatment stoppage because of symptoms of CNS toxicity or gastrointestinal upset, which occur at plasma concentrations slightly above therapeutic.

TOCAINIDE. Tocainide is a primary amine analog of lidocaine that emerged as the result of a systematic search for an "oral lidocaine." The cardiac actions of tocainide are similar to those of lidocaine and mexiletine. Tocainide and mexiletine can be used in patients with QT-interval prolongation. Tocainide has minimal hemodynamic effects, and can be used in patients with acute myocardial infarction. The usual dose is 200 to 600 mg three times daily. Doses are reduced with heart failure, hepatic dysfunction, or renal disease. Tocainide occasionally causes ventricular proarrhythmia or pulmonary fibrosis. Serious hematologic toxicity (agranulocytosis, thrombocytopenia, leukopenia, bone marrow depression, aplastic anemia) occurs in 0.2 percent of patients.[2,8] Otherwise, adverse effects are dose related and similar to those with lidocaine.

Encainide, Flecainide, Propafenone (Class 1C)

GROUP ACTIONS. Class 1C antiarrhythmic drugs compared to other class 1 drugs produce more pronounced use-dependent slowing of conduction in fast-response tissues, including accessory AV pathways. The long dissociation constant with these drugs likely explains QRS and occasional QT-interval prolongation, even at normal heart rates. APD and ERP typically shorten in Purkinje fibers, but may lengthen in ventricular muscle. High concentrations depress the slow-inward current, and therefore SA node automaticity and AV nodal conduction time. Although there is a lower incidence of noncardiac side effects with class 1C drugs as compared to other class 1 drugs, there is a much higher incidence of ventricular proarrhythmia. Long-term suppression of ventricular arrhythmias with class 1C drugs after myocardial infarction is associated with two to three-fold increased mortality from arrhythmias compared to placebo-treated controls.[1,37] Clinically important adverse cardiac effects of class 1C drugs are summarized in Table 5–16.

ENCAINIDE. Encainide is a structural analog of procainamide. While recently withdrawn from the market, the sponsor continues to

TABLE 5-16 *Clinically important adverse effects of class 1C antiarrhythmics and moricizine*

DRUG	CARDIAC EFFECTS	INTERACTIONS	CAUTIONS
Encainide	Proarrhythmia (VT–VF); SND; global depression of conduction; CHF	Levels ↑ by cimetidine/ inhibitors of cytochrome P-450; BB, CCB	Renal disease; SND or AV block; BB, CCB; LV dysfunction
Flecainide	Proarrhythmia (VT–VF); SND; AV heart block; negative inotrope	Levels ↑ by cimetidine/ inhibitors of cytochrome P-450; ↑ digoxin level	Renal disease; SND or AV block; BB, CCB; LV dysfunction
Moricizine	Proarrhythmia (VT–VF); CHF; ↓ AV node and contractility	Cimetidine can reduce clearance; ↑ clearance of theophylline	Hepatic or renal disease; drug- or disease-impaired conduction
Propafenone	Proarrhythmia (VT–VF); ↓ SA and AV node and contractility	Cimetidine ↑ levels; BB, CCB, antiarrhythmics; ↑ serum digoxin, warfarin	Hepatic disease; asthma and COPD, CHF; AV conduction defects

CHF, congestive heart failure; SND, sinus node dysfunction; AP, accessory pathway. COPD, chronic obstructive airways disease.

provide the drug to patients who previously required it for life-threatening arrhythmias.[8] Encainide has active metabolites (similar action to parent compound), metabolism is genetically determined, and the dose should be reduced in patients with renal dysfunction because of the reduced clearance of parent drug and metabolites. The usual daily dose is 25 to 50 mg three times daily. Adverse effects increase with increasing dose, and include dizziness, visual disturbances, headache, and gastrointestinal upset. Sinus arrest or AV heart block may occur with high doses. The incidence of ventricular proarrhythmia is approximately 10 percent. Ventricular proarrhythmia is more likely in patients with congestive heart failure, structural heart disease, or a history of sustained VT. Encainide is used to suppress recurrences of VT, AV reciprocating tachycardia, atrial flutter–fibrillation, and AV nodal reentrant tachycardia. It also prolongs accessory pathway conduction in WPW syndrome patients with atrial fibrillation.

FLECAINIDE. The actions of flecainide are typical of class 1C drugs (see group actions, earlier). Pacing thresholds are increased as much as 200 percent by flecainide,[8] so that the drug should be used with caution in pacemaker patients. In contrast to encainide, flecainide depresses cardiac performance, particularly in patients with impaired left ventricular function. Flecainide has active metabolites with similar but lesser effects than parent drug. Elimination is slower in patients with heart failure or renal dysfunction. The initial dose is 100 mg twice daily, which is increased to a maximum of 400 mg daily. The incidence of ventricular proarrhythmia ranges from 5 to 30 percent of patients.[2] The incidence is highest in patients with history of sustained VT, heart failure, or receiving high doses of flecainide. Proarrhythmic VT with flecainide is resistant to drugs and DC cardioversion, and carries a 10 percent mortality. Sinus arrest and AV heart block may also occur. Confusion and irritability are the most frequent noncardiac side effects. Flecainide has similar antiarrhythmic efficacy and use to that described for encainide.

PROPAFENONE. Propafenone's structure resembles propranolol and other BB, but its actions are more similar to those of encainide and flecainide. As a BB or CCB, it is about 1/40th and 1/100th as potent as propranolol and verapamil, respectively.[8] High doses of propafenone decrease contractility, and the drug may precipitate congestive heart failure in patients with impaired left ventricular function. This is not as common as with encainide or flecainide. Most patients respond to oral doses of 150 to 400 mg three times daily. Propafenone increases plasma concentrations of digoxin, warfarin, and metoprolol. Cimetidine increases plasma propafenone concentrations by about 20 percent. Oral bioavailability increases and metabolism decreases in patients with severe hepatic dysfunction or congestive heart failure, so that the propafenone dose is reduced by one-half in these patients. Since significant amounts of active metabolites are excreted by the kidney, dosage is reduced in these patients as well. CNS and gastrointestinal side effects are usually mild. Some amount of beta-blockade can be expected with high doses, and bronchospasm has been reported. The incidence of ventricular proarrhythmia with propafenone appears lower (about 5 percent) than with encainide or flecainide. Propafenone has similar use to encainide or flecainide.

Moricizine (Class 1A & 1B)

Moricizine, a phenothiazine derivative, has actions and kinetics of interaction with sodium channels characteristic of both 1A and 1B drugs (see Table 5–3). It also suppresses delayed afterpotentials and abnormal forms of automaticity in depolarized fibers, but has little effect on SA node or atrial tissue. Moricizine prolongs AV nodal conduction time and QRS duration. The drug is usually well tolerated, except with impaired ventricular function. Moricizine undergoes extensive hepatic metabolism. Less than 1 percent of the parent drug is excreted unchanged in the urine. Numerous metabolites, some active, are produced in small amounts, so that measurement plasma moricizine for therapeutic concentrations has relatively little meaning. The drug is administered in doses of 200 to 300 mg three times daily. The dose is reduced with hepatic or renal disease, or congestive heart failure. Moricizine may produce additive effects to other drugs that prolong AV nodal or ventricular conduction, and may worsen sinus node dysfunction. CNS and gastrointestinal side effects are relatively uncommon. The incidence of ventricular proarrhythmia is similar to that with encainide, and highest with impaired left ventricular function. The efficacy and use of moricizine is similar to that of class 1C drugs.

Beta-Adrenergic Blockers (Class 2)

The only BB currently approved for antiarrhythmic use or to prevent sudden death listed in Table 5–10. Except for esmolol, all are available for oral use. Propranolol and metoprolol are also approved for IV use but, because of their slower onset and long duration of action compared to esmolol, are used far less often for the acute management of tachycardia and arrhythmias. While other available BB (atenolol, nadolol, oxyprenolol, pindolol) may have antiarrhythmic efficacy, they are labeled only for use in the treatment of hypertension, angina pectoris, migraine, hypertrophic subaortic stenosis, essential tremor, or pheochomocytoma.

CARDIOVASCULAR EFFECTS. The electrophysiologic (Table 5-9) and hemodynamic effects of BB are essentially as described for esmolol. As with esmolol, effects are greatest when increased sympathetic tone, catecholamines, or digitalis excess cause or contribute to tachycardia and arrhythmias. Since catecholamines are increased with exercise, myocardial infarction and congestive heart failure, BB may be effective against supraventricular or ventricular arrhythmias in these circumstances. BB are also used to reduce the incidence of sudden death following myocardial infarction, and may be more effective than digitalis or verapamil for prophylaxis of SVT following coronary artery bypass surgery.[38] Some BB possess partial agonist activity (acetbutolol, labetalol, oxyprenolol, pindolol), but whether this confers any therapeutic advantage is uncertain. Perhaps, there might be less reduction in resting heart rate or cardiac output. Other BB can block sodium channels (acebutolol, labetalol, metoprolol, oxyprenolol, pindolol, propranolol) by a membrane-stabilizing or quinidine-like action. This property may also help reduce platelet aggregation.[8] Since BB reduce myocardial contractility, they can precipitate or worsen heart failure. By blocking only the beta-effects of adrenergic stimulation, alpha-effects are unopposed and could cause peripheral vasoconstriction or coronary vasospasm in some patients.

PHARMACOKINETICS AND DOSING. The pharmacokinetics of the various BB differ substantially. For example, propranolol has only about 25 percent bioavailability compared to 75 percent with pindolol.[39] More selective BB (atenolol, metoprolol, and acebutolol) have 40 to 50 percent bioavailability. The half-life in plasma for most BB ranges from 2 to 5 hours. Ranges for atenolol and nadolol are 5 to 8 and 10 to 20 hours, respectively. BB are administered orally or IV in doses required to produce the desired effect without adverse effects. Oral dosing can vary considerably, depending on bioavailability.[9,39] The initial IV dose for labetalol is 20 mg administered over 5 to 10 min, and the maximum daily IV dose is 300 mg.[8] For metoprolol and propranolol, the initial and daily IV doses are 5 and 15, and 1 to 3 and 10 to 15 mg, respectively. With propranolol, at least 4 hours should be allowed between successive IV doses.

CLINICAL USE. Supraventricular and ventricular arrhythmias provoked or aggravated by adrenergic stimulation (Table 5-17) or digitalis may be prevented by or respond to BB. They are also effective for noncompensatory sinus tachycardia and rate reduction with atrial

TABLE 5-17 *Conditions with excess adrenergic stimulation*

Anesthetic sensitization	Airway manipulation
Aortic dissection	Sternotomy; cardiotomy
Exercise; emotions	Inadequate anesthesia
Hyperthyroidism	Pain; awareness
Fever; shock states	Hypoxia, hypercarbia
Cocaine, amphetamines, etc.	Pheochromocytoma

flutter–fibrillation. BB occasionally convert the latter disturbances to sinus rhythm, especially if of recent onset. BB are also be used to prevent recurrences of paroxysmal (reentrant) SVT, or AV reciprocating tachycardia in WPW syndrome patients. Combining BB with digitalis may be more effective than using BB alone. Intravenous BB are effective against arrhythmias associated with digitalis toxicity because central sympathetic hyperactivity contributes to arrhythmias. However, if digitalis arrhythmias are associated with AV heart block, phenytoin or lidocaine are preferred to BB. Oral BB are used as prophylaxis for ventricular arrhythmias associated with the congenital long QT-interval or mitral valve prolapse syndromes. While BB effectively suppress frequent premature ventricular beats in 50 to 60 percent of patients, they are less effective for suppressing recurrences of sustained VT. In fact, BB are usually avoided in patients with recurrent sustained VT because of associated left ventricular dysfunction.[8] Finally, BB are sometimes prescribed to help reduce the incidence of overall mortality following myocardial infarction, although the mechanism for this salutary effect is not known.[2]

ADVERSE EFFECTS. Most of the adverse effects of BB (Table 5–18) result from beta-blockade or unopposed alpha-stimulation, and are more pronounced in patients with enhanced adrenergic tone. Too abrupt stoppage of BB has been associated with arrhythmias, hypertension, myocardial ischemia or infarction, and even death. In hypoglycemic diabetics, BB may mask related symptoms of tachycardia and diaphoresis.

Sotalol (Class 2 and 3)

Sotalol is a recently approved BB with prominent class 3 activity.[7,40,41] Sotalol is a nonselective BB with membrane-stabilizing and partial agonist activity. It also prolongs APD and refractoriness in all fast-response fibers by blocking potassium repolarization currents. Sotalol is available as a racemic mixture of its stereoisomers. The

TABLE 5-18 *Cardiovascular, CNS, and other adverse effects of beta-adrenergic blockers*

CARDIOVASCULAR	CNS	OTHER
Congestive heart failure	Mental depression	Worsen asthma or COPD
Untoward hypotension	Vivid dreams; insomnia	Nausea, vomiting, pain
Bradycardia; AV block	Hallucinations	Constipation; diarrhea
Intermittent claudication	Easy fatigability	Agranulocytosis (rare)
Raynaud's phenomenon	Sexual dysfunction	Hair loss; baldness

COPD, chronic obstructive pulmonary disease.

d-isomer possesses 1/50th the BB activity of the l-isomer, but both isomers have class 3 activity. At present, only oral sotalol is available in the United States, but the IV form is available in Europe. If the drug becomes available in IV form here, it might be useful in patients having cardiothoracic and vascular surgery, especially those with arrhythmias related coronary artery or chronic obstructive pulmonary disease.

CARDIOVASCULAR EFFECTS. The class 2 actions and side effects of sotalol are similar to those of other BB. Sotalol increases atrial, His–Purkinje, and ventricular refractoriness, as well as that of accessory AV pathways. It causes reverse use-dependent QTc-interval prolongation (i.e., more prolonged at slower rates). In isolated tissue, sotalol increases contractility, possibly because of increased APD and time for calcium influx.[41] While animal and clinical data confirm less reduction in contractility with sotalol compared to equivalent BB doses of propranolol, sotalol may still aggravate heart failure in some patients with compromised ventricular function.

PHARMACOKINETICS AND DOSING. After oral sotalol, bioavailability is high (≥ 90 percent). Peak plasma concentrations occur in 2 to 4 hours. There is no biotransformation, and elimination is by renal excretion (half-life 7 to 18 hours).[41] With moderate to severe renal disease, mean half-life increases to 24 to 41 hours.[41] Since higher sotalol doses are needed for class 3 effects, the QTc interval is monitored to prevent toxicity. Therapeutic sotalol (160 to 320 mg daily) increases the QTc interval by 40 to 100 msec, and QTc intervals ≥ 500 msec predispose to proarrhythmia.

CLINICAL USE. Sotalol appears less effective than other BB for reducing mortality after myocardial infarction, which is probably due to ventricular proarrhythmia.[41] Similar to other BB, sotalol reduces the incidence of reinfarction. Sotalol (IV bolus) terminates 33 and 20 percent, respectively, of episodes of acute atrial flutter–fibrillation. Efficacy increases with continuous infusion.[42] With atrial flutter–fibrillation after cardiopulmonary bypass, sotalol (bolus 1 mg/kg; infusion 0.2 mg/kg every 12 hours) was as effective as digoxin plus disopyramide[43]. Further, oral sotalol (40 mg every 6 hours) compared to placebo reduced the incidence of atrial flutter–fibrillation by one-half up to 6 days after coronary bypass surgery.[44] Sotalol is used to prevent recurrences of atrial fibrillation, and reentry tachycardia involving the AV node with or without accessory pathways.[41] Sotalol appears as or more effective than conventional antiarrhythmics for prevention of recurrences of symptomatic nonsustained or sustained ventricular arrhythmias.[41]

ADVERSE EFFECTS. Aside from adverse effects due to BB activity (Table 5-18), ventricular proarrhythmia or torsades de pointes VT (~ 2 percent incidence) are of most concern. Left ventricular dysfunction, hypokalemia, bradycardia, or concurrent use of drugs that prolong repolarization increase the risk of proarrhythmia.

References

1. Roden, D. Risks and benefits of antiarrhythmic therapy. N Engl J Med 1994; 331:785–791.
2. Zipes D. Management of cardiac arrhythmias: Pharmacological, electrical, and surgical techniques. In Braunwald E (ed): Heart Disease. 4th ed. Philadelphia: WB Saunders, 1992: pp. 628–666.
3. Vaughan Williams E. A classification of antiarrhythmic actions reassessed after a decade of new drugs. J Clin Pharmacol 1984;24: 129–147.
4. Harrison D. Antiarrhythmic drug classification: New science and practical applications. Am J Cardiol 1985;56:185–187.
5. Barber M. Class I antiarrhythmic agents. In Lynch C III (ed): Clinical Cardiac Electrophysiology. Philadelphia: JB Lippincott, 1994: pp. 85–111.
6. Josephson M. Evaluation of antiarrhythmic agents. In Clinical Cardiac Electrophysiology. Philadelphia: Lea & Febiger, 1994: pp. 630–682.
7. Bigger JJ, Hoffman B. Antiarrhythmic drugs. In Gilman A, Rall T, Nies A, Taylor P (eds): The Pharmacological Basis of Therapeutics. 8th ed. New York: Pergamon Press, 1990: pp. 840–873.

8. Murray K, Ramo B, Hurwitz J. Clinical pharmacology and use of antiarrhythmic drugs. In Waugh R, Ramo B, Wagner G, Gilbert M (ed) Cardiac Arrhythmias. 2nd ed. Philadelphia: FA Davis, 1994: pp. 347–391.
9. Tatro D, Olin B, Hebel S (eds). Drug Interaction Facts. 4th ed. St. Louis: Facts and Comparisons, 1994: p. 1068.
10. The Cardiac Arrhythmia Suppression Trial (CAST) Investigators: Preliminary report: Effect of encainide and flecainide on mortality in a randomized trial of arrhythmia suppression after myocardial infarction. N Engl J Med 1989;321:406–412.
11. The Cardiac Arrhythmia Suppression Trial II Investigators: Effect of the antiarrhythmic agent moricizine on survival after myocardial infarction. N Engl J Med 1992;327:227–233.
12. Atlee J. Adenosine, diltiazem, edrophonium, esmolol, magnesium sulfate, and other new antiarrhythmic drugs. Cardiothorac Vasc Anesth Update 1993;3:1–13.
13. Belardinelli L, Lerman B. Adenosine: Cardiac electrophysiology. PACE 1991;14:1672–1680.
14. Camm A, Garrat C. Adenosine and supraventricular tachycardia. N Engl J Med 1991;325:1621–1629.
15. Faulds D, Chrisp P, Buckley M. Adenosine. Drugs 1991;41:596–624.
16. Biaggioni J, Olafsson B, Robertson R, et al. Cardiovascular and respiratory effects of adenosine in conscious man: Evidence for chemoreceptor activation. Circ Res 1987;61:779–786.
17. Klein G, Gulamhusein S. Intermittent preexcitation in the Wolff–Parkinson–White syndrome. Am J Cardiol 1983;52:292–296.
18. Atlee J. Perioperative Cardiac Dysrhythmias. 2nd ed. Chicago: Year Book Medical Publishers, 1990.
19. Gilman A, Rall T, Nies A, Taylor P (eds). The Pharmacological Basis of Therapeutics. 8th ed. New York: Pergammon Press, 1990.
20. Hoffman B, Bigger JJ. Digitalis and allied glycosides. In Goodman A, Rall T, Nies A, Taylor P (eds). The Pharmacological Basis of Therapeutics. 8th ed. New York: Pergamon Press, 1990: pp. 814–839.
21. Esmolol Multicenter Research Group. Efficacy and safety of esmolol vs. propranolol in the treatment of supraventricular tachyarrhythmias: A multicenter, double-blind clinical trial. Am Heart J 1985; 110:913–922.
22. Esmolol Multicenter Research Group. Intravenous esmolol for the treatment of supraventricular tachyarrhythmia: Results of a multicenter baseline-controlled safety and efficacy study in 160 patients. Am Heart J 1986;112:498–505.
23. Brown J. Atropine, scopolamine, and related antimuscarinic drugs. In Gilman A, Rall T, Nies A, Taylor P (eds): The Pharmacological Basis of Therapeutics. 8th ed. New York: Pergammon Press, 1990: pp. 150–165.
24. Hoffman B, Lefkowitz R. Catecholamines and sympathomimetic drugs. In Gilman A, Rall T, Nies A, Taylor P (eds). The Pharmacologic Basis of Therapeutics. 8th ed. New York: Pergammon Press, 1990: pp. 187–220.

25. Eldor J, Frankel D. Use of low-dose neostigmine intravenously in the treatment of supraventricular tachycardia: An immediate bradycardic effect. Resuscitation 1989;18:103–110.
26. Moss A, Aledort L. Use of edrophonium (Tensilon) in the evaluation of supraventricular tachycardias. Am J Cardiol 1966;17:58–62.
27. Frieden J, Cooper J, Grossman J. Continuous infusion of edrophonium (Tensilon) in treating supraventricular arrhythmias. Am J Cardiol 1971;27:294–297.
28. Taylor P. Cholinergic agonists. In Gilman A, Rall T, Nies A, Taylor P (eds): The Pharmacological Basis of Therapeutics. 8th ed. New York: Pergammon Press, 1990: pp. 122–130.
29. Taylor P. Anticholinesterase agents. In Gilman A, Rall T, Nies A, Taylor P (eds): The Pharmacological Basis of Therapeutics. 8th ed. New York: Pergammon Press, 1990: pp. 131–149.
30. Mudge G, Weiner I. Agents affecting volume and composition of body fluids. In Goodman A, Rall T, Nies A, Taylor P (eds): The Pharmacological Basis of Therapeutics. 8th ed. New York: Pergammon Press, 1990: pp. 682–707.
31. De Carli C, Sprouse G, LaRosa J. Serum magnesium levels in symptomatic atrial fibrillation and their relation to rhythm control by intravenous digoxin. Am J Cardiol 1986;57:956–959.
32. Surawicz B. Is hypomagnesemia or magnesium deficiency arrhythmogenic? J Am Coll Cardiol 1989;14:1093–1096.
33. Gettes L. Electrolyte abnormalities underlying lethal and ventricular arrhythmias. Circulation 1992;85:70–76.
34. Tzivoni D, Banai S, Schuger C, et al. Treatment of torsades de pointes with magnesium sulfate. Circulation 1988;77:392–397.
35. Tzivoni D, Keren A. Suppression of ventricular arrhythmias by magnesium. Am J Cardiol 1990;65:1397–1399.
36. Emergency Cardiac Care Committee and Subcommittees AHA. Guidelines for cardiopulmonary resuscitation and emergency cardiac care. Part III. Adult advanced cardiac life support. JAMA 1992;268:2199–2241.
37. Epstein A, Hallstrom A, Rogers W, et al. Mortality following ventricular arrhythmia suppression by encainide, flecainide, and moricizine after myocardial infarction. JAMA 1993;270:2451–2455.
38. Andrews T, Reimold S, Berlin J, Antman E. Prevention of supraventricular arrhythmias after coronary artery bypass surgery: A meta-analysis of randomized controlled trials. Circulation 1991;84(Suppl III):236–244.
39. Hoffman B, Lefkowitz R. Adrenergic receptor antagonists. In Gilman A, Rall T, Nies A, Taylor P (eds): The Pharmacological Basis of Therapeutics. 8th ed. New York: Pergammon Press, 1990: pp. 221–243.
40. Singh B. Expanding clinical role of unique class III antiarrhythmic effects of sotalol. Am J Cardiol 1990;65:84A–88A.
41. Hohnloser S, Woosley R. Sotalol. New Engl J Med 1994;331:31–38.
42. Teo K, Harte M, Horgan J. Sotalol infusion in the treatment of supraventricular tachyarrhythmias. Chest 1985;87:113–118.

43. Campbell T, Gavaghan T, Morgan J. Intravenous sotalol for the treatment of atrial fibrillation and flutter after cardiopulmonary bypass: comparison with disopyramide and digoxin a randomized trial. Br Heart J 1985;54:86–90.
44. Suttorp M, Kingma J, Peels H, et al. Effectiveness of sotalol in preventing supraventricular tachyarrhythmias shortly after coronary artery bypass grafting. Am J Cardiol 1991;68:1163–1169.

6

Pacing and Cardiac Electroversion

Abbreviations Used in Chapter Six

AV	Atrioventricular
ECG	Electrocardiogram
ICD	Internal cardioverter-defibrillator
SA	Sinoatrial
SND	Sinus node dysfunction
SVT	Supraventricular tachycardia
VA	Ventriculoatrial
VF	Ventricular fibrillation
VT	Ventricular tachycardia

The purpose of this chapter is to provide the reader with background information on the design and operation of cardiac pacemakers and internal cardioverter-defibrillators (ICD), the hemodynamics of pacing, and indications for pacing and electroversion. Two subsequent chapters will focus on the more practical aspects of temporary pacing and perioperative management of patients with implanted pacemakers or ICD devices.

Perspectives

THE BEGINNINGS

External electrical stimulation of the heart for bradycardia was developed in the late 1920s, but it was not until the 1950s that implantable pacemakers were first used. Pacemakers of the 1950s and 1960s were large, had a short battery life (≤ 2 years), paced only one chamber, and provided no sensing. Therefore, they were asynchronous units that competed with the patient's spontaneous rhythm. Since the early pacemakers could not be programmed, they had predetermined stimulus characteristics and rate. Finally, most early pacemakers were implanted with epicardial as opposed to endocardial (transvenous) lead systems. Thus, a thoracotomy was required for lead placement.

ADVANCES IN PACEMAKER DESIGN

Numerous advances have been made in cardiac pacing since the 1960s. Batteries are smaller and now last for 4 to 12 years, depending on the complexity of circuitry and energy expended for pacing. Electronic circuitry inside the pacemaker "can" (i.e., housing or casing) now controls numerous functions besides pulse rate, duration, and output. External programming devices can noninvasively and reversibly alter a multitude of pacemaker functions. Dual-chamber pacing and sensing, as well as rate-adaptive (sensor-modulated) pacing using a variety of physiologic sensors (Table 6–1), are now commonplace.[1] In addition to a variety of pacing modes for bradycardia, some modern pacemakers also have provisions for antitachycardia pacing. Further, third- and fourth-generation ICD devices may feature back-up bradycardia and antitachycardia pacing. Significant improvements have also been made in the design of pacing leads and electrodes, including smaller, less thrombogenic and more reliable transvenous leads with steroid-eluting electrodes.[2] The latter substantially reduce pacing thresholds over time compared to earlier electrode designs. Since this

TABLE 6-1 *Types of physiologic sensors for sensor-modulated pacemakers*

Sinus node (atrial) rate*	Activity sensors (vibration, etc.)
QT interval; stimulus–T interval	Endocardial depolarization integral
Body (central venous) temperature	Minute ventilation (impedance)
Preejection interval	pH of mixed venous blood
Mixed venous oxygen saturation	Stroke volume (cardiac impedance)
Right ventricular dP/dt[†]	Magnetic ball inductance (motion)

*The ideal "sensor," but unsuitable with atrial tachyarrhythmias.
[†]dp/dt - change in pressure over time.

reduces stimulus current requirements, it also helps increase pacemaker battery longevity.

PREVALENCE

Somewhat over one million persons worldwide, with about one-half of these in the United States, have permanent pacemaker or antitachycardia ICD devices. The latter may comprise up to 10 percent of all implanted devices. All anesthesia and critical care practitioners will undoubtedly at some time encounter patients with pacemakers or ICD devices. Additionally, significant numbers of patients may require temporary cardiac pacing for transient conditions. This is increasingly likely given the advancing age of our surgical and critical care populations, the complexity and risks of modern surgical procedures, and the potential for adverse drug effects or interactions affecting cardiac automaticity or conduction with multiple-drug therapy.

SIGNIFICANCE

Physicians have long recognized bradycardia as a cause of heart failure and death, regardless of whether bradycardia was due to impaired conduction or impulse formation. However, well into the 20th century, physicians were powerless to offer more than symptomatic or supportive treatment. In contrast, effective medical treatment for many tachycardias (i.e., digitalis) has existed for several centuries. It is only over the past 20 years or so that cardiac pacing has assumed a prominent place among the options available for treatment of cardiac arrhythmias. In fact, cardiac pacing and other forms of "electrical" therapy are becoming more and more preferred to drugs because of the high incidence of untoward effects with drugs (see Chapter 5). Also, it is appreciated that temporary or permanent pacing can reduce the requirement for drugs.

Pacemaker Operation

PACEMAKER DESIGN

Temporary and permanent pacing systems consist of a battery-powered pulse generator that supplies stimuli conducted by pacing leads to electrodes situated inside (endocardial) or on (epicardial) the heart's surface. Circuitry within the hermetically sealed (to protect against body fluids) titanium pacemaker can regulates stimulus timing and characteristics. The insulated pacing lead may contain one or two conductors, depending on whether the pacemaker system is unipolar or bipolar. Each conductor is connected distally to an electrode, and proximally via a pin to the pacemaker itself. With a unipolar pacing system, a single myocardial electrode serves as cathode and the pacemaker can as anode (Fig. 6–1). With a bipolar system, both the anode and cathode are myocardial (Fig. 6–1). The distinction between unipolar and bipolar pacing systems is important, because unipolar systems are more susceptible to malfunction produced by sensed electromagnetic interference (see Chapter 8). This is because the large surface area of the pacemaker can (anode) encourages sensing of skeletal myopotentials, while the lead itself provides an antenna of sorts for sensing extraneous electrical noise.

All contemporary pacemakers are programmable, which means that it is possible to reversibly alter most pacemaker functions. Implanted pacemakers are commonly powered by lithium iodide or lithium cupric sulfide, which retain a satisfactory voltage for 90 percent of their life.[3,4] For single- or dual-chamber pacemakers this can be 7 to 12 or 4 to 8 years, respectively. Among other things, battery longevity will depend on the complexity of pacemaker function, time spent actually pacing with demand units, and electrode impedance.

PACEMAKER TERMINOLOGY AND OPERATION

Asynchronous or Synchronous Pacing

Pacemakers that deliver stimuli without regard to the patient's spontaneous rhythm are *asynchronous* pacers. They are also known as fixed-rate or competitive pacers. Pacemakers that sense atrial or ventricular myopotentials, and respond by inhibition or triggering of

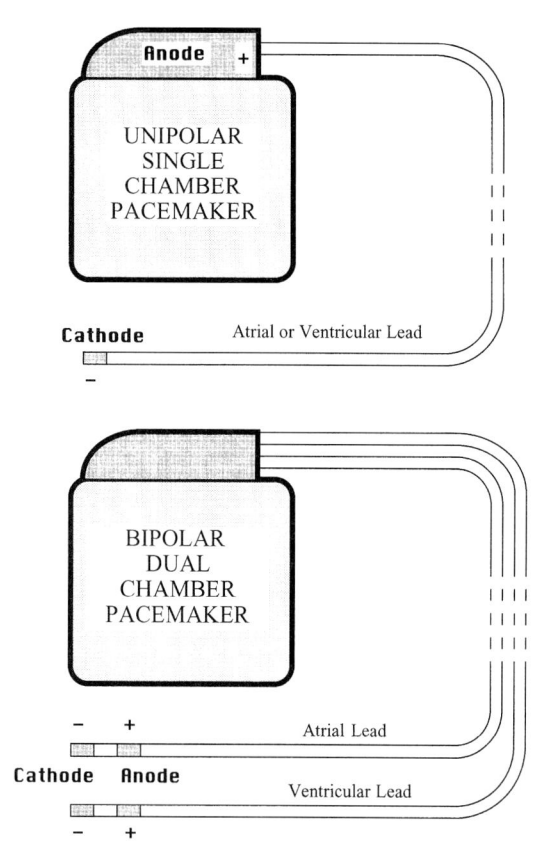

FIGURE 6-1 *Schematic of unipolar single-chamber and bipolar dual-chamber permanent pacing systems. With the unipolar system (top), there is only one lead and one myocardial electrode. The latter serves as cathode and the pacemaker can as anode. Since the unipolar system has only one lead, it can be used only for atrial or ventricular pacing. With the bipolar system (bottom), the distal bipolar electrode serves as cathode and the proximal electrode as anode. One bipolar lead is for atrial sensing and/or pacing, and the other for ventricular sensing and/or pacing.*

stimulus output, are termed *synchronous* pacers. They are also referred to as demand or noncompetitive pacers.

Pacing Rate and Atrioventricular Interval

The *rate* of a pacemaker is the frequency with which it stimulates the heart in the absence of sensed cardiac activity. If the device functions at only one rate, this is the *demand* or *back-up rate*. Synchronous or sensor-modulated (rate-adaptive) pacemakers have some *upper rate* that the pacemaker cannot exceed. That being so, the demand rate can also be referred to as the *lower rate*. Both the demand and upper rate limits are programmable in contemporary pacemakers. The *atrioventricular (AV) interval* in dual-chamber pacemakers is the maximum time interval between atrial and ventricular events. It is initiated by a paced or spontaneous atrial beat. After the predetermined (programmable) AV interval, the ventricular stimulus will be delivered if no prior spontaneous ventricular event has occurred. An optimal AV interval (~150 msec) provides adequate time for atrial systole to augment ventricular filling, which is most important in patients with reduced ventricular compliance. However, in patients with functional retrograde or VA (ventriculoatrial) conduction, a shorter AV interval reduces the risk of retrograde atrial activation and initiation of reentrant SVT.

Escape, Hysteresis, and Demand Intervals

The *escape interval* is the time after a paced or sensed beat that the pacemaker waits before delivering a pacing stimulus. Some pacemakers also have a programmed *hysteresis interval* to maximize the opportunity for continued spontaneous rhythm. It is longer than the escape interval. The *demand interval* determines the rate of paced rhythm, and may be the same as the escape interval. Hysteresis is commonly programmed for patients with sinus node dysfunction and ventricular demand pacemakers, because sinus rhythm is hemodynamically more effective than paced ventricular rhythm (see later discussion). For example, a pacemaker patient with sinus node dysfunction might normally have sinus rates between 50 and 90 beats/min (from Holter recordings) without undue fatigue or symptoms of heart failure, but only rare episodes of symptomatic sinus bradycardia below 50 beats/min. If so, a hysteresis interval would be programmed at 1,500 msec (40 beats/min) in case of a prolonged sinus pause or severe bradycardia. If a spontaneous beat did not occur before 1,500 msec, ventricular pacing would commence at 70 beats/min (Fig. 6–2). Once ventricular pacing commenced, the pacemaker would wait 860 msec (demand interval) before delivering the next pacing stimulus (Fig. 6–2).

Pulse Characteristics

Most pacemakers produce stimuli with constant voltage, typically in the range of 2.5 to 5.0 volts. Current that flows is determined by resistance of the lead and at the electrode–tissue interface. Because

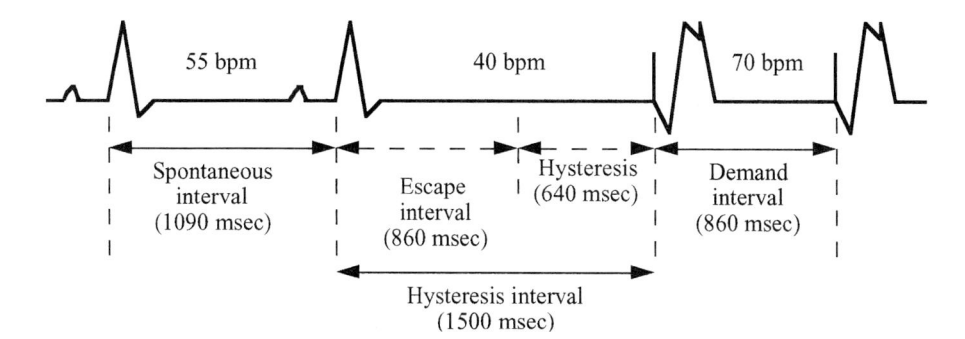

FIGURE 6-2 *Depiction of spontaneous and paced beats with a ventricular demand pacemaker that has been programmed with hysteresis (640 msec). Two spontaneous (sinus) beats at 55 beats/min are followed by sinus pause. The escape and demand intervals are both 860 msec, equivalent to a rate of 70 beats/min. However, 640 msec of hysteresis has been programmed to provide a hysteresis interval of 1,500 msec. This maximizes the opportunity for resumption of sinus rhythm. Since it doesn't, paced rhythm occurs at the demand rate of 70 beats/min.*

there is a component of capacitance at the latter, resistance is more properly referred to as *impedance*. Typically, lead–tissue impedance is in the range of 500 to 700 ohms.[2,3] Pacing pulse widths are commonly 0.5 to 1.5 msec.

Pacing Threshold

The minimum energy required to capture the atria or ventricles is the *pacing threshold*. It may be defined in terms of voltage, current, energy, or pulse width. When programming pacemakers, one goal is to minimize current to prolong battery life. This is done by adjusting pulse width and voltage. When the pacing lead is first implanted, the pacing threshold is measured with a pacing system analyzer, which must be matched by the manufacturer to the particular pacing system. The lowest voltage required for capture at a given pulse width is threshold voltage. Threshold voltage is lowest at implantation, and increases by 600 to 700 percent with solid electrodes, or 100 to 150 percent with steroid-eluting electrodes, over the next 1 to 3 weeks.[2] After 4 to 8 weeks for stabilization, thresholds return to 200 to 300 or 100 percent above initial values for solid and steroid electrodes, respectively.[2] Finally, a number of factors can influence pacing thresholds (Table 6–2).[3,5] However, despite the common notion to the contrary, clinically useful concentrations of inhalation anesthetics are not known to affect

TABLE 6-2 *Factors that can influence pacing thresholds*

INCREASE	DECREASE
Propranolol; verapamil	Exercise; stress
Mineralocorticoids	Glucocorticoids
Potassium and insulin	Potassium alone (brief ↓)
Hypothyroidism	Hyperthyroidism
Antiarrhythmics	Sympathomimetic drugs
Myocardial ischemia	Severe hypoxia

pacing thresholds. However, high systemic concentrations of local anesthetics may increase pacing thresholds.

Sensitivity

The intracardiac electrogram is transmitted to the pacemaker by the pacemaker lead to provide a sensed intracardiac electrogram. Pacemaker *sensitivity,* which is programmable, determines intracardiac electrogram amplitude required for sensing, which in turn causes inhibition or triggering of output. Typical atrial myopotentials range from 1 to 4 mV, and ventricular myopotentials from 4 to 25 mV. If sensitivity is programmed to high, or myopotentials have too low amplitudes, then the pacemaker functions as an *asynchronous* device, because there is no inhibition or triggering of output. Conversely, if sensitivity is programmed too low or myopotentials have too high amplitudes, then there is *inappropriate* inhibition or triggering of output.

Ventricular Refractory Periods

Refractory periods are programmed intervals during which the ventricular sensing circuit is temporarily disabled. In the case of a ventricular sensing pacemaker, the *ventricular (sensing) refractory period* begins with delivery of the ventricular pacing stimulus and continues for about 300 msec (Fig. 6–3). This is to prevent sensing of the T wave or premature beats, which could cause inappropriate inhibition of output. While the design of the ventricular refractory period varies among manufacturers,[6] there is commonly an absolute refractory period during which the pacemaker is nonreceptive to all incoming signals. There may also be a *noise sampling interval* or refractory period during which the frequency of incoming signals is evaluated. If continuous noise is detected (i.e., electrocautery inter-

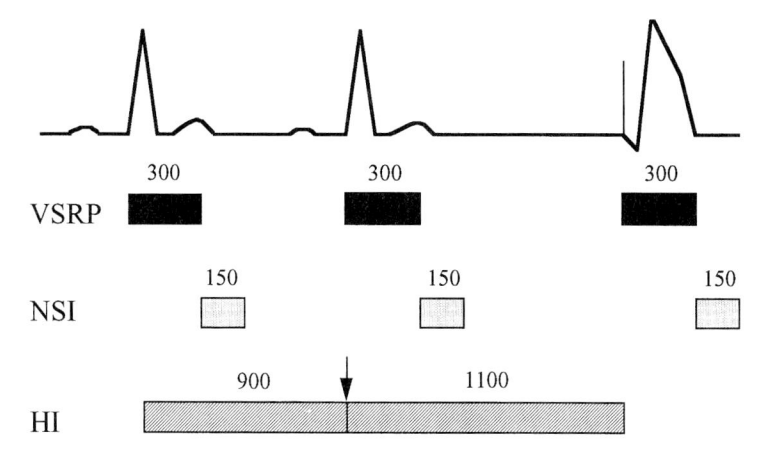

FIGURE 6–3 *Ventricular refractory periods. Shown are two spontaneous beats followed by a paced ventricular beat. The* **ventricular sensing refractory period (VSRP) begins with the R wave and extends to near the end of the T wave. The noise sampling interval (NSI) extends for 150 msec beyond the VSRP. Finally, a hysteresis interval (HI) of 1,100 msec is interrupted at 900 msec (arrow) by a spontaneous beat, thereby resetting this interval. See text for further discussion.**

ference), the pacemaker will pace at its programmed nominal or interference rate.

Dual-Chamber Refractory Periods

With dual-chamber pacemakers, both the atrial and ventricular channels have refractory periods. In addition to the ventricular refractory periods just discussed, it may also be necessary to program a *ventricular blanking refractory period* to prevent the ventricular channel from sensing atrial stimuli, thereby inhibiting ventricular output. This is known as *crosstalk*. The *atrial sensing refractory period* has two components: (1) an *AV interval* (already discussed); and (2) a *postventricular atrial sensing refractory period* initiated by a spontaneous or paced ventricular beat. The latter serves two purposes. First, it prevents sensing of retrograde P waves in patients with intact VA conduction, which could trigger paced ventricular beats and endless-loop tachycardia with some pacemakers (see Chapter 8). Second, it limits the rate of pacemaker-mediated tachycardia, where by atrial tracking, ventricular pacemakers track all atrial depolarizations with supraventricular tachycardia (SVT) (see

Chapter 8). Atrial refractory and blanking periods are illustrated in Figure 6–4.

Programmability and Telemetry

Programmability and telemetry are important features of modern pacemakers, because they permit the implanting physician to diag-

FIGURE 6–4 *Atrial refractory and blanking periods with a dual-chamber pacemaker. The ventricular sensing refractory period and noise sampling interval are omitted. The first beat is spontaneous. With all other beats, one or both chambers are paced. The atrial hysteresis interval (AHI) is 800 msec, and is initiated by a sensed spontaneous or paced ventricular beat. However, its duration is determined by whether or not a spontaneous atrial event (beat 2) occurs. If an atrial event is not sensed by the end of the AHI, atrial pacing occurs (beats 3 and 4). The atrial sensing refractory period (ASRP, 540 msec) includes the AV interval (AVI, 160 or 200 msec) and the postventricular atrial sensing refractory period, which is the difference between the ASRP and AVI. Note that the AVI is longer for the beats 2 and 4 because of AV hysteresis, whereby ventricular stimuli (arrows) are withheld for up to 200 msec to allow for conduction of paced or spontaneous atrial beats. Finally, a blanking period of 40 msec is provided after paced atrial beats to prevent the ventricular channel from sensing paced atrial beats, thereby possibly inhibiting ventricular output.*

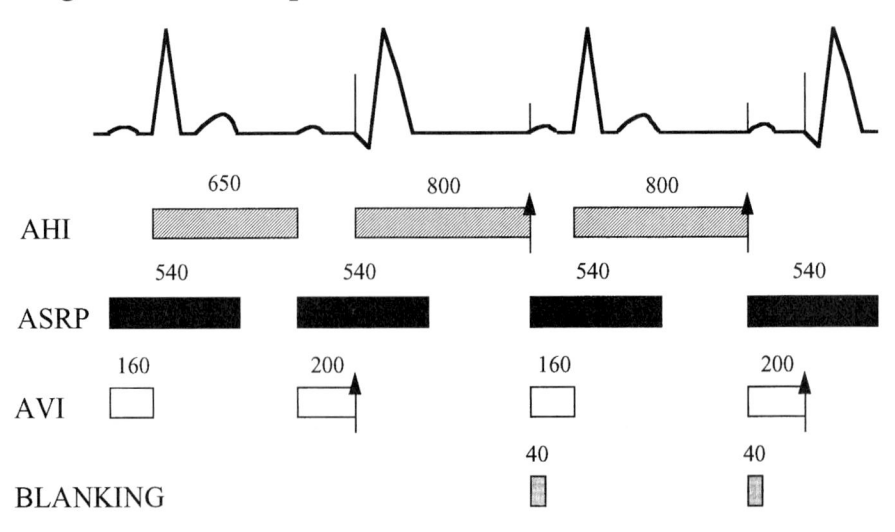

nose and correct many types of pacemaker malfunction noninvasively; that is, without having to resort to surgical pacemaker system revision. Included are over- and undersensing, inappropriate sensing (e.g., T waves, crosstalk), and loss of capture.[4,7,8] These and other types of pacemaker malfunction are discussed in Chapter 8. *Simple programmability* implies the ability to alter at least three of the four basic pacemaker functions: rate, current output, sensitivity, and refractory periods. *Multiprogrammability* implies the ability to alter more than three pacemaker functions, including all four basic functions and pacing mode, rate hysteresis, pulse width, lead polarity, voltage, AV delay, AV hysteresis, blanking period, upper rate limit, lower rate limit, interference modes, and rate-adaptive sensor variables. In short, multiprogrammability affords the implanting physician or pacemaker follow-up clinician the opportunity to tailor the pacemaker system for the individual patient's needs and lifestyle, as well as to accommodate changes in the underlying heart condition during the lifetime of the pacemaker. Radiofrequency signals are almost exclusively used today to communicate between the external programming device ("programmer") and pacemaker, although some devices may still require coded electromagnetic impulses. Another feature that has been incorporated into newer pacemakers is *telemetry*. This permits transcribing data via telephone from the pacemaker to the programmer and vice versa. Telemetered data may consist of current programmed parameters, functional characteristics of the pacemaker, lead impedance, and stored sensed intracardiac electrograms. The addition of telemetry has greatly improved the care of pacemaker patients, because with telemetry it may be possible to diagnose or confirm programmed pacemaker function or suspected malfunction that cannot be diagnosed by electrocardiography (ECG) or are of intermittent nature.

PACEMAKER IDENTIFICATION CODE

A five-position generic code is widely used as shorthand notation to designate pacemaker operation. The five positions are I, chamber paced; II, chamber sensed; III, response to sensed events; IV, programmability and rate responsiveness; and V, antitachycardia function (Table 6–3). To describe pacing modes for bradycardia, most practitioners use only the first three positions. The letter "O" in any position, which means *none* or *not applicable*, was added so that antitachycardia devices with no back-up bradycardia pacing could be described in code. Thus, a single-chamber pacemaker that paces and senses only the ventricle, and responds to sensed events by inhibition of pacing stimuli, would be designated a VVI pacemaker. A single-chamber

TABLE 6-3 *NASPE–BPEG codes to describe pacemaker functions or specify pacing modalities*

I PACING	II SENSING	III RESPONSE	IV PROGRAM- MABILITY	V TACHY- CARDIA
O = None	O = None	O = None	O = None	O = None
A = Atrium	A = Atrium	I = Inhibited	C = Communi- cating	P = Pacing
V = Ventricle	V = Ventricle	T = Triggered	P = S-Program- mable*	S = Shock
D = Dual- chamber	D = Dual- chamber	D = Dual (I, T)†	M = M-Program- mable*	D = Dual (P, S)

NASPE, North American Society of Pacing and Electrophysiology; BPEG, British Pacing and Electrophysiology Group.
*(S-, M-) Programmable, Simple or multiprogrammable; †Dual (I & T), Atrial triggered and ventricular inhibited.

ventricular pacemaker with no sensing would be VOO. Further, if this VVI pacemaker were multiprogrammable (e.g., rate, stimulus characteristics, refractory periods, etc.), it could be designated VVIM.

FIGURE 6-5 *Schematic of single-chamber pacing modes. Shown are the chambers (a, atrium; v, ventricle) paced (P) or sensed (S), as well as the response to sensed events. This could be inhibition (I) or triggering (T) of pacing stimuli. Atrial and ventricular events are identified as spontaneous (SA, SV) or paced (PA, PV). AOO, atrial asynchronous pacing. All atrial beats are baced, regardless of spontaneous atrial beats, and conducted normally to the ventricles. AAI, atrial-inhibited pacing. Sensed atrial events inhibit atrial pacing with the first two beats, but the third atrial beat is paced. All atrial beats are conducted normally to the ventricles. VOO, ventricular asynchronous pacing. All ventricular beats are paced, and bear no relation to spontaneous atrial beats. VVI, ventricular-inhibited pacing. The atrial rhythm is fibrillation and the first two ventricular beats are spontaneous. The third ventricular beat is paced after the programmed escape interval. VAT, atrial-triggered, ventricular pacing. All atrial beats are spontaneous and sensed. Each initiates an AV interval after which a ventricular stimulus will be delivered (second and third beats), unless a normally conducted, spontaneous ventricular beat intervenes (first beat).*

PACING AND CARDIAC ELECTROVERSION **217**

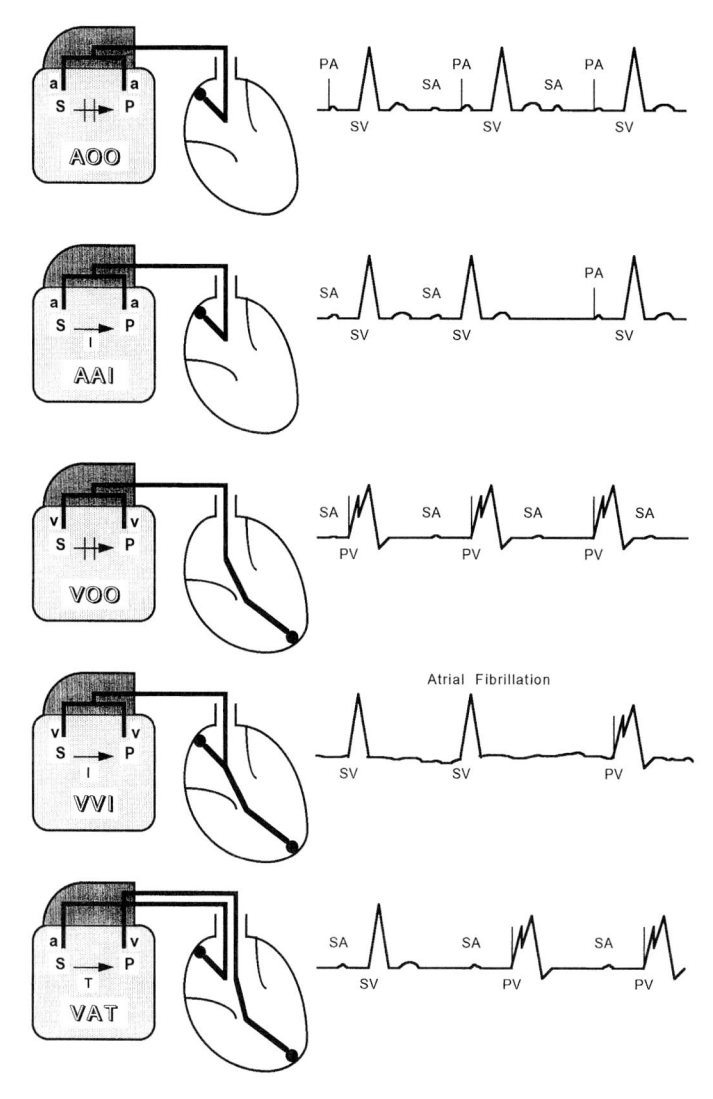

FIGURE 6–5 *See legend on opposite page*

Similarly, a multiprogrammable dual-chamber pacemaker that paced only the ventricle after being triggered by a sensed atrial event would be designated VATM. ICD, which are multiprogrammable but have no back-up bradycardia pacing, are designated OOOMS. An ICD with back-up demand ventricular pacing would be VVIMS, and so forth. However, virtually without exception, most modern pacemakers are multiprogrammable, so that feature can be assumed. Therefore, throughout this chapter and the remainder of the book, we will use only the first three letters of the pacemaker code to simplify matters, except that "R" may be used (VVIR, DDDR) sometimes to designate sensor-driven rate modulation.

PACING MODES FOR BRADYCARDIA

Single-Chamber Modes

Single-chamber pacing modes permit pacing in the atria or ventricles, although there can be sensing in the atria that inhibits or triggers ventricular pacing (Fig. 6–5). *Atrial or ventricular asynchronous* (AOO, VOO) pacing modes are rarely programmed for permanent pacemakers, but are commonly used for temporary pacing applications. *Atrial-inhibited* (AAI) pacing (also, atrial demand or noncompetitive pacing) is preferred for patients with bradycardia when feasible. With this mode, the atria are paced at the demand rate if no spontaneous atrial beats sensed during the atrial escape interval. Spontaneous atrial beats inhibit pacing and reset the timing of the atrial escape interval. The advantage of atrial compared to ventricular pacing is normal AV synchrony and ventricular activation. However, atrial pacing is not feasible with atrial flutter–fibrillation, or even the intermittent occurrence of these arrhythmias. Neither is it feasible in patients with advanced second- or third-degree AV heart block. *Ventricular-inhibited* (VVI) pacing (also, ventricular demand or noncompetitive pacing) is probably still the most commonly prescribed mode of pacing, and the only feasible one in patients with atrial flutter–fibrillation associated with bradycardia. The operation of VVI pacing is similar to that for AAI pacing, except that sensing and pacing take place in the ventricle. With *atrial-triggered ventricular* (VAT) pacing (also, atrial synchronous or tracking pacing), sensed atrial beats always trigger paced ventricular beats after the programmed AV interval (i.e., a "committed" response). This mode may be prescribed in patients with AV heart block, normal sinus node function, and little likelihood of atrial tachyarrhythmias.

Dual-Chamber Modes

Dual-chamber pacing modes permit both sensing and pacing with triggering and inhibition in one or both heart chambers (Fig. 6–6). *Dual-sequential asynchronous* (DOO) pacing (also, AV sequential asynchronous or fixed-rate pacing) is rarely programmed, except for temporary pacing applications. *Atrial-triggered, ventricular-inhibited* (VDD) pacing (also, atrial synchronous or tracking pacing) is similar to VAT pacing (Fig. 6–5), except that there is also sensing in the ventricles. As with VAT pacing, a sensed atrial event triggers ventricular pacing after a programmed AV interval. However, a sensed ventricular event during the AV interval inhibits ventricular pacing by resetting the demand interval (i.e., a "noncommitted" response). With *dual-sequential, ventricular-inhibited* (DVI) pacing (also, AV sequential demand pacing), there is pacing in both the atria and ventricles, but sensing only in the ventricle. Pacing in the atria occurs at the programmed demand rate, irrespective of spontaneous atrial activity. Pacing in the ventricle occurs after the programmed AV interval, but a sensed ventricular event within that interval inhibits delivery of the ventricular pacing stimulus. The principal disadvantage of the DVI pacemaker is the possibility of atrial competition and AV dyssynchrony if the patient's spontaneous atrial rate is faster than the paced or spontaneous ventricular rate. To achieve more effective AV synchronization with a DVI pacemaker, it is necessary to program the atrial demand rate faster than the patient's normal atrial rate to overdrive the spontaneous atrial rate. A useful modification of the DVI mode has been *dual-sequential, atrial–ventricular-inhibited* (DDD pacing) (also, dual-chamber, sequential demand pacing), in which the pacemaker also functions at a fixed rate but atrial sensing is added. Unlike DVI pacing, both atrial and ventricular events, are sensed during DDI pacing, so that it does not compete with spontaneous atrial beats when the patient's atrial rate exceeds the programmed demand rate. Finally, the most sophisticated pacing mode is *dual-chamber sequential, atrial-triggered–ventricular-inhibited* (DDD) pacing (also, AV universal pacing). The DDD pacer actually functions in one of two modes, depending on whether or not atrial activity is present at the programmed lower (demand) rate of the pacemaker. At this lower rate limit, in the absence of sensed spontaneous atrial activity, the pacemaker functions in the DVI mode. When atrial activity faster than the lower rate interval is detected, the pacemaker functions in the VAT mode (Fig. 6–5). The pacemaker continues to function in this mode up to the programmed upper rate limit, so as to avoid one-to-one tracking of noncompensatory atrial tachycardia. There are a number of ways this can be achieved (including pseudo-Wenckebach upper-rate behavior, fixed-ratio AV block, fallback, rate smoothing), which vary

220 PACING AND CARDIAC ELECTROVERSION

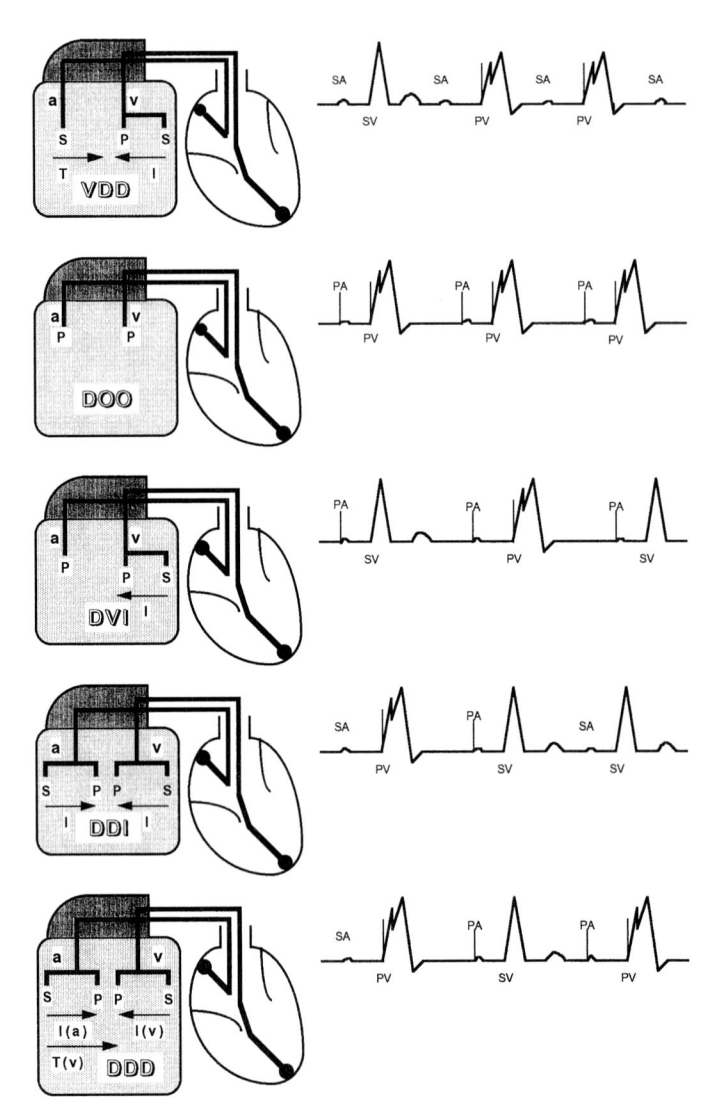

FIGURE 6–6 *See legend on opposite page*

among pacemaker devices and are beyond the scope of this discussion.[3,9] Generic codes for dual-chamber and single-chamber pacing modalities are summarized in Table 6-4.

PACING FOR TACHYARRHYTHMIAS

Temporary Pacing

Temporary pacing for tachycardia includes pacing to prevent bradycardia-dependent tachyarrhythmias and special pacing techniques to terminate reentrant tachyarrhythmias.[3,10-13] In patients

---

FIGURE 6-6 *Schematic of dual-chamber pacing modes. Shown are the chambers (a, atrium; v, ventricle) paced (P) or sensed (S), as well as the response to sensed events. This could be inhibition (I) or triggering (T) of pacing stimuli. Atrial and ventricular events are identified as spontaneous (SA, SV) or paced (PA, PV). VDD, atrial-triggered, ventricular-inhibited pacing. Atrial sensing will trigger ventricular pacing after the programmed AV interval (second and third beats) unless a spontaneous, sensed ventricular beat occurs (first beat). DOO, dual-sequential asynchronous pacing. All atrial and ventricular beats are paced. There is no sensing in either chamber. DVI, dual-sequential inhibited pacing. All atrial beats are paced, and initiate an AV interval after which a ventricular stimulus is delivered (second beat) unless spontaneous ventricular beats are sensed and inhibit ventricular pacing (first and third beats). DDI, dual-chamber, sequential demand pacing. Sensed, spontaneous atrial beats (first and third) inhibit atrial pacing. They do not trigger ventricular pacing. Instead, ventricular pacing is controlled by the programmed escape and demand intervals of the ventricular channel. If a spontaneous ventricular beat does not occur within this interval (second and third beats), then ventricular pacing will occur (first beat). The second atrial beat is paced since a spontaneous atrial beat does not occur within the programmed atrial escape (demand) interval. DDD, dual-sequential, atrial-triggered, ventricular-inhibited or AV universal pacing. Sensed (first) and paced atrial (second and third) beats trigger ventricular pacing (first and third beats) after the programmed AV interval, provided a spontaneous ventricular beat does not occur (second beat) to inhibit ventricular pacing. Atrial pacing is also inhibited by sensed atrial events (first beat).*

TABLE 6-4 *Generic codes for single- and dual-chamber pacing modalities*

AOO, VOO, DOO	Atrial asynchronous, ventricular asynchronous, or dual-sequential asynchronous pacing
AAI, VVI, DVI	Atrial-inhibited, ventricular-inhibited, or dual-sequential ventricular-inhibited pacing
VAT or VDD	Atrial-triggered ventricular, or atrial-triggered, ventricular-inhibited pacing
DDI or DDD	Dual-sequential, atrial–ventricular-inhibited, or dual-sequential, atrial-triggered–ventricular inhibited pacing

with sinus node dysfunction (SND) and bradycardia-dependent atrial tachyarrhythmias, atrial pacing to increase heart rate may prevent tachyarrhythmias. In patients with cardiomyopathies, bradycardia can increase dispersion of ventricular refractoriness, furthering possible predisposition to reentrant ventricular tachycardia (VT). In patients with acquired or congenital QT-interval prolongation and torsades de pointes VT, bradycardia promotes abnormalities of repolarization and refractoriness, thereby increasing the likelihood of torsades de pointes VT. Pacing to increase heart rate may oppose recurrences of torsades de pointes VT. Pacing to terminate reentrant tachyarrhythmias requires properly timed premature stimuli (extrastimulation), trains of rapid stimuli (burst pacing), or pacing at a rate in excess of the tachycardia (overdrive pacing). These methods are explained in Chapter 7 under Pacing for Specific Tachyarrhythmias. Paroxysmal (reentrant) SVT, slow atrial flutter (atrial rate ≤ 340 beats/min), and slow monomorphic VT are the arrhythmias most likely to be terminated by pacing, provided they are reasonably well tolerated and there is adequate time for attempts at pacing conversion. Otherwise, tachycardia is best terminated by DC cardioversion. Other tachyarrhythmias are not treated by pacing.

Implanted Pacemakers

Pacing with permanent devices for prevention or termination of tachycardia is feasible, but used in only small numbers of patients, perhaps only 1 percent of all pacemaker implants.[3,10] This is mostly due to the fact that catheter ablation or surgical treatment is curative in up to 95 percent of patients with tachyarrhythmias that might formally have been considered for long-term pacing therapy. Otherwise, ICD are more reliable for termination of tachycardia. The success of antitachycardia pacing is highly dependent on the accuracy of the detection algorithm. Only when drug therapy is ineffective or not tolerated, the patient has undergone unsuccessful curative ablation treatment or surgery, or such treatment is refused or contraindicated is a permanent antitachycardia pacemaker considered. Antitachycardia pacing for SVT has primarily been for termination AV nodal or AV reentry (i.e., AV node with accessory pathway). While up to 85 percent of patients initially have a favorable response, only 60 to 80 percent of pacemaker systems are effective at 5 years, and 40 to 50 percent of patients still require drugs.[3] Some slow VT is amenable to termination by pacing, but only with ICD backup. Fast VT requires a more aggressive pacing protocol associated with a greater incidence of acceleration and degeneration into ventricular fibrillation (VF). About 70 percent of patients will at least initially have a favorable response to pacing for VT.[3]

Physiologic Pacing: The Hemodynamics of Pacing

A physiologic pacemaker attempts to preserve normal synchrony between the atria and ventricles, as well as to adapt the heart rate to meet increased body needs with exercise or stress compared to rest. The earliest pacemakers were by no means physiologic, but refinements in component and sensor technology, as well as circuit miniaturization, have made physiologic pacing feasible in many patients with permanent pacemakers. Contemporary temporary pacing pulse generators make physiologic pacing possible for temporary pacing applications as well.[14-16]

HEMODYNAMICS OF PACING

Atrial Function

The importance of atrial function to ventricular filling was appreciated in the 17th century by William Harvey, but not experimentally confirmed until the early 20th century by Gesell.[13] Gesell demonstrated that properly timed atrial systoles could increase ventricular stroke volume by as much as 50 percent, and that randomly associated systoles produced large beat-to-beat fluctuations in systolic blood pressure. The atrial contribution to ventricular filling is both active (atrial systole) and passive (initial rapid then slow ventricular filling).[4,13,17] This means that both the *force of atrial contraction* and *atrial compliance* affect ventricular filling and stroke

TABLE 6-5 *Function of properly synchronized atrial systoles*

Atrial systole is important for normal mitral valve function.
Permit optimal LV filling without high mean LA pressure.
Fiber stretch just before systole augments LV stroke volume.

LV, left ventricular; LA, left atrial.

volume. Properly timed atrial systole, or *AV synchrony*, provides several important functions (Table 6–5). Low atrial compliance (increased stiffness) also has an important effect on ventricular filling, since it impedes venous return and limits the increase in levels of peak and mean atrial pressure during passive ventricular filling.[17] Low atrial compliance can result from chronic valvular insufficiency, chronic atrial fibrillation, intrinsic atrial disease, and chronic pacing with modes that do not preserve AV synchrony.

Ventricular Function

It is now widely appreciated that *ventricular diastolic dysfunction* can give rise to heart failure independent of decreased systolic function. Diastolic dysfunction is defined as a restriction to filling of one or both ventricles, and can be due to impaired active relaxation or reduced compliance and passive filling. Ventricular diastolic dysfunction occurs with cardiomyopathies (e.g., ischemic, dilated, hypertrophic) and the aging process itself. Because impaired active relaxation and reduced compliance (stiff ventricle) both impede passive atrial filling, patients with ventricular diastolic dysfunction are more dependent on atrial systole for adequate ventricular filling. Indeed, properly timed atrial systole may contribute as much as 30 to 40 percent to end-diastolic volume and cardiac output at rest in these patients.[3] Clinical confirmation of this is observation of the effect of AV junctional rhythm on arterial blood pressure in patients with presumed normal or abnormal ventricular diastolic function (Fig. 6–7). Indeed, we have observed more than doubling of cardiac output with atrial pacing for treatment of AV junctional rhythm in patients with ischemic cardiomyopathy.[18]

PHYSIOLOGIC PACING MODES

There are two requirements for physiologic pacing: (1) AV synchronization for optimum ventricular filling and to prevent valvular insufficiency in patients with retrograde atrial activation during ventricular pacing; and (2) the ability to increase heart rate to meet increased

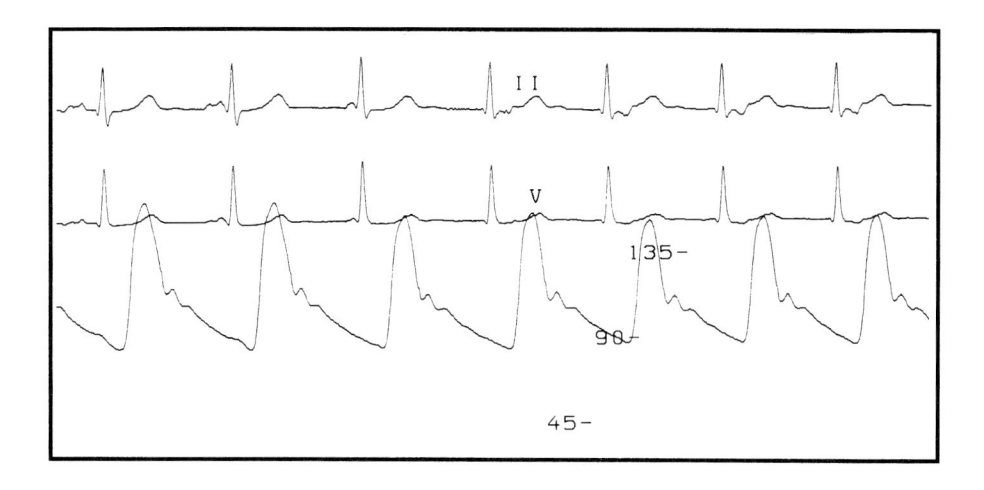

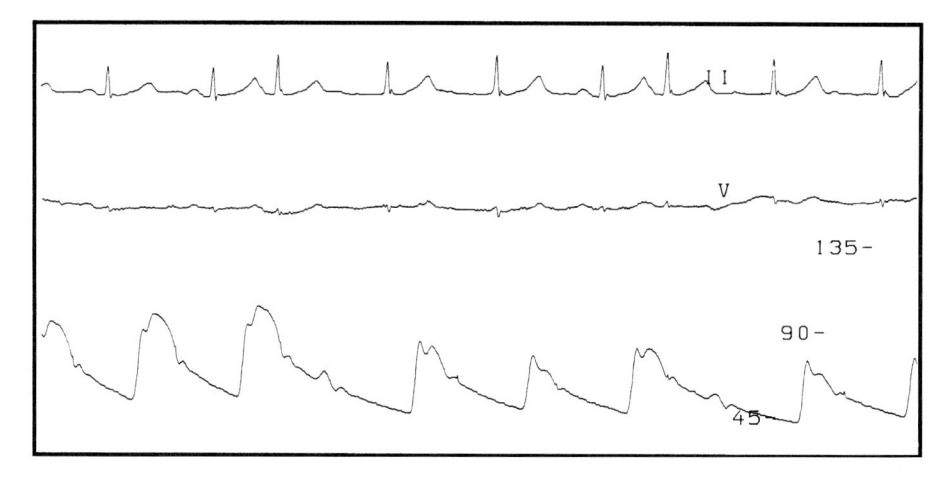

FIGURE 6–7 (Top) *Hemodynamic changes with AV junctional rhythm in a patient with presumed normal ventricular diastolic function. Note approximate 10-mmHg decrease in systolic blood pressure. (Bottom) Elderly patient with hypertensive and ischemic cardiomyopathy undergoing right thoracotomy. ECG V lead placed on back. Intermittent AV junctional rhythm coincided with dissection adjacent to the pericardium, and caused an approximate 35-mmHg decrease in systolic blood pressure. The decrease in systolic blood pressure with junctional rhythm at other times during the case varied from 25 to 50 mmHg, presumably because of minute-to-minute changes in intravascular volume and venous return.*

physical or metabolic needs, or rate responsiveness.[3,4,19] Provision of physiologic pacing can improve the quality of life and reduce morbidity, and may even increase survival in patients with physiologic permanent pacing systems.[4,19-21] However, it remains to be shown whether physiologic pacing modes can improve outcomes or reduce requirements for other types of circulatory support (drugs or devices) in surgical or critical care patients who require temporary pacing.

Atrioventricular Synchrony

Pacing modes that preserve AV synchrony include any that pace the atria—AOO, AAI, DOO, DVI, DDI, DDD—or in which sensing of spontaneous atrial events triggers ventricular pacing—VAT, VDD, DDD (Figs. 6-5 and 6-6). Any of these "physiologic" pacing modes avoids potential disadvantages of single-chamber ventricular pacing: reduced stroke volume, and cardiac output, AV valvular insufficiency, beat-to-beat variations in systemic arterial pressure, predisposition to reentrant tachycardia with functional retrograde (VA) conduction, and symptoms of the *pacemaker syndrome*.[3,4,19] Symptoms of the latter consist of weakness, fatigue, lassitude, apprehension, cough, exercise intolerance, pulsations in the abdomen or neck, dizziness, near-syncope, syncope, dyspnea, cold extremities, and other manifestations of low cardiac output, including congestive heart failure. The worst symptoms of the pacemaker syndrome occur in patients with functional VA conduction, in which paced ventricular beats result in atrial contraction after ventricular systole. Besides the loss of atrial synchronization, cannon A waves produced by atrial systole against closed AV valves activate vasomotor reflexes and create unpleasant sensations in some patients. Patients at greatest risk of adverse effects from single-chamber ventricular pacing are those with functional VA conduction or impaired ventricular diastolic function.

Rate Responsiveness

In patients with sinus node chronotropic competence (i.e., sinus rate can increase to meet increased metabolic needs) and without atrial fibrillation, pacing modes that track atrial activity (VAT, VDD, DDD) will provide physiologic pacing. The major limitation to use of these modes is the possibility of one-to-one tracking of noncompensatory sinus tachycardia or other nonphysiologic SVT, although this can be ameliorated by programming an upper rate limit for ventricular pacing. While the sinus node with chronotropic competence is the best physiologic sensor, in patients with SND, especially those with the bradycardia-tachycardia syndrome (see Chapter 9), sensor-modulated, rate-adaptive pacing is prescribed. Possible sensing algorithms for sensor-modulated pacing were listed in Table 6-1.

Pacing Indications

In a nutshell, temporary or permanent pacing is indicated for any symptomatic or hemodynamically disadvantageous bradycardia (defined later), whether due to SND or AV heart block. Pacing may also be effective for some reentrant tachyarrhythmias. Temporary pacing is used for urgent treatment and as a bridge to permanent pacing. Permanent pacing is prescribed for chronic symptomatic arrhythmias.

PERMANENT PACING INDICATIONS

Definition of Symptomatic or Disadvantageous Bradycardia

Symptomatic or *disadvantageous bradycardia* refers to manifestations of cerebral insufficiency attributable to slow heart rate (transient dizziness, light-headedness, near syncope, or frank syncope), or to more generalized symptoms such as severe exercise intolerance or congestive heart failure.[22] Hemodynamically disadvantageous bradycardia in unconscious patients is bradycardia that compromises vital organ perfusion through inadequate cardiac output or reduced perfusion pressure.

Indications for Implantation of Pacemakers or Antitachycardia Devices

INDICATIONS AND DEFINITIONS. The American College of Cardiology/American Heart Association Task Force Committee on Pacemaker Implantation has grouped indications for permanent pacemakers and antitachycardia devices into three classes: *class I*, conditions for which there is general agreement that permanent pacemakers or antitachycardia devices should be implanted; *class II*, conditions for which permanent pacemakers or antitachycardia devices are frequently used, but about which there is divergence of opinion with respect to the necessity of their insertion; and *class III*, conditions for which there is general agreement that pacemakers or antitachycardia devices are unnecessary.[22,23] Indications for implantation of permanent bradycardia pacemakers in adults and children, as well antitachycardia pacing devices, are summarized in Tables 6–6, 6–7, and 6–8.[22] AV heart block is defined as follows: (1) first-degree AV block is PR-interval prolongation without dropped beats; (2) type I (Wenckebach) second-degree AV block is increasing PR-interval prolongation with dropped beats; (3) type II (Mobitz) second-degree AV block is intermittent dropped beats without PR-interval prolongation; (4) advanced second-degree AV block is two or more successive dropped beats with some conducted beats; and (5) third-degree or

TABLE 6-6 *Indications for implantation of permanent pacemakers for bradycardia in adults*

ACQUIRED AV HEART BLOCK*

Class I: Permanent or intermittent third-degree block with symptomatic bradycardia or congestive heart failure. Ectopic rhythms or medical conditions requiring bradycardic drugs. Asystole ≥ 3.0 second or escape rate < 40 beats/min without symptoms. Post AV junctional ablation, or myotonic dystrophy. Type I or II, second-degree AV block with symptomatic bradycardia. Atrial flutter–fibrillation or SVT with advanced second or third-degree AV block and symptomatic bradycardia not due to drugs.

Class II: Asymptomatic third-degree AV block with rates > 40 beats/min. Asymptomatic type II, second-degree AV block. Asymptomatic type I, second-degree AV block at or below the common (His) bundle.

Class III: Asymptomatic first-degree AV block. Type I, second-degree AV block at the AV node.

AV BLOCK AFTER MYOCARDIAL INFARCTION

Class I: Persistent advanced second- or third-degree AV block with block in the His–Purkinje system. Patients with transient advanced second-degree AV block and bundle branch block.

Class II: Patients with persistent advanced second-degree AV block at the AV node.

Class III: Transient AV conduction disturbances without intraventricular conduction defects. Transient AV block with isolated left anterior hemoblock, or the latter without AV block. Persistent first-degree AV block in the presence of bundle branch block not demonstrated previously.

CHRONIC BIFASCICULAR AND TRIFASCICULAR BLOCK*

Class I: Bifascicular or trifascicular block with intermittent third-degree AV block and symptomatic bradycardia or intermittent type II, second-degree AV block with symptoms attributable to heart block.

Class II: Bifascicular or trifascicular block with syncope that cannot be attributed to third-degree AV block or other causes. Prolonged HV interval† (≥ 100 msec) or pacing-induced infra-His block.

Class III: Fascicular block (± first-degree AV block) without type II second-degree AV block or symptoms.

SINUS NODE DYSFUNCTION

Class I: SND wth documented symptomatic bradycardia, including that consequent to chronic, essential drug therapy for which there are not acceptable alternatives.

Class II: Spontaneous or drug-induced SND with heart rates ≤ 40 beats/min when there is no clear association between symptoms of bradycardia and the occurrence of bradycardia.

Class III: SND without symptoms, including with heart rates ≤ 40 beats/min or drug-induced. SND in patients with symptoms suggestive of bradycardia, but shown not due to bradycardia.

TABLE 6-6 *Indications for implantation of permanent pacemakers for bradycardia in adults* Continued

HYPERSENSITIVE CAROTID SINUS AND NEUROVASCULAR SYNDROMES

Class I: Recurrent syncope associated with clear, spontaneous events provoked by carotid sinus stimulation. Minimal carotid sinus pressure induces asystole > 3 seconds in the absence of drugs that depress sinus or AV node function.

Class II: Recurrent syncope without clear, provocative events, and with a hypersensitive cardioinhibitory response. Syncope with associated bradycardia reproduced by provocative maneuvers (e.g., head-up tilt ± isoproterenol), and in which temporary pacing and a second provocative test establish the likely benefits of permanent pacing.

Class III: Hyperactive cardioinhibitory response with or without vague symptoms such as dizziness or light-headedness or both. Recurrent syncope, dizziness, light-headedness in the absence of a cardoinhibitory response.

*AV, intraventricular, and fascicular heart block are defined in text. †HV interval, onset of His deflection to beginning of ventricular electrogram in His bundle electrogram (see Fig. 2–1). (Adapted from Dreifus et al.,[22] with permission.) See text for additional discussion.

complete AV block is no conducted beats from the atrium. *Intraventricular heart block* is the term used to denote conduction block within or anywhere below the common (His) bundle, and fascicular heart block to denote conduction block occurring the right bundle branch or the two major divisions of the left bundle branch (Fig. 6–8). In patients being considered for permanent pacing devices, the decision to implant the device might also be influenced by other factors (Table 6–9).[22]

CLARIFICATION. Some of the categories of pacing indications listed Table 6–6 require further explanation.[22] For patients with *AV block after myocardial infarction* (Table 6–6), pacing indications are related primarily to the presence of intraventricular conduction disturbances, and not necessarily to the presence of symptoms. Also, the need for temporary pacing with acute myocardial infarction does not by itself constitute an indication for permanent pacing. Although complete heart block is most often preceded by *bifascicular block*, the evidence is impressive that the rate of progression to complete heart block is quite low. Further, no single clinical or laboratory variable, including bifascicular block, identifies patients at high risk of death from future bradycardia due to bundle branch block. Some investigators suggest that asymptomatic patients with bifascicular block and HV-interval (His–Purkinje conduction time, Fig. 2–1) prolonga-

TABLE 6-7 *Indications for pacing in children with bradycardia or AV heart block*

CLASS I INDICATIONS

1. Second- or third-degree AV heart block, or SND, with symptomatic bradycardia.
2. Advanced second- or third-degree AV block with moderate exercise intolerance.
3. Congenital AV block and wide QRS escape rhythm or intraventricular block.
4. Advanced second- or third-degree AV block 10 to 14 days following cardiac surgery.

CLASS II INDICATIONS

1. Brady–tachy syndrome if digitalis or phenytoin does not control arrhythmias.
2. Second- or third-degree AV block within common bundle in asymptomatic patient.
3. Transient surgical second- or third-degree AV block that reverts to bifascicular block.
4. Asymptomatic second- or third-degree AV block and ventricular rate < 45 beats/min (awake).
5. Complete AV block with average ventricular rate < 50 beats/min (awake).
6. Asymptomatic neonate, congenital third-degree AV block and bradycardia.*
7. Complex ventricular arrhythmias with second- or third-degree AV block or sinus bradycardia.
8. Congenital long-QT syndrome for prophylaxis of torsades de pointes VT.

CLASS III INDICATIONS

1. Asymptomatic, postoperative bifascicular block with or without first-degree AV block.
2. Transient surgical AV block that returns to normal conduction in < 1 week.
3. Asymptomatic congenital heart block without profound bradycardia.*

See text for further discussion. *Bradycardia in relation to normal values for children with congenital heart block and same age. (Adapted from Dreifus et al.,[22] with permission.)

tion ≥ 100 msec be considered for prophylactic permanent pacing. However, while the prevalence of prolonged HV is high, the incidence of progression to complete heart block is low. Also, while HV prolongation accompanies most advanced heart disease and is asso-

TABLE 6-8 *Indications for permanent antitachyarrhythmia pacing devices*

DEVICES THAT AUTOMATICALLY DETECT AND PACE TO TERMINATE TACHYCARDIAS
Class I: Symptomatic recurrent SVT when drugs fail to control the arrhythmia or produce intolerable side effects, and catheter or surgical ablation failed or refused. Symptomatic recurrent VT with ICD back-up if recurrent VT is not prevented by drugs and no other therapy is available. *Class II:* Pacing for recurrent SVT in place of drugs or other treatment. *Class III:* Tachycardias that accelerate/convert to fibrillation with pacing.
EXTERNAL, MANUALLY ACTIVATED DEVICES TO TERMINATE TACHYCARDIA
Class I: Recurrent symptomatic VT uncontrolled by drugs when surgery, catheter ablation or ICD/automatic device implantation is not indicated. *Class III:* Recurrent SVT or VT that produces syncope.
OVERDRIVE OR ATRIAL SYNCHRONOUS PACEMAKERS TO PREVENT TACHYCARDIA
Class I: AV or AV node reentrant SVT not responsive to medical therapy. *Class II:* Sustained VT if other therapies are ineffective or inapplicable and efficacy of pacing is thoroughly documented. Long-QT syndrome. *Class III:* Frequent or complex ventricular ectopy without sustained VT associated with coronary artery disease, cardiomyopathy, mitral valve prolapse, or abnormal heart in the absence of the long-QT syndrome. Long-QT syndrome due to remediable causes.

See text for further discussion. (Adapted from Dreifus et al.,[22] with permission.)

ciated with increased mortality, death is not sudden and is due to the underlying disease rather than to complete heart block. *Sinus node dysfunction* (sick sinus syndrome) constitutes a wide spectrum of arrhythmias, including sinus bradycardia, sinus pause or arrest, sinoatrial block, paroxysms of SVT (including atrial flutter–fibrillation), and paroxysmal SVT with bradycardia (bradycardia–tachycardia syndrome). For pacing to be indicated, it is necessary that symptoms be correlated with specific arrhythmias, but this may be difficult because of the intermittent nature of arrhythmias. Also, resting sinus bradycardia ≤ 50 beats/min, or rates of 30 to 40 beats/min with type I, second-degree AV block producing asystolic intervals of nearly 2 seconds while asleep, is common in trained athletes. The *hypersensitive carotid sinus syndrome* is defined as syncope resulting from an exaggerated, reflex response to carotid

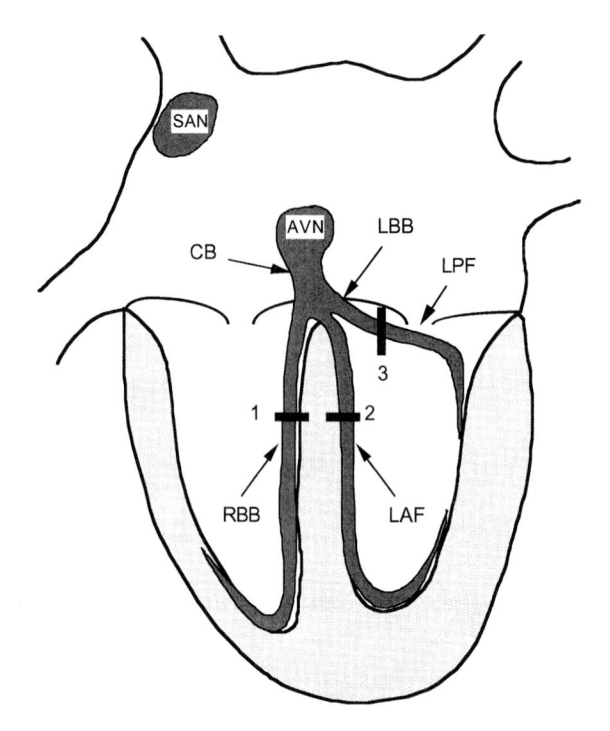

FIGURE 6-8 *Intraventricular heart block. Intraventricular block can occur anywhere below the AV node (AVN), including the common bundle (CB), left or right bundle branch (LBB, RBB), the left anterior and posterior fascicles (LAF, LPF), the distal His–Purkinje network, or ventricular myocardium itself.* **Fascicular heart block** *refers to conduction block in the RBB (1), LAF (2), or LPF (3). Block within any two of these fascicles (e.g., RBB-LAF, RBB-LPF, or LBB) is bifascicular block. Trifascicular block is usually considered synonymous with complete heart block, although the term is sometimes used to denote block of the septal branch of the LAF (not shown) with any two of the other three fascicles.*

sinus stimulation. There are two components to the reflex: (1) *cardioinhibitory*, vagally mediated slowing of sinus rate or PR-interval prolongation and advanced AV block, alone or in combination; and (2) *vasodepressor*, vasodilation with hypotension due to reduced sympathetic tone. Before permanent pacemaker implantation, it is necessary to determine the relative contribution of both components to the patient's symptoms. A hyperactive response to carotid sinus stimulation is defined as asystole due to sinus arrest or AV block > 3 seconds, a substantial symptomatic decrease in blood pressure, or both.

TABLE 6-9 *Additional factors that can influence the decision to implant a pacemaker*

1. Overall physical and mental status of the patient, including associated diseases that may result in a limited quality or prognosis for life. Desires of the patient and family.
2. Presence of underlying structural heart disease that may be affected adversely by bradycardia (e.g., dilated cardiomyopathy).
3. Desire of the patient to operate a motor vehicle or the need to use hazardous tools and operate machinery.
4. Remoteness of medical care, including patients who travel widely or live alone who therefore may be unable to seek medical help if serious symptoms arise.
5. Necessity for administering medication that may depress escape heart rates or aggravate AV heart block. Slowing of basic escape rates due to whatever cause.
6. Significant cerebrovascular disease that might result in a stroke if cerebral perfusion were to suddenly decrease.

(Adapted from Dreifus et al.,[22] with permission.)

PACING IN CHILDREN. Although the indications for pacing in children (Table 6–7) are similar to those in adults, there are some special considerations.[22] As in adults, concurrence of symptoms with bradycardia provides the optimal indication for pacemaker implantation. Such concurrence may be determined by Holter monitoring or transtelephonic electrocardiography. SND is not by itself an indication for pacing, and even greater emphasis than in adults is placed on the concurrence of specific arrhythmias related to SND with symptoms. Alternative causes for symptoms, including seizures, breath-holding, infantile apnea, and dysautonomia, must be excluded. Finally, the bradycardia–tachycardia (brady–tachy) syndrome is frequently an indication for pacing in children, particularly when antiarrhythmic drugs other than digitalis must be prescribed. The use of quinidine, other class 1 drugs, amiodarone, and propranolol is especially dangerous in children with the brady–tachy syndrome. Any can severely depress SA node function, and their use may necessitate pacing in children with the brady–tachy syndrome.

ANTITACHYCARDIA PACING. The decision to implant a pacemaker for control of tachyarrhythmias is made only after careful observation and electrophysiologic study.[22] Potential recipients of these devices should undergo extensive electrophysiologic testing before implantation to ensure that the device can reliably terminate tachycardia without accelerating it or causing fibrillation. Candidates for antitachycardia pacing (Table 6–8) usually have been unresponsive to antiarrhythmic drug therapy, do not tolerate such drugs, and are not suitable for or refuse catheter or surgical ablation therapy. Reentrant SVT or VT may be interrupted by a variety of pacing techniques, including programmed extrastimulation, overdrive pacing, or short bursts of rapid pacing. Antitachycardia pacemakers may automatically detect tachycardia and initiate a pacing sequence, or they may respond only after external instruction. This could be the application of a magnet.

TEMPORARY PACING INDICATIONS

Temporary pacing indications for bradycardia among anesthesia and critical care practitioners vary greatly, and depend to a large extent on the type of equipment available, familiarity with use, how aggressive the practitioner is with use of invasive pacing, and the type of practice. Thus, a cardiothoracic and vascular anesthesiologist intensivist is more likely than the generalist to be familiar with and routinely use temporary transvenous or epicardial pacing in his or her practice. While noninvasive transcutaneous indirect ventricular pacing is available, it is not always feasible, effective or hemodynamically advantageous for patients with bradyarrhythmias (see Chapter 7). However, noninvasive transesophageal pacing overcomes many of the obstacles of invasive or transcutaneous pacing (see Chapter 7), and will undoubtedly see increasing use in the years to come. If so, indications for temporary pacing will evolve considerably from those today.

Indications for pacing during anesthesia and surgery or in critical care units, collectively "perioperative settings," might also be considered as class I, II, and III. These have similar meaning to the three classes of indications for permanent pacemakers, except that rather than a consensus recommendation, (has yet to be formulated) they are based on the author's experience, perception of current anesthesia and critical care practice, and available technology.

Perioperative Temporary Pacing Indications

CLASS I PACING INDICATIONS. Any class I indication for permanent pacing in patients with bradycardia should be considered a class I indication for temporary pacing in patients without a pacemaker and facing anesthesia and surgery or in intensive care units. Multiple causes for physiologic imbalance under these circumstances have recognized potential to aggravate bradycardia and bradycardia-dependent arrhythmias.[24] Temporary pacing may be required before implantation of a permanent pacing system to stabilize patients with bradycardia, since it is preferred to perform the implantation under controlled circumstances.[22]

CLASS II PACING INDICATIONS. Hemodynamically disadvantageous bradycardia in perioperative settings should be considered a class II indication, since while drugs are commonly employed, they are not necessarily safe, reliable, or efficient for increasing the rate of automaticity in the SA node or latent pacemakers, or improving AV conduction with heart block (e.g., Tables 1–8 and 5–12). Also, the probability of using pacing for disadvantageous bradycardia will depend on the whether pacing is feasible, equipment availability, and operator familiarity. If the patient already has a pacing catheter or wires, or if transesophageal pacing is feasible, pacing is definitely preferred to drugs. However, transcutaneous pacing, which may not even be practical or effective, is not preferred to drugs because it is a nonphysiologic pacing mode. If drugs have failed and no other pacing means is available, transcutaneous pacing may be life-saving and should be attempted. Another class 2 indication is the prophylactic use of epicardial pacing wires following cardiac surgery for prevention of tachyarrhythmias and overdrive pacing for ectopic rhythms.[11] While a routine practice in some centers, it is not in others.

CLASS III PACING INDICATIONS. Class III indications include prophylactic invasive pacing for the patient with asymptomatic or minimally symptomatic SND based on the assumption that the patient is likely to develop drug-induced hemodynamic instability with bradycardia.[18,25] Similarly, patients with bifascicular block have never been shown likely to develop higher block during anesthesia and surgery, so they should not require prophylactic pacing without evidence of symptoms due to bradycardia. However, with increasing availability of noninvasive, disposable transesophageal pacing products, either of these groups of patients might be considered as having a class II indication for routine prophylactic temporary pacing. Further, prophylactic transesophageal atrial pacing might come to be used in patients with dilated cardiomyopathy or heart failure to optimize hemodynamic profiles.

Cardiac Electroversion

The term *electroversion* includes both direct current (DC) cardioversion and defibrillation. Both techniques use high-energy capacitor discharges to simultaneously depolarize a sufficient mass of myocardium to terminate an abnormal rhythm and allow resumption of normal sinus rhythm. Standard external defibrillators operate in a synchronized or nonsynchronized mode. *Cardioversion* with synchronized shocks is used for termination of tachyarrhythmias when defibrillator capacitor discharge can be synchronized with QRS complexes. In the synchronized mode, the defibrillator monitors the patient's QRS complexes and automatically times delivery of the electrical shock to occur during the QRS complex. This prevents the induction of VF due to delivery of the shock during ventricular repolarization, the so-called vulnerable period. With some arrhythmias, such as VF and torsades de pointes VT, there are no discreet QRS complexes with which to synchronize defibrillator discharge. Therefore, *defibrillation* with nonsynchronized shocks must be used.

CARDIOVERSION VERSUS DRUGS FOR TACHYARRHYTHMIAS

Cardioversion has several potential advantages over drugs for treatment of tachyarrhythmias.[3] First, a precisely regulated amount of current will often immediately restore sinus rhythm. Second, distinction between SVT and VT, sometimes next to impossible, is not critical for success of treatment. Third, the adverse cardiac and side effects of antiarrhythmic drugs (see Chapter 5), and sometimes time-consuming titration to effect, is avoided with electroversion. However, as with antitachycardia pacing therapy, drugs may improve success with cardioversion or be required to prevent recurrences of tachyarrhythmias.

INDICATIONS FOR CARDIOVERSION

Reentrant Tachycardia

Cardioversion is used to terminate reentrant arrhythmias (Table 6–10), regardless of the site for reentry. Cardioversion terminates reentrant arrhythmias by depolarizing all excitable myocardium, including automatic foci and the circuit(s) sustaining reentry. With resulting electrical homogeneity, the substrate for reentry is removed,

TABLE 6-10 *Reentry arrhythmias terminated by cardioversion*

Atrial flutter–fibrillation	AV node reentry (PSVT)†
AV reciprocating tachycardia*	SA node reentry (PSVT)†
SA node reentry (PSVT)†	PSVT with Wolfe–Parkinson–White syndrome‡
VT with ischemia or infarction	Bundle branch reentry

*AV node and concealed accessory pathway reentry (see Chapter 9). †Paroxysmal SVT, can be due to reentry at any of these sites. ‡Orthodromic or antidromic tachycardia with manifest accessory pathways (see Chapter 10).

at least temporarily. However, the tachyarrhythmia may recur if the imbalance or conditions that provoked it in the first place are not corrected or removed. Also, antiarrhythmic drugs or pacing may be needed to prevent recurrences.

Use for Other Tachyarrhythmias

Direct current cardioversion is not effective or indicated for terminating automatic or triggered arrhythmias (Table 6–11). One reason for this is that cardioversion merely resets the cycle of automaticity or triggered activity, so that the arrhythmia promptly resumes following cardioversion. Also, with tachyarrhythmias due to digitalis toxicity, severe hypokalemia or alkalosis, and especially combinations of these, cardioversion has the potential to initiate VF. Finally, some acute tachyarrhythmias due to enhanced automaticity, especially accelerated AV junctional or idioventricular rhythm, are better managed with atrial overdrive pacing. With restoration of AV synchrony and hemodynamic improvement, the arrhythmia may resolve spontaneously after weaning from pacing.

PROCEDURE FOR CARDIOVERSION

Prevention of Equipment Failure

The following applies to DC cardioversion and defibrillation. External defibrillators should be in good working order and potential operators familiar with their use. Evidence reviewed by the Defibrillator Working Group (DFW) indicates that equipment failures due to operator or maintenance errors compared to malfunction are more

TABLE 6-11 *Automatic or triggered arrhythmias not terminated by DC cardioversion*

AUTOMATIC	TRIGGERED
Ectopic atrial tachycardia ± AV block	Digitalis tachyarrhythmias (SVT, VT)
Multiform ectopic atrial tachycardia	Torsades de pointes VT with CLQTS or ALQTS
Accelerated AV junctional rhythm	VT with acute myocardial infarction
Accelerated idioventricular rhythm	Due to myocardial reperfusion injury

CLQTS, congenital long-QT-interval syndrome.
ALQTS, acquired long-QT interval syndrome.

common than previously suspected.[26] DFW-recommended standards include daily checklists for equipment, prescribed periodic care and maintenance, and adoption of requirements for initial training and continuing education. Another authority states that the most common cause for equipment failure in treatment of VF is for the defibrillator to be set in the synchronized mode when nonsynchronized shocks are required.[12] Without a sensed QRS for delivery of synchronized shocks, defibrillator discharge cannot occur.

Monitoring for Cardioversion

The ECG lead selected for monitoring during cardioversion should be one that produces the largest R- or S-wave and smallest T-wave amplitude. The defibrillator should be checked for proper synchronization to the R or S wave, and the 12-lead ECG should be recorded before after cardioversion if possible. Ideally, pulse oximetry should be used during the cardioversion procedure. In addition, blood pressure should be recorded before and after cardioversion.

Electrode Positions

Electrode paddles for cardioversion or defibrillation should be coated with a thin layer of electrode gel. Too generous application can provide a low-resistance pathway between the paddle electrodes. This may shunt current away from the heart, thereby increasing the energy requirements for cardioversion or defibrillation. Either the *anterolateral* or *anteroposterior paddle positions* are satisfactory. With the former, one paddle is placed in the fifth left intercostal space in the midclavicular line (lateral electrode position), and the other paddle in the second intercostal space to the right of the sternum (anterior electrode position). With the latter, one paddle is placed underneath the patient's left clavicle (posterior electrode position), and the other in the anterior electrode position. Alternatively, the anterior electrode can be used with a second electrode positioned at the cardiac apex *(anteroapical paddle position)*. The objective is to have as much myocardial mass as possible between the paddle electrodes (i.e., in the current pathway). If self-adhesive electrode pads are used in place of paddles, they should be checked frequently for damage to foil and patient contact.

Cardioversion With a Permanent Pacemaker or Internal Cardioverter–Defibrillator Device

Pacemakers should be programmed to asynchronous operation by a cardiologist or the pacemaker clinic before external cardioversion.

Following cardioversion, the device must be checked for proper function and reprogrammed to an appropriate mode. Similarly, ICD devices should also be deactivated prior to elective cardioversion. For patients with permanent pacemakers or ICD, electrode pads or paddles should be positioned at least 12 cm (5 inches) from the pacemaker or ICD pulse generator to prevent damage to it. Usually, the anteroposterior position is used, but this may not be possible in some patients.

Energy for Cardioversion

Because myocardial damage is directly proportional to the energy used for cardioversion, only the lowest possible energies should be used. Except for atrial fibrillation–flutter, external shocks in the range of 25 to 50 joules (J) will terminate most SVT and VT. For internal paddles, 10 to 20 J may suffice. For external or internal cardioversion of atrial fibrillation–flutter, 50 to 100 J or 20 to 50 J, respectively, is usually required. When there is extreme urgency for terminating tachycardia, the higher suggested initial current values can be used.

COMPLICATIONS OF CARDIOVERSION AND THEIR PREVENTION

Digitalized Patients

It has long been believed that there is increased risk of inducing ventricular arrhythmias with DC cardioversion in digitalized patients. In practice, this does not seem to be a problem, provided the patient has therapeutic concentrations of digitalis.[12] However, elective cardioversion of atrial fibrillation should not be attempted in patients with known or suspected digitalis toxicity, or with any digitalis in association with acute acid–base, potassium, or magnesium imbalance, because of increased risk of inducing VF.

Nondigitalized Patients

In nondigitalized patients, attention should be paid prior to cardioversion to correcting or treating any obvious imbalance that contributes to or aggravates arrhythmias (see Chapter 3). This will increase the likelihood of success with cardioversion, and also reduce current requirements and need for repeated shocks.

Prior Treatment With Quinidine or Procainamide

Quinidine or procainamide are sometimes prescribed before elective cardioversion to increase the chances of success with cardioversion for atrial fibrillation–flutter, and to reduce the incidence of recurrences. However, some authors caution against this practice because of the risk of ventricular proarrhythmia with these drugs (see Chapter 5).[12]

Ventricular Fibrillation

There is some risk of inducing VF with cardioversion, even with properly synchronization of shocks and other precautions. Therefore, the practitioner must be prepared to immediately recharge the defibrillator and deliver a nonsynchronized shock.

Postshock Bradycardia or Atrial Asystole

Bradycardia and asystole are more likely in patients with SND and atrial fibrillation. These are usually transient occurrences, and related to intense vagal stimulation with cardioversion. If prolonged, they usually respond to atropine. Temporary pacing may be required for some patients, thus there should be provision for back-up noninvasive pacing (see Chapter 7) following cardioversion.

Anticoagulation

A requirement for routine anticoagulation in all patients prior to elective conversion of chronic atrial fibrillation has not been established.[12] However, in those at increased risk for systemic embolism from mural thrombi (see Chapter 9), there is general agreement that anticoagulation with warfarin for 2 to 3 weeks, or heparin in emergencies, is desirable to minimize the risk of thromboembolism with atrial contractions after restoration of sinus rhythm.

Pain and Burns

Other complications with cardioversion include pain associated with the shock and skin burns from excessive heat build-up under improperly applied electrodes. The former is relieved by use of intravenous anesthesia (short-acting barbiturates, etomidate, propofol), and the latter by adequate skin preparation and application of sufficient electrode gel to maximally reduce skin resistance.

DEFIBRILLATION

With defibrillation compared to cardioversion, current requirements are much larger. This is because a significantly larger amount (critical mass) of myocardium is required to sustain VF because of multiple microreentry circuits. In order to terminate fibrillation, this critical mass of myocardium must be simultaneously depolarized by capacitor discharge.

Factors Affecting Success With Defibrillation

Factors that can affect the success of defibrillatory shocks are summarized in Table 6–12.[27] Transthoracic resistance is the major one. It is determined by intrathoracic constitutive properties, body habitus, chest width and configuration, ventilatory phase, electrode–skin interface, electrode position, electrode area, force of electrode application, and the time between and number of shocks.[27] Electrode gels are more conductive than pastes, creams, or saline-soaked sponges, and there is no evidence that the anterolateral, anteroposterior, or anteroapical paddle position is superior for success with defibrillation. For most cardioversion–defibrillation, paddle diameter is 8.0 to 8.5 cm, although transthoracic impedance may be ~ 30 percent lower with 13-cm-diameter paddles.[27]

Suggested Procedure

There has been some controversy regarding optimal energy requirements for defibrillation.[27,28] Too high energy levels increase the risk of myocardial damage. Too low levels reduce the likelihood of success, prolong ischemic time, and increase the need for repeated shocks. The current Adult Advanced Cardiac Life Support (ACLS) recommendations for energy and timing of shocks are summarized in Figure 6–9.[30] Early defibrillation is the major determinant of survival in cardiac arrest due to VF. Because of this, shocks should be administered to patients in VF as soon as a defibrillator is available and working. The energy for the first defibrillation attempt is 200 J, the second shock 200 to 300 J, and the third shock 360 J. These shocks are delivered in succession (if needed), as fast as the defibrillator recharges. It has been shown that successive shocks are more important than adjunct drug therapy, and that delays between shocks

TABLE 6-12 *Factors that can affect the efficacy of defibrillation*

Transthoracic resistance	Long duration of fibrillation (↓)
Acidosis and hypoxia (↓)	Class 1A antiarrhythmics (↓)
Amiodarone, phenytoin (↓)	Lidocaine (±)
Volatile anesthetics (±)	Morbid obesity (↓)
Autonomic constraints	Hypothermia (↓)

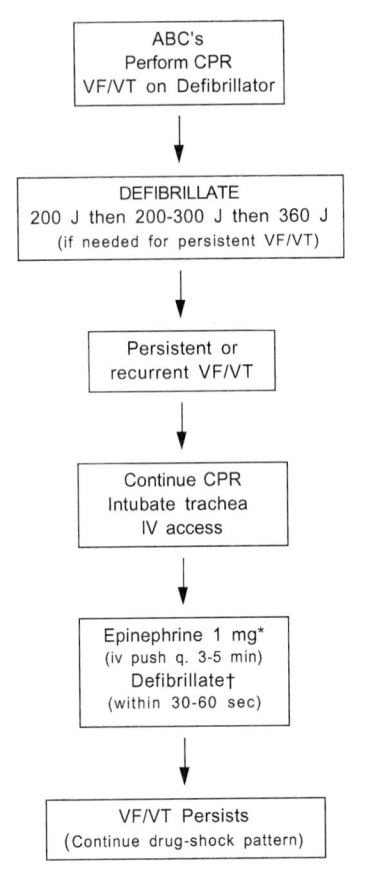

```
                    ┌─────────────────────┐
                    │       ABC's         │
                    │    Perform CPR      │
                    │ VF/VT on Defibrillator │
                    └──────────┬──────────┘
                               ↓
                ┌──────────────────────────────┐
                │         DEFIBRILLATE         │
                │ 200 J then 200-300 J then 360 J │
                │  (if needed for persistent VF/VT) │
                └──────────────┬───────────────┘
                               ↓
                    ┌─────────────────────┐
                    │    Persistent or    │
                    │   recurrent VF/VT   │
                    └──────────┬──────────┘
                               ↓
                    ┌─────────────────────┐
                    │    Continue CPR     │
                    │  Intubate trachea   │
                    │     IV access       │
                    └──────────┬──────────┘
                               ↓
                    ┌─────────────────────┐
                    │  Epinephrine 1 mg*  │
                    │ (iv push q. 3-5 min) │
                    │     Defibrillate†   │
                    │  (within 30-60 sec) │
                    └──────────┬──────────┘
                               ↓
                    ┌─────────────────────┐
                    │    VF/VT Persists   │
                    │ (Continue drug-shock pattern) │
                    └─────────────────────┘
```

FIGURE 6-9 *Advanced cardiac life support (ACLS) algorithm for defibrillation with VF or pulseless VT. ABC (airway–breathing–circulation) and CPR (cardiopulmonary resuscitation) require no further explanation. *Epinephrine is repeated if VF/VT persists and administered 30 to 60 seconds before subsequent shocks. †This can be either 360 J or multiple sequenced shocks (200 J → 200 to 300 J → 360 J). (Adapted from "Guidelines for Cardiopulmonary Resuscitation and Emergency Cardiac Care,"[29] with permission.)*

to deliver medications can be detrimental.[29] The reason for specifying a range (200 to 300 J) for the second shock is that for any given energy level there is a probability that defibrillation can be achieved. Thus, for repeated shocks, the probability should be additive. Also, since transthoracic impedance declines (modestly) with repeated shocks, somewhat higher current will be generated by subsequent shocks with the same energy. This would favor repeating the second shock at the same energy as the first, if it fails to terminate fibrillation. However, a greater and more predictable increase in current will occur if the shock energy is raised; hence, specifying up to 300 J for the second shock. Finally, if the first two shocks fail, the third shock of 360 J should be delivered immediately. If VF terminates initially but recurs, additional shocks should be at the energy level that first terminated VF. Shock energies should be increased only if a shock fails to terminate VF.

INTERNAL CARDIOVERSION–DEFIBRILLATION

Internal cardioverter–Defibrillator device malfunction and perioperative management is discussed in Chapter 8. Addressed below are the rationale for ICD use, device description and prevalence, and indications.

Rationale

There has been increasing concern among physicians about use of antiarrhythmic drugs in asymptomatic patients with coronary artery disease to prevent VT–VF and sudden death, especially since drugs have been shown to increase mortality when used for this purpose (see Chapter 5). Even so, the prognosis of patients with untreated or drug-resistant, recurrent ventricular tachyarrhythmias is poor, and such patients frequently suffer sudden death. By comparison, survival in patients treated with ICD is quite favorable.[22,30] For this reason, and the absence of other therapeutic options, there is considerable current interest in ICD devices for preventing sudden death from ventricular tachyarrhythmias.

Device Description and Prevalence

Over the past 10 years or so ICD devices have rapidly evolved from relatively simple devices that recognized only VF to extremely sophisticated devices that are currently being implanted or undergoing evaluation. These feature back-up bradycardia pacing, stimulation algorithms for treatment or prevention of tachycardia, low- and high-amplitude shocks, improved tachycardia detection algorithms, refinements in lead systems, including ones that do not require thoracotomy, programmability, and telemetry.[30] While it is difficult to estimate the numbers of patients currently with these devices (probably > 40,000 in the United States), one company's device (CPI, St. Paul, MN) had been used for 50,000 implants by 1994, and two other companies had approved devices (Medtronic, Minneapolis, Mn; Ventritex, Sylmar, CA). Several other companies have devices under evaluation.[30]

Indications

Before a patient is considered a candidate for implantation of an ICD device, the arrhythmia in question must be shown to be life-threatening, and capable of producing sudden death, syncope, or severe hemodynamic compromise.[22] Remediable causes for the arrhythmia, including acute myocardial infarction, myocardial ischemia, electrolyte imbalance, and drug toxicity, must have been excluded. The appropriate ICD device is prescribed only after careful electrophysiologic investigation. While the current consensus indications are shown in Table 6-13, these remain evolutionary and controversial.[30]

TABLE 6-13 *Indications for implantation of automatic cardioverter-defibrillator devices*

CLASS I INDICATIONS

A. Documented occurrence(s) of disadvantageous VT or VF when EP testing or ambulatory monitoring cannot be used to predict efficacy of drug therapy.
B. Documented occurrence(s) of disadvantageous VT or VF in a patient in whom no currently available and appropriate drug is effective or tolerated.
C. Continued inducibility of disadvantageous VT or VF, despite the best available drug therapy, or surgery or catheter ablation if drug therapy has failed.

CLASS II INDICATIONS

A. Documented occurrence(s) of disadvantageous VT or VF in a patient in whom drug efficacy testing is possible.
B. Recurrent syncope of undetermined origin in a patient with disadvantageous VT or VF induced at EP study, but for whom no effective or tolerated drug can be found.

CLASS III INDICATIONS

A. Recurrent syncope of undetermined cause without inducible tachyarrhythmias.
B. Arrhythmias other than disadvantageous VT or VF.
C. Incessant (i.e., virtually uninterrupted) VT or VF.

EP, electrophysiologic. *Disadvantageous VT* means hemodynamically significant VT. (Adapted from Dreifus et al.,[22] with permission.)

References

1. Furman S. Rate modulated pacing. In Furman S, Hayes D, Holmes D (eds): A Practice of Cardiac Pacing. 3rd ed. Mount Kisco, NY: Futura Publishing, 1993: pp. 401–463.
2. Furman S. Basic concepts. In Furman S, Hayes D, Holmes D (eds): A Practice of Cardiac Pacing. 3rd ed. Mt. Kisco, NY: Futura Publishers, 1993: pp. 29–88.
3. Barold S, Zipes D. Cardiac pacemakers and antiarrhythmic devices. In Braunwald E (ed): Heart Disease. 4th ed. Philadelphia: WB Saunders, 1992: pp. 726–755.
4. German L. Cardiac pacing for bradycardia. In Waugh R, Ramo B, Wagner G, Gilbert M (eds): Cardiac Arrhythmias. 2nd ed. Philadelphia: FA Davis, 1994: pp. 392–411.
5. Furman S. Physiologic basis of cardiac pacing. In Varriale P, Naclerio E (eds): Cardiac Pacing. Philadelphia: Lea & Febiger, 1979: pp. 59–72.
6. Brinker J, Platia E. Bradyarrhythmias and pacemaker therapy. In Platia E (eds): Management of Cardiac Arrhythmias. Philadelphia: JB Lippincott, 1987: pp. 156–200.
7. Hayes D. Programmability. In Furman S, Hayes D, Holmes D (eds): A Practice of Cardiac Pacing. Mt. Kisco, NY: Futura Publishing, 1993: pp. 635–663.
8. Furman S. Telemetry. In Furman S, Hayes D, Holmes D (eds): A Practice of Cardiac Pacing. Mt. Kisco, NY: Futura Publishing, 1993: pp. 605–633.
9. Hayes D. Pacemaker electrocardiography. In Furman S, Hayes D, Holmes D (eds): A Practice of Cardiac Pacing. Mt. Kisco, NY: Futura Publishing, 1993: pp. 309–359.
10. Holmes D. Pacing for tachyarrhythmias. In Furman S, Hayes D, Holmes D (eds): A Practice of Cardiac Pacing. Mt. Kisco, NY: Futura Publishing, 1993: pp. 509–535.
11. Waldo A, Wells J, Cooper T, Maclean W. Temporary cardiac pacing: Applications and techniques in the treatment of cardiac arrhythmias. Prog Cardiovasc Dis 1981;23:451–474.
12. German L. Nonpharmacologic therapy of tachyarrhythmias. In Waugh R, Ramo B, Wagner G, Gilbert M (eds): Cardiac Arrhythmias. 2nd ed. Philadelphia: FA Davis, 1994: pp. 412–424.
13. Atlee J. Cardiac pacing and electroversion. In Kaplan J (ed): Cardiac Anesthesia. 3rd ed. Philadelphia: WB Saunders, 1993: pp. 877–904.
14. Donovan K, Dobb G, Lee K-Y. Hemodynamic benefit of maintaining atrioventricular synchrony during cardiac pacing in critically ill patients. Crit Care Med 1991;19:320–326.
15. Wallenhaupt S, Rogers A. Intraoperative use of dual-chamber demand pacemakers for open heart operations. Ann Thorac Surg 1989;48:579–581.
16. Ferguson T, Cox J. Temporary external DDD pacing after cardiac operations. J Thorac Surg 1991;51:723–732.

17. Baig M, Perrins E. The hemodynamics of cardiac pacing. Clinical and physiological aspects. Prog Cardiovasc Dis 1991;33:283–298.
18. Atlee J, Pattison C, Mathews E, Hedman A. Transesophageal atrial pacing for intraoperative sinus bradycardia or AV junctional rhythm: Feasibility as prophylaxis in 200 anesthetized adults and hemodynamic effects of treatment. J Cardiothorac Vasc Anesth 1993;7(4):436–441.
19. Hayes D, Holmes D. Hemodynamics of cardiac pacing. In Furman S, Hayes D, Holmes D (eds): A Practice of Cardiac Pacing. 3rd ed. Mt. Kisco, NY: Futura Publishing, 1993: pp. 195–218.
20. Buckingham T, Janosik D, Pearson A. Pacemaker hemodynamics: Clinical implications. Prog Cardiovasc Dis 1992;34:347–366.
21. Hedman A. Rate-responsive cardiac pacing. In Atlee J, Gombotz H, Tscheliessnigg K (eds): Perioperative Management of Pacemaker Patients. Berlin: Springer-Verlag, 1992: pp. 47–52.
22. Dreifus L, Fisch C, Griffen J, et al. Guidelines for implantation of cardiac pacemakers and antiarrhythmia devices. J Am Coll Cardiol 1991;18:1–13.
23. Frye R, Collins J, DeSanctis R, et al. Guidelines for permanent cardiac pacemaker implantation, May 1984. Circulation 1984;70:A331–A339.
24. Atlee J, Bosnjak Z. Mechanisms for cardiac dysrhythmias during anesthesia. Anesthesiology 1990;72:347–374.
25. Pattison C, Atlee J, Krebs L, et al. Transesophageal indirect atrial pacing for drug-resistant sinus bradycardia. Anesthesiology 1991;74:1141–1144.
26. Cummins R, Chesmore K, White R, and the Defibrillator Working Group. Defibrillator failures. JAMA 1990;264:1019–1025.
27. Lerman B. Electrical cardioversion and defibrillation. In Platia E (ed): Management of Cardiac Arrhythmias. Philadelphia: JB Lippincott, 1987: pp. 236–271.
28. Ewy G. Energy requirements for defibrillation. Circulation 1986;74 (Suppl 4):111–116.
29. Emergency Cardiac Care Committee and Subcommittees, American Heart Association. Guidelines for cardiopulmonary resuscitation and emergency cardiac care, III: Adult advanced cardiac life support. JAMA 1992;268:2199–2241.
30. Holmes D. The implantable cardioverter defibrillator. In Furman S, Hayes D, Holme D (eds): A Practice of Cardiac Pacing. Mt. Kisco, NY: Futura Publishing, 1993: pp. 465–508.

7

Temporary Cardiac Pacing: Practical Aspects

Abbreviations Used in Chapter Seven	
AV	Atrioventricular
AVJT	Atrioventricular junctional tachycardia
ECG	Electrocardiogram
NCST	Noncompensatory sinus tachycardia
PA	Pulmonary artery
SND	Sinus node dysfunction
SVT	Supraventricular tachycardia
TCP	Transcutaneous pacing
TE(A/V)P	Transesophageal (atrial/ventricular) pacing
TEVP	Transesophageal ventricular pacing
VA	Ventriculoatrial
VT	Ventricular tachycardia

This chapter discusses the practical aspects of temporary cardiac pacing, including equipment, methods, limitations, and indications for each of the four conventional routes used for temporary pacing: epicardial, transvenous endocardial, transcutaneous, and transesophageal. Another section deals with pacing methods to suppress or terminate specific cardiac rhythm disturbances. Transthoracic pacing, whereby intracardiac pacing wires are passed through the chest wall into the right ventricle, is not discussed because the technique is no longer recommended.[1] Transthoracic pacing was rarely successful and carried with it significant potential risks, including coronary artery laceration and pneumothorax.

An overview of indications for temporary cardiac pacing was provided in Chapter 6. Also discussed in Chapter 6 were pacing modes used for bradycardia and the hemodynamics of pacing. The North American Society of Pacing and Electrophysiology–British Pacing and Electrophysiology Group (NASPE–BPEG) code for various bradycardia pacing modalities (see Tables 6–3 and 6–4) will be used as shorthand notation in this and subsequent chapters.

Temporary Pacing Versus Drugs for Bradycardia

Either drugs or temporary cardiac pacing may be used for the initial management of bradycardia due to atrioventricular (AV) heart block or sinus node dysfunction (SND). Below, the pros and cons of each are discussed, with argument made for increased use of temporary pacing. This, in turn, is followed by the suggested use of temporary cardiac pacing in emergency and perioperative settings.

DRUGS TO INCREASE HEART RATE OR SPEED CONDUCTION

Drugs that affect heart rate or conduction are known as *positive* or *negative chronotropes* or *dromotropes*, respectively. Positive chronotropes and dromotropes increase heart rate and speed conduction, while negative chronotropes or dromotropes do just the opposite. Available positive chronotropes or dromotropes are mostly muscarinic blockers or beta-1 adrenergic agonists. Their effects are most pronounced where parasympathetic or sympathetic innervation is most dense. Consequently, sinus rate is increased most, followed by that of subsidiary atrial and AV junctional pacemakers, and lastly ventricular pacemakers. Similarly, sinoatrial and AV node conduction time is most affected by muscarinic blockers or beta-1 adrenergic agonists. These drugs have little significant effect on atrial or ventricular specialized conduction. Therefore, no positive chronotrope or dromotrope should be relied upon to significantly increase the rate of ventricular pacemakers or speed His–Purkinje or ventricular conduction with advanced second-degree or complete AV heart block.

Specific Drugs

Clinical use of positive chronotropes and dromotropes was discussed in Chapter 5 under Adjunct Parenteral Drugs for Treatment of Arrhythmias. Discussion here focuses more on mechanism of effect and potential for adverse effects or interactions with other drugs.

ANTIMUSCARINICS. Muscarinic blockers such as atropine and glycopyrrolate block the effects of acetylcholine on M_1 (ganglionic) and M_2 (cardiac effectors).[2] Small intravenous doses of these drugs (atropine < 0.4 mg) often produce paradoxical initial slowing (< 10 beats/min) of sinus rate. This is not due to central vagal stimulation, as earlier believed, but rather to preferential initial block of M_1 compared to M_2 vagal receptors. Subsequently, atropine-like drugs produce a dose-related increase in heart rate and shortened PR interval by blocking effects of vagal stimulation on M_2 receptors at the sinus or AV nodes. These effects are more pronounced in healthy young adults and trained athletes with high resting vagal tone. Even large doses of atropine may have negligible effects on sinus rate or AV node conduction in infants or the elderly. With atropine and other antimuscarinic drugs, the effect on bradyarrhythmias depends on sinus node function and the balance between vagal and adrenergic tone. Thus, atropine may not be effective in patients with intrinsic or extrinsic SND, or receiving beta-blockers. Also in patients with high adrenergic tone, atropine may cause excess tachycardia, ventricular arrhythmias, or hypertension because of the removal of vagal tone. Antimuscarinics are most effective for reversing the muscarinic cardiac effects of anticholinesterase drugs. They are also useful if bradycardia or heart block is due to vagal stimulation (e.g., oculocardiac reflex, hypersensitive carotid sinus reflex).

DOBUTAMINE. Compared to isoproterenol, dobutamine has relatively more potent inotropic than chronotropic effects. At equipotent inotropic doses, isoproterenol increases sinus rate more than dobutamine, but improvement in AV nodal and ventricular conduction is comparable. Racemic dobutamine has alpha-1 and beta-2 agonist activity. Consequently, in patients receiving beta-blockers, dobutamine can increase systemic resistance and blood pressure. Hypertensive patients appear at greatest risk for an exaggerated pressor response. In patients with atrial fibrillation, dobutamine can markedly increase ventricular rate. With SND, it may accelerate the rate of secondary pacemakers more than the sinus node to cause ectopic rhythms.

EPHEDRINE. Ephedrine is a mixed adrenergic agonist. Additionally, it enhances release of norepinephrine from adrenergic neurons. Ephedrine increases heart rate and blood pressure with bradycardia. It is probably safer and more reliable for reversing bradycardia with hypotension than atropine, since effects do not rely on removal of vagal tone. Ephedrine is commonly used to reverse bradycardia and hypotension with anesthetic overdose and high spinal or epidural anesthesia. It may cause tachycardia and arrhythmias in some patients, but is less likely than atropine to do so. Arrhythmias are more likely in patients with SND because of the increase in latent pacemaker automaticity.

ISOPROTERENOL. Isoproterenol is a mixed beta adrenergic agonist with low affinity for alpha-adrenergic receptors. It has strong positive chronotropic, dromotropic, and inotropic actions (beta-1), and lowers systemic resistance (beta-2). Therefore, while isoproterenol increases heart rate and cardiac output, systolic blood pressure remains unchanged or rises only modestly. Isoproterenol may cause sinus tachycardia, tachyarrhythmias, and myocardial ischemia. In patients with SND, isoproterenol is more likely than dobutamine or ephedrine to accelerate the rate of latent pacemakers. Despite its limitations, however, isoproterenol is still indicated as a precautionary drug for management of bradycardia due to pacemaker malfunction in pacemaker-dependent patients with SND or AV heart block.

Pros and Cons of Drugs

PROS. Without doubt, drugs are more convenient and easier to use than any form of temporary pacing, and there is a low risk of sepsis with proper precautions. Further, initial treatment cost with drugs is less than with invasive or noninvasive pacing, unless pacing has previously been instituted. However, this cost does not include the cost of treatment for drug-related complications, including tachycardia, arrhythmias, myocardial ischemia, inadequate or adverse effects, or requirement for other drugs or pacing.

CONS. Drugs require time to produce their effects, although this is less than 5 minutes for all of the drugs discussed above. However, the effect with antimuscarinics and ephedrine may last longer than desired, and it may be difficult to titrate the desired effect with these drugs. In contrast, dobutamine and isoproterenol infusions have a more prompt onset and offset of action. Regardless, the chief drawback to use of positive chronotropic or dromotropic drugs is the risk of causing excessive tachycardia, tachyarrhythmias, or myocardial ischemia. When this happens, it may be necessary to administer additional drugs, with toxicity of their own, to treat complications. Furthermore, if a drug produces evidence of myocardial ischemia, especially in an unconscious patient with or at presumed risk for coronary disease, it is probably necessary to rule out myocardial infarction. At a minimum, this requires serial electrocardiography (ECG) and enzyme levels, and a cardiology consult. Based on results of these tests, more extensive work-up and hospitalization may be required.

TEMPORARY PACING TO INCREASE HEART RATE

Selection of Method

Of the available methods, only invasive epicardial and transvenous endocardial pacing are suitable for both single- and dual-chamber pacing modes (see Figs. 6–5 and 6–6). With current technology, noninvasive transcutaneous (TCP) and transesophageal pacing (TEP) are suitable only for indirect ventricular or atrial pacing, respectively. Thus, TCP can serve only as interim pacing method for the patient who requires atrial synchrony, and TEP will not be effective for the patient with atrial fibrillation or complete AV heart block. Other factors that affect the selection of a temporary pacing method are summarized in Table 7–1.

Pros and Cons of Pacing Compared to Drugs

PROS.   The chief advantage of temporary pacing compared to drugs for treatment of bradycardia due to SND or AV heart block is that once electrodes are properly situated, pacing can be turned on or off at will. Additionally, the optimum heart rate for hemodynamic effectiveness can be selected. With epicardial and transvenous pacing,

TABLE 7-1   *Factors that affect selection of a temporary pacing method*

Chest open and heart accessible?	Is there central venous access?
Operator proficiency and experience	Expected duration of pacing?
Patient position and sterile fields	Available pacing equipment
Sterile facility? Fluoroscopy?	Adequate technical support?

a physiologic pacing mode can also be selected, although TEP (atrial pacing) will also provide physiologic pacing in patients without atrial fibrillation or third-degree AV heart block. Newer, temporary pulse generators for use with epicardial or endocardial leads can be programmed with any available asynchronous or synchronous (demand) pacing mode (see Figs. 6–5 and 6–6). Also, appropriate refractory periods, hysteresis, upper and lower rate limits, and escape intervals can be programmed. Other advantages of pacing compared to drugs for treatment of bradycardia include less risk of provoking new or worse arrhythmias and less risk of myocardial ischemia, provided appropriate rates of stimulation are used.

CONS. *Epicardial pacing* is the most costly and invasive route for temporary pacing. Risks include direct damage to the heart, infection, hemorrhage, and mechanical stimulation of arrhythmias, so the technique is reserved for cardiac surgery following the completion of cardiopulmonary bypass. Therefore, a cardiothoracic surgeon, adequate technical support, and fully equipped operating room are required. *Transvenous endocardial pacing* is also costly and invasive. Risks include infection, myocardial perforation, direct injury to the heart, stimulation of arrhythmias, third-degree AV block in patients with left bundle branch block, and hemorrhage. Institution of transvenous pacing requires a properly trained physician, technical support, sometimes fluoroscopy, and an adequately equipped special procedure facility. *Transcutaneous pacing* can be instituted by trained nurses, technicians, or paramedical personnel, although it is not reliable or effective in some patients and circumstances. It may be difficult to obtain pacing capture in patients with morbid obesity, emphysema, or pneumothorax. Also, it may not be possible to apply cutaneous patch electrodes for prophylactic pacing with some surgical procedures or sterile fields must be broken down for application of electrodes in emergencies. Finally, TCP may be hemodynamically ineffective in patients with heart failure, especially if due to diastolic ventricular dysfunction. Available *transesophageal pacing* products are intended only for atrial pacing (TEAP), although feasibility of ventricular pacing (TEVP) has been demonstrated (see later discussion). TEAP is ineffective in patients with atrial fibrillation, unless they are candidates for elective DC cardioversion. Neither is TEAP effective in patients with advanced second-degree or complete AV heart block. Also, TEAP or TEVP may not be feasible in some patients with esophageal disease.

SUMMARY: DRUGS VERSUS TEMPORARY PACING

The pros and cons of drugs or temporary pacing for treatment of disadvantageous bradycardia due to AV heart block or SND are summarized in Figures 7–1 and 7–2. Concerning drugs, it should be recognized that complications often require additional treatment or intervention, which adds to the cost of treatment and may produce further complications. Concerning temporary pacing, while more predictable and associated with fewer complications, available technology is often too costly, high-tech, or invasive, which discourages routine use. And, less costly noninvasive methods have yet to be perfected to encourage such use. Nevertheless, on the balance, even with available technology, temporary pacing should be considered superior to drugs for treating most disadvantageous bradyarrhythmias in perioperative circumstances (Fig. 7–3). New TEP technology now under development will make TEP a complete (TEAP, TEVP) and relatively inexpensive noninvasive temporary pacing method, and one that is also easy to use in emergencies. Customary uses for the four usual temporary cardiac pacing routes are summarized in Table 7–2.

Epicardial Pacing

Epicardial temporary pacing systems are used almost exclusively in patients undergoing cardiac surgery. In some centers, atrial and/or

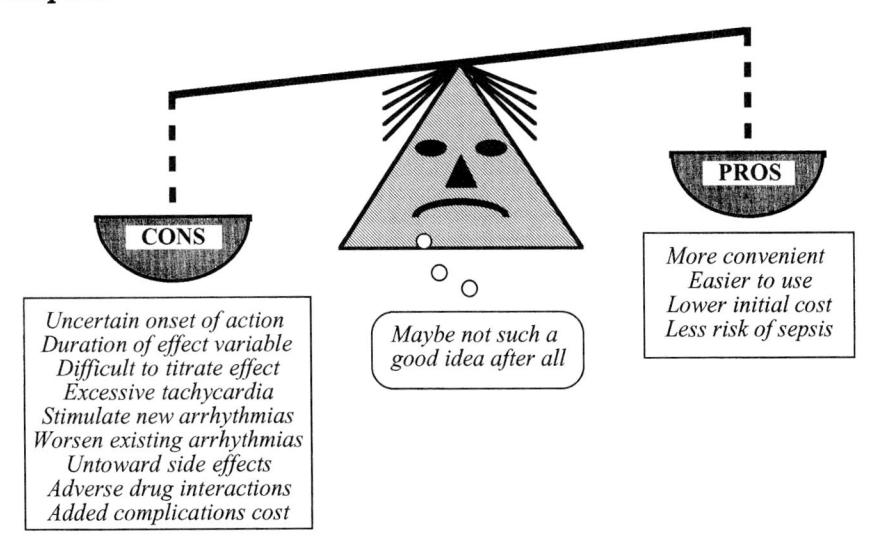

FIGURE 7–1 *Cartoon depicting pros and cons of using drugs to treat disadvantageous bradycardia. The cons with drugs are believed to outweigh the pros of convenience, lower cost and asepsis.*

CONS
*Uncertain onset of action
Duration of effect variable
Difficult to titrate effect
Excessive tachycardia
Stimulate new arrhythmias
Worsen existing arrhythmias
Untoward side effects
Adverse drug interactions
Added complications cost*

Maybe not such a good idea after all

PROS
*More convenient
Easier to use
Lower initial cost
Less risk of sepsis*

254 TEMPORARY CARDIAC PACING: PRACTICAL ASPECTS

CONS
High initial cost
Maybe invasive*
Possibly sepsis*
Relatively hi-tech

*Transvenous & epicardial pacing

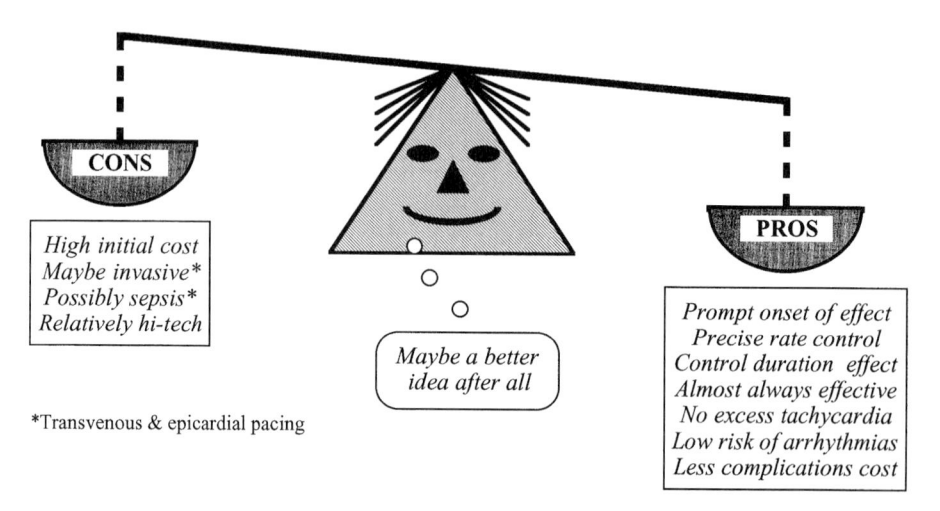

Maybe a better idea after all

PROS
Prompt onset of effect
Precise rate control
Control duration effect
Almost always effective
No excess tachycardia
Low risk of arrhythmias
Less complications cost

FIGURE 7-2 *Cartoon depicting pros and cons of using temporary pacing to treat disadvantageous bradycardia. The pros with pacing are believed to outweigh the cons of higher cost, technical sophistication, and invasiveness or sepsis with epicardial or transvenous compared to noninvasive TCP or TEP.*

ventricular pacing wires are placed prophylactically in all patients following completion of cardiopulmonary bypass. In others, epicardial pacing wires are placed only if the patient develops AV heart block or bradyarrhythmias during the procedure.

EQUIPMENT AND METHODS

Pulse Generators

The same pulse generators are used with temporary epicardial and endocardial pacing leads. Nonprogrammable—or programmable without special diagnostic features—single-chamber or AV sequential demand devices (Fig. 7-4) are often used for their simplicity of operation. However, newer multiprogrammable DDD devices (Fig. 7-5), while more complex, provide atrial tracking modes, and, in some cases, antitachycardia pacing function as well. Cardiac anesthesiologists or critical care specialists who regularly care for cardiac surgical patients with epicardial temporary pacing wires will probably want to know how to employ these newer devices without consulting a cardiologist. However, the diagnostic features of some devices may be of more interest to cardiac electrophysiologists or pacemaker specialists. Among the special features are atrial burst pacing for tachyarrhythmia termination, histograms for assessment of heart rate

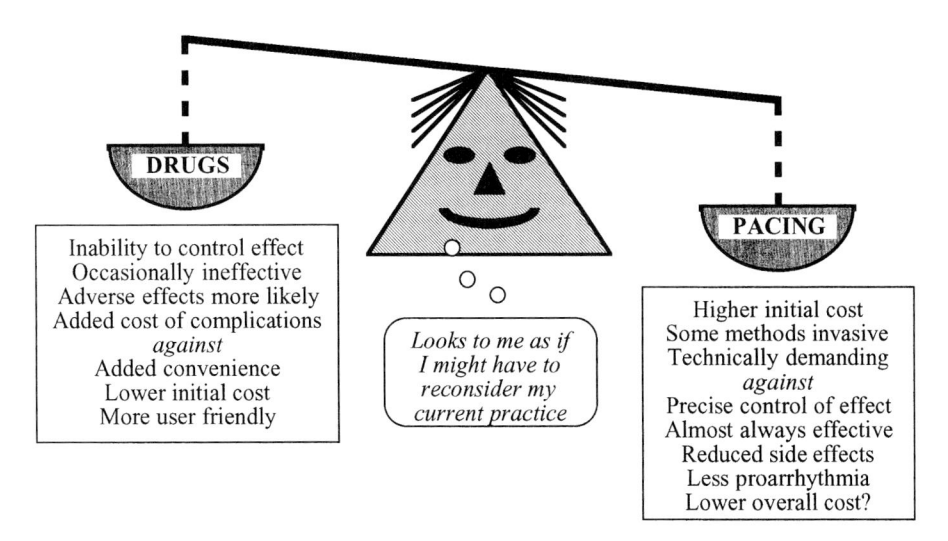

DRUGS		PACING
Inability to control effect Occasionally ineffective Adverse effects more likely Added cost of complications *against* Added convenience Lower initial cost More user friendly	*Looks to me as if I might have to reconsider my current practice*	Higher initial cost Some methods invasive Technically demanding *against* Precise control of effect Almost always effective Reduced side effects Less proarrhythmia Lower overall cost?

FIGURE 7-3 *Cartoon depicting comparison of drugs and temporary pacing for treatment of disadvantageous bradycardia. Pacing is preferred to drugs for the stated reasons, except that it is underutilized because of the increased cost (unless cost of complications with drugs are factored in), because transvenous and epicardial pacing are invasive, and because TCP or transesophageal noninvasive pacing with today's technology are suitable only for ventricular (V) or atrial (A) pacing, respectively.*

distribution and arrhythmia therapies, means to determine retrograde (ventriculoatrial, VA) conduction times, and blanking.

Pacing Leads

The leads used for temporary epicardial pacing are usually Teflon-coated, unipolar stainless steel wires that are sutured loosely to the epicardium and brought out through the chest wall (Fig. 7-6). Usually, pairs of electrodes are put on the atrium and ventricle, and one or more skin ground wires may be placed. The atrial and ventricular wires must be carefully distinguished, and carefully fixed to the skin to prevent inadvertent traction or displacement. As with transvenous pacing leads, the exposed proximal ends of pacing wires should be insulated when not in use.

NUMBER AND PLACEMENT OF ELECTRODES. It is recommended that at least one pair of temporary wire electrodes be placed on the high right atrium and also the right ventricle following completion of cardiopulmonary bypass.[3] In patients with the Wolff-Parkinson-

TABLE 7-2 *Customary uses for four available temporary cardiac pacing routes*

EPICARDIAL	TRANSVENOUS
Atrial, ventricular, sequential pacing	Atrial, sequential, ventricular pacing
Cardiac surgery following sternotomy	Extended pacing in conscious patients
Usually preferred in infants and children	Before elective pacemaker implantation

TRANSCUTANEOUS	TRANSESOPHAGEAL
Initial pacing with brady-systolic arrest	Initial pacing with intact AV conduction*
Bradycardia with atrial fibrillation*	Transient perioperative bradyarrhythmias†
Bradycardia with third-degree AV heart block*	Prophylaxis for sinus node dysfunction

*Until transvenous or epicardial pacing can be established. †Provided the patient is not in atrial fibrillation.

White syndrome who have undergone surgical ablation of an accessory AV connection for arrhythmias, placement of four pairs of electrodes is recommended, one on each of the four heart chambers for electrophysiologic testing in the postoperative period. For the same reason, three pairs of electrodes (right atrium and ventricle, left ventricle) are recommended for patients having surgery for recurrent ventricular tachycardia.

PATIENT MANAGEMENT. Patients with temporary epicardial pacing wires are monitored whenever leads are connected to an external pulse generator. If the pulse generator is disconnected before the wires are removed, monitoring is not required. In contrast to patients with temporary transvenous pacing leads, those with disconnected temporary epicardial leads can ambulate normally without movement restrictions. The exit sites for epicardial wires should be redressed daily with an antiseptic or antibiotic ointment. Stimulation thresholds with some epicardial wires may increase rapidly, and the result may be failure to pace.[1] Sensing and pacing thresholds should be checked and noted daily in patients who are pacemaker dependent, and early conversion to a permanent pacing system should be considered. Finally, during atrial pacing, a ventricular wire should never be used as the anodal ground.[1]

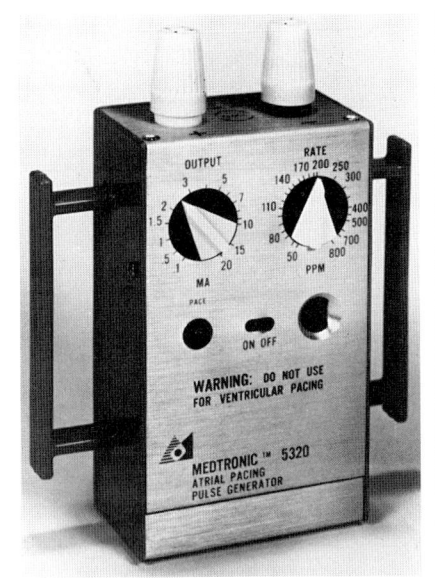

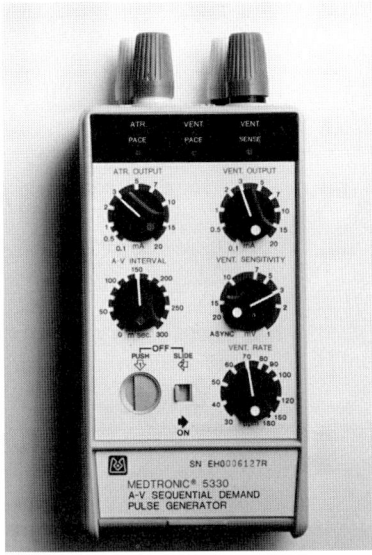

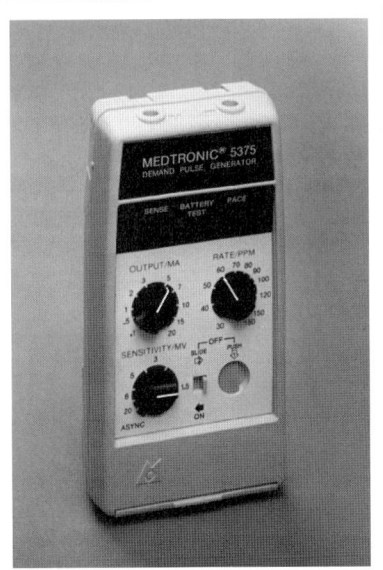

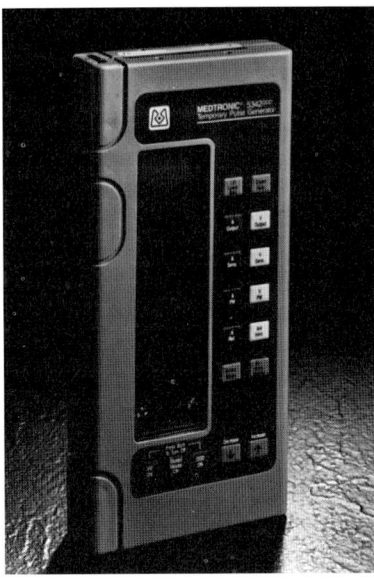

TEMPORARY CARDIAC PACING: PRACTICAL ASPECTS **257**

FIGURE 7-4   *Temporary external pulse generators for use with epicardial or transvenous endocardial pacing leads.* (Top left) *Medtronic Model 5348, asynchronous atrial pulse generator.* (Top right) *Medtronic Model 5330 AV sequential demand pulse generator.* (Bottom left) *Medtronic Model 5375 ventricular demand pulse generator.* (Bottom right) *Medtronic 5342 temporary DDD pulse generator. (Courtesy of Medtronic, Inc., Minneapolis, MN.)*

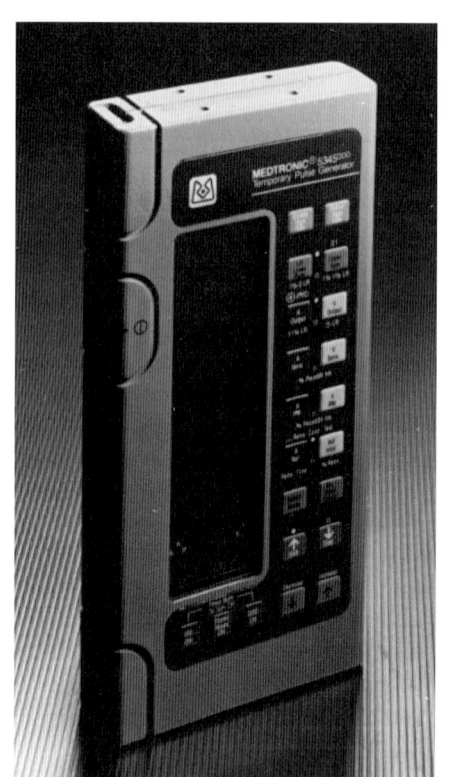

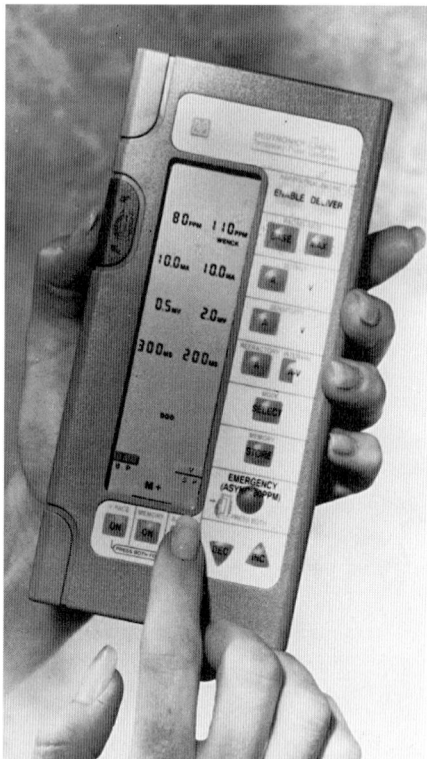

FIGURE 7-5 Programmable AV universal (DDD) temporary external pulse generators for use with epicardial wires or transvenous endocardial pacing leads. (Top left) Medtronic 5345 programmable temporary DDD pulse generator with special diagnostic functions. (Courtesy of Medtronic, Inc., Minneapolis, MN.) (Top right) Medtronic 5346 programmable temporary DDD pulse generator. (Courtesy of Medtronic, Inc., Minneapolis, MN.)

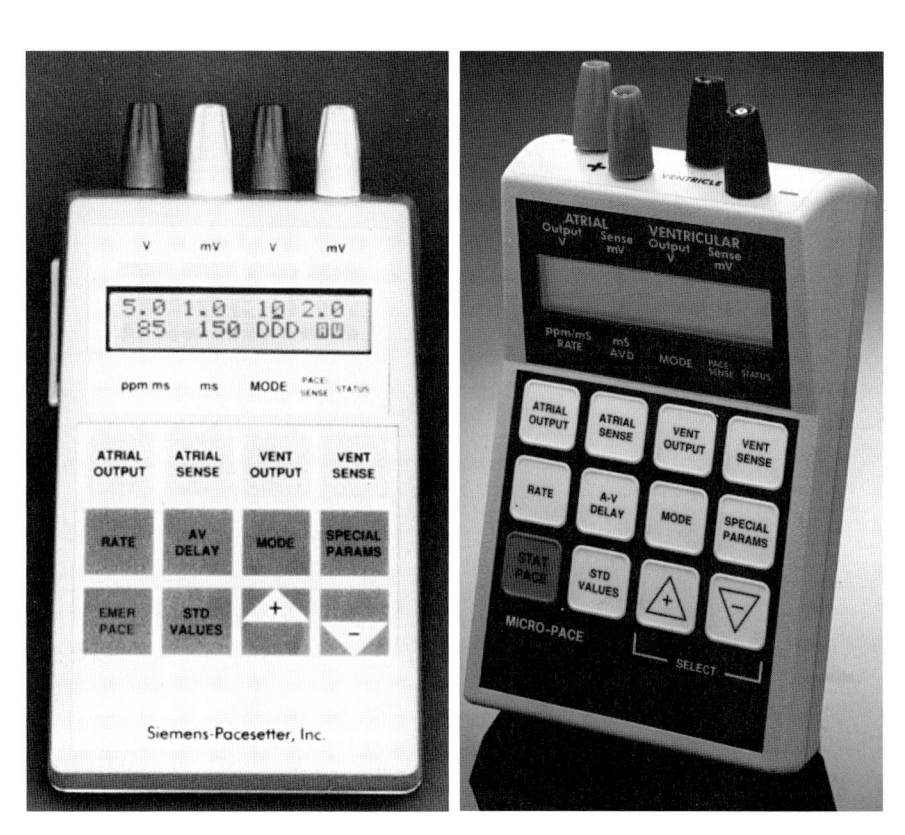

FIGURE 7–5 *Continued* **(Left)** *Siemens Pacesetter programmable temporary DDD pulse generator. (Courtesy of Siemens Pacesetter, Inc., Sylmar, CA.)* **(Right)** *Telectronics programmable temporary DDD pulse generator. (Courtesy of Telectronics Pacing Systems, Inc., Englewood, CO.)*

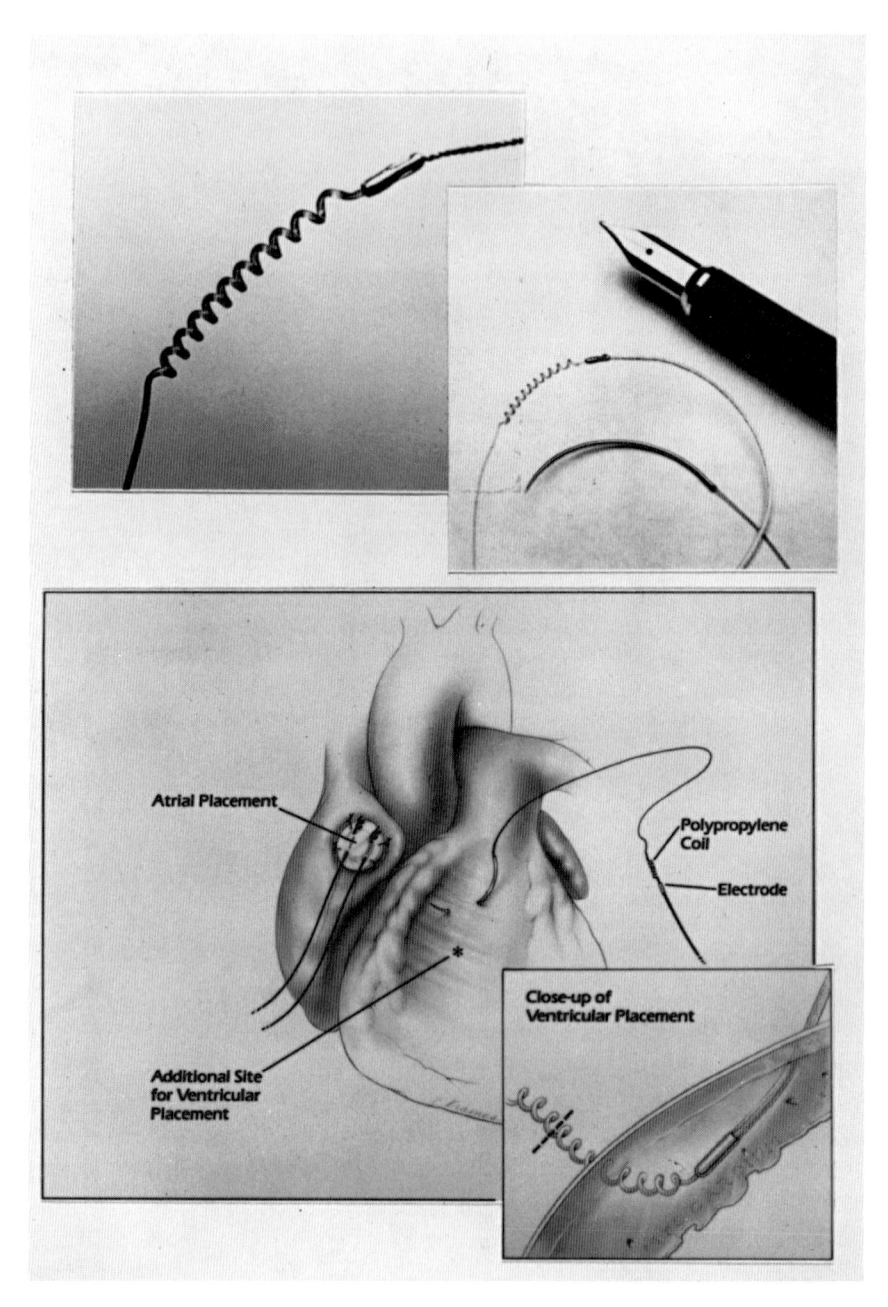

FIGURE 7-6 *Epicardial wire temporary pacing lead. (Top left) Unipolar electrode element of Medtronic 6500 temporary ventricular epicardial wire pacing lead. (Top right) Same lead with proximal suture needle in scale. (Bottom) Schematics showing placement of atrial and ventricular epicardial wire pacing leads. (Courtesy of Medtronic, Inc., Minneapolis, MN.)*

Applications of Temporary Epicardial Pacing

DIAGNOSIS. Atrial pacing wires can be used for diagnosis of arrhythmias in two ways. *First,* they are used to record atrial electrograms to establish the relation between atrial and ventricular activation with complex arrhythmias, or the atrial mechanism for arrhythmias. Atrial activity in the surface electrocardiogram (ECG) (P waves) may be nonapparent or only partially so, so that it may be difficult or impossible to determine the mechanism for wide-QRS tachycardia or supraventricular tachycardia (SVT) (e.g., paroxysmal SVT, atrial ectopy, flutter, or fibrillation). *Second,* atrial wires can be used for pacing to assist in the diagnosis of arrhythmias and conduction disturbances. For example, the effect of atrial overdrive pacing during SVT of 150 beats/min with 1 : 1 AV conduction may help to differentiate sinus tachycardia from other mechanisms for tachycardia. Also, atrial pacing may be used to assess sinus node function or AV conduction, including sinus node recovery time or Wenckebach cycle length.

PACING. In patients with functional AV conduction, atrial pacing can be used to increase heart rate with bradyarrhythmias; suppress frequent atrial or ventricular premature beats, bradycardia-dependent tachyarrhythmias with SND, or QT-interval prolongation; overdrive suppress AV junctional or idioventricular rhythms and tachycardia; and interrupt reentrant SVT, type I atrial flutter (≤ 340 beats/min) or slow ventricular tachycardia (VT). Pacing techniques for termination or suppression of specific arrhythmias are discussed later in this chapter. Also, temporary pacing modes that preserve AV synchrony may used to optimize heart rate and improve hemodynamics in patients with heart failure and/or reduced ventricular compliance.[4]

Transvenous Endocardial Pacing

EQUIPMENT

Transvenous Pacing Leads

The temporary pulse generators used for temporary transvenous pacing are the same ones as those used for epicardial pacing. A number of different types of transvenous catheter pacing leads are available for atrial and/or ventricular pacing (Fig. 7–7). Although unipolar and multipolar leads are available, the vast majority of transvenous pacing leads are bipolar. Catheter leads vary in stiffness, some have an internal guidewire, some are more flexible balloon flotation devices, and others have a lumen for simultaneous pressure

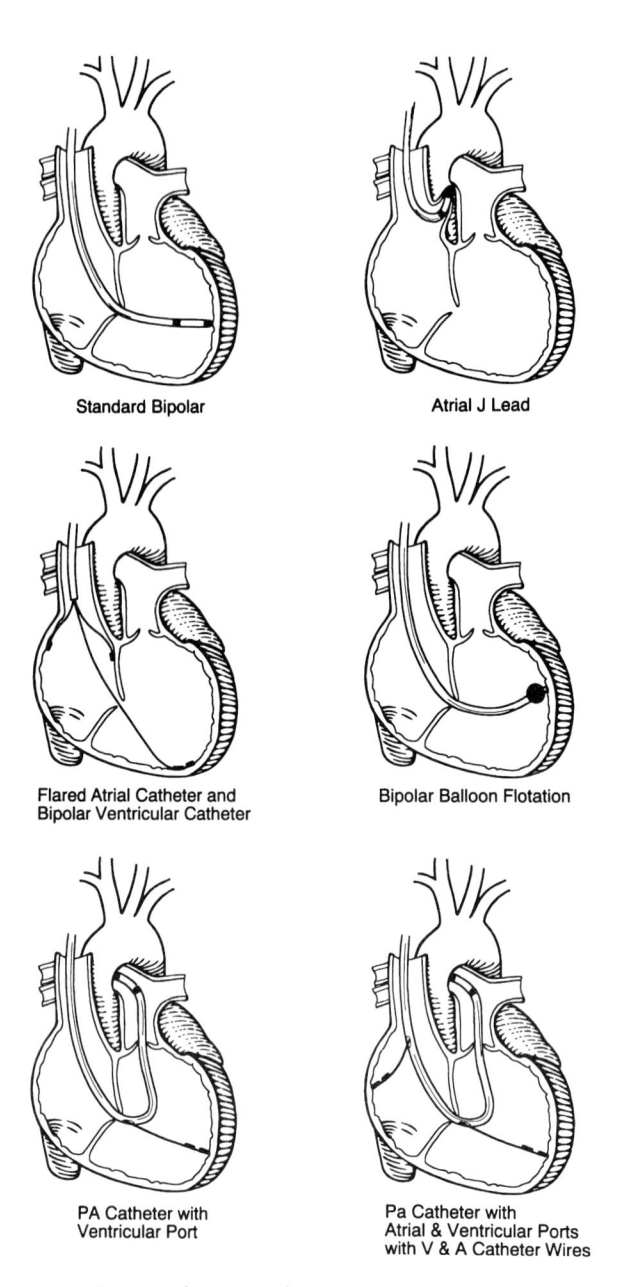

FIGURE 7-7 Schematic showing representative available types of transvenous catheter pacing leads. **(Top left)** Standard bipolar pacing catheter positioned in the right ventricle. **(Top right)** Atrial J lead positioned in the right atrial appendage. **(Middle left)** Flared atrial catheter lead with two contact points and bipolar ventricular catheter lead. **(Middle right)** Bipolar balloon flotation electrode in right ventricle. **(Bottom left)** PA catheter with bipolar ventricular pacing wire. **(Bottom right)** PA catheter with bipolar atrial and ventricular pacing wires.

monitoring. The type of probe chosen will depend on the anticipated pacing mode(s), the urgency of pacing, whether the patient has intact AV conduction or chronic atrial fibrillation, and operator preferences.

Balloon Flotation Catheters

Balloon flotation catheters (Fig. 7–8) are more flexible than standard pacing catheters. They have a balloon between the distal and proximal bipolar electrodes which provides flow-guided access to the heart, but which is deflated once the lead is positioned for pacing. These catheters do not require fluoroscopy for insertion, and are therefore often preferred for pacing emergencies. It is recommended that intracardiac ECG be recorded during positioning of balloon flotation leads.

Standard Bipolar Pacing Catheters

Standard pacing catheters (Fig. 7–8) are more rigid than balloon-tipped catheters. Except for semiflotation versions, these catheters usually require fluoroscopic imaging for optimal positioning. However, because the catheters remain somewhat firmer after placement, they are generally less likely to dislodge during pacing. In emergencies if fluoroscopy is not available, and a standard catheter lead is the only type of pacing lead available, intracardiac electrograms can be used to position the lead (Fig. 7–9). A unipolar intracardiac electrogram is recorded by substituting the distal catheter electrode for the V position of a five-lead ECG monitoring system. A bipolar intracardiac electrogram is recorded by substituting the proximal and distal catheter electrode pins for the right and left arm positions, and selecting ECG lead I. Bipolar electrograms are less affected by motion artifact produced by respiratory excursions. When the lead is in the right atrium, atrial deflections (P waves) are usually larger than accompanying QRS complexes (Fig. 7–9). As the lead is advanced across the tricuspid valve, the P waves become smaller and QRS complexes larger (Fig. 7–9). When the electrode contacts ventricular myocardium, prominent ST-segment elevation occurs as a result of current of injury (Fig. 7–9).

Atrial J Catheters and Flared Leads

The atrial J lead (Fig. 7–8), similar to permanent atrial pacing leads, provides reliable pacing because the electrode tip is in the right atrial appendage (Fig. 7–7) instead of floating freely in the atrial chamber. Another design provides for the introduction of a thin atrial lead, which, on entry into the atrium and withdrawal of the accompanying introducer sheath, can flare and provide at least two contact

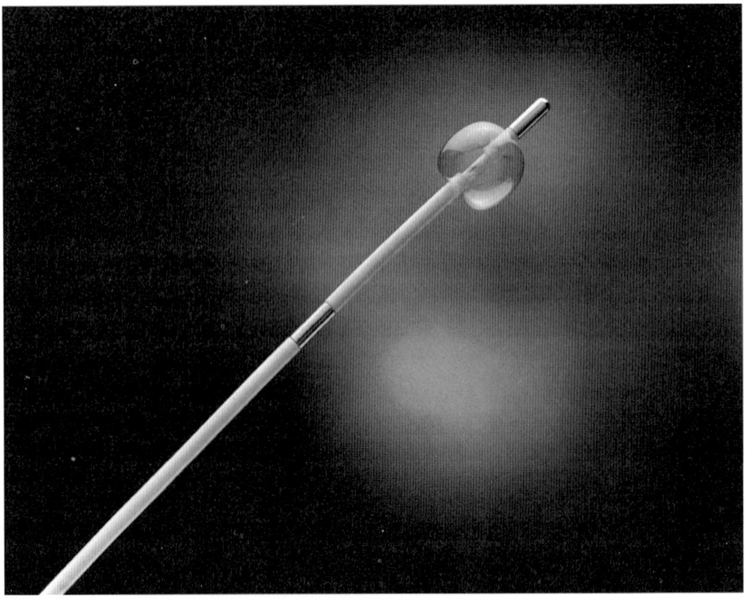

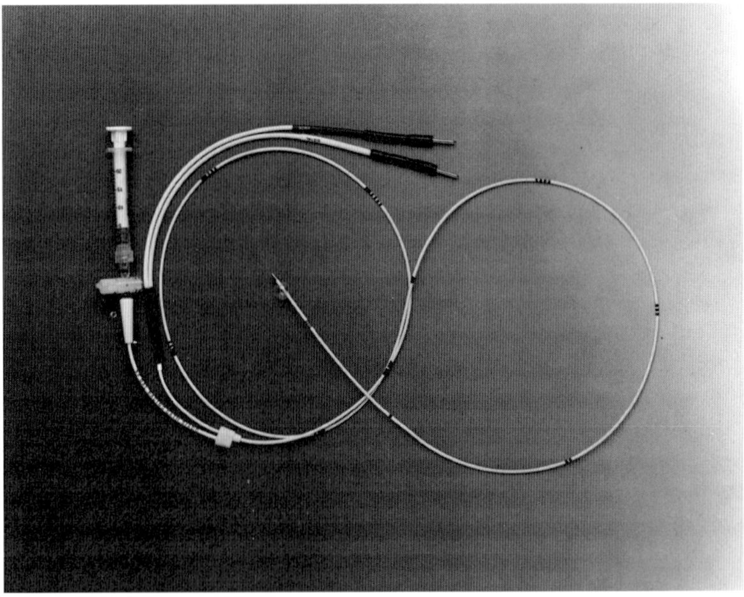

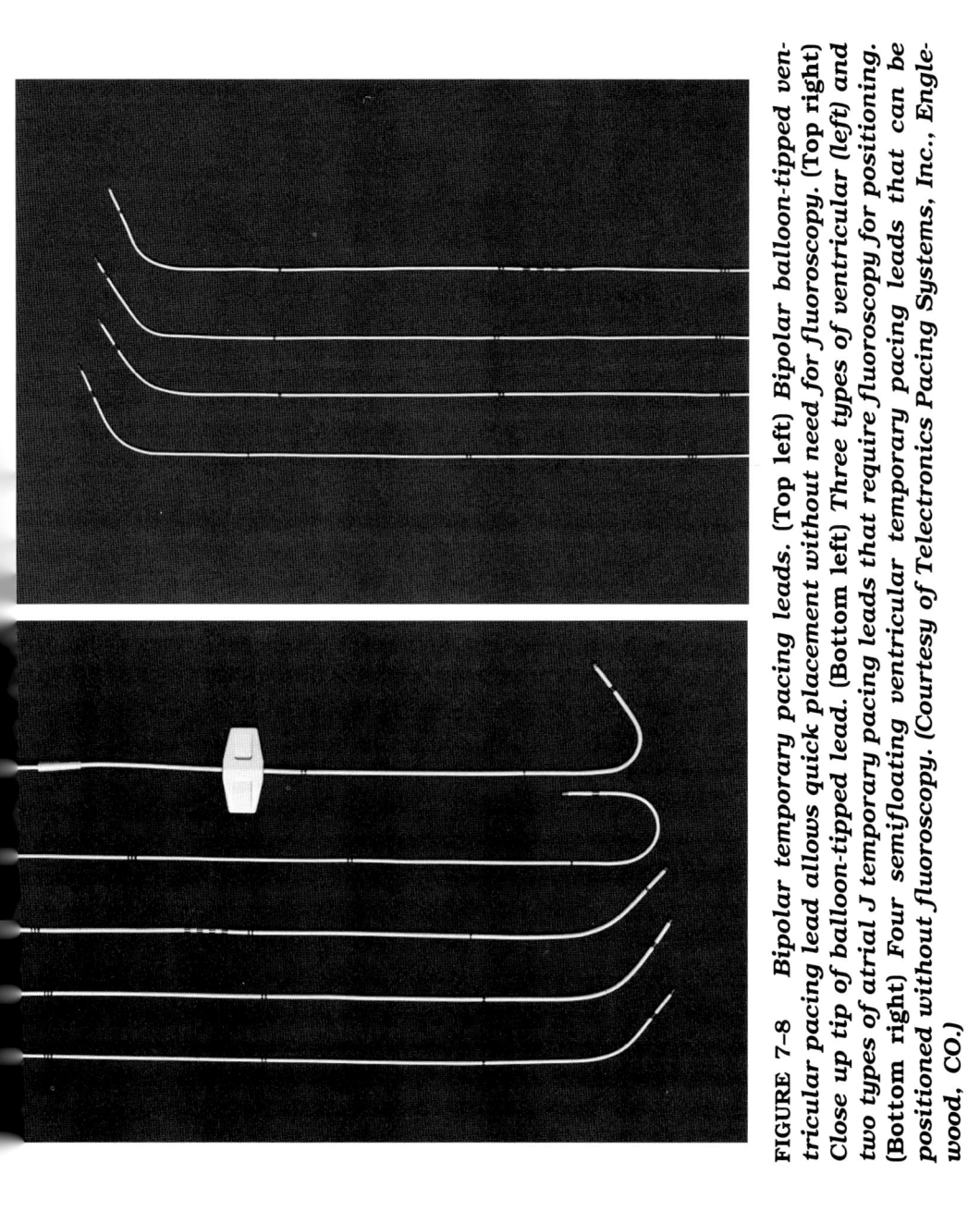

FIGURE 7-8 Bipolar temporary pacing leads. (Top left) Bipolar balloon-tipped ventricular pacing lead allows quick placement without need for fluoroscopy. (Top right) Close up tip of balloon-tipped lead. (Bottom left) Three types of ventricular (left) and two types of atrial J temporary pacing leads that require fluoroscopy for positioning. (Bottom right) Four semifloating ventricular temporary pacing leads that can be positioned without fluoroscopy. (Courtesy of Telectronics Pacing Systems, Inc., Englewood, CO.)

265

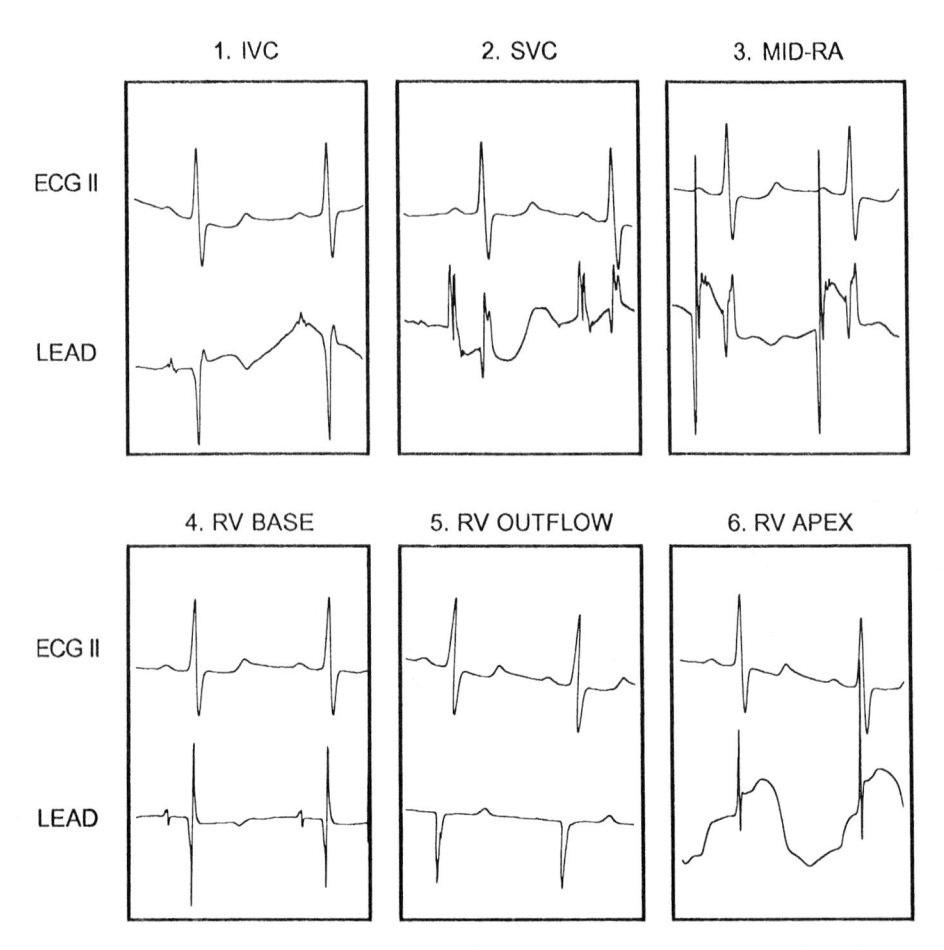

266 TEMPORARY CARDIAC PACING: PRACTICAL ASPECTS

FIGURE 7–9 *Bipolar intracardiac electrograms recorded during insertion of an endocardial pacing lead. In all panels, the top tracing is surface ECG lead II (ECG II) and the bottom one from the bipolar pacing lead (Lead). IVC/SVC, inferior/superior vena cava; MID-RA, mid-right atrium; RV BASE/OUTFLOW/APEX, base, outflow tract or apex of right ventricle, respectively. See text for discussion. (Tracings supplied by William T. Pochis, M.D.)*

points in the atrium (Fig. 7–8).[4] The introducer also accommodates a small-gauge ventricular pacing catheter, so that dual-chamber pacing can be accomplished using the same introducer.

Pacing Pulmonary Artery Catheters

Three types of pacing pulmonary artery (PA) catheters are available (Fig. 7–10). The first pacing PA catheter was pentapolar

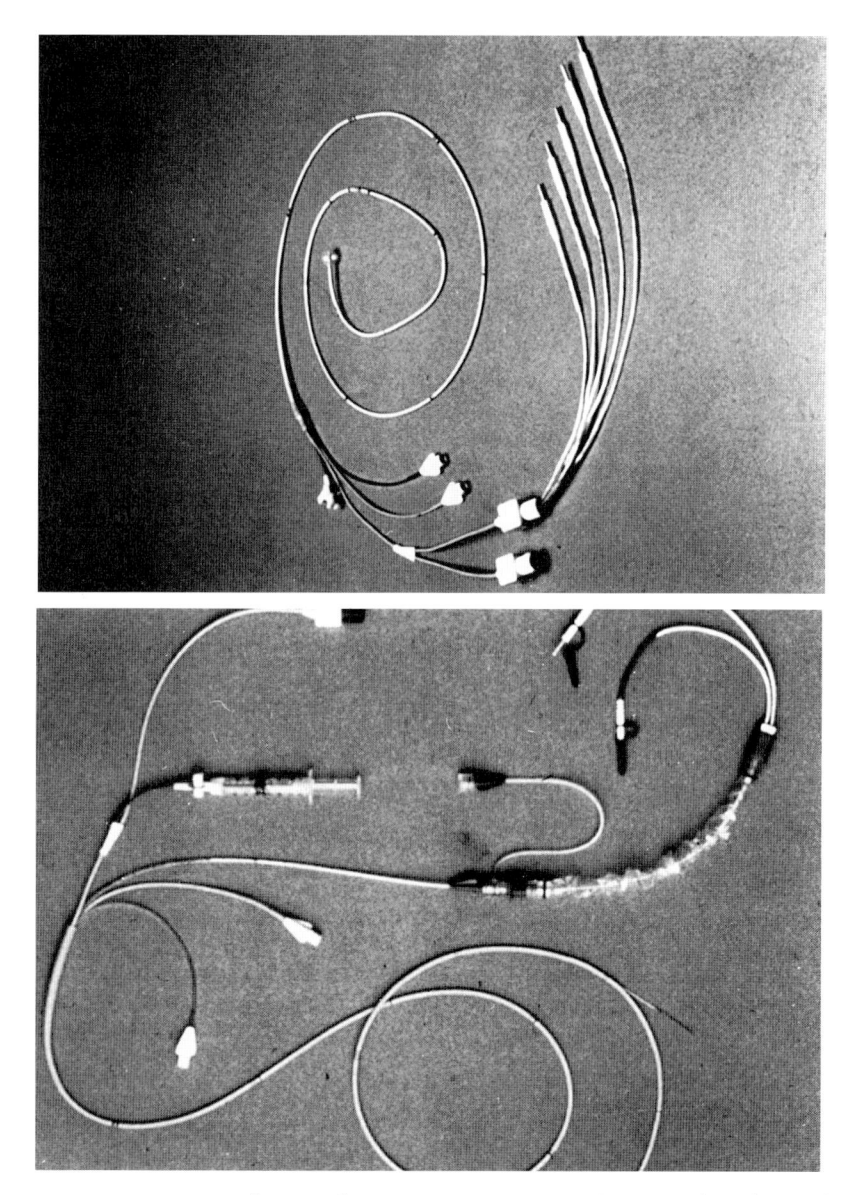

FIGURE 7-10 *Pacing pulmonary artery catheters.* (Top) *Pacing TD^{TM} catheter with three atrial and two ventricular electrodes.* (Bottom) *Paceport^{TM} catheter with Chandler^{TM} ventricular pacing wire.*

Illustration continued on following page

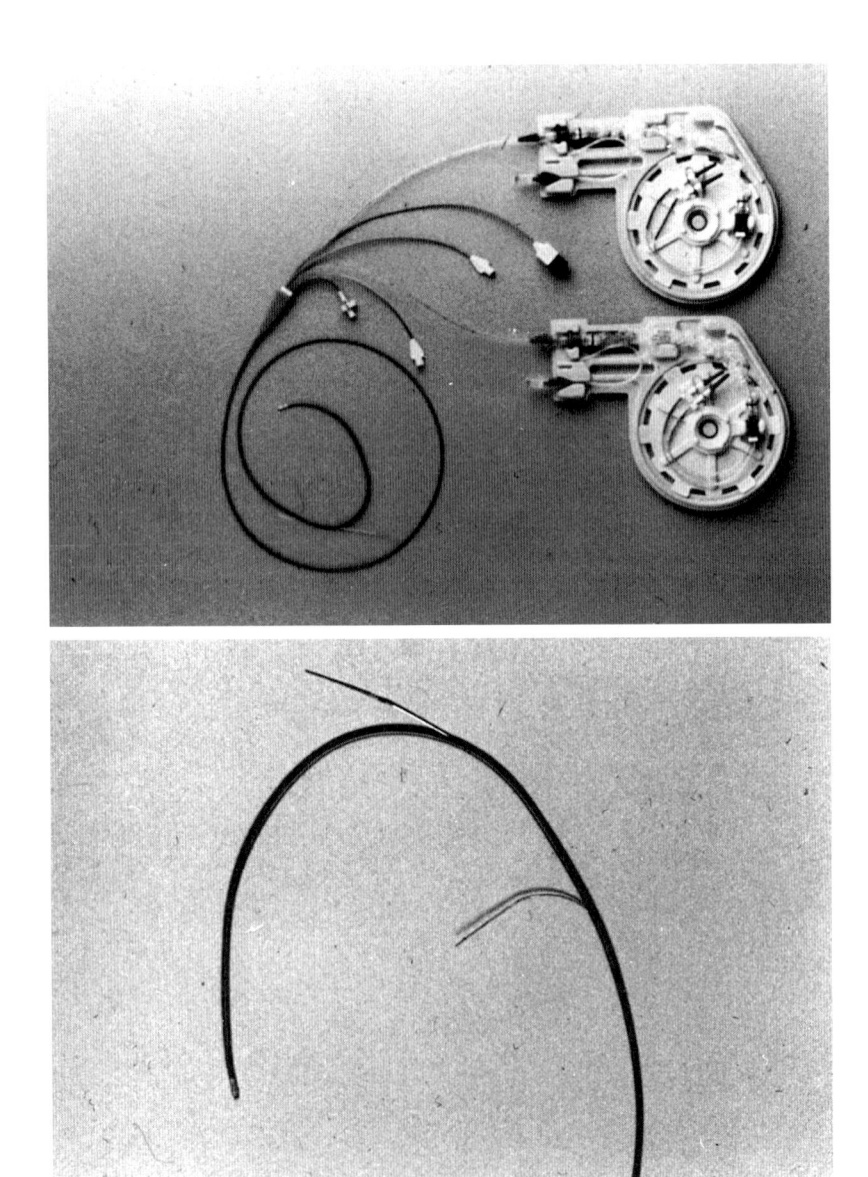

FIGURE 7-10 *Continued* **(Top)** *A-V Paceport™ catheter with Chandler™ ventricular and Flex-Tip™ atrial pacing wires.* **(Bottom)** *Distal A-V Paceport™ catheter with atrial and ventricular pacing wires extended. (Courtesy of Baxter Healthcare Corporation, Cardiovascular Group, Edwards Critical-Care Division, Irvine, CA.)*

(Pacing TD™, Baxter Healthcare, Irvine, CA): two of three proximal electrodes are used for atrial and two distal electrodes for ventricular pacing. However, this catheter is less used today because it is often difficult to obtain reliable pacing capture and record PA wedge pressures at the same time. Another pacing PA catheter features a separate ventricular port for the introduction of a bipolar pacing wire into the right ventricle (Paceport™, Baxter Healthcare). The pacing wire is positioned with intracardiac ECG guidance (Fig. 7–9). Finally, the newest pacing PA catheter features atrial and ventricular ports for introduction of pacing wires (A–V Paceport™, Baxter Healthcare). These too are positioned with intracardiac ECG.

LEAD INSERTION AND PLACEMENT

Access to the central venous system for placement of temporary pacing leads is possible from the internal or external jugular, subclavian, axillary, brachial, or femoral veins. The selection of one or another approach depends on operator preference, the temporary pacing system being installed, and patient access. As a rule, a central location is preferred because pacing leads are less easily dislodged with flexion or extension of the extremities. The femoral vein route is preferred in catheterization laboratories, but not for emergency temporary pacing. Rapid access to the right ventricle from the femoral vein is not possible without fluoroscopy. However, temporary atrial pacing with rigid catheters is more easily performed from the femoral vein. Nevertheless, a limitation to the femoral approach may be a somewhat higher incidence of infection and venous thrombosis.[4] ECG monitoring during insertion of temporary pacing leads is required because of the danger of inducing serious arrhythmias. An external cardioverter–defibrillator and a resuscitation cart should also be available.

APPLICATIONS

Transvenous endocardial pacing is preferred for most temporary pacing outside of cardiac surgery, especially if pacing will be needed for longer than several hours. It is also used prior to sternotomy with cardiac surgery in patients considered at high risk for disadvantageous bradycardia due to SND or AV heart block. Transvenous pacing leads are never inserted solely for the purpose of intracardiac ECG diagnosis, but once inserted can be used for this purpose, much as with atrial or ventricular epicardial pacing wires. Transvenous pacing applications are the same as with epicardial wires.

Transcutaneous Pacing

Transcutaneous pacing (TCP) is one of the two noninvasive routes for temporary cardiac pacing. Since institution of TCP is fairly easy and prompt, and can be performed by nonphysician medical personnel, the technique is well suited for use in medical emergencies when invasive pacing is not available or practical. In fact, the current Adult Advanced Cardiac Life Support Guidelines (1992) put more emphasis on TCP compared to transvenous pacing in emergency cardiac care.[5] TCP is considered more suitable than transvenous pacing because electrodes are easier to position, and pulse generators simpler to operate and more widely available.

PERSPECTIVES AND INDICATIONS

Noninvasive TCP was first used to resuscitate patients with recurring asystole in 1952.[6] However, early TCP suffered from many problems, the most significant of which were severe pain and strong muscular contractions caused by the large currents required for TCP capture. Also, the large artifacts produced by TCP stimulation and muscular contractions distorted the QRS complexes during TCP, so that it was difficult to ascertain pacing capture. These problems led to abandonment of TCP and substitution of transvenous or transthoracic pacing for use in emergencies outside of cardiac surgery. Improvements in TCP technology in the 1980s, including larger surface area electrodes, longer stimulus durations, uniform current strength, and stimulus artifact suppression, however, have increased physician and patient acceptance of TCP.[7] In fact, today TCP is the preferred pacing modality for emergency and standby pacing in a number of circumstances (Table 7–3), especially when transvenous pacing is not practical or cost effective, or could take some time to institute.[5] Disadvantageous bradyarrhythmias (Table 7–3) are defined as those associated with a systolic blood pressure < 80 mmHg, change in mental status, myocardial ischemia, or pulmonary edema.[5] If standby TCP is to be used, a brief trial of pacing should be attempted to determine if capture can be achieved, and if the patient can tolerate pacing.

EQUIPMENT

Transcutaneous pacing devices may be packaged separately or combined with a DC cardioverter–defibrillator–ECG monitor/strip chart recorder in a single unit. TCP units are available from a number of manufacturers; the units of one manufacturer are shown in Figure 7–11. All TCP devices can be used with paddle or TCP pacing elec-

TABLE 7-3 *Indications for emergency or standby transcutaneous pacing*

EMERGENCY	STANDBY
Hemodynamically disadvantageous bradyarrhythmias as defined in text	Stable bradyarrhythmias that are not disadvantageous (see text)
Bradycardia with malignant escape rhythms unresponsive to drugs	Acute myocardial infarction with symptomatic SND
Overdrive pacing of SVT or some VT refractory to drugs or cardioversion	Type II (Mobitz) second-degree AV heart block with acute myocardial infarction
Bradysystolic arrest if pacing can be instituted early (≤ 5 minutes)	Acute myocardial infarction with third-degree AV or new bifascicular heart block

(Adapted from Adult Advanced Cardiac Life Support guidelines,[5] with permission.)

trodes, or multifunctional, anterior–posterior chest wall electrodes for "hands off" pacing, cardioversion–defibrillation, and ECG monitoring.

LIMITATIONS, SAFETY, AND PRECAUTIONS

Failure to Capture

Failure to capture with TCP may be related to electrode placement or patient size (e.g., morbid obesity). Patients with pulmonary emphysema and barrel-shaped chests conduct electricity poorly and may be refractory to TCP capture. A large pericardial effusion or tamponade can increase TCP threshold current. Pneumothorax or hemothorax will also increase TCP thresholds or prevent capture. Finally, some surgical procedures, because of the location of the operative site and sterile field precautions, may preclude prophylactic use of TCP.

Discomfort

Transcutaneous pacing is associated with some discomfort due to muscle contractions in most conscious patients, and this may be intolerable in some. This can be reduced by placing TCP electrodes over areas of least skeletal muscle, such as the midline anterior chest and just below the left clavicle.[8] Also, sedative-hypnotics (benzodiazepines) and/or analgesia (opiates) will reduce discomfort with TCP, at least making it more tolerable until temporary transvenous pacing can be instituted.

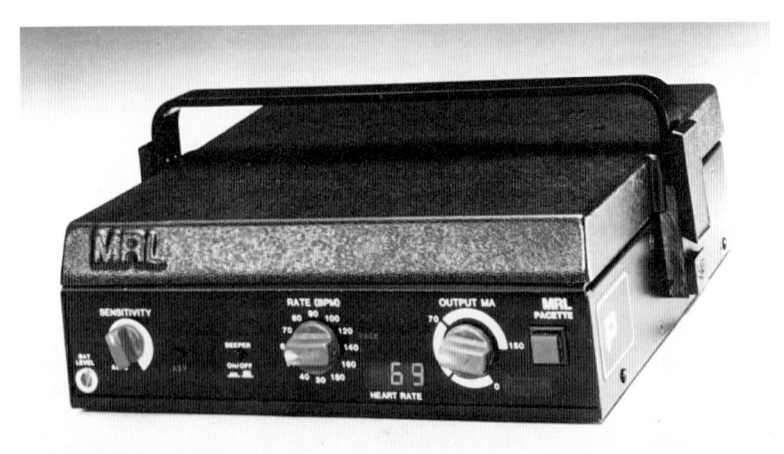

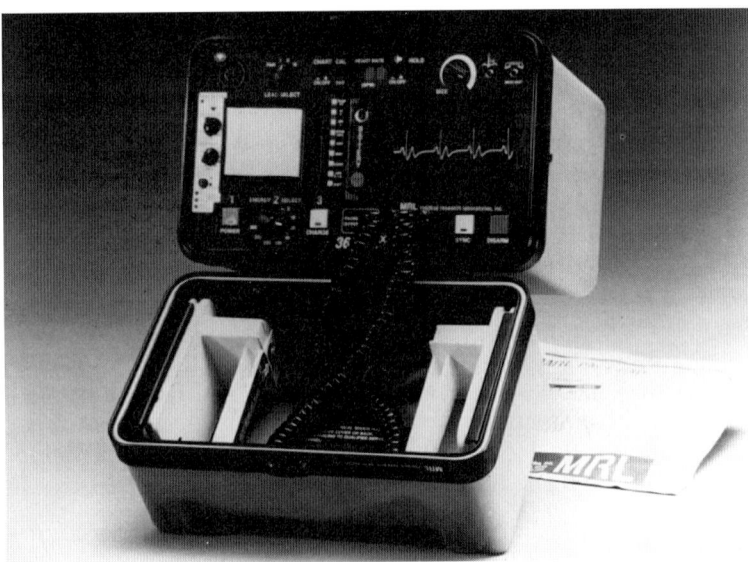

FIGURE 7-11 *Transcutaneous pacing (TCP) devices.* (Top) *Portable asynchronous or demand TCP pulse generator.* (Bottom) *The TCP pulse generator is part of a stand-alone cardioverter–defibrillator–ECG monitoring system suitable for field use by trained rescue personnel. (Courtesy of Medical Research Laboratories, Inc., Buffalo Grove, IL.)*

Safety

Numerous animal and human studies attest to the safety of TCP.[7-9] Induction of R-on-T ventricular arrhythmias in animals requires 10 to 12 times threshold current for TCP, although comparable studies have not been performed in humans. Neither has histopathologic, echocardiographic, or enzymatic evidence of myocardial pacing injury been found in animals or humans following TCP. Local skin irritation and erythema can develop under the pacing electrodes in a small number of patients, but thermal lesions are rare and occur with improper application of pacing electrodes or continuous TCP with high currents for many hours, especially in premature infants or newborns.[6]

HEMODYNAMICS

Studies, reviewed elsewhere,[7-9] suggest that TCP can produce at least equivalent hemodynamics to those with right ventricular endocardial pacing. However, because of loss of AV synchrony, blood pressure and cardiac output are reduced compared to pacing modes that preserve AV synchrony. Reduction in cardiac performance is expected to be greatest in patients with decreased ventricular compliance (see Chapter 6). TCP may produce simultaneous four-chamber activation in some patients, but usually the current for atrial capture is much higher than that needed for ventricular pacing capture.[10] However, in patients with intact retrograde (VA) conduction, TCP may produce atrial contractions after ventricular systole, with further reduction in cardiac output and activation of vasomotor reflexes (i.e., the pacemaker syndrome; see Chapter 6).

INDICATIONS

Bradyasystolic Arrest

The results of TCP for bradyasystolic arrest during advanced cardiac life support have been disappointing, especially when TCP is instituted more than 15 minutes after cardiac arrest.[5,7-9] It appears that the greatest likelihood of successful resuscitation is in patients receiving TCP within 5 minutes of cardiac arrest.[11,12] Concerning use of TCP for bradyasystolic arrest, it is suggested that TCP is most useful in patients whose primary problem is a disorder of impulse formation or conduction in the presence of preserved myocardial function.[5]

Tachyarrhythmias

Transcutaneous pacing can be used to terminate reentrant SVT and VT using single or multiple extrastimuli, or overdrive pacing.[7] Although TCP shows promise for terminating these arrhythmias, drug therapy is still the preferred initial treatment in patients with reasonable hemodynamics. DC cardioversion is always the preferred initial treatment in hemodynamically unstable patients.[5]

Transesophageal Pacing

Transesophageal pacing (TEP) was first attempted in dogs by Zoll in 1952, and performed in humans by Shafiroff and Linder in 1957.[13] However, there was little interest in the method because of discomfort with pacing, and no further development until the late 1970s. One reason for this was the lack of suitable animal models. Except for humans and several of the higher great apes, most large animal species have too great a distance between the esophagus and posterior heart and/or interposed lung tissue. Important past restrictions to more widespread acceptance of TEP have been the inability to do reliable ventricular pacing from the esophagus, the relative high cost of products, and the lack of clinical application and outcome studies—especially in anesthesia, critical care, and emergency medicine, where TEP appears well-suited for most emergency pacing.

PRECEDENT

Atrial Pacing

The principal use of atrial TEP (TEAP) has been in cardiology for noninvasive cardiac electrophysiologic testing, termination of reentrant SVT and atrial flutter, temporary pacing of bradycardia in patients with intact AV conduction, and stress atrial pacing for diagnosis of coronary artery disease.[13] Until recently, there were only sporadic reports of the use of TEAP or transesophageal ECG recording in the anesthesiology literature,[14] mainly because of the unavailability of suitable pacing probes. However, probes designed for TEAP were tested and became commercially available in the early 1990s, so that now there are several reports of TEAP for the treatment of sinus bradycardia and AV junctional rhythms in perioperative settings,[15-19] including two that clearly demonstrate the advantages of TEAP compared to drugs for treatment of sinus bradycardia and bradyarrhythmias.[18,19]

Ventricular Pacing

Indirect ventricular TEP (TEVP) has been more problematic because of increased esophageal–left ventricular (1.5 to 2.0 cm) compared to esophageal–left atrial distance (0.5 to 1.0 cm) in humans. Because of this, successful TEVP capture was obtained in only one-third of patients using an available TEP stethoscope and a custom stimulator that supplied up to 100 mA.[20] One approach to reduce the esophageal–ventricular distance has been to use inflatable balloon electrodes.[21,22] However, there seems to have been little interest in pursuing this method, possibly because of its cost and because balloon inflation causes overpressure on the esophageal mucosa, with the risk of tissue necrosis during protracted pacing. Another approach has been to construct an electrode that projects toward the ventricle within the esophageal lumen.[23] While this permitted sustained TEVP capture in 11 successive adult patients, pacing thresholds were unacceptably high (range 22 to 77 mA). The threshold for perception of TEP in conscious patients is 15 to 20 mA, which can only be increased by 5 to 10 mA with sedative-analgesics (unpublished observations of the author). Nevertheless, it appears that TEVP thresholds are substantially reduced by prototype TEP probes now being tested. Therefore, it is expected that TEP will become a practical, effective, and complete noninvasive pacing method within the next five years or so.

EQUIPMENT

Only one U.S. company marketed approved TEP products in mid 1995, although at least two other U.S. companies had products under development. TEP products are available from several companies in Europe.

Pulse Generators

Two transesophageal pulse generators are available (Fig. 7–12). One (Arzco Model 2A) supplies variable current (1 to 40 mA) with a fixed pulse duration (10 msec), and the other (Arzco Model 7A) variable current and pulse duration (1 to 40 mA and 1 to 10 msec). The 10-msec pulse duration, however, is standard for most TEP applications, since at least atrial current requirements increase with pulse durations below 6 msec.[24] Both TEP pulse generators are asynchronous atrial pacing devices (AOO), although the Model 7A can be triggered by external impulses for programmed extrastimulation. The Model 2A pulse generator paces the atria between 50 and 200 beats/min. The Model 7A stimulator can pace the atria between 60 and 300 beats/min. The higher rates can be used for overdrive pacing of SVT or slow atrial

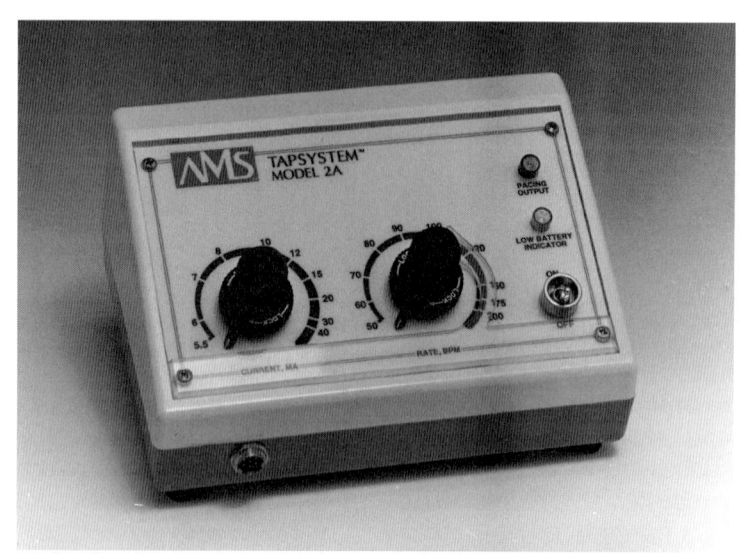

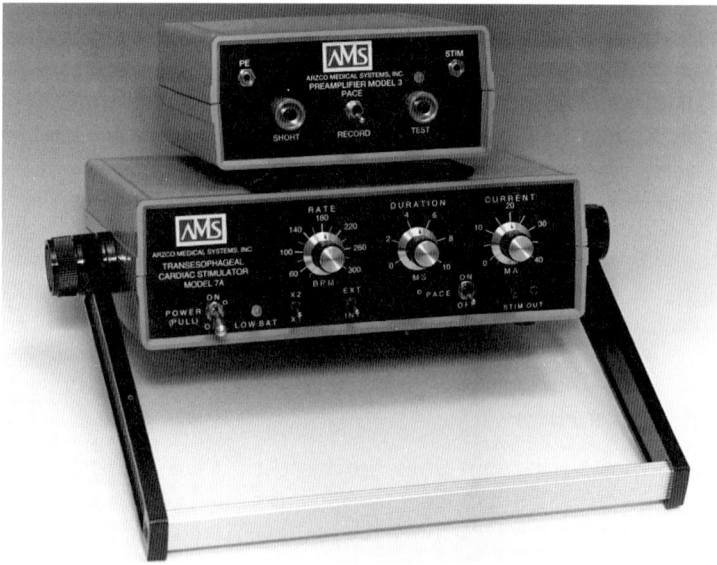

FIGURE 7-12 *Available transesophageal pacing stimulators.* **(Top)** *Arzco Model 2A stimulator. This stimulator does not feature an ECG preamplifier to aid in arrhythmia or ischemia diagnosis, or for optimal positioning of pacing electrodes.* **(Bottom)** *Arzco 7A stimulator, which does feature an ECG preamplifier. (Illustrations kindly furnished by Arzco Medical Systems, Inc., Tampa, FL.)*

flutter. The selected pacing rate can also be temporarily doubled to 120 to 600 beats/min by depressing the "X2" toggle switch (Fig. 7–12). This feature is used for fast atrial flutter, burst pacing, or induction of atrial fibrillation during bedside cardiac electrophysiologic testing.

Pacing Probes

Electrodes suitable for TEAP or ECG recording in conscious or unconscious patients are shown in Figure 7–13. These probes permit practitioners to perform TEAP or transesophageal ECG recording in a variety of patients and circumstances, including infants, children, and patients having transesophageal echocardiographic studies. None of these probes are suitable for TEVP, except that sustained or intermittent TEVP capture may be possible in most neonates or infants, and perhaps up to 50 to 60 percent of adults.[20,23]

METHODS

Positioning Probes

Transesophageal atrial pacing can be instituted in adults in under 1 minute by any person experienced with esophageal intubation. In an emergency, reliable TEAP can be achieved in ≥ 90 percent of adults by positioning the bipolar electrode center point 30 to 31 or 32 to 33 cm (females and males, respectively) from the inferior alveolar ridge and setting current at 25 mA with a pulse duration of 10 msec.[15–19] Proximal markings on TEAP probes facilitate positioning. When time permits, the probe can repositioned at the point of minimum pacing threshold, determined by advancing and retracting the probe by 1-cm amounts. For more extended pacing (more than several minutes), to reduce the possibility of current injury to the esophagus, the minimum TEAP threshold position should be located. A similar procedure for positioning TEAP probes in emergencies can be used in infants and children, except that the distances will be smaller. However, a table of TEAP distances for different age groups was not available at this writing. Time permitting, the preferred method for positioning TEAP or TEVP probes is to position electrodes at the point of maximum-amplitude P waves (Pmax) or QRS complexes (Vmax), as shown in Figure 7–14. The point of minimum TEAP or TEVP thresholds will usually be at or 1 cm beyond Pmax or Vmax, respectively.[15,16,20,23] In the absence of type I (Wenckebach), second-degree AV block (Fig. 7–15), TEAP capture is recognized by a distinct and fairly constant stimulus-to-R interval (Fig. 7–16). In contrast, TEVP capture is recognized by no distinct stimulus-to-R interval in association with QRS aberration (Fig. 7–16).

278

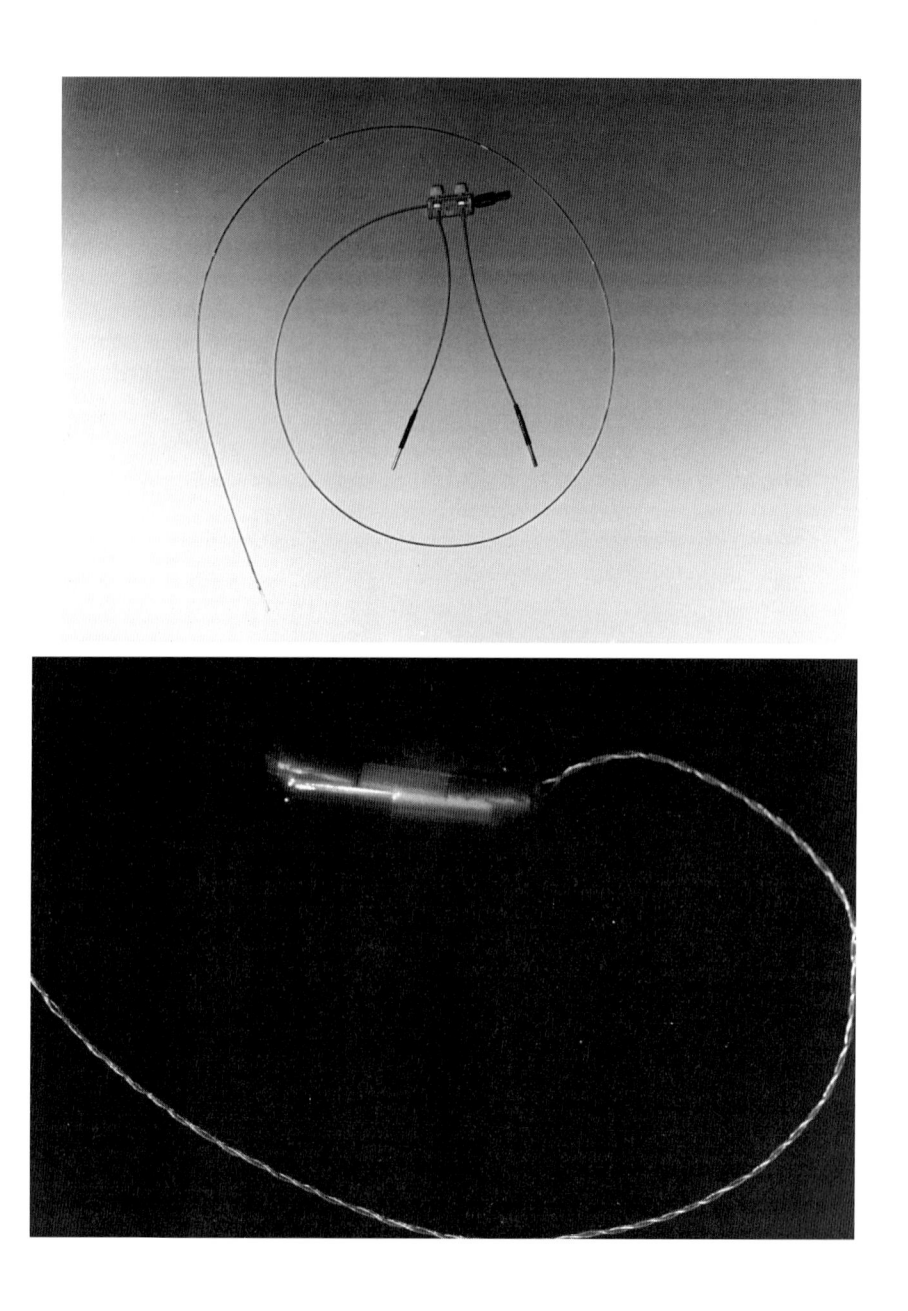

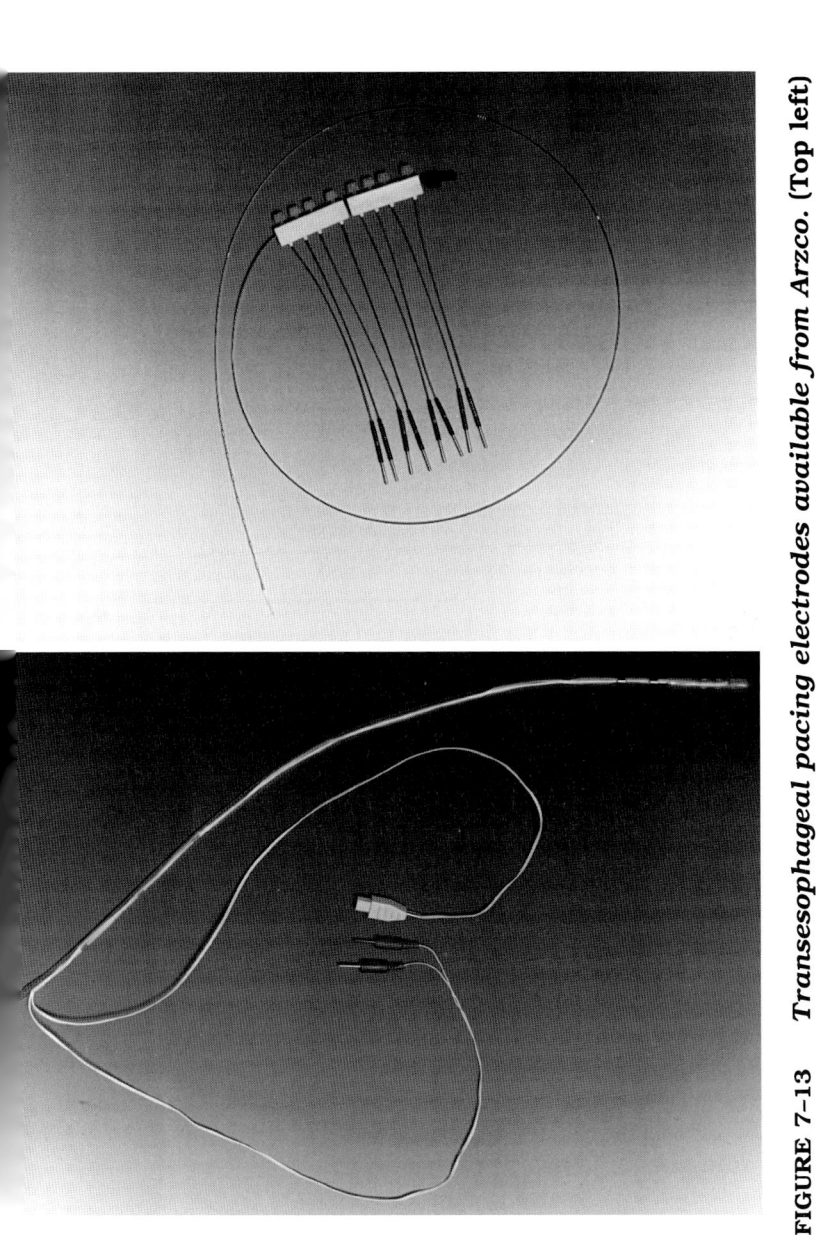

FIGURE 7-13   Transesophageal pacing electrodes available from Arzco. (Top left) Bipolar pill electrode for atrial pacing and recording. (Top right) Bipolar catheter electrode (4 Fr) for atrial pacing or recording, especially useful in neonates and small children. A wire stylet facilitates insertion. (Bottom left) 18 Fr, bipolar pacing esophageal stethoscope for intraoperative ECG recording or atrial pacing in adults. (Bottom right) Octapolar catheter electrode (4 Fr) for atrial pacing or recording with transesophageal echocardiography probe. (Illustrations kindly furnished by Arzco Medical Systems, Inc., Tampa, FL.)

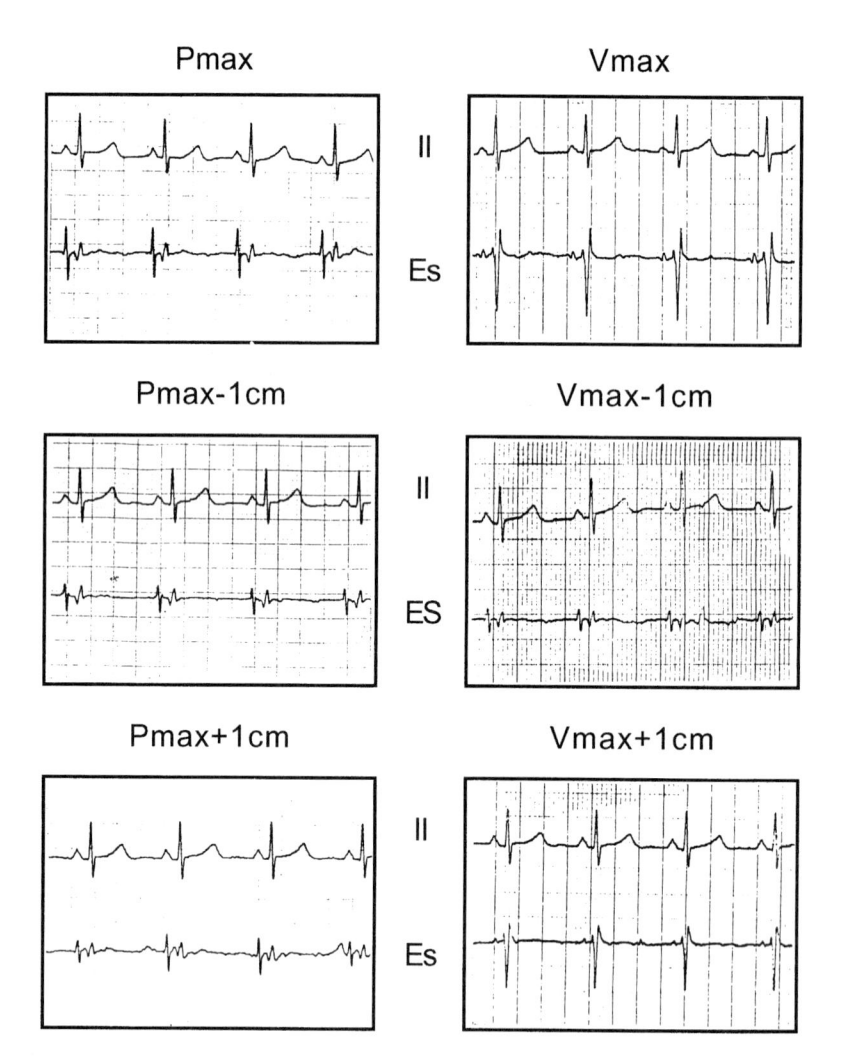

FIGURE 7-14 *Esophageal ECG (Es) at the position of a maximum amplitude P wave (Pmax) or QRS complex (Vmax), and points 1 cm proximal (Pmax − 1 cm, Vmax − 1 cm) or distal (Pmax + 1 cm, Vmax + 1 cm). Surface ECG lead II is shown above Es.*

Pacing Technique

Transesophageal pacing will most commonly be used for management of transient, disadvantageous sinus bradycardia, AV junctional rhythm disturbances, or heart block in place of atropine or other chronotropic drugs. It is recommended that the point of minimum pacing thresholds (A-Thmin or V-Thmin) be identified, and the probe be positioned there. While no thermal injury has been reported with

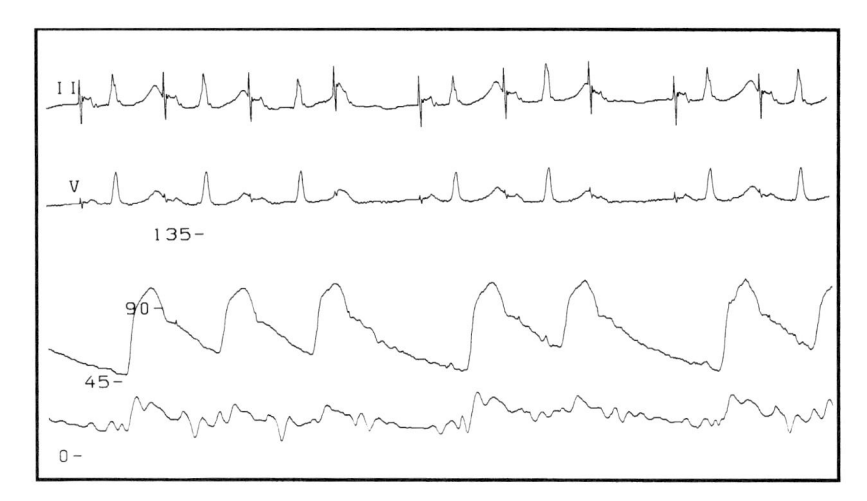

FIGURE 7-15 *Varying (4:3 and 3:2) AV nodal Wenckebach block during atrial epicardial pacing. The same phenomenon could occur with atrial endocardial or esophageal pacing, and could easily be misdiagnosed as failure to capture. Note, however, that all pacing stimuli produce P waves.*

TEAP, or for that matter TEVP, current above 15 to 20 mA may be perceived by conscious or lightly sedated patients and there is risk of simultaneous atrial and ventricular or ventricular activation with high currents. This is more likely with probes with electrode spacing more than 2.0 cm since V-Thmin is within 4 to 5 cm from A-Thmin.[20,23] Once A(V)-Thmin has been identified, current for TEA(V)P is set at 1.5 to 2.0 times A(V)-Thmin. A(V)-Thmin is determined by decreasing current until capture is just lost. The rate is set at 70 to 80 beats/min for most bradycardia, and just above that of AV junctional or idioventricular rhythm to overdrive the disturbance. TEAP can be used to overdrive ventricular escape beats and idioventricular rhythm with intact AV conduction. Pulse duration for TEAP or TEVP is 10 msec. While A-Thmin is fairly constant for pulse durations above 6 msec,[24] the strength–duration relation for TEVP has not been reported. Nevertheless, it should be similar to that with TEAP, provided the esophageal–ventricular distance is 1.0 cm or less and electrode spacing is no more than 2.0 cm.[25]

LIMITATIONS AND PRECAUTIONS

The most important limitation to TEP with available devices is the inability to pace the ventricles, except in infants and small children. Because of this, there has been a less than enthusiastic reception to TEP among practitioners as an alternative to drugs or other forms of

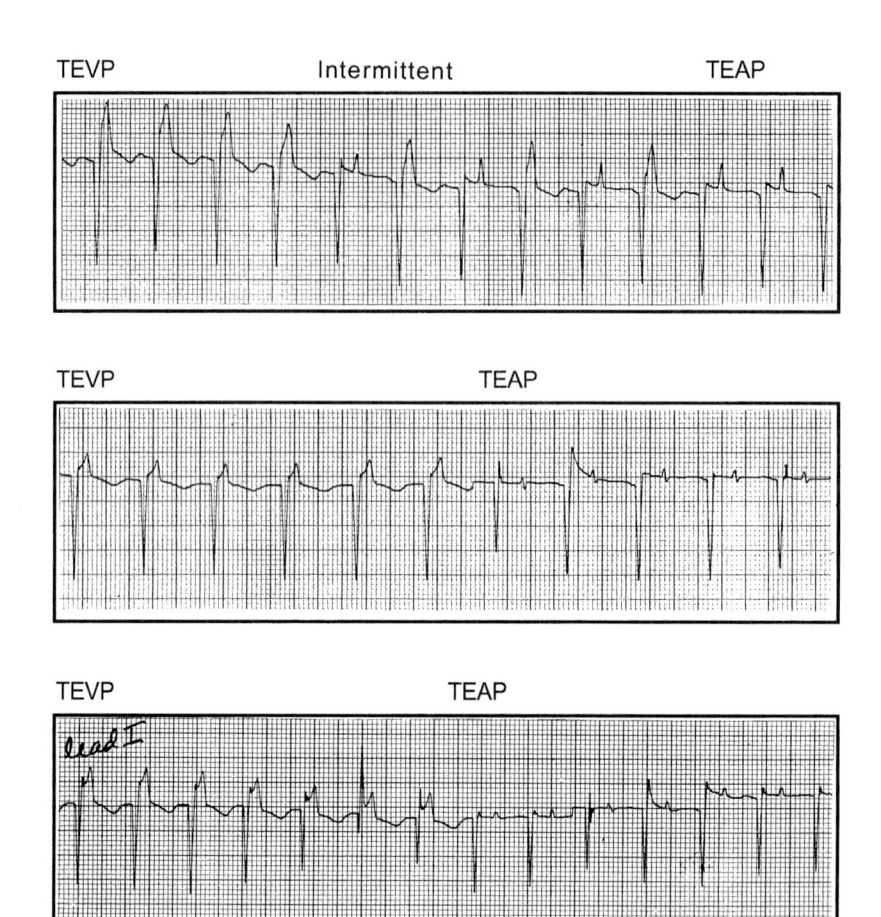

FIGURE 7-16   *Differentiation of transesophageal ventricular (TEVP) and atrial pacing capture (TEAP) in three patients.*[23] *The electrode spanned the AV groove, so that atrial or ventricular pacing was possible in all patients, depending on current supplied. All surface ECG tracings are lead I to reduce the amplitude of stimulus artifacts. To produce TEAP (all panels), current was decreased to loss of TEVP capture. In all tracings, with TEVP or TEAP, the amplitude of QRS complexes (upward deflections) is small in comparison to that of stimulus artifacts (downward deflections). Note that TEVP capture beats show no discernible S-to-R interval, while TEAP beats have a distinct S-to-R interval.* **(Top)** *Note intermittent TEVP capture as pacing current is reduced.* **(Middle and Bottom)** *There is a smooth transition to TEAP as current is reduced.*

pacing for disadvantageous bradyarrhythmias, even though available TEAP probes are relatively inexpensive and disposable, and can meet most needs for temporary perioperative pacing. However, it is recognized that TEVP will be required for many temporary pacing indications in cardiology and emergency medicine, where there is a higher proportion of patients with high-degree AV heart block or significant bradycardia in association with atrial fibrillation. Probes suitable for TEAP or TEVP, or monitoring probes that can easily be adapted for TEVP, were under development or being tested at this writing. Finally, a *relative* contraindication to TEP, or any esophageal intubation for that matter, is the presence of esophageal disease or strictures. Nevertheless, in emergencies, if TEP is the only pacing method available or that can be instituted rapidly, it should not necessarily be withheld in favor of drugs in such patients. However, for obvious reasons, the TEP probe should be inserted with particular caution, and not advanced beyond a position that will assure pacing with reasonable thresholds, not necessarily at A-Thmin or V-Thmin.

Pacing Methods for Specific Rhythm Disturbances

Unless otherwise noted, any of the temporary pacing methods discussed above, including noninvasive TCP and TEP, can be used for pacing with most of the rhythm disturbances discussed later in this section. However, methods that pace only the ventricle may provide inadequate hemodynamics in patients with heart failure, and atrial pacing is not feasible with chronic atrial fibrillation or complete AV heart block. Concerning temporary pacing for interruption of tachyarrhythmias, it is cautioned that pacing is rarely a first-choice therapy, even for disturbances known to be easily pace terminable (e.g., reentry SVT). Certainly, pacing should not be used as the initial treatment for tachyarrhythmias with severe circulatory compromise. Instead, DC cardioversion and drugs are preferred treatment. Also, when pacing is used for interruption or management of tachyarrhythmias, drugs may also be needed to achieve the desired effect or to prevent recurrences. Finally, with any antitachycardia pacing, it is mandatory that a back-up, functioning, DC cardioverter–defibrillator be physically available.

BRADYCARDIA, ESCAPE RHYTHMS AND ATRIOVENTRICULAR HEART BLOCK

The goal is to relieve disadvantageous hemodynamics produced by bradycardia, loss of AV synchrony, or both. If there is high-degree AV

284 TEMPORARY CARDIAC PACING: PRACTICAL ASPECTS

1. AV Junctional Rhythm (50 bpm) 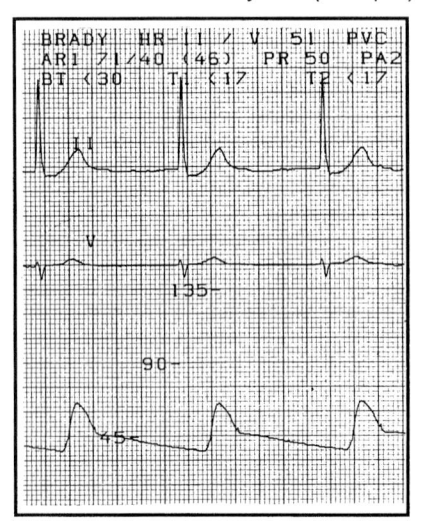
2. Following Atropine (0.4 mg) 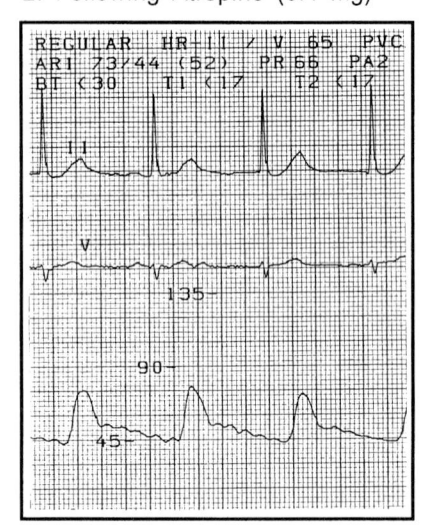
3. Following Ephedrine (10 mg) 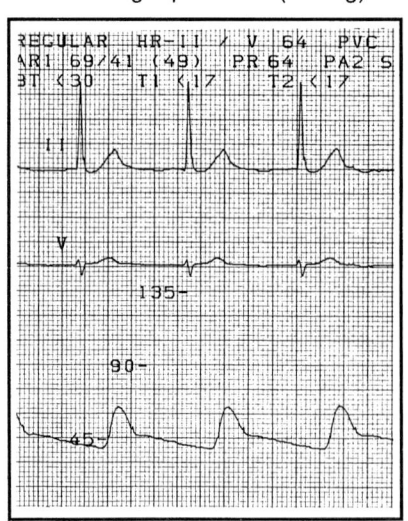
4. During Atrial Pacing (80 bpm)

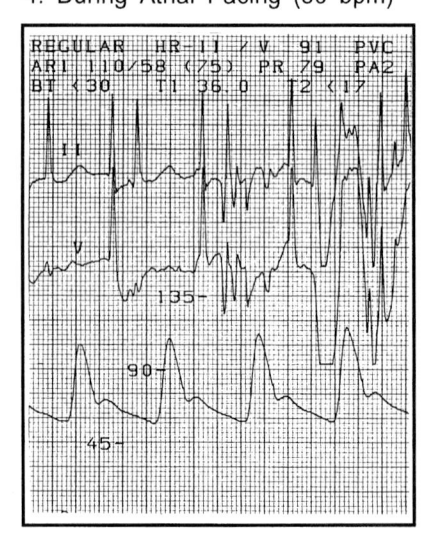

FIGURE 7–17 *See legend on opposite page*

conduction block, and the atria are not fibrillating, then synchronized atrial or AV sequential pacing is preferred to ventricular pacing. If conduction is intact, as it usually is with AV junctional and ventricular escape rhythms, then atrial overdrive pacing will suppress arrhythmias and restore hemodynamics (Fig. 7–17). The rate of atrial pacing is that which overdrives the disturbance and provides optimal hemodynamics. However, in patients with sinus bradycardia, even though cardiac output is the product of heart rate and stroke volume, too great an increase in heart rate may produce myocardial ischemia or shorten diastolic time. In patients with coronary artery disease, rates above 120 beats/min increase the risk of ischemia, although this can vary considerably among patients. Cardiac output will increase in most between 60 and 100 beats/min. Above this, there is little further increase in cardiac output, or even a decrease due to diastolic encroachment or ischemia. Finally, in patients with disadvantageous bradycardia and in need of temporary pacing, if the patient has epicardial or endocardial leads and a programmable temporary pulse generator is available (Fig. 7–5), selection of the appropriate pacing mode will depend on the nature of bradycardia (AV heart block or SND), whether the patient has atrial fibrillation, and whether the patient is susceptible to atrial tachycardia (Fig. 7–18).

SUPPRESSION OR TERMINATION OF TACHYARRHYTHMIAS

Pacing may be used to overdrive frequent premature atrial or ventricular beats, particularly following open heart surgery and

---

FIGURE 7–17   *Transesophageal atrial overdrive pacing for disadvantageous AV junctional rhythm unresponsive to drugs.* (Top left) *AV junctional rhythm at 50 beats/min (bpm) with an average blood pressure of 65/36 mmHg.* (Top right) *Only the rate of AV junctional rhythm (65 beats/min) has increased significantly by 1 minute after atropine, since average blood pressure increased transiently to 75/44 mmHg but declined after 1 minute.* (Bottom left) *Ephedrine was administered next, with no improvement in heart rate or blood pressure.* (Bottom right) *Transesophageal atrial overdrive pacing restored AV synchrony and produced an immediate increase in average blood pressure to 112/57 mmHg. Pacing was required for the duration of anesthesia and surgery, but sinus rhythm was restored during emergence from anesthesia (not shown).*

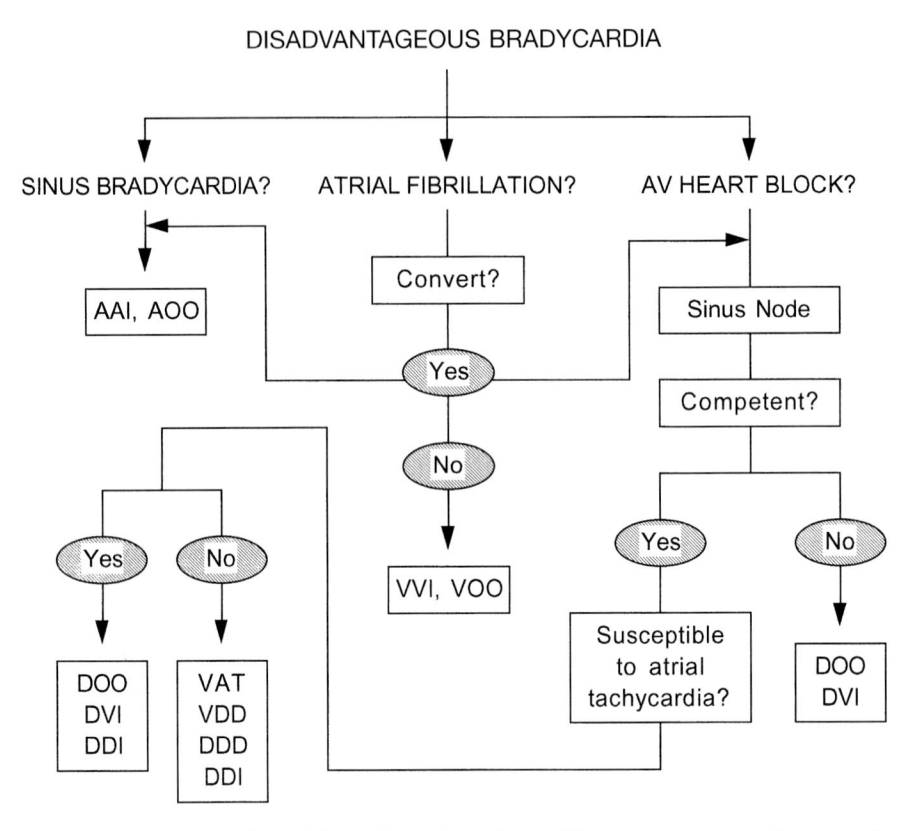

286 TEMPORARY CARDIAC PACING: PRACTICAL ASPECTS

```
                    DISADVANTAGEOUS BRADYCARDIA
                                 │
          ┌──────────────────────┼──────────────────────┐
          ▼                      ▼                      ▼
   SINUS BRADYCARDIA?    ATRIAL FIBRILLATION?      AV HEART BLOCK?
          │                      │                      │
          ▼                   Convert?              Sinus Node
       AAI, AOO                  │                  Competent?
                               Yes                      │
                                │                  ┌────┴────┐
                               No                 Yes        No
                                │                  │          │
                                ▼              Susceptible   DOO
                            VVI, VOO          to atrial      DVI
                                               tachycardia?
       Yes    No
        │      │
        ▼      ▼
      DOO    VAT
      DVI    VDD
      DDI    DDD
             DDI
```

FIGURE 7–18 *Algorithm for selection of temporary pacing mode in patients with bradycardia due to SND or AV heart block. Atrial tracking pacing modes, whereby ventricular pacing is triggered by sensed atrial events, are not appropriate for patients with susceptibility to atrial tachyarrhythmias because of the risk of one-to-one tracking of tachycardia. Code for NASPE–BPEG pacing modes is explained in Table 6–3.*

especially when these reduce cardiac output or trigger more bothersome arrhythmias.[3,26,27] The rate may need to be as fast as 100 to 110 beats/min. As discussed earlier, patients with SND or acquired long-QT-interval syndrome may benefit from pacing at faster rates (80 to 100 beats/min) to reduce the likelihood of bradycardia-dependent SVT or torsades de pointes VT.

Atrial Flutter

There are two types of atrial flutter, slow (type I) atrial flutter with an atrial rate of 230 to 340 beats/min, and fast (type II) atrial flutter with an atrial rate of 340 to 430 beats/min.[28] Type I flutter is, and type II flutter is not, terminated by rapid atrial pacing at a rate faster than the spontaneous flutter rate for a sufficient duration of time (≥ 10 seconds). Also, the current required for pacing atrial flutter (two to four times threshold) is greater than for other atrial pacing applications in order to assure atrial capture. Waldo recommends a ramp atrial pacing technique for terminating type I atrial flutter.[3,26,27] Atrial pacing is begun at a rate 10 beats/min faster than the spontaneous flutter rate while ECG lead II is continuously recorded. When it is shown that the atrial rate has increased to the pacing rate (e.g., an increase in the ventricular rate in presence of 2:1 AV block, or decrease in rate with higher degree block), the pacing rate is gradually increased until flutter waves in lead II, which were previously negative, become positive. This almost invariably indicates interruption of flutter. Alternatively, pacing may be begun at a rate that is 120 to 130 percent of the flutter rate and continued for 30 seconds or until the flutter waves become positive. If this fails, the rate is increased by 5- to 10-beats/min increments. When flutter has been interrupted, pacing may be terminated abruptly or first slowed gradually to about 100 beats/min. Prolonged sinus pause or asystole may occur in patients with SND after too abrupt termination of pacing. This is due to overdrive suppression of the sinus node by atrial flutter and rapid atrial pacing.

Regardless of which method is used for pacing, rapid atrial pacing may produce atrial fibrillation in some patients. This may terminate spontaneously within several minutes, or persist. If atrial fibrillation persists, this may be preferable to atrial flutter because the ventricular rate with atrial fibrillation is more easily controlled by drugs. Finally, for patients in whom atrial flutter recurs despite interruption by pacing, continuous atrial pacing at rates of 400 to 450 beats/min to precipitate sustained atrial fibrillation may be indicated.

Atrioventricular Nodal and Atrioventricular Reentry Tachycardia

In the author's experience, neither of these types of reentry SVT involving the AV node with or without an accessory AV bypass pathway is common in anesthetized patients. They are more commonly observed in emergency departments, in anxious patients in preoperative holding areas, and in postanesthesia or critical care units. Perhaps this is because anesthetic drugs and/or the anesthetic state, as a result of the relative vagotonia with increased AV refractoriness, are less conducive to reentry SVT involving the AV node. Evidence for this is presented or discussed elsewhere.[29,30] AV nodal and AV reentry tachycardia are probably the easiest tachyarrhythmias to interrupt with atrial pacing. Should either occur in a patient with atrial pacing leads (epicardial wires, transvenous pacing, or TEAP), pacing is considered by some the initial treatment of choice.[3,26,27] While these arrhythmias may be interrupted by appropriately timed premature extrastimulation, this is beyond the capability of available temporary external pulse generators. However, a simple modification of extrastimulation is to pace the atria (or ventricles in patients with intact VA conduction) at a rate slower than that of SVT (e.g., 100 beats/min) until a paced beat randomly occurs at an appropriate interval after a spontaneous beat of tachycardia and interrupts the tachycardia. However, since this technique ("underdrive pacing") does not work predictably, and reentry SVT can always be interrupted by pacing at rates faster than the rate of tachycardia, overdrive pacing at a rate 5 to 15 beats/min faster than the tachycardia rate is recommended.[3,26,27] In some patients, rates 20 to 50 beats/min faster than the tachycardia rate may be required, especially if the slower rate only transiently entrains reentry SVT.[3,26,27] For those patients in whom tachycardia recurs, despite successful interruption by atrial overdrive pacing, indicated drugs may be added to help prevent recurrences (see Chapter 5). Finally, continuous rapid atrial pacing techniques, such as deliberate induction and maintenance of atrial fibrillation (discussed earlier) or pacing at 200 to 220 beats/min and maintaining 2:1 AV conduction, may be required to suppress reentry SVT and control the ventricular rate.

Ectopic (Nonparoxysmal) Atrial Tachycardia

Ectopic atrial tachycardia may be an automatic or triggered disturbance, with uniform (nonparoxysmal atrial tachycardia, with or without AV block) or multiform atrial complexes (multiform atrial tachycardia). The atrial rates with ectopic atrial tachycardia range from 130 to 240 beats/min, with the slower rates more characteristic of the multiform variant. Uniform ectopic atrial tachycardia with 2:1 AV block is a common manifestation of digitalis toxicity. The ventricular rate with 2:1 AV block may be clinically acceptable, so that no treatment is indicated. Some atrial ectopic tachycardia is due to intraatrial reentry, and therefore potentially interrupted by atrial pacing similar to that for atrial flutter (discussed earlier), except that slower rates are used. During pacing the rhythm is transiently entrained to match the pacing rate until, at a sufficiently fast pacing rate, the rhythm is interrupted.[3,26,27] Finally, for some patients, continuous rapid atrial pacing may be required to achieve and maintain 2:1 AV conduction and a slower ventricular rate.

Noncompensatory Sinus and Atrioventricular Junctional Automatic Tachycardias

Neither of these rhythm disturbances are amenable to temporary pacing, although pacing may be useful in differential diagnosis and management. Noncompensatory sinus tachycardia (NCST) (i.e., not due to hypovolemia) is more often than not a manifestation of too light anesthesia, venodilation or vasodilation, or pain and anxiety. Therefore treatment is to correct the cause as appropriate. While NCST can be overdriven by atrial pacing at a rate faster than tachycardia, following cessation of pacing the tachycardia resumes after a gradual "warm-up" period. AV junctional tachycardia (AVJT) is AV junctional rhythm above 80 beats/min, which is tachycardia for the junctional pacemakers. Rarely is AVJT faster than 130 beats/min in adults. AVJT is also easily overdriven by atrial or ventricular pacing, but the disturbance usually recurs following cessation of pacing unless the cause has been removed. In some patients with AVJT and severe hemodynamic compromise, it may be necessary to provide atrial pacing to restore hemodynamics, even if the rate of pacing would normally be considered tachycardia. In fact, the risk of ischemia due to inadequate coronary perfusion with AVJT may be greater than that with pacing at 120 to 130 beats/min to overdrive AVJT. With restoration of adequate hemodynamics and coronary perfusion, it is frequently possible to wean the patient from pacing over a period of minutes to hours. Since AVJT in perioperative settings is often caused by myocardial ischemia, drugs to treat ischemia and improve coronary perfusion with pacing may correct the disturbance. Sometimes, AVJT is associated with a significant degree of antegrade AV block (e.g., following valvular or congenital heart surgery). If so, atrial pacing at a rate faster than the AV junctional pacemaker will result in high-degree AV block and not overdrive AVJT. In this case, sequential AV pacing (DOO, DVI, DDI, DDD) at a rate appropriately faster than the AV junctional pacemaker is required.

Atrioventricular Junctional Tachycardia in Neonates and Infants

Atrioventricular junctional tachycardia in neonates and infants can be much faster than in adults (e.g., 250 to 260 beats/min), and sometimes produces life-threatening hemodynamic compromise. In this case, a special pacing technique known as *atrial* or *ventricular paired pacing* is used to halve the effective mechanical ventricular rate. With paired pacing, a paced premature atrial or ventricular beat is coupled to each paced overdrive beat or spontaneous beat of AVJT. The premature beats result in electrical, but not mechanical, responses, thereby improving hemodynamics. Disadvantages of the technique include increased metabolic demand of the heart, the requirement for a programmable external stimulator that can deliver extrastimuli, a knowledgable user, and risk of inducing ventricular fibrillation. An alternative technique for pacing rapid AVJT using a conventional external pulse generator (Medtronic 5330 AV sequential demand pacemaker, Fig. 7–4) was described by Sluysmans and coauthors.[31] One of the ventricular electrodes was connected to the negative poles of both the atrial and ventricular channels, and the other to the positive poles of the atrial and ventricular channels. This enabled stimulation of the ventricle with an atrial stimulus (S_1) followed by paired ventricular stimulation (S_2) after the selected AV delay of 220 msec. The S_1 rate was 136 beats (cycle length = 440 msec), providing ventricular capture at a rate of 272 beats/min. Then, the S_1–S_2 interval was reduced to 180 msec, which was short enough to produce an electrical response without a mechanical response, thereby halving the effective mechanical rate to 136 beats/min and increasing systolic blood pressure from 60 to 100 mmHg. The intervals 180 and 260 msec (summed = 440 msec "atrial" rate) were short enough to suppress AVJT (cycle length 245 to 265 msec = 245 to 226 beats/min). After 12 hours, paired pacing could be discontinued with an adequate atrial rhythm, and normal sinus rhythm was restored by discharge on the fifth day.

Ventricular Tachycardias

Intravenous drug treatment and DC cardioversion–defibrillation are preferred initial treatment for most VT, especially with severe circulatory instability. However, without circulatory compromise and with reentry VT, rapid ventricular and sometimes even atrial pacing may interrupt tachycardia, as with reentry SVT. Atrial pacing will be effective only if there is 1:1 conduction of paced atrial beats so as to permit entrainment of VT. The pacing methods are similar to those used for type I atrial flutter and reentry SVT (discussed earlier). As with pacing for these disturbances, pacing must be sufficiently faster than the VT rate for entrainment, pacing must be continued for a sufficient time, and pacing to terminate VT must achieve a critical rate, which is usually greater than the entrainment rate. Finally, as with AVJT (discussed earlier), ventricular paired pacing may be required to terminate some reentrant VT.

References

1. Hayes D, Holmes D. Temporary cardiac pacing. In Furman S, Hayes D, Holmes D (eds): A Practice of Cardiac Pacing. 3rd ed. Mt. Kisco, NY: Futura Publishing, 1993: pp. 231–260.
2. Brown J. Atropine, scopolamine, and related antimuscarinic drugs. In Gilman A, Rall T, Nies A, Taylor P (eds): The Pharmacological Basis of Therapeutics. 8th ed. New York: Pergammon Press, 1990: pp. 150–165.
3. Waldo A, Wells J, Cooper T, MacLean W. Temporary cardiac pacing: Applications and techniques in the treatment of cardiac arrhythmias. Prog Cardiovasc Dis 1981;23:451–474.
4. Luceri R, Stafford W, Castellanos A, Myerburg R. The temporary pacemaker. In Platia E (ed): Management of Cardiac Arrhythmias. Philadelphia: JB Lippincott, 1987: pp. 219–235.
5. Emergency Cardiac Care Committee and Subcommittees AHA. Guidelines for cardiopulmonary resuscitation and emergency cardiac care, III: Adult advanced cardiac life support. JAMA 1992;268:2199–2241.
6. Zoll P. Noninvasive cardiac stimulation revisited. PACE 1990;13:2014–2016.
7. Birkui P, Trigano J, Zoll P (eds). Noninvasive Transcutaneous Pacing. Mount Kisco, NY: Futura Publishing, 1993.
8. Bocka J. External transcutaneous pacemakers. Ann Emerg Med 1989;18:1280–1286.
9. Kelly J, Royster R. Noninvasive transcutaneous pacing. Anesth Analg 1989;69:229–238.
10. Altamura G, Toscano S, Bianconi L, et al. Transcutaneous cardiac pacing: Evaluation of cardiac activation. PACE 1990;13:2017–2021.
11. Syverud S, Dalsey W, Hedges J. Transcutaneous and transvenous cardiac pacing for early bradyasystolic cardiac arrest. Ann Emerg Med 1986;15:121–124.
12. Zoll P, Zoll R, Falk R, et al. External noninvasive temporary cardiac pacing: Clinical trials. Circulation 1985;71:937–944.
13. Benson DJ. Transesophageal electrocardiography and cardiac pacing: State of the art. Circulation 1987;75(Suppl III):86–90.
14. Atlee J. Transesophageal and other new pacing modalities. In Kaplan J (ed): Cardiothoracic and Vascular Anesthesia Update. Vol. 3, Chapter 3. Philadelphia: WB Saunders, 1993: pp. 1–9.
15. Pattison C, Atlee J, Mathews E, et al. Atrial pacing thresholds measured in anesthetized patients with the use of an esophageal stethoscope modified for pacing. Anesthesiology 1991;74:854–859.
16. Atlee J, Pattison C, Mathews E, et al. Evaluation of transesophageal atrial pacing stethoscope in adult surgical patients under general anesthesia. PACE 1992;15:1515–1525.
17. Atlee J, Pattison C, Mathews E, Hedman A. Transesophageal atrial pacing for intraoperative sinus bradycardia or AV junctional rhythm:

Feasibility as prophylaxis in 200 anesthetized adults and hemodynamic effects of treatment. J Cardiothorac Vasc Anesth 1993;74: 436–441.
18. Pattison C, Atlee J, Krebs L, et al. Transesophageal indirect atrial pacing for drug-resistant sinus bradycardia. Anesthesiology 1991; 74:1141–1144.
19. Smith I, Monk T, White P. Comparison of transesophageal atrial pacing with anticholinergic drugs for the treatment of intraoperative bradycardia. Anesth Analg 1994;78:245–252.
20. Atlee J, Bilof R. Feasibility of transesophageal indirect ventricular pacing with a pacing esophageal stethoscope. Anesthesiology 1992; 77:A66.
21. Andersen H, Pless P. Transesophageal pacing. PACE 1983;6:674–679.
22. Andersen H, Pless P. Transesophageal dual-chamber pacing. Int J Cardiol 1984;5:745–748.
23. Atlee J, Bilof R. Transesophageal ventricular pacing in anesthetized adults. Anesthesiology 1993;79:A75.
24. Chung D, Townsend G, Kerr C. The optimum site and strength–duration relationship of transesophageal indirect atrial pacing. Anesthesiology 1986;65:428–431.
25. Crawford T, Dick MI, Bank E, Jenkins J. Transesophageal atrial pacing: Importance of the atrial-esophageal relationship. Med Instrument 1986;20:1280–1286.
26. Waldo A, Biblo L, Carlson M. Temporary pacing in diagnosis and treatment of arrhythmias after open-heart surgery. In Barold S, Mugica J (eds): New Perspectives in Cardiac Pacing. 2. Mt. Kisco, NY, Futura Publishing, 1991: pp. 339–357.
27. Waldo A, Henthorn R, Plumb V. Temporary epicardial wire electrodes in the diagnosis and treatment of arrhythmias after open heart surgery. Am J Surg 1984;148:275–283.
28. Wells J, MacLean W, James T, Waldo A. Characterization of atrial flutter. Studies in man after open heart surgery using fixed atrial electrodes. Circulation 1979;60:665–673.
29. Atlee J, Yeager T. Electrophysiologic assessment of the effects of enflurane, halothane, and isoflurane on properties affecting supraventricular reentry in chronically instrumented dogs. Anesthesiology 1989;71:941–952.
30. Atlee J, Bosnjak Z. Mechanisms for cardiac dysrhythmias during anesthesia. Anesthesiology 1990;72:347–374.
31. Sluysmans T, Moulin D, Jaumin P, et al. Ventricular paired pacing to control intractable junctional tachycardia following open heart surgery in a child. Intens Care Med 1989;15:203–205.

8

Management of Patients with Pacemakers or ICD Devices

Abbreviations Used in Chapter Eight

AV	Atrioventricular
CMOS	Complementary Metal Oxide Semiconductor
ECG	Electrocardiogram (cardiography)
ECT	Electroconvulsive therapy
EMI	Electromagnetic interference
ESWL	Extracorporeal shock wave lithotripsy
ICD	Internal cardioverter–defibrillator
MRI	Magnetic resonance imaging
PAC	Pulmonary artery catheter
PDF	Probability density function
SVT	Supraventricular tachycardia
TENS	Transcutaneous electrical nerve stimulation
VA	Ventriculoatrial
VT/VF	Ventricular tachycardia/fibrillation

Pacemakers and internal cardioverter–defibrillators (ICD) are highly sophisticated devices that are especially susceptible to system malfunction or failure in hospital environments. Also, these devices are implanted in patients with severe cardiac disease, often with significant concurrent major systemic disease. Therefore, there is recognized potential for malfunction and complications with pacemaker or ICD devices. Discussion of these, along with suggested prevention and management, is the purpose of this chapter. Also, because anesthesia practitioners may on occasion provide anesthesia or monitored care for patients undergoing pacemaker or ICD system revision or implantation, perioperative management is also discussed. As in the previous two chapters, North American Society of Pacing and Electrophysiology–British Pacing and Electrophysiology Group codes (Table 6–3) will be used in this chapter to designate pacing modes.

Pacemaker Complications

Early (≤ 1 month) and late complications of pacemaker or ICD implantation are summarized in Table 8–1.[1-5] Some are of little importance to physicians who do not see patients with pacemakers, but others do have relevance to anesthetic and critical care management.

EARLY COMPLICATIONS

TABLE 8-1 *Early and late complications associated with pacemakers and ICD devices*

EARLY	LATE	EARLY OR LATE
Pneumo(hemo)thorax	Pulse generator erosion	Lead dislodgement
Subcutaneous emphysema	Thromboembolism	Pacemaker arrhythmias
Myocardial perforation	Lead defects	Pacemaker infection
Arterial lead placement	High-pacing thresholds	Pacemaker syndrome
Brachial plexus injury	Battery depletion	Generator malfunction
Operative complications	Twiddler's syndrome	Extracardiac stimulation
Pulmonary complications	Pacemaker allergy	Loose connections

Hemothorax or Pneumothorax

The subclavian vein is commonly used for implantation of permanent transvenous pacemaker leads. Since the vein is usually approached blindly, there is risk of subclavian arterial or venous laceration, or lung puncture, with hemothorax or pneumothorax. These are more likely in patients with unusual chest wall or sternoclavicular anatomy, in which case leads are best positioned with fluoroscopic guidance.[1] Pneumothorax or hemothorax may manifest as late as 48 hours after pacemaker implantation as respiratory distress, chest pain, or hypotension. A chest tube is indicated for pneumothorax greater than 10 percent, hemothorax, or respiratory distress.

Subcutaneous Emphysema

Subcutaneous emphysema is also a complication of subclavian puncture, and a patient with this condition should be evaluated for associated pneumothorax. If subcutaneous emphysema extends to the pacemaker pocket with a unipolar device, air accumulation in the pacemaker pocket can insulate the unipolar (anodal) pacemaker can and cause pacemaker malfunction (i.e., failure to pace or sense). If the polarity of pacing and sensing can be programmed independently, it is possible to see failure of pacing or sensing. Gentle pressure on the pacemaker site to express air surrounding the pulse generator may help to restore normal pacemaker function.

Arterial Lead Placement

While inadvertent subclavian artery puncture is usually recognized during attempts at vein puncture, it occasionally may be unnoticed until positioning of the pacing leads in the left ventricle is detected.[1] Left ventricular placement can also occur with pacing lead positioning via the right subclavian vein in patients with unsuspected atrial or ventricular septal defects. While left ventricular pacing can function well, it has been associated with thromboembolism and stroke. For this reason, early removal of the left ventricular pacing lead is advised.

Myocardial Perforation

Lack of any symptoms after ventricular perforation by a lead is not uncommon. The only sign may be an increase in pacing thresholds. Symptoms include pericardial pain and friction rub; other signs are a change in the ventricular activation pattern during pacing, cardiac tamponade, pericardial effusion, pericarditis, and intercostal muscle or diaphragmatic stimulation. Roentgenography, electrocardiography (ECG), and two-dimensional echocardiography are used to confirm the diagnosis. Once perforation is confirmed the lead must be removed, which is usually uncomplicated. Pericardial bleeding or tamponade are said to be rare.[1]

LATE COMPLICATIONS

Thromboembolism

Fortunately, thromboembolic complications following permanent pacemaker implantation are rare. If thrombosis involves the subclavian vein, superior vena cava, right atrium, or ventricle, it can cause superior vena cava occlusion, reduced cardiac output and hypotension secondary to impaired venous return, pulmonary embolism, or an edematous and painful upper extremity. Venous obstruction as the result of a chronically implanted pacing lead can be relieved by balloon venoplasty.[1]

Lead Insulation Defects and Fracture

Polyurethane and silicone are used as insulation for most permanent pacing leads. The former is more susceptible to lead insulation defects.[1] These occur at points of stress, crush injury, and ligature sites. Lead fracture, common in the early years of pacing, has become less common with improvements in conductor technology. Lead fractures commonly occur adjacent to the pulse generator or near the venous access site, points of most shear stress. Direct trauma to pacing leads is an uncommon cause. When unipolar lead fracture occurs, it is usually necessary to replace the lead. With bipolar leads and a polarity-programmable pacer, it may be possible to temporarily restore function by reprogramming the device to the unipolar configuration.[1]

High Pacing Thresholds Due to Exit Block

Extrinsic causes for increased pacing thresholds are discussed later under Drug Device Interactions. An unusual intrinsic cause is exit block, which is persistent, often progressive, high pacing thresholds after the usual acute rise in pacing thresholds between the first 3 and 6 weeks.[1] High thresholds are not explained on the basis of lead perforation or migration. Rather, the cause is related to lead design or excessive tissue reaction surrounding the electrode. Reprogramming the pacemaker with higher outputs may not solve the problem, since required current may exceed the capacity of the pacemaker. Newer steroid-eluting leads have helped to prevent exit block.[1]

Premature Battery Depletion

Battery depletion is expected eventually, so it is not an unexpected occurrence or necessarily considered a complication. However, if battery depletion occurs much earlier than expected, it is considered a complication and potential causes should be explored. Among the causes is improper programming of pacing parameters so that more energy than necessary is consumed. For example, a dual-chamber pacing mode might be programmed when a single-chamber mode would suffice. Another cause for premature battery depletion could be excessive energy drain due to loss of lead integrity.

Twiddler's Syndrome

Purposeful or absentminded manipulation ("twiddling") of the pulse generator by the patient is termed *twiddler's syndrome*. Such manipulation can cause axial rotation of the pulse generator and twisting of the lead, resulting in lead fracture or dislodgement with consequent pacemaker malfunction. The problem is most likely to occur when the pacemaker pocket is too large or because the pacemaker has migrated.

Pacemaker Allergy

Allergy to the pacemaker can or other system components is a very rare but reported complication.[1] Materials in the pacemaker system that are most commonly responsible for allergy include titanium, epoxy cement, silicone rubber, and polyurethane. Some apparent cases of allergy are in fact low-grade *Staphylococcus epidermidis* infections.

EARLY OR LATE COMPLICATIONS

Lead Dislodgement and Migration

Active and passive fixation devices with contemporary pacing leads have significantly reduced the incidence of lead dislodgement. Secondary intervention rates for these complications should be well below 2 and 5 percent for ventricular and atrial leads, respectively.[1] Lead dislodgement and migration is among the causes for failure to pace and under- or oversensing (discussed later). Proximal dislodgement can be prevented by use of a snugly fitting polyester pouch at the time of system implantation to encase the pulse generator and leads within the pacemaker pocket.[6] This pouch reduces the likelihood of significant torsion of the proximal lead connections and pulse generator.

Pacemaker-Related Arrhythmias

LEAD INSERTION AND MANIPULATION. Supraventricular and ventricular arrhythmias may be produced during lead insertion and manipulation for proper electrode positioning (Fig. 8-1).

TIP EXTRASYSTOLES. Tip extrasystoles may be seen in the early (≤ 48 hours) postoperative period.[1] These are ventricular-origin beats with the same morphology as paced ventricular beats, but not preceded by a pacing stimulus. They originate at the electrode–tissue interface, presumably a result of local "irritation" produced by the newly implanted lead. The ventricular beats in the bottom panel of Figure 8-1 can be considered examples of tip extrasystoles, except that the lead had only just been secured.

PACEMAKER RUNAWAY. Pacemaker runaway is a rare complication with modern pacemakers because of mandated incorporation of runaway protection circuitry,[7] and other technologic improvements. These are designed to limit the upper rate of stimulation during runaway to under 140 beats/min. With pacemaker runaway and more rapid rates, stimulation is either ineffectual or occurs intermittently, producing bursts of tachycardia.[1,8] Runaway is due to circuit malfunction, and might occur following exposure to therapeutic ionizing radiation or strong electromagnetic interference.

VENTRICULAR PACING-INDUCED ARRHYTHMIAS. While ventricular pacing may be used to suppress ventricular arrhythmias, it may also induce them. This can occur if a demand (VVI) pacemaker is programmed so fast that the patient's intrinsic rhythm is not adequately suppressed and there is competition between pacemakers (Fig. 8-2). Asynchronous ventricular pacing into the ventricular vulnerable period in patients with increased susceptibility to arrhythmias (Table 8-2) may induce serious ventricular arrhythmias. Similarly, asynchronous atrial pacing might also result in atrial extrasystoles or tachyarrhythmias.

ENDLESS-LOOP TACHYCARDIA. Endless-loop tachycardia is another well-recognized arrhythmic pacemaker complication. Endless-loop tachycardia is the pacemaker analog of AV reciprocating tachycardia (see Chapter 9).[9] Endless-loop tachycardia is most commonly initiated by a ventricular extrasystole that is conducted back to the atria to produce a retrograde P wave. This is sensed by the pacemaker as a spontaneous atrial event and tracked by atrial-triggered, ventricular pacing modes (VAT, VDD, and DDD). The triggered, paced ventricular beat, in turn, is conducted back to the atria to sustain AV

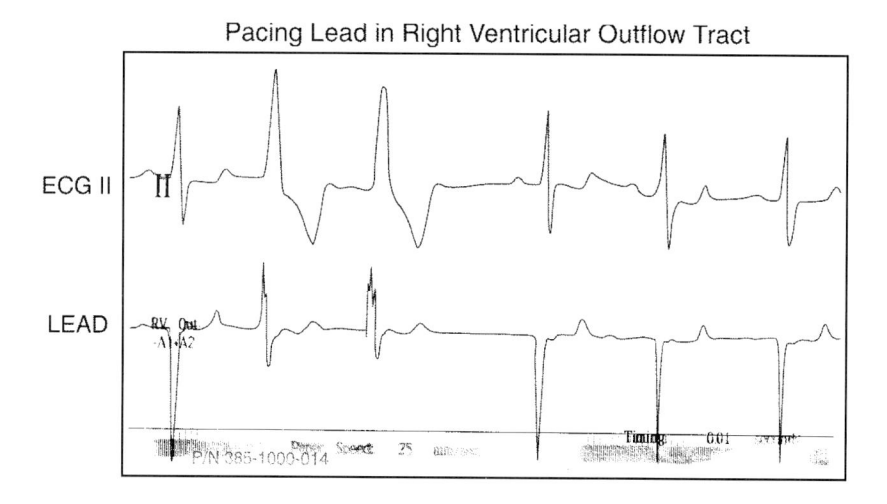

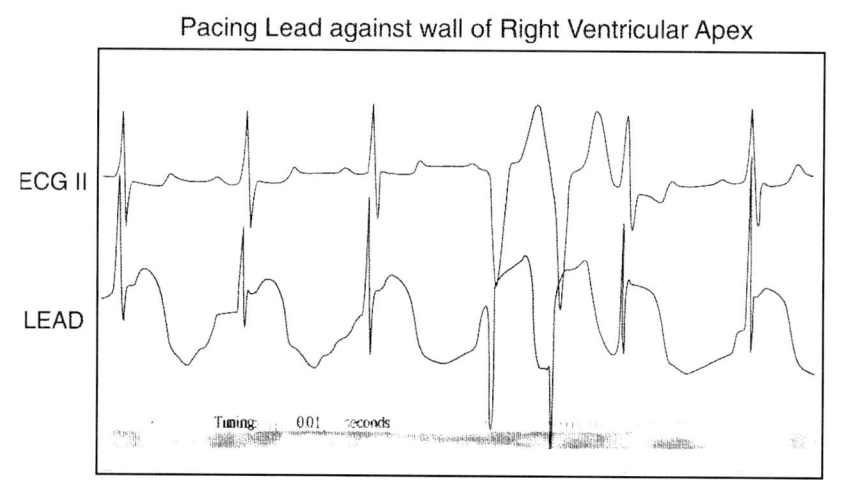

FIGURE 8-1 *Ventricular arrhythmias recorded during insertion of a bipolar, ventricular, endocardial pacing lead. In both panels the top tracing is surface ECG lead II (ECG II), and the bottom tracing the intracavitary electrogram from the pacing lead (LEAD). (Top) Ventricular extrasystoles when the tip of the pacing lead was in the right ventricular outflow tract. (Bottom) "Tip" ventricular extrasystoles with the tip of the pacing lead against the wall of the right ventricular apex. Paper speed = 25 mm/sec. (Recordings furnished by William T. Pochis, M.D.)*

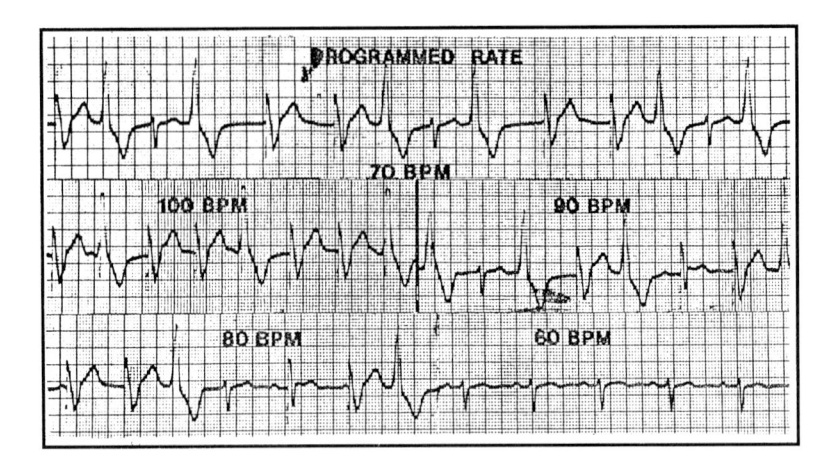

FIGURE 8-2 *Ventricular extrasystoles induced by ventricular pacing stimulation. At programmed VVI rates of 70, 100, 90, and 80 beats/min, there are frequent ventricular extrasystoles as well as paced ventricular or spontaneous beats. With VVI pacing at 60 beats/min, the rate is slow enough to allow the patient's spontaneous rhythm to predominate. (From Hayes,[1] with permission.)*

TABLE 8-2 *Factors that increase the risk of ventricular tachyarrhythmias with asynchronous pacing stimulation during the period of increased vulnerability*

Myocardial ischemia	High catecholamines	Acute potassium imbalance
Myocardial infarction	Digitalis toxicity	Hypomagnesemia
Hypermetabolic states	Long QT interval	Hypothermia
Myocarditis/pericarditis	Cardiomyopathies	Autonomic dysfunction

reciprocating tachycardia. Thus, with this type of AV reciprocation, the pacemaker itself is part of the reentry circuit.

Pacemaker Infection

Management of patients with pacemaker-related infections is the province of implanting physicians.[1] Prophylactic use of antibiotics for pacemaker implantation or system revision is controversial. Obviously, pacemaker infections are serious because of the potential for sepsis, endocarditis, or myocarditis. Pacemaker infection may be recognized as local inflammation or abscess formation in the area of the pulse generator pocket. It could also present as erosion of part of the pacing system through the skin with secondary infection, or as fever with positive blood cultures without an obvious focus of infection. Early infections are usually caused by *S. aureus*, are aggressive, and are often associated with fever and sepsis. Late infections are more indolent and commonly caused by *Staphylococcus epidermidis*. Treatment is removal of the entire infected pacing system and replacement with a new system.[1]

Pacemaker Syndrome

The pacemaker syndrome was mentioned in Chapter 6 under Hemodynamics of Pacing. It occurs most commonly in patients with normal or near-normal left ventricular function and retrograde (ventriculoatrial, VA) conduction. It results from contraction of the atria against closed AV valves as well as valvular regurgitation with ventricular contractions, all the result of retrograde atrial activation by nonsynchronous ventricular pacing modes (VOO, VVI). Symptoms and signs of the pacemaker syndrome are summarized in Table 8–3.

Generator Malfunction

Causes for pulse generator malfunction include (1) improper programming of parameters; (2) intrinsic component failure, battery depletion, or a defective magnetic reed switch; (3) extrinsic causes such as defibrillation shocks, ionizing radiation, or surgical electrocautery in immediate proximity to pacemaker leads or the pulse generator; and (4) poor anodal contact with unipolar pacemakers due to air in the pacemaker pocket or dry pocket.[8] Manifestations of pulse generator malfunction include failure to pace, undersensing, oversensing, and pacing at an altered rate. These are discussed later under Pacemaker Malfunction.

TABLE 8-3 *Symptoms and signs with the pacemaker syndrome*

SYMPTOMS	SIGNS
Weakness, lethargy, lassitude	Orthostatic hypotension; ↓ BP
Near-syncope or syncope	Cannon A waves; MI and TI*
Light-headedness, apprehension	Abnormal venous pulsations
Cough, chest pain, dyspnea	↓ CO; congestive heart failure

*Mitral and tricuspid insufficiency with ventricular contraction and open valves. BP, blood pressure; CO, cardiac output.

Extracardiac Stimulation

Extracardiac stimulation usually involves the diaphragm or pectoral muscles.[1,8] That involving the former is due to direct stimulation of the left hemidiaphragm or indirect (phrenic nerve) stimulation of the right hemidiaphragm. The potential for diaphragmatic stimulation is tested at time of system implantation, with the leads repositioned if necessary. If a late complication, diaphragmatic stimulation may be corrected by reducing pacemaker output. If due to lead migration or perforation, the pacing system may have to be revised. Pectoral muscle stimulation may also be caused by an insulation break from the extravascular portion of the pacing leads, current leakage from the connector or sealing plugs, erosion of the pacemaker's protective coating, or too high atrial output with a unipolar dual-chamber pacemaker. Pectoral muscle stimulation is less common with bipolar stimulators. If it occurs with a polarity-programmable device, reprogramming to bipolar pacing may solve the problem. Otherwise, the defective portion of the system must be replaced.

Loose Connections

Intermittent or complete failure to deliver stimuli or sense can occur as a result of a loose connection at the pacing lead–connector interface. When there is a loose connection, manipulating the pacemaker may reproduce the problem.

Pacemaker Malfunction

Pacemaker malfunction is the failure to deliver pacing stimuli at the programmed time, or the delivery of stimuli at an inappropriate rate. With asynchronous pacing modes, the cause for malfunction must be the battery itself, output circuitry, connectors, pacing leads, or the electrode–tissue interface. With demand pacers, in addition to the foregoing, there may also be sensing malfunction as under- or oversensing. The causes for pacemaker malfunction are considered in this section,[8,10,11] followed by a brief discussion of assessment of pacemaker function. Much of what follows concerning pacemaker malfunction also applies to temporary pacemakers for use with endocardial or epicardial leads (see Figs. 7–4 and 7–5). While the diagnosis of permanent pacemaker malfunction is usually made from rhythm strips and a 12-lead surface ECG,[10] temporary or permanent pacemaker malfunction is also diagnosed or suspected from arterial pulse waveform analysis (direct or oximetric) along with monitored ECG or strip-chart recordings.

FAILURE TO CAPTURE

If each pacemaker stimulus is not followed by a P wave or QRS complex, failure to capture may exist (Fig. 8–3). Causes for failure to capture are summarized in Table 8–4. Lead dislodgement or incorrect positioning of leads is the most common cause. Lead wire fracture or insulation defects, lead migration, and increased pacing thresholds (discussed later) are also causes. Absence of pacing stimuli is usually due to pulse generator failure or to interruption of the current circuit with no current flow. Exit block, discussed earlier under Late Pacemaker Complications, is another cause for failure to capture. The

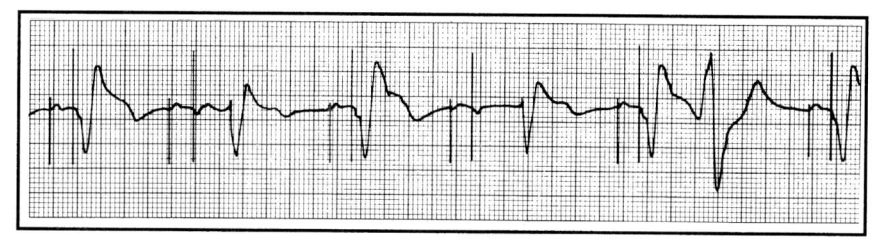

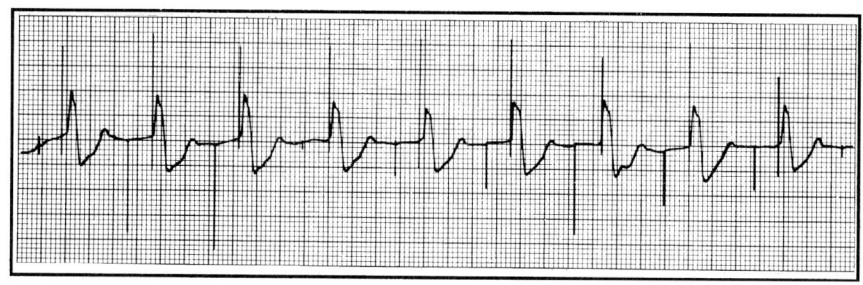

FIGURE 8–3 *Failure to capture. (Top) DDD pacemaker. With paced complexes 2 and 5, there is loss of ventricular capture. Complexes 3, 6, and 8 demonstrate appropriate ventricular sensing. Atrial pacing capture is apparent except possibly for complex 5, although other leads are required to ascertain this. Atrial sensing function cannot be determined from this recording since there are no spontaneous P waves. (Bottom) DDD pacemaker. There are no sensed atrial or ventricular events. In this recording, there is no evidence of atrial pacing capture, although other leads are required to confirm this diagnosis. (Tracings kindly furnished by Medtronic, Inc., Minneapolis, MN.)*

TABLE 8-4 *Common causes for failure to capture*

MALFUNCTION	PSEUDOMALFUNCTION
Lead dislodgement	Low-energy output settings
Lead insulation defect	Stimulus in refractory period
Battery depletion; exit block	
Increased pacing thresholds	

misdiagnosis of failure to capture, a type of pacing "pseudomalfunction," may be made if inappropriately low pacemaker output was programmed or if the pacemaker stimulus falls in the myocardial refractory period.

OUTPUT FAILURE

Output Failure Due to Oversensing

Failure to deliver a stimulus, or output failure, can have several causes (Table 8-5). Oversensing is the most common cause for failure to output (Fig. 8-4). Inappropriate sensing can lead to inhibition or triggering of stimulation, depending on the pacing mode selected. By way of example, ventricular pacing modes may sense T waves if the ventricular sensing amplifier is too sensitive or its refractory period programmed too short. Additionally, it may sense peaked or delayed T waves caused by hyperkalemia or hypocalcemia, respectively. A dislodged or misplaced ventricular lead in the right ventricular outflow tract may lead to inappropriate sensing of P waves. Atrial sensing modes may sense QRS activity if P waves are too small to be sensed, with consequent failure to initiate appropriate atrial refractory periods (see Chapter 6). Sensing of atrial stimuli by the ventricular sensing amplifier, or crosstalk (see discussion of dual-chamber refractory periods in Chapter 6), inhibition of output by electromagnetic interference (EMI, discussed further later), and skeletal myopotential inhibition (mechanical interference, discussed later) are also examples of oversensing. The pacemaker itself can generate signals that are sensed and inhibit delivery of pacing stimuli. For example, the electrode–tissue interface can act as a capacitor that generates polarization potentials (afterpotentials) that dissipate slowly and may be sensed by the pacemaker. Also, "make–break" signals may be generated by defective pacing leads or loose connections and sensed by the pacer.

MANAGEMENT OF PATIENTS WITH PACEMAKERS OR ICD DEVICES   **305**

TABLE 8-5   *Common causes for output failure*

MALFUNCTION	PSEUDOMALFUNCTION
Oversensing	Invisible stimulus artifact
Lead fracture/disconnection	Crosstalk; normal inhibition
Power source failure	
Component failure (rare)	

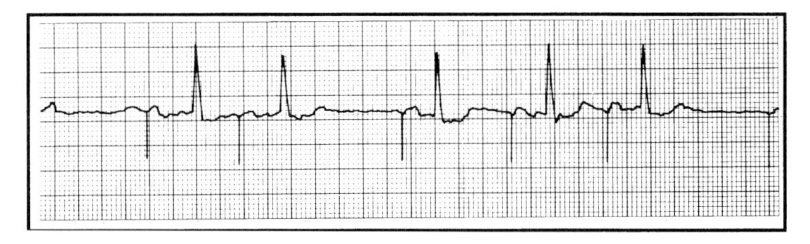

FIGURE 8–4   *Ventricular oversensing with DVI pacemaker. Oversensing must be considered as the cause for the unexpected pause after QRS complexes 2 and 5. It could be that the ventricular sensing amplifier was programmed too responsive, or sensing refractory period too short, causing the T waves after these beats to be sensed to inhibit atrial and ventricular output. (Tracing kindly furnished by Medtronic, Inc., Minneapolis, MN.)*

Misdiagnosis of Output Failure

Output failure might also be misdiagnosed (pseudomalfunction) if the patient's spontaneous rate is faster than the programmed pacing rate. Output failure with sensed EMI or skeletal myopotentials, which can appropriately inhibit pacemaker output, is more likely with unipolar compared to bipolar pacemaker systems. This is because the large interelectrode distance serves as an antenna of sorts and the large surface area of the pacemaker can encourage sensing of pectoral muscle potentials. Finally, ventricular activity may originate in different foci within the ventricle. These may be sensed by the ventricular sensing amplifier, leading to appropriate inhibition of output. However, the same ventricular potentials could be isoelectric on the surface ECG, giving the observer the impression of oversensing malfunction, when in fact the pacemaker was functioning normally. Similarly, invisible stimulus artifacts in the surface ECG, when in fact the unit is functioning normally, are yet another potential type of output

306 MANAGEMENT OF PATIENTS WITH PACEMAKERS OR ICD DEVICES

pseudomalfunction. Finally, multiple ECG leads and a pacing system analyzer may be required to make the diagnosis of normal function, malfunction, or pseudomalfunction.

IMPROPER SENSING

Undersensing

The occurrence of stimulus artifacts at an unexplained time suggests the failure to sense properly. If the interval between the preceding QRS complex and the paced beat is shorter than the programmed automatic interval, undersensing is likely (Fig. 8–5). Similar to failure to capture, undersensing is usually caused by lead dislodgement or incorrect positioning of leads (Table 8–6). Undersensing is often seen in conjunction with failure to capture (Fig. 8–6), but the two can occur

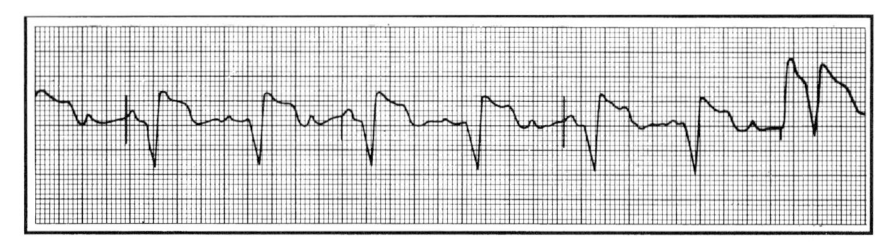

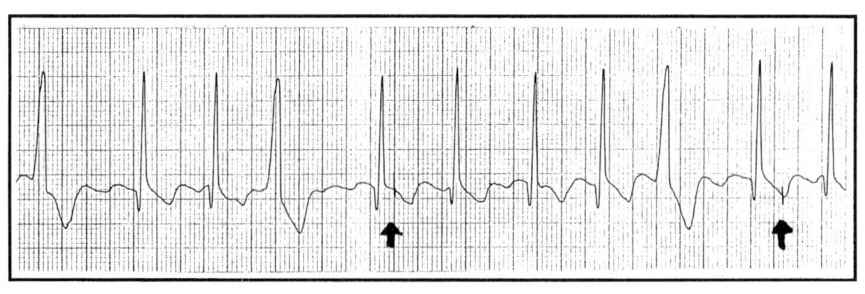

FIGURE 8–5 *Undersensing. (Top) Intermittent atrial undersensing with DDD pacemaker. All ventricular beats are spontaneous, but conducted with ventricular aberration. However, there is intermittent atrial sensing, so that only every other spontaneous P wave is detected. The other P waves are atrial capture beats. (Bottom) Undersensing with a VVI pacemaker. All QRS complexes result from spontaneous beats. Beats 1, 4, and 9 are ventricular extrasystoles. Note the small ventricular pacing artifacts after beats 5 and 10 (arrows). These beats should have been detected and reset the pacemaker. (Tracings kindly furnished by Medtronic, Inc., Minneapolis, MN.)*

TABLE 8-6 *Common causes of undersensing*

MALFUNCTION	PSEUDOMALFUNCTION
Lead dislodgement	Magnet application
Incorrect lead position	Pacer in interference mode
Lead insulation defect	Monitor artifacts
Low-amplitude myopotentials	Fusion/pseudofusion beats

separately. Since the pacemaker sensing amplifier directly senses cardiac activity, it is not possible to know from the surface ECG when the cardiac electrogram actually began and, therefore, whether proper sensing occurred. For example, the sensing amplifier might not detect all ventricular extrasystoles from several different foci. Low-amplitude myopotentials leading to undersensing might result from improper lead placement and changes in myocardial activation patterns caused by ischemia, fibrosis, or the effects of drugs and electrolyte imbalance. Undersensing can be caused by improper programming of amplifier sensitivity, refractory periods, or pacing modes.

Misdiagnosis of Undersensing

Undersensing may be misdiagnosed if the pacemaker has been unknowingly converted to asynchronous operation by EMI (see discussion, later) or uncharted reprogramming. Monitor artifacts and fusion beats may also be misinterpreted as malfunction. Fusion beats are the result of simultaneous myocardial activation by paced and spontaneous beats (Fig. 8–7). Pseudofusion occurs when the pacing stimulus artifact coincides with the QRS complex, but does not alter its appearance (Fig. 8–7). Neither fusion or pseudofusion beats are necessarily the result of sensing malfunction.

PACING AT AN INAPPROPRIATE RATE

Causes for pacing at an inappropriate rate are listed in Table 8–7. As discussed earlier, oversensing may lead to inappropriate inhibition or triggering of output, and pacing at an inappropriate rate. Rate drift is a gradual shift in pacemaker rate due to the effects of component aging, and was most common in older pacemakers without digital timing circuits. In contrast, end-of-life rate reduction is normal operation in most pacemakers, indicating impending battery depletion. Finally, component failure can lead to no output or pacemaker runaway (see Pacemaker Arrhythmias, earlier in this chapter).

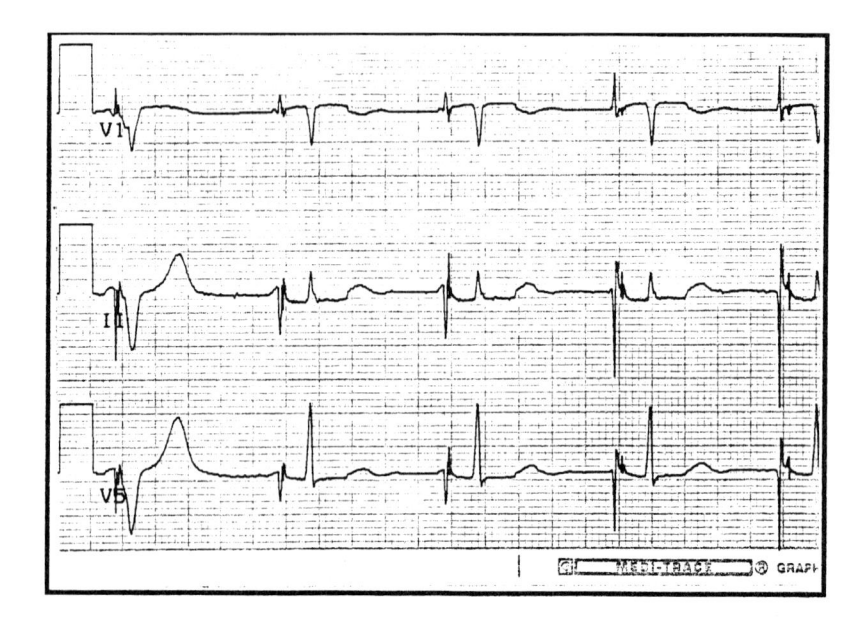

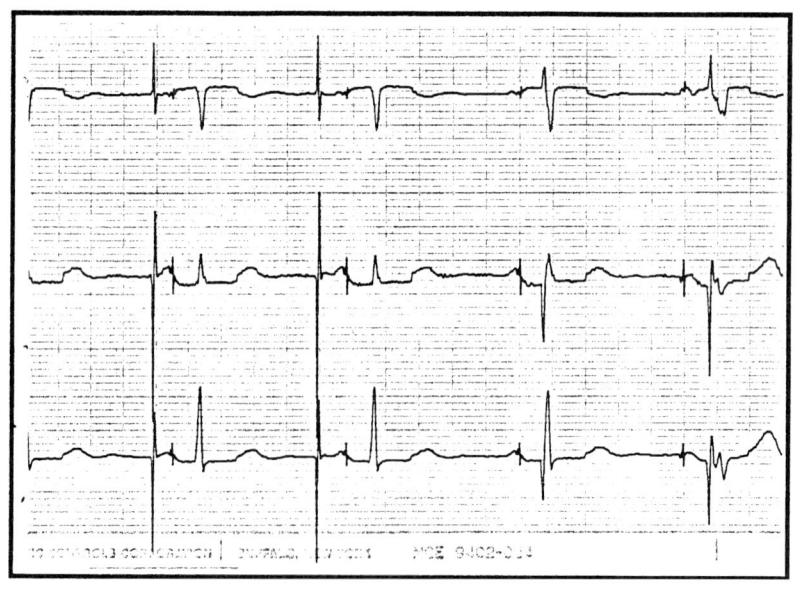

FIGURE 8-6 *Sensing and output failure. Contiguous tracings from patient with malfunctioning DDD pacemaker. The underlying rhythm is normal sinus rhythm at 60 beats/min. Note that atrial and ventricular pacing artifacts are not necessarily in proper sequence, and produce no atrial or ventricular capture beats.*

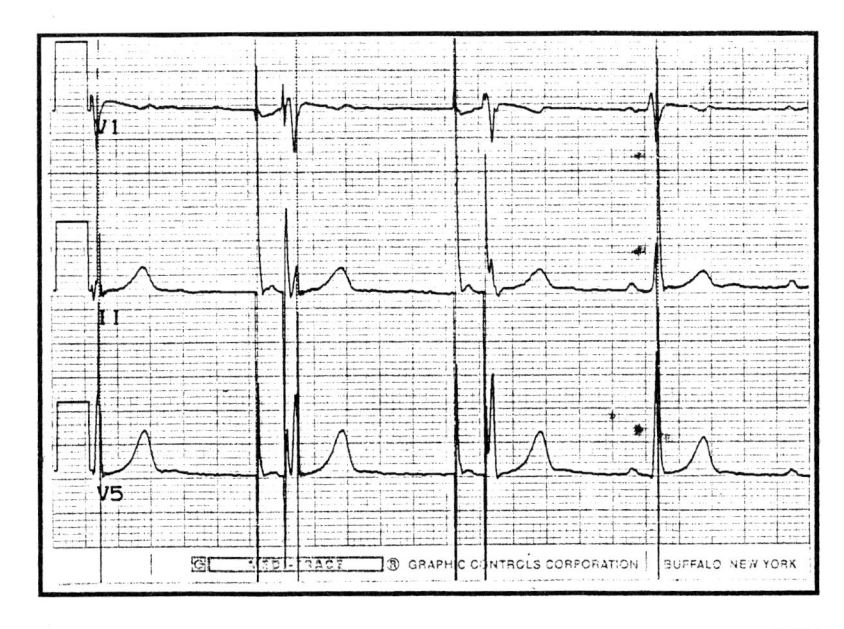

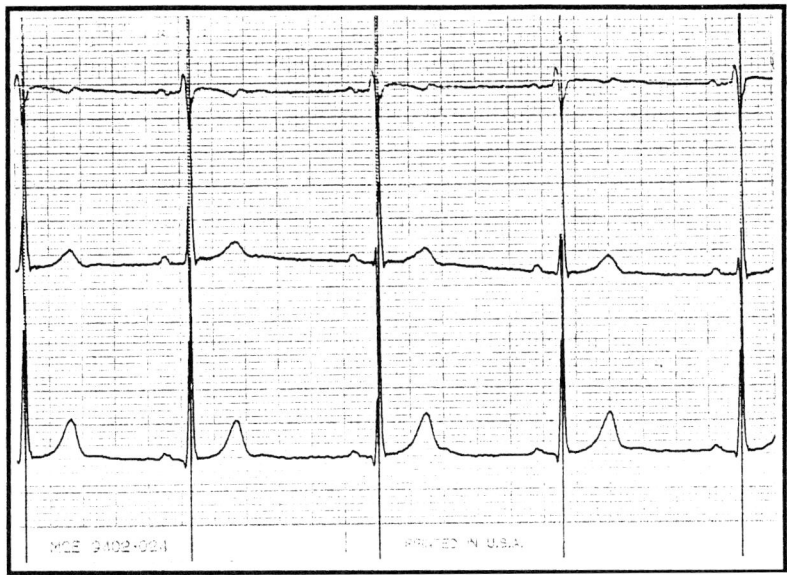

FIGURE 8-7   *Fusion and pseudofusion beats in a patient with a DDD pacemaker. Contiguous tracings. The first two beats are paced atrial beats with capture; all other atrial beats are spontaneous and properly sensed. The first two paced ventricular beats are probably fusion beats. Note that at least the initial QRS deflection arises from the pacing stimulus, in comparison to all other QRS complexes, which are merely distorted by the pacing stimulus, and therefore pseudofusion beats.*

TABLE 8-7 *Common causes of pacing at an inappropriate rate*

MALFUNCTION	PSEUDOMALFUNCTION
Oversensing	Programmed rate hysteresis
Rate drift	Unfamiliarity with device
Rate reduction	Tracking increased atrial rate
Component failure	

ASSESSMENT OF PACEMAKER FUNCTION

Because of stress anxiety and other factors common to perioperative and critical care environments, it is common for demand pacemakers to be suppressed by adequate spontaneous rates. Therefore, it cannot be known whether the device is functioning properly or not. Ideally, time permitting, the patient should be referred to a pacemaker clinic or implanting physician for assessment of pacemaker function and programmed parameters, with proper notation made in the patient's chart. However, this is not always practical or feasible. Therefore, it may be necessary to ascertain proper pacemaker function at the bedside. "Vagal maneuvers," including carotid sinus massage or administration of drugs (edrophonium, adenosine) to transiently slow spontaneous rate, are employed for this purpose by the author (Fig. 8–8). Additionally, the response of a suppressed demand pacemaker to a magnet should be checked (Fig. 8–8).

Electromagnetic Interference

TYPES AND SOURCES OF ELECTROMAGNETIC INTERFERENCE

Extraneous electromagnetic signals from the patient's environment (EMI) can affect pacemaker function.[1,8,12,13] EMI can be classified as galvanic, electrically coupled, or magnetic. *Galvanic interference* requires direct contact with current (e.g., electrocautery, DC cardiac electroversion, diathermy). *Electrically coupled interference* does not require direct contact with current (e.g., electrical appliances, radio frequencies, metal detectors, therapeutic radiation). *Magnetic interference* occurs when the patient comes into close contact with a strong magnetic field (e.g., magnetic resonance imaging). Specific, hospital-related sources of EMI are discussed later. Nonhospital sources of EMI

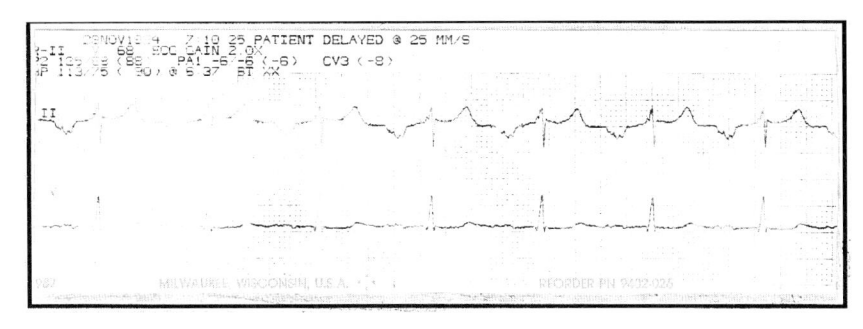

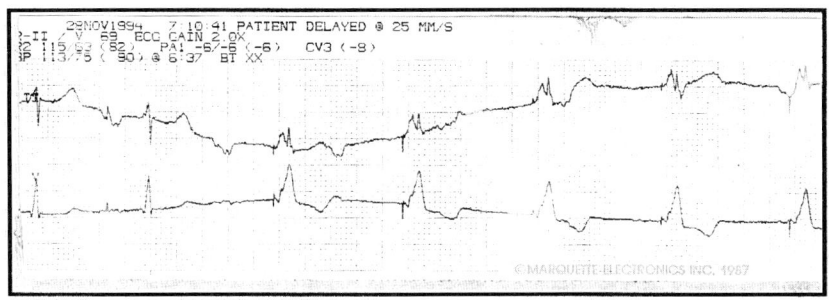

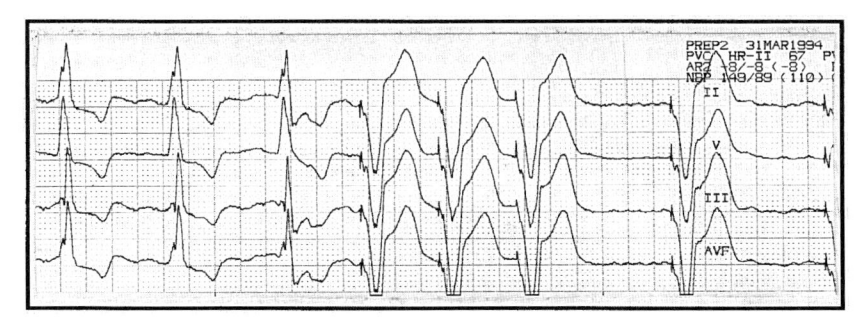

MANAGEMENT OF PATIENTS WITH PACEMAKERS OR ICD DEVICES **311**

FIGURE 8-8 *Bedside assessment of demand pacemaker function. (Top) VVI pacemaker suppressed by spontaneous, atrial ectopic rhythm at 72 beats/min in the preoperative holding area. (Middle) Spontaneous rate is slowed by edrophonium (5 mg + 5 mg), so that VVI pacing at 60 beats/min occurs. (Bottom) Another patient with a VVI pacemaker suppressed by spontaneous rhythm at 71 beats/min (beats 1 to 3). Holding a magnet over the pacemaker causes initial asynchronous pacing at 100 beats/min (beats 4 to 6), followed by slower pacing at 60 beats/min (magnet reversion mode).*

are not likely to affect pacemaker function, and include metal detectors, washers and dryers, televisions and radios, microwaves, hair dryers, heating pads, electric blankets, electric razors, and vibrators. Nonetheless, moving a razor or vibrator directly over the pacemaker pulse generator could affect its function.

PACEMAKER RESPONSE TO ELECTROMAGNETIC INTERFERENCE

Most energy of intracardiac signals lies in the frequency range of 10 to 100 Hz. Selective bandpass filtering by the pacemaker's sensing circuitry attenuates, but does not totally eliminate, signals with frequencies above and below this range. The response of the pacemaker to EMI depends on the EMI source, its strength and duration, and the pacing mode and polarity. Intense, direct EMI in the immediate vicinity of the pacemaker, leads, or electrode–tissue interface could produce damage to the pulse generator circuitry or leads, or tissue necrosis. There may be no pacemaker response to sensed EMI, or it may cause inappropriate inhibition or triggering of output, more commonly the former. Additionally, EMI may alter pacemaker function through reprogramming of pacing and sensing parameters. EMI is of most concern for the pacemaker-dependent patient, in whom EMI-caused pacemaker inhibition could produce asystolic cardiac arrest.

SPECIFIC SOURCES OF ELECTROMAGNETIC INTERFERENCE

Electrocautery and Cardiac Electroversion

PRECAUTIONS. Prior to any procedure involving surgical electrocautery or direct current cardioversion or defibrillation (DC electroversion), it is important to know how the pacemaker is programmed so that correct parameters can be restored should the device be reprogrammed by the procedure. Further, the pacemaker device should be interrogated by a pacing system analyzer following the procedure for changes in programmed parameters or malfunction. Bipolar cautery is encouraged whenever possible, and the electrode should be kept at least 4 to 6 inches from the pulse generator. The grounding plate of unipolar cautery units should be far removed from the pulse generator (e.g., buttocks). For DC electroversion, the paddles should be perpendicular to the axis of the pulse generator and leads. Therefore, the anteroposterior as opposed to the anteroapical or anterolateral paddle positions are recommended. During surgical procedures that require electrocautery, the arterial pressure waveform should be monitored continuously by pulse oximetry or direct recording, since EMI from the cautery will interfere with interpretation of the ECG.

DAMAGE TO THE PULSE GENERATOR. The extremely high transthoracic currents used with cardiac electroversion can damage pacemakers. Capacitor discharge induces an electromagnetic field which, in a unipolar system, could shunt significant current through the electrode.[13] This could damage tissue under the electrode tip, resulting in temporary or permanent sensing malfunction. If induced current is shorted over a protection circuit inside the pacer, it can still create significant voltage there which could reprogram or damage the pulse generator.

EFFECT ON PACEMAKER FUNCTION. The most common problem with electrocautery is inhibition of pacemaker output. Provided inhibition is only brief (seconds), it should not produce disadvantageous hemodynamics in most patients. More prolonged cautery may cause the pacemaker to revert to the asynchronous "noise reversion mode".[12] This could be asynchronous atrial, ventricular, or dual-chamber pacing at some nominal rate (e.g., 70 beats/min). Characteristics of this mode will be known by a consulting pacemaker physician or the pacemaker clinic, so the practitioner should not confuse its presence with pacemaker malfunction. If it is known before surgery that there will be extensive or uninterrupted use of electrocautery, consideration should be given to programming the pacemaker to asynchronous operation to avoid intermittent inhibition. In non-programmable pacemakers (rare today), a magnet can be placed and left over the device to convert it to asynchronous operation. *This should not be done with programmable devices, because it may activate the unit to receive EMI as erroneous programming information.* Rather, programming the pacemaker to asynchronous operation is recommended in pacemaker-dependent patients. This is usually done in the pacemaker clinic or by the implanting physician. Usually, the pacemaker can easily be programmed back to its former operation after the surgical procedure, but some devices may require special access codes for reprogramming out of asynchronous operation.

MISCELLANEOUS EFFECTS OF ELECTROCAUTERY EMI. Finally, electrocautery impulses might trigger rapid paced rates in patients with atrial-triggered, ventricular pacing modes (VAT, VDD, and DDD). Also, electrocautery EMI can produce detrimental effects at the electrode–tissue interface. Although unusual, electrocautery in close proximity to pacing leads can be transmitted directly to the heart, where it can trigger arrhythmias or produce local tissue necrosis. The latter could be the cause for increased pacing thresholds or poor sensing.

Magnetic Resonance Imaging

Magnetic resonance imaging (MRI) is a commonly used diagnostic tool. MRI, with its powerful static magnetic, time-varying gradient, and radiofrequency fields, can greatly alter normal pacemaker operation and function.[12,14] In fact, manufacturers of MRI scanners and pacemakers advise that MRI of pacemaker patients is contraindicated. Nevertheless, MRI results may be needed for planning oncologic or surgical interventions, and there is no alternative diagnostic procedure that can provide the same information.

PACEMAKER RESPONSE TO MRI. At the very least, exposure to MRI causes all pacemakers to revert to an asynchronous interference or magnet-response mode. This can be avoided only in pacemakers in which the magnet response can be programmed to "off." Investigations have shown that MRI does not permanently damage pulse generator components. Radiofrequency artifacts do not alter acutely programmed variables, change the normal magnet reversion rate, or induce pacing in most pacemaker devices tested. In animal studies, certain pacemakers exposed to MRI have paced at the radiofrequency pulse period, which could be up to 3,000 beats/min for 20-msec pulse period intervals.[12]

SUGGESTED PATIENT MANAGEMENT. No generalizations can be made about which pacemaker patients can be safely exposed to MRI. If possible, MRI should be avoided in patients with pacemakers. However, if required, the following are recommended.[12,14] In non-pacemaker-dependent patients, the pacemaker should be programmed to a stimulus output (volts) at which capture is no longer possible. This will effectively protect the patient from extremely rapid pacing rates equal to the radiofrequency pulse period. If the pacemaker can be programmed "off," the non-pacemaker-dependent patient can probably be scanned safely. Alternatively, the pacemaker can be explanted for the duration of MRI, again provided the patient is not pacemaker dependent. The pacemaker-dependent patient should be informed of the risk of MRI-induced pacemaker failure and the possibility of immediate need for resuscitation and pacemaker system revision. Also, prior to MRI investigation, the following should be documented in the patient's chart: (1) spontaneous heart rate, (2) pacemaker status, (3) response to positive chronotropic and dromotropic drugs, and (4) results of routine preoperative evaluation for monitored anesthesia care or general anesthesia. If unexpected difficulties do occur during MRI, the patient should be removed from the static magnetic field to at least 10 meters from the scanner.

Extracorporeal Shock Wave Lithotripsy (ESWL)

PACEMAKER RESPONSE TO ESWL. Extracorporeal shock wave lithotripsy is used frequently for the treatment of nephrolithiasis, but less frequently for cholelithiasis. However, the numbers of pacemaker patients undergoing ESWL worldwide is probably under 5,000/year.[15] Nonetheless, ESWL can cause problems with pacemakers.[12,15] Shock waves produced by the lithotripter are usually synchronized to the patient's QRS complex or the pacing stimulus artifact. Testing of pacemakers in vitro and limited patient experience has shown that ESWL does not interfere with fixed-rate VVI pacing as long as the lithotripter focal point is at least 6 inches from the pacemaker. In patients with dual-chamber pacemakers, synchronization of the lithotripter with atrial output can result in inhibition of ventricular output. This is because the lithotripter shock is delayed by up to 160 msec from the atrial stimulus, and could be detected by the ventricular channel as a ventricular event leading to inhibition of output.[15]

SUGGESTED PATIENT MANAGEMENT. The pacemaker should be reprogrammed VOO or VVI for the duration of ESWL, and shocks always triggered by the QRS potential. In patients with activity-sensing, rate-adaptive pacemakers, sensing of lithotripter shock waves can result in increased pacing rates and damage to the activity sensor crystal if placed near the focal point of the lithotripter. As a precaution, rate-adaptive pacemakers should be programmed to their non-rate-sensing mode to avoid rate alterations with ESWL. Finally, it is necessary that both ECG and arterial pulse waveform or heart sounds be monitored during ESWL, and there should be back-up temporary cardiac pacing for patients who are pacemaker dependent. All patients should be checked for proper pacemaker function following ESWL.

Therapeutic Radiation

POTENTIAL FOR PACEMAKER MALFUNCTION. Diagnostic x-rays do not interfere with pacemaker function. Modern pacemakers with complementary metal oxide semiconductors (CMOS) for integrated circuitry, compared to transistors of older pacemaker devices, are more sensitive to the effects of ionizing radiation. Specifically, ionizing radiation damages the silicon and silicon oxide insulators within the metallic oxide semiconductors. Damage to pacemaker electronics varies, is sometimes transient but more often permanent, and *always is cumulative*. Therapeutic radiation may be of sufficient strength to result in complete system failure, or it may produce only random damage to circuit components. Sudden output failure or pacemaker runaway may occur. As the damage is random and cumulative, no specific prediction as to damage relative to dose can be made. There have been reports of CMOS damage in some pacemaker devices following exposure to as little as 1,000 rads, while with other devices, 3,000 to 15,000 rads have been required.[12] The cumulative effect of repeated exposure to therapeutic radiation is particularly important in patients undergoing radiation treatment for thoracic or chest wall malignancies.

SUGGESTED PATIENT MANAGEMENT. For patients whose pacemaker will be in the field of radiation, it may be necessary to relocate the pulse generator. If the pacemaker is not directly in the field of radiation, it is still necessary to shield the pulse generator to prevent damage. Regardless, pacemaker function should be monitored during treatments (heart sounds, pulse oximetry, ECG). For pacemaker-dependent patients, temporary pacing should be available for sudden system failure. Finally, pacemaker function should be checked following treatment, and system revision may be required.

Transcutaneous Electrical Nerve Stimulation

Transcutaneous electrical nerve stimulation (TENS) is used to treat musculoskeletal and neurologic disorders, and appears to be safe in most patients with permanent pacemakers.[12] TENS rarely causes pacemaker inhibition, reprogramming, or interference. It is not known how close to the pacemaker the TENS unit can be placed, and it is recommended that the TENS stimulator not be applied to a vector or path parallel to the pacing leads.[12] Pacemaker-dependent patients should be monitored for proper pacemaker function during initial TENS treatment to be certain that no inhibition occurs. Finally, in patients with atrial tracking modes (VAT, VDD, DDD), TENS can potentially cause an increase in the rate of ventricular stimulation if noise from TENS were interpreted as atrial activity.

Diathermy

Some types of diathermy equipment can cause inappropriate inhibition or triggering of ventricular pacing output, depending on whether the pacemaker operates as a demand or atrial tracking device.[12,13] Bipolar diathermy is preferred for the same reasons given earlier for electrocautery. Diathermy in the immediate vicinity of the pulse generator or leads may heat components or the insulation to a temperature sufficient to destroy the device or lead to sensing malfunction or ineffective stimulation. As with electrocautery, monitoring of the patient's arterial pulse waveform and heart sounds is recommended during diathermy procedures.

RADIOFREQUENCY CATHETER ABLATION

There has been a substantial increase in the use of radiofrequency catheter ablation for interruption of supraventricular tachycardia (SVT) and even ventricular tachycardia (VT). If this procedure is performed on patients with permanent pacemakers, the pacemaker might be inappropriately triggered, inhibited, or reprogrammed by radiofrequency exposure.[12] A pacemaker programmer should be available during the procedure. To be sure that previously programmed parameters have not been altered by radiofrequency catheter ablation, the pacemaker should be interrogated following the ablation procedure.

Electroconvulsive Therapy

Electroconvulsive therapy (ECT) in the patient with a permanent pacemaker should not be associated with malfunction or damage to the system. It is possible that EMI from ECT could reprogram a pacemaker. Therefore, the device should be interrogated if malfunction is suspected. A more likely type of malfunction with ECT is inappropriate triggering or inhibition of output with muscle movement in incompletely paralyzed patients. Pacemaker function should be monitored by pulse oximetry during ECT treatments.

Nonmedical Equipment and Devices

Permanent damage to implanted pacemakers by nonmedical electrical equipment has not been reported and is unlikely.[12] Transient interference with pacemaker function is possible if the patient is subjected to sustained EMI. This could produce inappropriate inhibition or triggering of output, but will not damage the pacemaker system itself. There are restrictions, however, for patients who work in close proximity to large electrical generators, motors, or arc welding equipment. These are more the concern of the implanting pacemaker physician. While it is sometimes asked whether microwave ovens or airport metal detectors interfere with pacemaker function, these cause only transient (several beats at most) inhibition of pacemaker output.

Mechanical Interference

MYOPOTENTIALS

Myopotential interference, the oversensing of skeletal muscle potentials, remains the most common cause of transient pacemaker inhibition, and occurs almost invariably with unipolar pacemaker devices.[8] Although myopotential interference can be demonstrated in up to 50 percent of patients with unipolar pacemakers, only 10 percent report symptoms and require system revision or reprogramming. Oversensing of diaphragmatic myopotentials provoked by deep inspirations is uncommon, but an atrial J-wire lead in the right atrial appendage may sense intercostal myopotentials with deep inspiration.[8] Myopotentials generated by involuntary muscle contractions may also interfere with unipolar pacemaker function.[11] Examples include fasciculations with depolarizing muscle relaxants, myoclonic movements, seizures, direct muscle stimulation, and large respiratory excursions with controlled or mechanical ventilation.

LEAD DISLODGEMENT

It is possible that large and sudden muscle movements might dislodge newly implanted pacemaker leads, especially those without some type of active fixation device (e.g., myocardial screw-in lead). Nonfixed endocardial leads might also be dislodged during pulmonary artery catheter flotation. This should not be a problem with actively fixed electrodes 4 to 6 weeks following implantation (fixation stabilization period).

Adverse Pacemaker Interactions

Adverse interactions with permanent pacemakers fall into two categories: (1) Device–device interactions between separate implanted devices, one for control of bradycardia and the other for tachyarrhythmias; and (2) drug–device interactions between drugs the patient may be receiving and the implanted pacemaker system.[5,12]

DEVICE–DEVICE INTERACTIONS

There are two potential device combinations: an ICD device with a bradycardia pacemaker, and an ICD device with a pacemaker that has bradycardia and antitachycardia pacing modes. Now, with technology advances and further down-sizing of circuitry and other components, there is a move to incorporate all of these functions in a single device (see discussion later in this chapter).

Internal Cardioverter–Defibrillator Device–Bradycardia Pacing Device

BRADYCARDIA INCIDENCE. In patients with ICD devices, the incidence of symptomatic bradycardia requiring permanent pacing is believed to be around 10 percent.[5] Up to 25 percent of patients with ICD devices may require bradycardia pacing for several minutes following ICD shock delivery.[5] However, this may be a high estimate, because it is based on data from the 1980s, when ICD devices were restricted to patients meeting rather strict implantation criteria. Many of these had poor ventricular function and were receiving antiarrhythmic drugs associated with bradycardia (e.g., amiodarone).

TYPES OF INTERACTION. The interaction between ICD devices and bradycardia pacemakers can be lethal, based on consideration of the sensing algorithms used.[5] Since detection algorithms for ventricular tachycardia and fibrillation (VT/VF) are constantly evolving, and vary among manufacturers, what follows is intended only as an illustration of what might happen. A weak signal with "fine" VF is not be sensed by the bradycardia pacemaker, so that there is pacemaker escape and ineffective stimulation. In turn, the ICD device misinterprets the ineffective stimuli as spontaneous rhythm and withholds or delays shocks. The ICD device might also double-count the pacemaker stimuli and evoked myopotentials as tachycardia, causing inappropriate discharge. This can be prevented by programming the pacemaker to less than one-half the ICD cutoff rate, or increasing the cutoff rate. If there is dual-chamber bradycardia pacing, then there is the possibility of triple- or quadruple-counting of atrial and ventricular pacing stimuli and myopotentials, with inappropriate ICD discharge. ICD discharge might also cause an inhibited pacemaker (VVI, DDD) to revert to asynchronous pacing (VOO, DOO). This would necessitate subsequent reprogramming. In the patient with an ICD device and a permanent pacemaker, transcutaneous cardioversion–defibrillation may alter the function of both devices, so that function needs to be tested as soon as possible following the procedure. Programming a pacemaker may cause inappropriate ICD discharge or deactivate the device,[2] and ICD discharge may cause temporary loss of sensing or pacing, or increased pacing thresholds.

Internal Cardioverter–Defibrillator Device–Bradycardia–Antitachycardia Device

It would be unusual today for a patient to have both an antitachycardia pacemaker and an ICD device. The two functions are more likely combined in the same ICD device, with the ICD device serving as backup for failed pacing conversion of tachycardia. Nevertheless, with an ICD device and antitachycardia pacemaker, several possible interactions exist: (1) antitachycardia pacing stimuli are sensed by the ICD device, causing inappropriate discharge or inhibition, depending on the ICD cutoff rate; (2) antitachycardia pacing accelerates tachycardia and it is poorly tolerated, but since the rate is less than the ICD cutoff rate, shocks are not delivered; (3) atrial or ventricular fibrillation is induced by antitachycardia pacing, and ICD shocks may or may not be delivered; (4) antitachycardia pacing successfully terminates tachycardia, yet the ICD device still discharges, triggering another episode of tachycardia that is not terminated by pacing or ICD discharge; and (5) regardless of the effect of pacing on tachycardia, the antitachycardia pacing method used causes the ICD device to discharge inappropriately.[5]

DRUG–DEVICE INTERACTIONS

Whenever a new drug or an anesthetic is prescribed for a patient receiving other medications, thought is always given to the potential for adverse interactions. The same consideration must be provided for patients with pacemakers. Although drug effects on pacemaker function are usually thought of in terms of altered pacing thresholds, with the newer rate-adaptive pacemakers, whether atrial-triggered or sensor-modulated, there may be other types of malfunction with far more serious consequences.

Bradycardia Pacemakers

DRUGS AND FACTORS THAT INCREASE PACING THRESHOLDS. All antiarrhythmic drugs, with the exception of calcium-channel blockers and digitalis, have the potential to increase pacing thresholds. The greatest increase (up to 200 percent) is seen with class 1C drugs (flecainide-like).[12] Therefore, class 1C drugs are rarely prescribed for pacemaker-dependent patients, and then only with extreme caution and frequent checking of pacing thresholds. The increase in pacing thresholds with class 1A drugs (quinidine-like) is not usually a problem with therapeutic drug concentrations, but may be with toxic concentrations. Class 1B drugs (lidocaine-like) have no appreciable effect on pacing thresholds. Beta-blockers may increase pacing thresholds somewhat, especially if previous thresholds were low because of high sympathetic tone. Amiodarone may increase pacing thresholds in some patients.[5] Finally, there is some controversy regarding the effect of anesthetic drugs on pacing thresholds. Zaidan and coworkers have reported that potent inhalation anesthetics (enflurane, halothane, isoflurane) produce an acute increase in pacing thresholds.[16] The increase was small, however, and probably clinically insignificant, except that it might become so with obvious anesthetic overdose. The effects of other anesthetic drugs on pacing thresholds have not been reported. However, most anesthetic drugs produce direct myocardial depression, which probably correlates with increased pacing thresholds. However, systemic vasodilation, preload reduction, and decreased blood pressure with anesthesia, with a secondary increase in sympathetic tone, likely oppose any direct increase in pacing thresholds with anesthetics. Drugs and factors that may increase pacing thresholds are summarized in Table 8–8.

DRUGS AND FACTORS THAT LOWER PACING THRESHOLDS. Drugs and other factors can also lower pacing thresholds. Corticosteroids are perhaps the most important of these, and advantage of this has been taken by manufacturers of permanent pacing leads with the introduction of steroid-eluting leads. These permit local effects of steroids at the tissue–electrode interface, which is expected to persist for the lifetime of the patient. Human studies have shown that steroid-eluting leads prevent the usual increase in pacing thresholds over the first 4 to 6 weeks following pacemaker implantation. Also, sympathomimetics, hyperadrenergic and hypermetabolic states, and hyperthyroidism lower pacing thresholds.

DRUGS THAT AFFECT HEART RATE OR ATRIOVENTRICULAR CONDUCTION. The consequences to the pacemaker patient of chronotropic and dromotropic drug intervention depend on the pacing system and programmed operation. A negative chronotrope will enhance the

TABLE 8-8 *Factors that increase pacing thresholds*

First 1 to 6 weeks following pacemaker implantation
Antiarrhythmic drugs (especially class 1C drugs)
Myocardial ischemia and acute myocardial infarction
Acute electrolyte imbalance (especially potassium)
Local anesthetic toxicity (especially bupivacaine)
Miscellaneous (hypothermia, hypothyroidism)

occurrence of lower-rate pacing. While this may have little effect in a patient with an atrial or dual-chamber pacemaker, it could have an effect in the patient with sinus bradycardia and a VVI pacemaker. Loss of atrioventricular (AV) synchrony with ventricular pacing, or symptoms from retrograde atrial activation (pacemaker syndrome), could be quite bothersome in patients who rarely require pacing at the programmed low rate. Drugs that prolong or shorten AV node conduction might necessitate reprogramming of atrial refractory periods. Those that facilitate retrograde (VA) conduction might increase the likelihood of pacemaker-mediated tachycardia.

DRUGS AND RATE-ADAPTIVE OR SENSOR-MODULATED PACING. Drugs that slow atrial rate will reduce the effectiveness of atrial tracking pacing modes (VAT, VDD, DDD). Drugs that affect a physiologic sensor can alter the rate of pacing with sensor-modulated, rate-adaptive pacing. For example, drugs that cause muscle tremors or fasciculations may increase the rate of activity-sensing pacemakers. A respiratory minute-volume sensor might initiate faster than needed pacing in patients on mechanical respirators being hyperventilated. Further, any drug that affects ventricular function, depolarization, or repolarization can potentially affect sensors that modulate the rate of pacing based on measurements of the QT interval, change in pressure over time, or other parameters (Table 6–1).

Antitachycardia Pacemakers

Antiarrhythmic drugs, if effective, reduce the need for antitachycardia pacing. However, drugs might also affect antitachycardia pacing by slowing the rate of tachycardia. While such slowing might enhance termination, it could also prevent tachycardia recognition. Because antiarrhythmics also affect cardiac electrophysiologic properties, it may be necessary to reprogram antitachycardia pacing functions to account for changes in the behavior of clinical tachycardia. Finally, proarrhythmia with drugs may make it more difficult for the pacemaker to detect and terminate tachycardia.

Internal Cardioverter–Defibrillator Device Complications and Malfunction

The potential for complications and malfunction with ICD devices depends on system complexity and the algorithms used for detection of VT and VF. The first clinical device (1980; AID™, Intec Systems, Minneapolis, MN) identified and treated only VF. Second-generation devices also identified and treated VT. Third- and fourth-generation devices feature bradycardia pacing, and may also include antitachycardia pacing functions.

ARRHYTHMIA SENSING FUNCTIONS

Tachycardia or fibrillation sensing algorithms vary depending on the device and manufacturer.[2,8] Several functions or parameters for recognizing tachycardia or fibrillation might be programmable in a single device, including probability density function (PDF), rate, fibrillation interval, amplitude and stability of electrograms, duration of intracardiac signals, suddenness of tachycardia onset, the presence or absence of AV dissociation, and hemodynamic sensors. PDF determines the amount of time the ECG waveform is around baseline (i.e., isoelectric). VF or fast VT spend very little time there. Such potential complexity in tachycardia–fibrillation detection algorithms greatly increases the possibilities for ICD device complications and malfunction.

PERIOPERATIVE AND LATE COMPLICATIONS

Hospital mortality from ICD device implantation can be as high as 4 to 5 percent, and is related to severe cardiopulmonary functional impairment, complications of additional surgery such as coronary artery bypass and ventricular aneurysectomy, arrhythmias, sepsis, and congestive heart failure.[2,8] Causes for morbidity and mortality with ICD devices are listed in Table 8–9. Many of the complications with ICD devices are similar to those with pacemakers, except that instead of affecting pacing function, there is risk of failure to deliver shocks or inappropriate delivery of shocks. With regard to surgical complications and related morbidity or mortality, these are expected to decrease with increased use of transvenous ICD lead systems. A particularly

TABLE 8-9 *Morbidity and mortality with ICD devices*

Pericarditis and infection	Postoperative stroke
Atrial flutter or fibrillation	Congestive heart failure
Lead migration or fracture	Lead erosion or extrusion
Myocardial infarction	Early battery depletion
Component failure	Under- or oversensing
Inappropriate shocks	Emotional stress, anxiety

distressing (painful) complication for the patient is spurious ICD discharge, which could be triggered by extraneous events similar to those described for pacemakers earlier under Electromagnetic Interference and Mechanical Interference. Complications with combined ICD device–pacemaker systems were also discussed earlier under Device–Device Interactions.

ALTERED DEFIBRILLATION THRESHOLDS

Drugs and factors that may affect ICD thresholds or the rate cutoff algorithm for tachycardia detection are listed in Table 8–10. Class 1B and 1C drugs and amiodarone are the most significant of these, since they are often prescribed in patients with ICD devices. There is conflicting evidence whether anesthetic drugs affect ICD thresholds, which has importance for threshold testing during system implantation. Even if they do, the effect is probably quite small (< 5-J increase). More important, however, is the possible effect of drugs on VT/VF rate or morphology, which would interfere with detection and therefore delivery of shocks. Unfortunately, this has not yet been fully assessed.

DEVICE ACTIVATION–DEACTIVATION

Interaction with ICD devices is through external programmers or magnets. Concerning the latter, while a donut-shaped (toroid) magnet has been used, any sufficiently strong magnet should also suffice. Using the programmer, it is possible to activate or deactivate the device, as well as program arrhythmia detection parameters, shock energy levels, sequence of shocks, tachycardia rate cutoff, tiered therapy (differential responses to specific tachyarrhythmias), and backup bradycardia pacing functions. Application of a strong magnet will inactivate all contemporary ICD devices. Simply holding the

TABLE 8-10 *Drugs and factors that affect function of ICD devices*

Class 1C drugs (flecainide)*†	Aniodarone and sotalol*†
Class 1B drugs (lidocaine)*†	Beta-blockers, verapamil, diltiazem†
Magnesium sulfate*†	Hypothermia, hypothyroidism†
Sedative-hypnotics, anxiolytics†	Opioids (except meperidine)†

*Increase defibrillation thresholds.
†Affect detection algorithms.

magnet over the upper one-third of a CPI device (Cardiac Pacemakers, Inc., St. Paul, Mn) for 30 seconds will deactivate the unit, signaled by a continuous audible tone. Similarly, CPI devices are activated by application of the magnet for 30 seconds, signaled by a beeping tone corresponding to spontaneous heart beats. Output of the PCD (Pacer–Cardioverter–Defibrillator, Medtronic, Inc., Minneapolis, MN) and Ventritex, Sunnyvale, CA devices is inhibited so long as a magnet is held in place over the device. Otherwise, the devices will produce shocks in response to sensing VT/VF anytime after initial programming.

Patient Transport and Positioning

Care must be taken when transporting or positioning patients with temporary transvenous pacing leads to prevent accidental electrode dislodgement and pacing failure. This is most likely with extremity or neck leads because of flexion or extension at the lead insertion site. Electrode pins of any temporary pacing lead should be handled with latex or rubber gloves and insulated when not in use to protect from microshock. The pulse generator should be accessible to someone familiar with device operation during transport and positioning, and ECG and heart sounds or pulse waveform should also be monitored. Positive chronotropic and dromotropic drugs (atropine, isoproterenol) should be available in case of pacing system failure, but they cannot be relied on to produce an adequate increase in heart rate or improve conduction, and may provoke ectopic rhythm disturbances. Finally, for pacemaker-dependent patients, there should be some provision for backup noninvasive pacing.

Management of System Implantation or Revision

Patients requiring permanent pacemakers or ICD devices have significant cardiac disease. Often, this is associated with heart failure, renovascular, cerebrovascular, pulmonary, and other significant systemic disease. Cardiopulmonary and major organ system function requires thorough assessment by anesthesia or critical care practitioners responsible for the care of these patients in the perioperative period.

PACEMAKER IMPLANTATION OR SYSTEM REVISION

Anesthesia

Most permanent pacing systems today employ transvenous leads. These and the pulse generator can be implanted using local or regional anesthesia techniques.[6,17,18] Except in neonates, infants, and small children in whom epicardial lead systems requiring thoracotomy are used, general anesthesia has been discouraged by many authorities. Nevertheless, this might not be optimal, especially if the patient has a functioning temporary pacing system. Contemporary anesthetic drugs and techniques do not have clinically important depressant effects on automaticity or conduction, and do not significantly increase pacing thresholds. Further, they can be safely administered to most patients requiring pacemaker implantation or system revision. Advantages of a well-managed general or regional-sedation anesthesia technique include less stress for the patient and more ideal operating conditions for the implanting physician. Additionally, a knowledgeable and capable person is available to monitor and maintain the integrity of vital functions, while the implanting physician focuses on pacemaker system implantation or revision. However, a limitation to use of regional or general anesthesia may be availability of anesthesia coverage and reimbursement.

Other Considerations

If general, regional, or local anesthesia with monitored care is selected for pacemaker implantation or revision, the following is recommended. Pacemaker-dependent patients or those with symptomatic bradycardia should have a functioning temporary pacing system. While the patient may have adequate spontaneous rhythm at the moment, drugs should not be relied upon with asystole or disadvantageous bradycardia. The anesthesia practitioner should be familiar with operation of the temporary pulse generator. At least one and preferably two ECG leads should be monitored, one for detection of P waves and the other for ischemia. Peripheral intravenous access is required and central access preferred for sedation and cardiac drugs. Central access is usually available from the implanting physician. Pulse oximetry and noninvasive blood pressure are standard monitoring, but direct arterial pressure monitoring is preferred for patients who are hemodynamically unstable or on vasoactive drugs. Finally, the drugs selected for general anesthesia are not so important as their proper use. The goal is to maintain adequate sedation and analgesia with hemodynamic stability.

INTERNAL CARDIOVERTER–DEFIBRILLATOR DEVICE IMPLANTATION

Up until recently, the implantation procedure for ICD devices has required thoracotomy. However, now there is a move to nonthoracotomy lead systems employing one transvenous electrode with a subcutaneous patch electrode.[2,8,19] Also, there is accumulating experience with totally transvenous electrode systems. Therefore, anesthesia for ICD device implantation could be general, regional, or local with monitored care. Against regional or local anesthesia, however, could be the need for large amounts of local anesthetics and possibly an acute increase in defibrillation thresholds.

Monitoring and Precautionary Measures

Minimum monitoring is as described earlier for patients having permanent pacemaker implantation. Additionally, direct arterial pressure monitoring is necessary. This is because ICD patients often have severely compromised cardiovascular function, tend to be hemodynamically quite labile, may require inotropic and/or vasodilator support, and will undergo repeated induction of VT/VF with brief periods of profound circulatory collapse. Direct arterial pressure monitoring provides the anesthesia practitioner with a better idea of the adequacy of recovery from induced arrhythmias, and whether the patient will tolerate further threshold testing. While some might also routinely place a pulmonary artery catheter (PAC), the author does not unless there is severely compromised cardiac function and information gained from the PAC would be critical for management. Cutaneous cardioversion–defibrillation pads are placed in case the patient requires cardioversion–defibrillation prior to placement of ICD leads, and as a backup during defibrillation threshold testing. The external cardioverter–defibrillator should be tested for proper function prior to ICD implantation or operative system revision.

THORACOTOMY IMPLANTATION AND TESTING PROCEDURE. The agents and techniques used for anesthesia vary considerably among institutions, but often include a sedative-hypnotic, short-acting opiate, and a nondepolarizing muscle relaxant, since these are least likely to affect defibrillation thresholds or the characteristics of spontaneous or induced arrhythmias. It should be noted that volatile anesthetics have been shown to affect the inducibility of VT related to myocardial infarction in animal models.[20,21] However, if volatile anesthetics are used, the author's practice is to use them in substantially reduced inspired concentrations (typically, isoflurane < 0.5 percent). The use of antiarrhythmic drugs is discouraged unless absolutely required, since many of these drugs affect defibrillation thresholds or VT/VF detection algorithms (Table 8–10). Once the ICD system is installed, intraoperative testing of the device is performed in concert with a cardiac electrophysiologist. The sensing system must be assessed for satisfactory intracardiac signals during induced VT/VF for proper activation of the ICD device. Subsequently, energy requirements for termination of VT/VF are determined. Extrastimulation and alternating current or rapid pacing are used to induce VT and VF, respectively. An external defibrillator is used with the newly implanted ICD leads to test energy requirements for terminating VT/VF. These should be 20 J or less. The external defibrillator can also be used with the cutaneous pads or internal paddles for "rescue" cardioversion–defibrillation in case of ICD lead failure. Once it has been established that the ICD lead system is satisfactory, the ICD device itself is connected to the leads, activated, and programmed with an external programming device. Following programming, VT/VF may be induced again to test the complete system. If everything is satisfactory, the surgical wounds are closed. Since closure usually requires electrocautery, which could trigger inappropriate ICD discharge, the ICD device should be deactivated during wound closure.

References

1. Hayes D. Pacemaker complications. In Furman S, Hayes D, Holmes D (eds): A Practice of Cardiac Pacing. 3rd ed. Mt. Kisco, NY: Futura Publishing, 1993: pp. 537–569.
2. Holmes D. The implantable cardioverter defibrillator. In Furman S, Hayes D, Holmes D (eds): A Practice of Cardiac Pacing. 3rd ed. Mt. Kisco, NY: Futura Publishing, 1993: pp. 465–508.
3. Maloney J, Vanerio G, Pashkow F. Single-chamber rate-modulated pacing, AAIR–VVIR: Follow-up and complications. In Barold S, Mugica J (ed): New Perspectives in Cardiac Pacing. 2. Mt. Kisco, NY: Futura Publishing, 1991: pp. 429–458.
4. Hayes D, Higano S. DDDR pacing: Follow-up and complications. In Barold S, Mugica J (eds): New Perspectives in Cardiac Pacing. 2. Mt. Kisco, NY: Futura Publishing, 1991: pp. 473–491.
5. Luceri R, Brownstein S, Habal S, Castellanos A. Device-device and drug-device interactions. In Barold S, Mugica J (eds): New Perspectives in Cardiac Pacing. 2. Mt. Kisco, NY: Futura Publishing, 1991: pp. 527–544.
6. Hayes D, Holmes D, Furman S. Permanent pacemaker implantation. In Furman S, Hayes D, Holmes D (eds): A Practice of Cardiac Pacing. 3rd ed. Mt. Kisco, NY: Futura Publishing, 1993: pp. 261–307.
7. Leitgeb N. Safety standards for cardiac pacemakers. In Atlee J,

Gombotz H, Tscheliessnigg K (eds): Perioperative Management of Pacemaker Patients. Berlin: Springer-Verlag, 1992: pp. 27–32.

8. Barold S, Zipes D. Cardiac pacemakers and antiarrhythmic devices. In Braunwald E (ed): Heart Disease. 4th ed. Philadelphia: WB Saunders, 1992: pp. 726–755.

9. Furman S. Comprehension of pacemaker timing cycles. In Furman S, Hayes D, Holmes D (eds): A Practice of Cardiac Pacing. 3rd ed. Mt. Kisco, NY: Futura Publishing, 1993: pp. 135–194.

10. Hayes D. Pacemaker Electrocardiography. In Furman S, Hayes D, Holmes D (eds): A Practice of Cardiac Pacing. 3rd ed. Mt. Kisco, NY: Futura Publishing, 1993: pp. 309–359.

11. Atlee J. Perioperative Cardiac Dysrhythmias. 2nd ed. Chicago: Year Book Medical, 1990: p. 443.

12. Hayes D. Electromagnetic interference, drug-device interactions, and other practical considerations. In Furman S, Hayes D, Holmes D (eds): A Practice of Cardiac Pacing. 3rd ed. Mt. Kisco, NY: Futura Publishing, 1993: pp. 665–684.

13. Bourgeois I. Electromagnetic interference and cardiac pacemakers. In Atlee J, Gombotz H, Tscheliessnigg K (eds): Perioperative Management of Pacemaker Patients. Berlin: Springer-Verlag, 1992: pp. 70–82.

14. Iberer F, Justich E, Tscheliessnigg K, Wasler A. Nuclear magnetic resonance imaging in pacemaker patients. In Atlee J, Gombotz H, Tscheliessnigg K (eds): Perioperative Management of Pacemaker Patients. Berlin: Springer-Verlag, 1992: pp. 86–90.

15. Irnich W, Lazica M, Gleissner M. Extracorporeal shock wave lithotripsy in pacemaker patients. In Atlee J, Gombotz H, Tscheliessnigg K (eds): Perioperative Management of Pacemaker Patients. Berlin: Springer-Verlag, 1992: pp. 98–103.

16. Zaidan J, Curling P, Craver J. Effect of enflurane, isoflurane and halothane on pacing stimulation thresholds in man. PACE 1985;8: 32–34.

17. Martin R, Dupuis J, Tetrault J-P. Regional anesthesia for pacemaker insertion. Reg Anesth 1989;14:81–84.

18. Raza S, Vasireddy A, Candido K, et al. A complete regional anesthesia technique for cardiac pacemaker insertion. J Cardiothorac Vasc Anesth 1991;5:54–56.

19. Chapman P. Implantable cardioverter-defibrillators. In Atlee J, Gombotz H, Tscheliessnigg K (eds): Perioperative Management of Pacemaker Patients. Berlin: Springer-Verlag, 1992: pp. 62–69.

20. Atlee J, Bosnjak Z. Mechanisms for cardiac dysrhythmias during anesthesia. Anesthesiology 1990;72:347–374.

21. Deutsch N, Hantler C, Tait A, et al. Suppression of ventricular arrhythmias by volatile anesthetics in a canine model of chronic myocardial infarction. Anesthesiology 1990;72:1012–1021.

9

Recognition and Management of Supraventricular Arrhythmias

Abbreviations Used in Chapter Nine

AAT	Automatic atrial tachycardia
AES/VES	Atrial/ventricular extrasystole
AV	Atrioventricular
AVJR	AV junctional rhythm
CAD	Coronary artery disease
ECG	Electrocardiogram (-cardiography)
HCSS	Hypersensitive carotid sinus syndrome
PSVT	Paroxysmal SVT
SA	Sinoatrial
SND	Sinus node dysfunction
SVT	Supraventricular tachycardia
VA	Ventriculoatrial
VT/VF	Ventricular tachycardia/fibrillation
WPW	Wolff–Parkinson–White (syndrome)

The final two chapters deal with recognition and management of specific cardiac rhythm disturbances. Supraventricular arrhythmias are discussed in this chapter, and arrhythmias with ventricular preexcitation, ventricular arrhythmias, and atrioventricular (AV) and fascicular heart block in the final chapter. The electrocardiographic (ECG) diagnosis of cardiac arrhythmias was discussed in Chapter 4, although liberal use of ECG examples of arrhythmias is made in these final chapters.

Overview and Perspective

As discussed in Chapter 3, new or worsening arrhythmias in perioperative and critical care settings are often triggered or aggravated by the effects of imposed physiologic imbalance, rather than due primarily to underlying structural heart disease per se. Therefore, the diagnosis and treatment of cardiac arrhythmias in these settings is usually urgent and not continued on a long-term basis. In contrast, in the practice of cardiology, except for patients in medical intensive care or coronary care units, more attention is given to long-term prevention and management, including the treatment of underlying heart disease. Consequently, these final two chapters deviate somewhat from standard cardiology reference works on the subject.[1-3] The emphasis here is more on mechanisms, identification and correction of imbalance, parenteral drugs, and electrical therapy, compared to oral drugs, catheter or surgical ablative therapy, permanent pacemakers, or internal cardioverter-–defibrillator devices. The author has drawn heavily on his own clinical experience and selected published works,[4-20] as well as standard cardiology works on cardiac arrhythmias and electrophysiology.[1-3,21,22] Unless indicated otherwise, drug doses are those suggested in the product literature or the 1995 Physicians' Desk Reference.

Sinus Node Dysfunction

Possible manifestations of sinus node dysfunction (SND), which could be due to disease affecting the sinus node (intrinsic) or caused by drugs and other imbalance (extrinsic), include disorders of automaticity, conduction, or both. Because the sinus node is richly innervated by both the parasympathetic (vagus) and sympathetic nervous system, autonomic dysfunction must be considered as a major or at least contributing cause of arrhythmias with SND. However, this does mean that drugs to counteract excessive vagal (atropine) or adrenergic tone (beta-blockers) are necessarily appropriate treatment. This will depend on the contribution of dysautonomia to the disturbance, which may be difficult to determine or even estimate. Additionally, effects of autonomic agonists or antagonists are often imprecise (minimal, excessive), sometimes untoward, often long-lasting, and not always easily reversed. Disturbances of SND include sinus bradycardia, sinus arrhythmia, wandering atrial pacemaker, sinus pause and arrest, sinoatrial block, noncompensatory sinus tachycardia, bradycardia–tachycardia syndrome, and the hypersensitive carotid sinus syndrome.

SINUS BRADYCARDIA

Recognition

Normal sinus rhythm in adults is recognized by normal P waves (i.e., upright with rounded contour in lead II; inverted or biphasic in V_1), PR interval ≤ 0.12 second, and rate between 60 and 100 beats/min (Fig. 9–1). Sinus rhythm ≤ 60 beats/min is sinus bradycardia (Fig. 9–2), although ≤ 100 beats/min is bradycardia in newborns and infants. From birth to 3 months of age, the mean upper rate increases from 140 to 160 beats/min.[23] Thereafter, it decreases to 120 or 100 beats/min by 3 and 5 years of age, respectively. In conditioned athletes and adolescents, the rate during sleep may be < 40 beats/min. Aside from age and physical status, other factors that may affect the rate of normal sinus rhythm include gender, emotions, and body temperature.

Significance and Causes

Sinus bradycardia rarely causes hemodynamic embarrassment. In fact, low heart rates increase diastolic time and improve ventricular filling in many patients, and reduce the likelihood of myocardial ischemia in others with coronary artery disease (CAD). However, in patients with heart failure, whether due to systolic or diastolic dysfunction, and especially those with dilated cardiomyopathy, sinus bradycardia may be extremely disadvantageous. This is because the ability to increase heart rate may be the major adaptive mechanism for maintenance of adequate cardiac output. Sinus bradycardia has many possible causes (Table 9–1). Removal or correction of these should be considered in addition to providing drug or temporary pacing treatment.

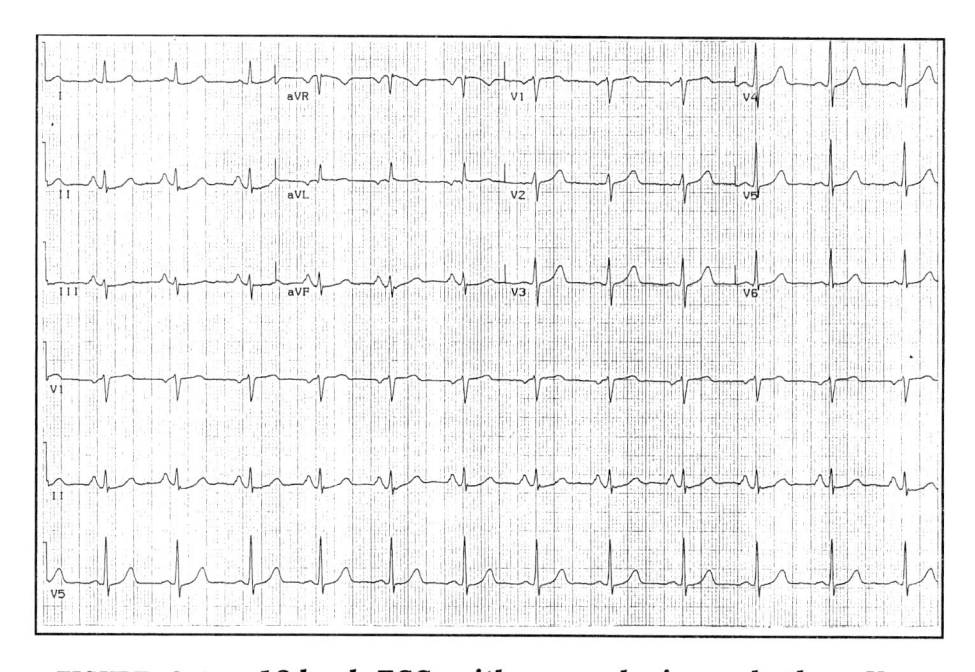

RECOGNITION/MANAGEMENT OF SUPRAVENTRICULAR ARRHYTHMIAS   **333**

FIGURE 9-1   *12-lead ECG with normal sinus rhythm. Note rounded, upright P waves in lead II, and negative (sometimes biphasic—Figs. 9-2 and 9-4) ones in V_1. The PR interval is 0.12 second, and rate 75 beats/min. The large P waves (II, III, aVF) suggest right atrial enlargement.*

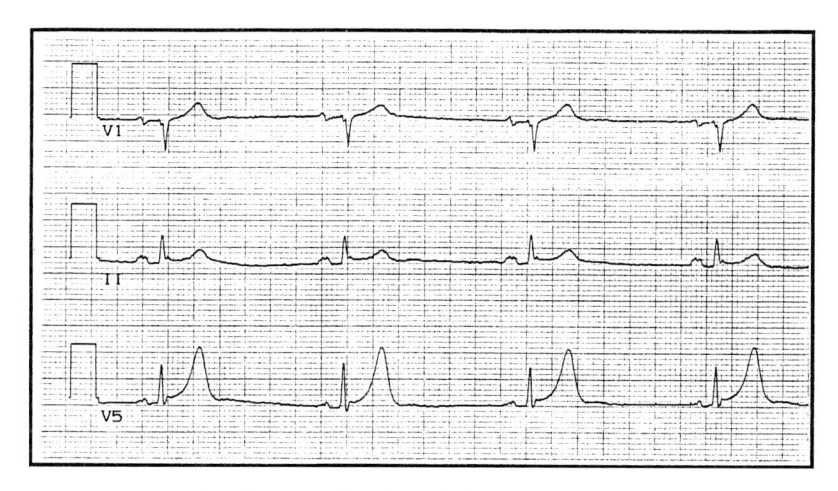

FIGURE 9-2   *Rhythm strip showing marked sinus bradycardia (42 beats/min).*

TABLE 9-1 *Some causes of sinus bradycardia in perioperative and critical care settings*

Increased vagal tone	Reduced sympathetic tone	Insecticides, poisons
Beta-blockers	Calcium-channel blockers	Central alpha-2 agonists*
Hypothermia	Hypoxia (later stages)	Myocardial infarction
↑ intracranial pressure	Hypothyroidism	Oculocardiac reflex
Procainamide	Quinidine	Anticholinergic drugs

*Clonidine; dexmedetomidine.

Drug Treatment

Sinus bradycardia requires no special treatment unless it produces severe hemodynamic compromise (mean arterial pressure < 60 mmHg), or is believed to threaten vital organ perfusion in patients with hypertension, or central nervous system, renal, or coronary disease (i.e., mean pressure < 70 to 80 mmHg; coronary perfusion pressure < 40 to 50 mmHg). If increased vagal tone is believed to be the cause, atropine may be effective treatment. However, a problem with atropine and other anticholinergics is that effects may outlast transient vagotonia, causing excess tachycardia or arrhythmias requiring further treatment. Ephedrine is also useful, particularly since it also increases cardiac output and blood pressure. Isoproterenol may also be used to increase heart rate and contractility, but is more likely than atropine or ephedrine to cause excess tachycardia or arrhythmias. Doses for drugs used to increase heart rate or speed AV node conduction (i.e., positive chronotropes or dromotropes) are provided in Table 9–2.

Pacing Treatment

Because drugs used to treat sinus bradycardia can cause excessive or adverse effects, temporary pacing is the safest and most reliable treatment, especially with the recent availability of noninvasive transesophageal atrial pacing products (see Chapter 7). However, with temporary pacing, one must optimize paced rates for each patient, since too great an increase in paced rate may reduce blood pressure as a result of encroachment on diastolic filling time (Fig. 9–3).

SINUS ARRHYTHMIA

Sinus arrhythmia is phasic variation in sinus rate, in which the maximal cycle length exceeds the minimum cycle length by at least 120

TABLE 9-2 *Suggested intravenous doses for positive chronotropes and dromotropes*

DRUG	BOLUS	INFUSION
Atropine (A)	0.4–1.0 mg (repeat × 2–5)*	—
Ephedrine	5–10 mg (up to 50 mg)	—
Glycopyrrolate (G)	0.2–0.5 mg (repeat × 2–5)	—
Isoproterenol	2–5 µg	1–3 µg/min

*Accepted vagal blocking dose in adults is 2.0 mg (A) or 1.0 mg (G).

msec (Fig. 9–4). The morphology of P waves is constant during cycle length variation. Sometimes cycle length variation is so extreme as to lead a casual observer palpating the pulse to diagnose atrial fibrillation or frequent extrasystoles. With *respiratory sinus arrhythmia,* the cycle length shortens with inspiration. Respiratory sinus arrhythmia is common in the young. Cycle length variability decreases with advancing age or autonomic dysfunction, as with diabetic neuropathy. It also decreases or becomes absent with general anesthesia. With *nonrespiratory sinus arrhythmia,* cycle length variation is not linked to respiration. It may result from intrinsic sinus node dysfunction or digitalis intoxication. Sinus arrhythmia rarely requires treatment. If it does, treatment is as for sinus bradycardia.

WANDERING ATRIAL PACEMAKER

Wandering (shifting) atrial pacemaker (Fig. 9–5) is a variant of sinus arrhythmia in which there is cyclical variation in P-wave morphology as well as cycle length. It may result from transfer of pacemaker dominance from the classic sinus node region (superior vena cava–right atrial junction) to the more caudally located subsidiary atrial pacemakers along the sulcus terminalis and other atrial sites.[10,11,13,14] Treatment for wandering atrial pacemaker is rarely required; otherwise, it is the same as for sinus bradycardia.

SINUS PAUSE OR ARREST

Sinus pause or arrest is recognized by an unexplained pause between P waves, or cessation of sinus rhythm and absent P waves. With sinus pause (Fig. 9–6), the P–P interval delimiting the pause is not a multiple of the basic P–P interval with normal sinus rhythm. With sinus arrest, there are no sinus P waves (Fig. 9–7) and asystole, unless a lower pacemaker escapes to control the heart (i.e., "a friend in need is a friend indeed" pacemaker). Escape beats or rhythm may originate in atrial,

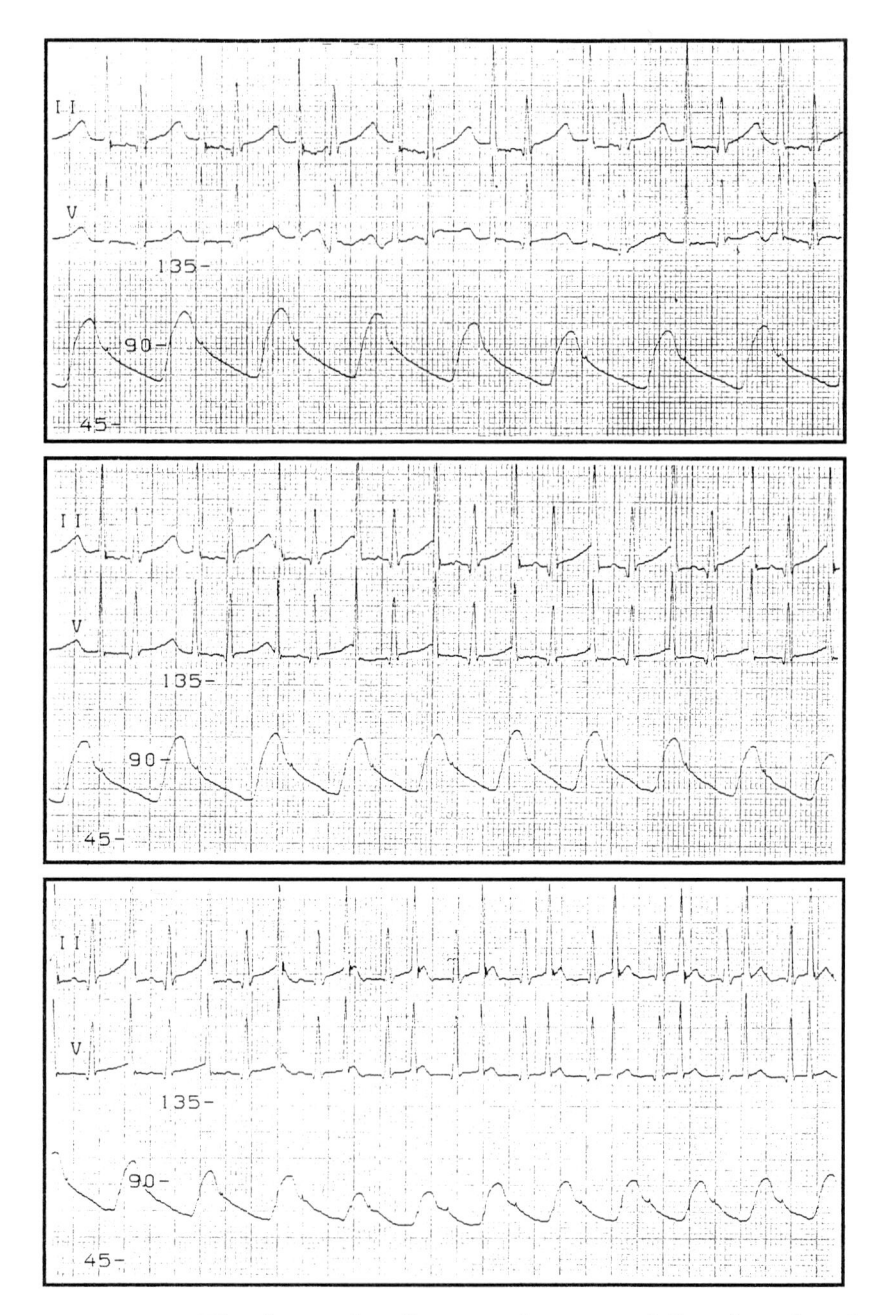

FIGURE 9-3 *Rhythm strips from patient paced for sinus bradycardia of 40 beats/min and hypotension 75/35 (56) mmHg. (Top) Transesophageal atrial pacing at 80 beats/min increases blood pressure to 108/72 (83) mmHg. (Middle) Pacing at 98 beats/min produces a similar blood pressure. (Bottom) However, when the paced rate is further increased to 115 beats/min, there is a decrease in blood pressure to 92/69 (76) mmHg due to diastolic encroachment.*

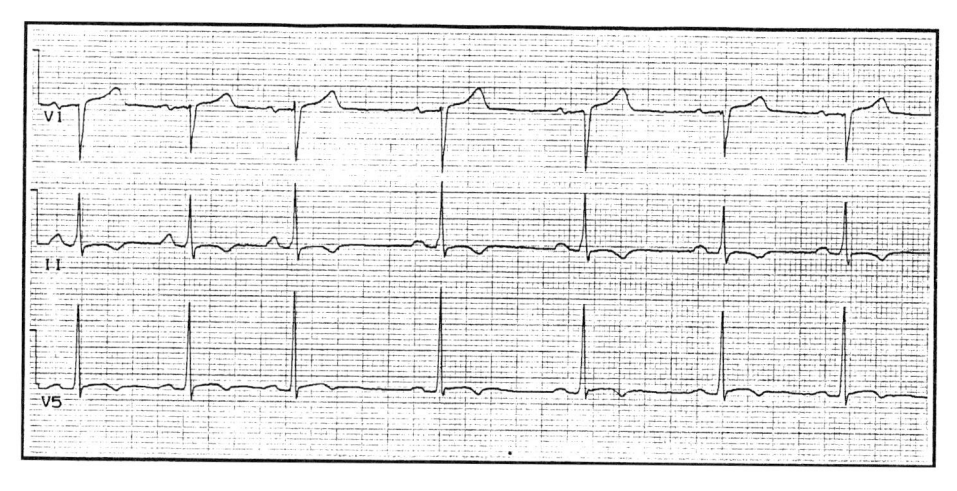

FIGURE 9-4 Rhythm strip showing sinus arrhythmia. The P waves are essentially unchanged despite cycle length variation of 820 to 1140 msec (73 to 53 beats/min).

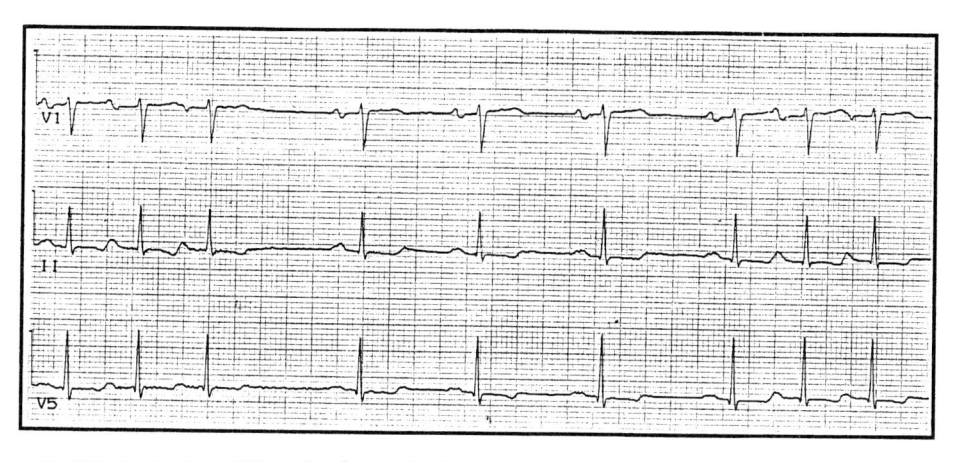

FIGURE 9-5 Wandering atrial pacemaker. Note cyclical variation in heart rate (51 to 111 beats/min) along with varying P-wave morphology. Three distinct P-wave morphologies are seen in lead II: upward notched (beats 1 and 4); tented (beats 2, 3, 8, and 9); and flattened notched (beats 5, 6, and 7).

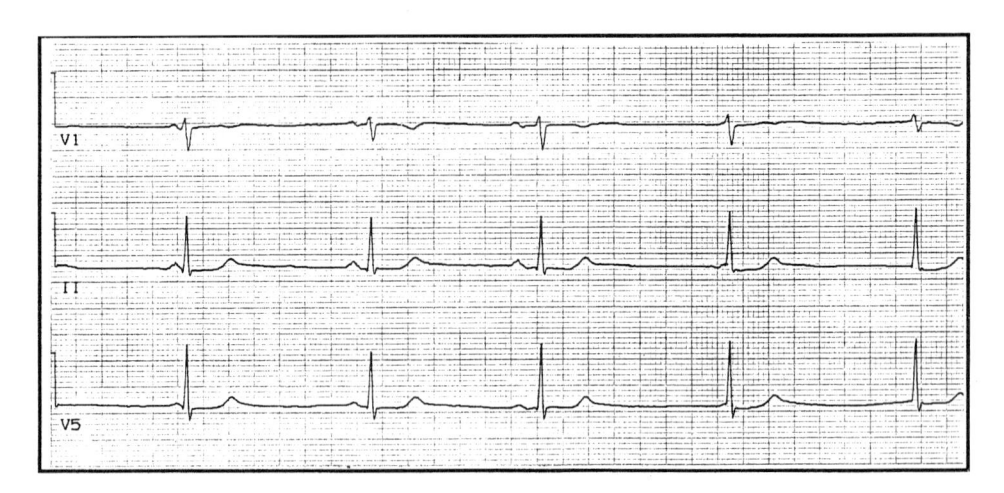

338 RECOGNITION/MANAGEMENT OF SUPRAVENTRICULAR ARRHYTHMIAS

FIGURE 9-6 *Sinus pause. The first three beats are sinus origin. The sinus node then fails to discharge at the expected time, so that the fourth and fifth beats are junctional escape beats. The sixth and succeeding beats (not shown) were of sinus origin.*

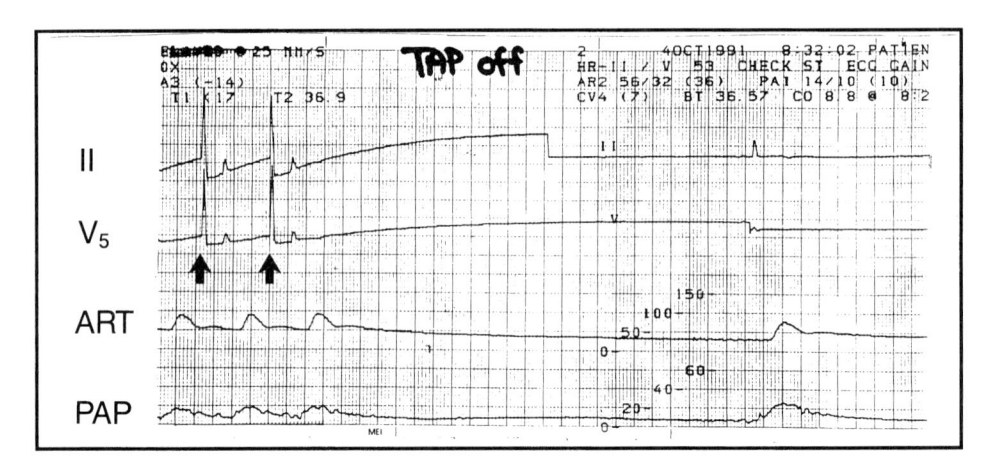

FIGURE 9-7 *Transient sinus arrest due to overdrive suppression of automaticity. Sinus arrest followed abrupt cessation of transesophageal atrial pacing for disadvantageous bradycardia in a patient with SND. A junctional escape beat ("a friend in need is a friend indeed pacemaker") occurs after nearly 5 seconds of asystole. Sinus arrest can also occur following spontaneous or electrical termination of tachycardias. (From Atlee et al.[19], with permission.)*

AV junctional, or ventricular secondary pacemakers. Sinus pause or arrest are due to defective or suppressed impulse generation within the sinus node. The former is caused by disease. The latter results from the effects of drugs (e.g., digitalis toxicity, beta-blockers), vagal stimulation, or overdrive suppression of automaticity by artificial pacing (Fig. 9–7) or sustained tachyarrhythmias. Failure of sinus node discharge without escape of secondary pacemakers can result in ventricular asystole or the genesis of lethal ventricular tachyarrhythmias. Treatment of sinus pause and arrest is as for sinus bradycardia. Temporary pacing is preferred to drugs because of the risk of accelerating lower pacemakers to cause ectopic tachycardia. Either sinus pause or arrest with symptomatic bradycardia and/or arrhythmias in patients with SND is a common indication for permanent pacemaker implantation.

SINOATRIAL BLOCK

With this rhythm disturbance there are also absent P waves at the expected time, except that the interval between dropped P waves is a multiple or nearly so of the basic P–P interval. With type II second-degree sinoatrial (SA) block, the interval without P waves is some whole-number multiple of the basic interval. With type I (Wenckebach) second-degree SA block, the P–P interval progressively shortens prior to the pause, and the duration of the pause is less than two basic P–P intervals (Fig. 9–8). The diagnosis of first- and third-degree SA block

FIGURE 9–8 *Sinus node (SA) exit block. Note that the P–P intervals progressively shorten before the dropped P wave, and the duration of the pause between dropped P waves (1,040 msec) is less than two P–P intervals (1240 msec).*

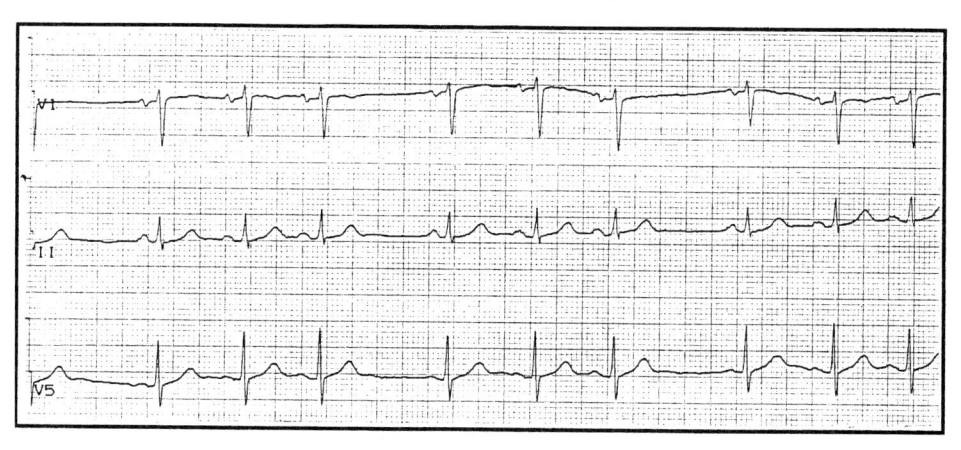

cannot be made from the surface ECG, but requires recording of sinus node electrograms. Causes and treatment for SA block are similar to those for sinus bradycardia.

NONCOMPENSATORY SINUS TACHYCARDIA

Noncompensatory sinus tachycardia is sinus rhythm at a rate exceeding 100 beats/min in adults or rates up to 160 beats/min in infants and children (see Sinus Bradycardia, earlier). By *noncompensatory* is meant that tachycardia is not secondary to hypovolemia, hemorrhage, sepsis, or shock. It may be the result of fear, anxiety, pain, awareness during anesthesia, stress, hypermetabolic states, pheochromocytoma, or nonapparent causes, any of which are associated with exaggerated sympathetic tone. Because tachycardia might be hemodynamically disadvantageous in some patients, or associated with myocardial ischemia in others, it may be necessary to treat the disturbance. After correction or removal of obvious causes, esmolol or a longer-acting beta-blocker may be used (Table 9-3). If there is concern for further hemodynamic compromise with beta-blockers, edrophonium (5 to 10 mg) may be used to establish the benefit of rate reduction, since it has no effect on ventricular contractility. If there is substantial hemodynamic improvement following rate reduction with edrophonium, then it is probable that beta-blockers can be safely used for continued treatment.

BRADYCARDIA–TACHYCARDIA SYNDROME

The bradycardia–tachycardia (brady–tachy) syndrome is yet another manifestation of SND. It is alternation of paroxysms of atrial tachyarrhythmias with periods of sinus rhythm or bradycardia, or slow ectopic rhythms (Figs. 9–9 and 9–10). These may occur in association

TABLE 9-3 *Recommended drugs and doses for noncompensatory sinus tachycardia*

DRUG	BOLUS	INFUSION
Esmolol	0.5–1.0 mg/kg	50–300 µg/kg/min*
Propranolol	0.5–1.0 mg/min*	—
Edrophonium	5–10 mg/1–2 min*†	—

*Titrate to desired heart rate.
†No more than 25 mg in adults.

RECOGNITION/MANAGEMENT OF SUPRAVENTRICULAR ARRHYTHMIAS **341**

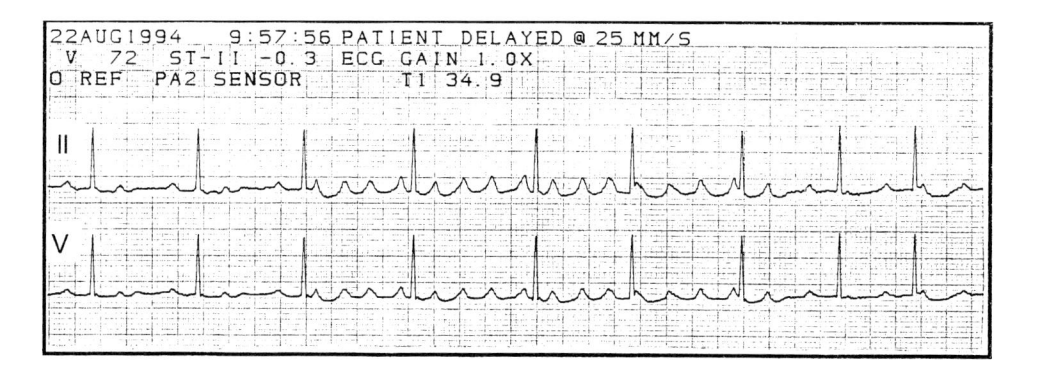

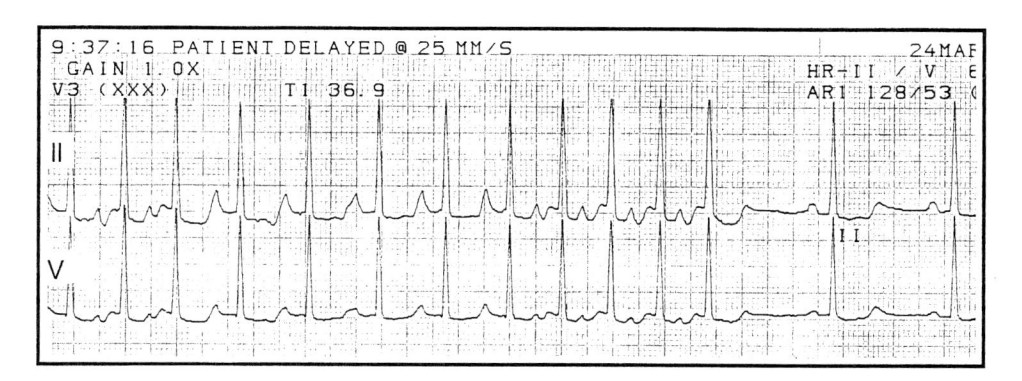

FIGURE 9–9 *Manifestations of bradycardia–tachycardia syndrome with sinus node dysfunction (SND). Top. The basic rhythm is sinus rhythm at 73 beats/min. This is interrupted by a paroxysm of atrial flutter with variable (4:1 and 3:1) AV block, which terminates spontaneously. Bottom. A paroxysm of multiform ectopic atrial tachycardia terminates spontaneously in slow sinus rhythm (62 beats/min). Both tracings were from anesthetized patients with known intrinsic SND.*

with sinoatrial or AV conduction disturbances, and in patients without obvious heart disease. Histologic findings include inflammatory changes or fibrous degeneration within the sinus node and at its atrial margins, the autonomic nerves and ganglia surrounding the sinus node, and also the atrial wall. Treatment of bradycardia is usually with pacing, since chronotropic drugs may have unpredictable and untoward effects on tachycardia or escape rhythms. Treatment of tachycardia is that indicated for the specific rhythm disturbance (discussed later).

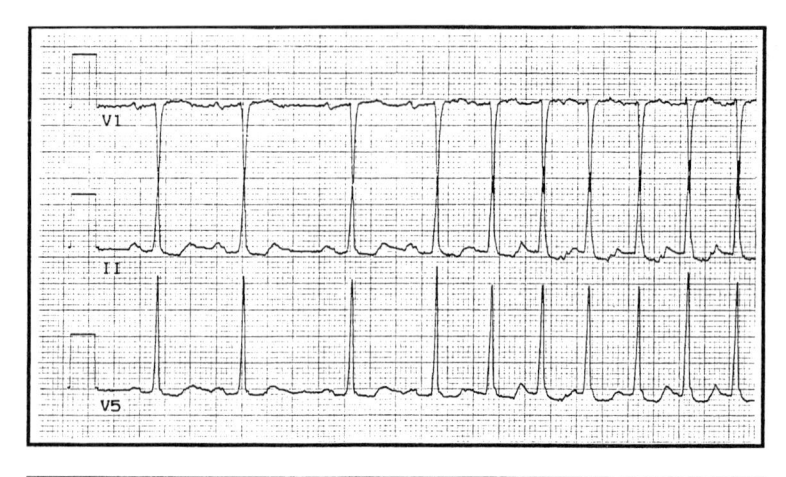

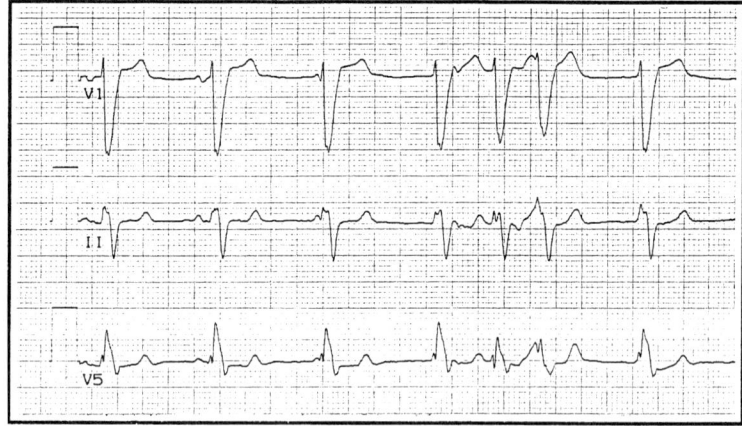

FIGURE 9-10 *Manifestations of bradycardia-tachycardia syndrome with sinus node dysfunction (SND). (Top) Rhythm strip from conscious patient with SND. Sinus arrhythmia is interrupted by a paroxysm of coarse atrial fibrillation with a ventricular rate of 143-171 beats/min. (Bottom) Rhythm strip from another conscious patient with SND, and also left bundle branch block. Slow sinus rhythm (65 beats/min) with two junctional escape beats followed by two premature atrial beats. The last beat is of junctional origin.*

HYPERSENSITIVE CAROTID SINUS SYNDROME

Recognition

The hypersensitive carotid sinus syndrome (HCSS) is manifest by cardioinhibitory or vasodepressor responses (see Chapter 6). On the ECG, cardioinhibitory HCSS is recognized by asystole secondary to sinus arrest or SA exit block. AV heart block is observed less frequently, possibly because the absence of atrial activity precludes diagnosis of AV heart block. Perhaps if atrial activity was maintained by pacing, manifestations of AV heart block would be present. In symptomatic patients, AV junctional or ventricular escape beats generally do not occur, suggesting that increased vagal tone or withdrawal of sympathetic tone can suppress latent pacemakers in the AV junctional tissues and ventricles.[3] HCSS commonly occurs in association with CAD, although the mechanism for HCSS in this context is not known.[3]

Management

Patients with symptomatic HCSS (syncope, near syncope) will likely have a permanent pacemaker. This should be capable of dual-chamber demand pacing, both to preserve atrial function and to provide for ventricular pacing with high-degree AV heart block. If a patient with symptoms of bradycardia and a hyperactive response to carotid sinus massage (asystole > 3 seconds; systolic blood pressure decrease > 50 mmHg) faces nonemergent surgery, consultation with a cardiologist and further work-up is advised. It is possible in patients with HCSS, especially with treated or untreated hypertension, that there could be exaggerated bradycardia or asystole with airway or surgical stimulation. Atropine or other positive chronotropes (Table 9–1) used to treat bradycardia or asystole might either be ineffective or produce excess tachycardia and arrhythmias with withdrawal of carotid sinus stimulation. In patients with HCSS having emergent surgery, adequate anesthesia, direct arterial vasodilators (e.g., nicardipine) as prophylaxis for hypertension, and prophylactic transesophageal atrial pacing are advised.

Ectopic Atrial Rhythm Disturbances

Ectopic atrial beats and tachycardia arise in sites other than the sinus node. They may be triggered or automatic, but differentiation between these mechanisms for supraventricular tachycardia (SVT) is sometimes difficult or even impossible in perioperative and critical care settings. Neither is it clinically important, since treatment is the same. However, the distinction between automatic-triggered (nonparoxysmal) and reentrant (paroxysmal) SVT is important for therapeutics. For example, direct current (DC) cardioversion is not effective for terminating the former. In fact, it may accelerate ectopic SVT or cause fibrillation. In contrast, cardioversion is highly effective for reentrant SVT. ECG features that suggest reentrant as opposed to ectopic SVT are listed in Table 9–4. However, none of these are "cast in stone." The clinical circumstance and patient history must also be considered. For example, SVT with chronic pulmonary or structural heart disease is more likely to be automatic, while SVT in an adult with no apparent heart disease is more likely to be reentrant. Also, SVT in patients under general anesthesia is more likely to be automatic. This is because drugs used for anesthesia tend to be vagotonic and/or increase supraventricular refractory periods (see Chapter 3), and should therefore oppose sustained reentrant SVT.

ATRIAL EXTRASYSTOLES AND ECTOPIC PACEMAKER RHYTHM

Extrasystoles

Atrial extrasystoles (AES) can originate from the sinus node, but are more likely to originate elsewhere in the atria. Therefore, the P-wave morphology with AES usually differs from that with sinus

TABLE 9-4 *Automatic-triggered compared to reentrant supraventricular tachycardia*

AUTOMATIC-TRIGGERED	REENTRANT
1. Gradual (nonparoxysmal) onset	1. Abrupt (paroxysmal) onset
2. Not initiated by a premature beat	2. Initiated by a premature beat*
3. Cycle length of tachycardia may vary	3. Cycle length of tachycardia constant
4. Small or minimal variation in P waves	4. P wave morphology fairly constant†
5. PR interval may vary somewhat	5. PR or RP interval fairly constant
6. Gradual slowing with termination	6. Abrupt termination with sinus pause

*Normal–premature beat interval is characteristically less than premature–first tachycardia beat interval.
†P wave of first beat of SVT differs from subsequent beats.

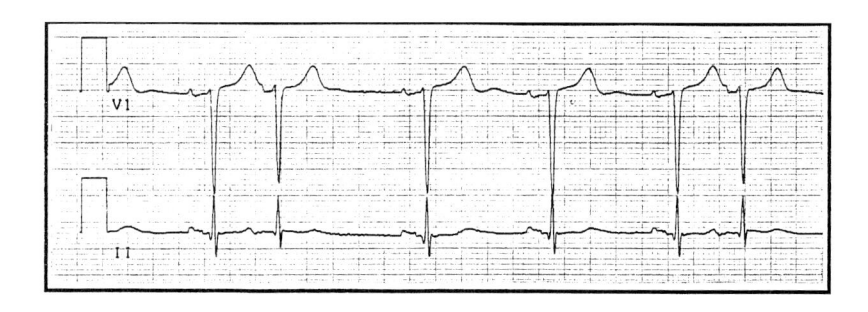

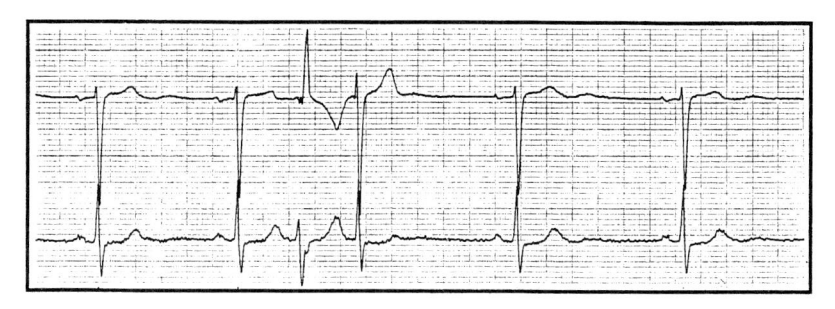

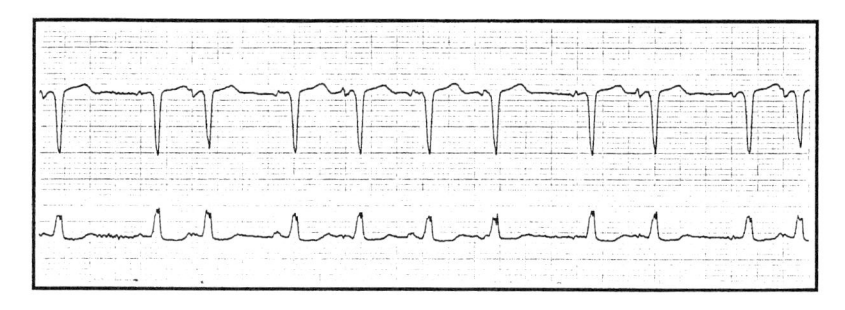

FIGURE 9-11 *ECG manifestations of atrial extrasystoles (AES). Same ECG leads and order in all panels. (Top) Normal sinus rhythm interrupted by two AES (beats 2 and 6) with PR intervals longer than for sinus beats. Note that P waves with AES have a different morphology from sinus beats, which is most evident in lead II. Also, note that AES "reset" automaticity of the sinus node due to penetration of the node. This accounts for the less than fully compensatory pause following AES. (Middle) An interpolated AES, conducted with right bundle branch block pattern aberration, occurs between beats 2 and 4. It is completely interpolated because it fails to penetrate the perinodal tissues and reset sinus node automaticity. As in the previous example, the PR interval with the AES is longer than that with sinus beats. (Bottom) Frequent, multiform AES (beats 3, 5, possibly 7, 9, and 11) interrupting probable ectopic atrial rhythm. The patient also appears to have incomplete left bundle branch block.*

rhythm (Fig. 9-11), although it may be difficult to detect AES P waves if they are "buried" in the T wave of the preceding beat. Multiple ECG leads and careful searching of the R wave to detect subtle T-wave distortion may be required. Additionally, the PR interval with AES is usually longer than that of sinus beats (Fig. 9-11), because of AV nodal delay caused by prematurity of the AES. If the AES reaches the ventricular conducting system before it has fully recovered from refractoriness, there may be ventricular conduction delay as well. This is the cause for ventricular aberration with some AES. Aberration is commonly with a right bundle branch pattern because of the longer refractoriness of the right compared to left bundle branch (Fig. 9-11). The significance of AES is that they may be so frequent as to produce tachycardia or to initiate reentrant SVT or atrial flutter–fibrillation. Acute treatment for significant AES is with beta-blockers (Table 9-3) or a calcium-channel blocker (Table 9-5). Otherwise, AES are not treated with specific drugs. However, identifiable acute imbalance that might cause or aggravate AES should be corrected.

Ectopic Atrial Pacemaker Rhythm

The P waves with ectopic atrial rhythm, as with AES, differ from those of normal sinus rhythm, and may display a variety of characteristics (notched, flattened, biphasic, etc.). The P waves and PR intervals, in contrast to wandering or shifting atrial pacemaker, are uniform. The rate of ectopic atrial rhythm is < 100 beats/min, and unless severely bradycardic, it rarely produces hemodynamic embar-

TABLE 9-5 *Calcium-channel blockers for ectopic–reentrant supraventricular arrhythmias*

DRUG	BOLUS	INFUSION
Diltiazem	0.25 mg/kg (20 mg avg. adult) or 0.15–0.35 mg/kg (25 mg)*	5–15 mg/hr beginning after bolus dosing for ≤ 24 hours*†
Verapamil	5–10 mg (0.075–0.15 mg/kg); repeat (10 mg) after 30 minutes*	2.5–5 µg/kg/min (approx. 10–20 mg/hr in avg. adult)*†

*Lower mg/kg (or µg/kg/min) dose suggested with potent volatile anesthetics, and higher dose as repeat dose after 15 minutes; additional doses must be individualized based on response.

†Higher rates or longer duration of infusion not recommended.

rassment because atrial function and AV synchrony are preserved. Treatment for disadvantageous bradycardia with atrial ectopic rhythm is as for sinus bradycardia.

AUTOMATIC ATRIAL TACHYCARDIA

Before discussing automatic atrial tachycardia (AAT), it is necessary to comment on terminology. First, all AAT is nonparoxysmal. Namely, AAT is not initiated by a premature beat and it gradually increases its rate to the rate of sustained tachycardia ($\leq$ 200 beats/min). Thus, as with sinus tachycardia and accelerated junctional rhythm (discussed later), there is a so-called warm-up phase with AAT. As the rate of AAT increases, there may be development of AV heart block, particularly with digitalis toxicity, in which case other manifestations of digitalis toxicity (e.g., ventricular extrasystoles) may also be present (Fig. 9–12). Finally, while AAT with block has in the past been referred to as "paroxysmal atrial tachycardia with block," or PAT, this is now considered incorrect.[1-3,24]

Recognition

The atrial rate of AAT is usually between 150 and 220 beats/min, and the P-wave contour is different from that with normal sinus rhythm, but uniform (Fig. 9–12). Some refer to the disturbance as *uniform or unifocal atrial tachycardia*, to distinguish it from multiform or multifocal atrial tachycardia (discussed later).[24] The PR interval is directly influenced by the rate of AAT, and AV block can exist without affecting the tachycardia. That is, AAT continues uninterrupted, in contrast to reentrant SVT. Vagal maneuvers and edrophonium generally do not terminate AAT, although they may produce or increase AV block. In contrast to reentrant SVT, the first P wave of AAT is the same as subsequent P waves of tachycardia (Fig. 9–12).

Management

Automatic atrial tachycardia occurs in all age groups, and occurs in association with chronic pulmonary disease (especially with acute inflammatory processes), acute ethanol intoxication, myocardial infarction, digitalis intoxication, and metabolic derangements such as hyperthyroidism. Hypokalemia, alkalosis, and hypomagnesemia may precipitate AAT in susceptible patients, particularly those receiving digitalis. Anesthetic drugs are not known

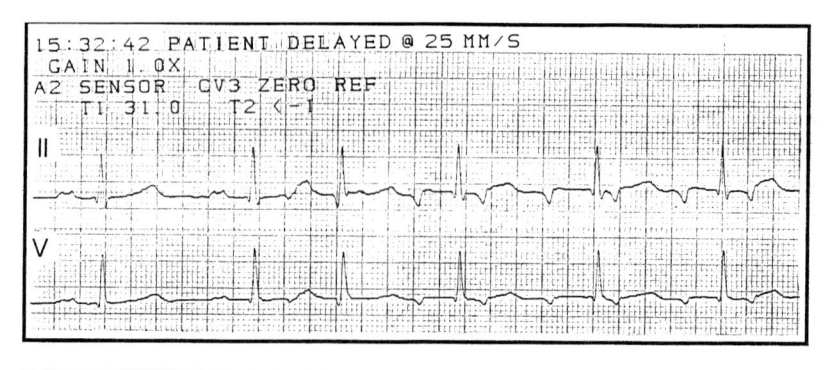

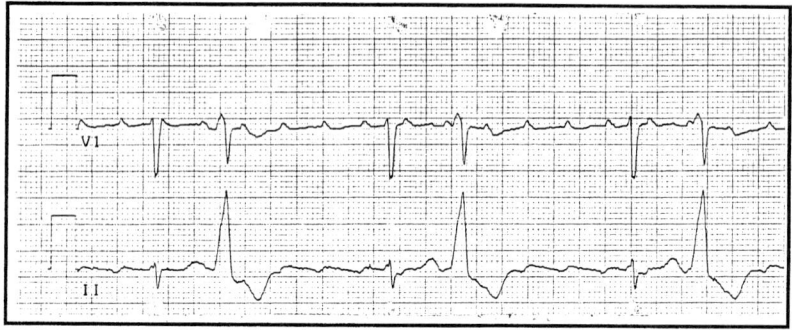

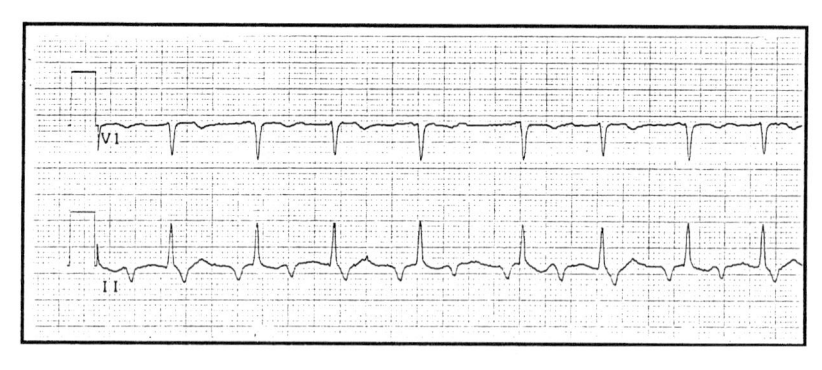

FIGURE 9-12 *Automatic atrial tachycardia (AAT). (Top) Onset of AAT in anesthetized patient with dilated cardiomyopathy and pulmonary hypertension. Note that the initial P wave of tachycardia, which distorts the T wave of the second sinus-origin beat, has the same direction and morphology of subsequent beats of AAT, which is not the case with reentrant (paroxysmal SVT). Also note variable (2:1, 3:1) AV block during tachycardia. The patient was not receiving digitalis, but had received moderate dose opiates. (Middle) AAT and ventricular extrasystoles in a bigeminal pattern in a patient receiving digitalis. (Bottom) AAT with variable (2:1, 3:1) AV heart block in patient not receiving digitalis.*

to either oppose or facilitate AAT. However, they may increase AV heart block with AAT because of increased AV nodal refractoriness.[7,16] Where possible, correction of imbalance is an important part of treatment, for AAT is difficult to treat with drugs. While AAT may be overdriven by pacing at a rate faster than tachycardia, it is not terminated. However, rapid atrial pacing may increase AV block and effectively slow the ventricular rate compared to AAT. AAT is not terminated by DC cardioversion. In fact, cardioversion may accelerate the rate of AAT, precipitate atrial fibrillation, or trigger ventricular tachyarrhythmias. The latter is more likely in patients with digitalis toxicity. Beta-adrenergic blockers, diltiazem or verapamil, and potassium and magnesium replacement (if indicated) may be effective in suppressing AAT. If AAT is due to digitalis, simply withholding the drug may be the only required treatment. Otherwise, class 1B antiarrhythmic drugs (i.e., phenytoin, lidocaine; see Chapter 5) are often effective.

MULTIFORM ATRIAL RHYTHM OR TACHYCARDIA

In contrast to wandering atrial pacemaker, where there is a cyclic variation in P-wave morphology and heart rate, with multiform (chaotic) atrial rhythm there is beat-to-beat variation in P-wave morphology, as well as in the PR and P-P intervals (Fig. 9–13). By convention, at least three distinct P-wave morphologies must be seen. Most or all P waves are conducted to the ventricles, but with some variation in the PR interval. When the ventricular rate of the disturbance exceeds 100 beats/min (seldom > 180 beats/min), it is termed *multiform (chaotic) atrial tachycardia* (Fig. 9–13). This is an automatic or triggered as opposed to reentrant rhythm disturbance. Triggering must be suspected because verapamil, which blocks calcium channels fundamental to this mechanism, often suppresses ectopic beats with multiform atrial tachycardia.[1] This disturbance is common in acutely ill elderly patients, and 60 percent of patients have associated pulmonary disease.[24] Initial treatment should be directed at improving the cardiac, pulmonary, infectious, or metabolic conditions responsible for the disturbance. Vagal maneuvers or edrophonium will transiently slow the atrial rate and ventricular response. Magnesium and potassium replacement may be useful when deficiencies of these ions are present or suspected. However, most success appears to be with beta-1-selective blockers and verapamil (diltiazem should be similarly effective), although beta-blockers should be used with caution in patients with reactive airways or heart failure.

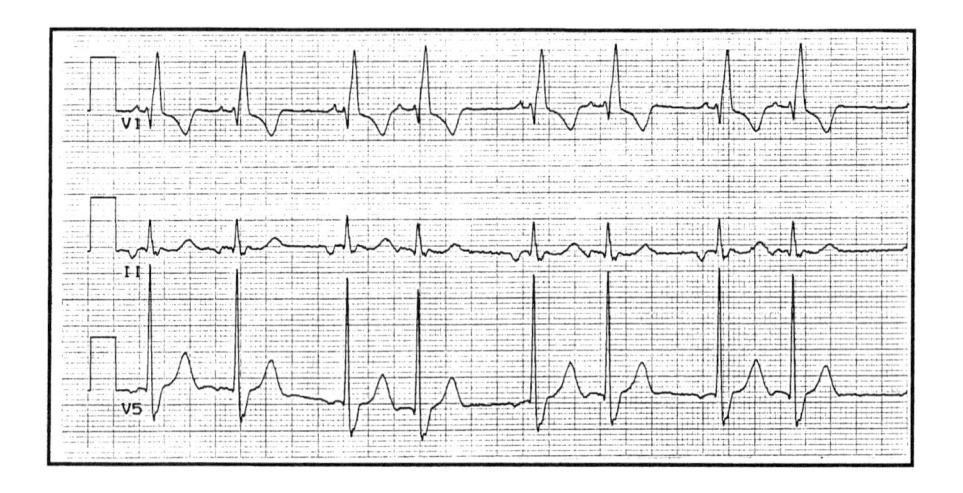

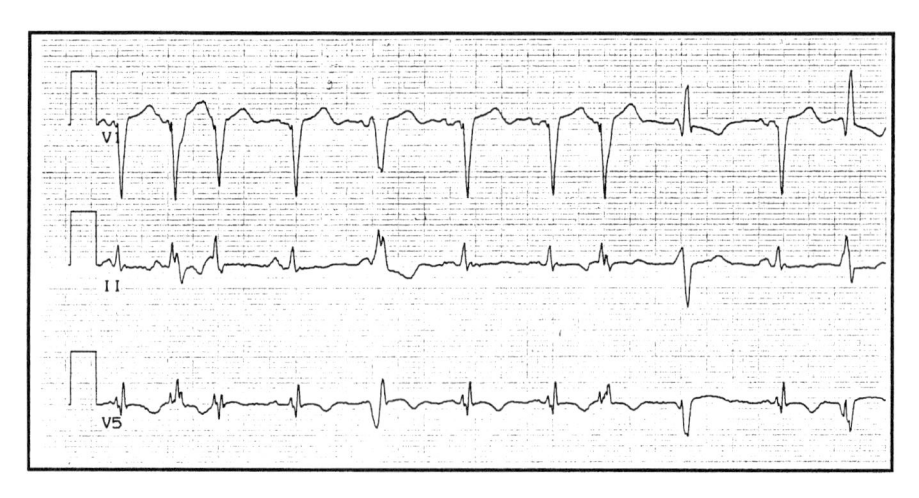

FIGURE 9-13   *Multiform atrial rhythm and tachycardia.* (Top) Multiform (chaotic) atrial rhythm at 81 beats/min. Note at least three different P wave morphologies (leads V_1 and II), and variation in the P-P and PR intervals. (Bottom) Multiform (chaotic) atrial tachycardia at 104 beats/min. Note at least five different P wave morphologies (lead II), and variation in the P-P and PR intervals.

Reentrant Supraventricular Tachycardia

Supraventricular tachycardia is any tachyarrhythmia that requires atrial or AV junctional tissue for its initiation and maintenance.[24] Reentrant SVT, in contrast to automatic-triggered SVT, is caused by AV node, AV, SA node, or atrial reentry. The latter two mechanisms account for only 10 to 15 percent electrophysiologically studied cases of reentrant SVT, while AV node or AV reentry account for an almost equal proportion of the rest.[1,3,24] Reentrant SVT is characterized by its abrupt onset and termination following a premature beat; hence the use of the term *paroxysmal SVT* (PSVT) to refer to this type of tachycardia. In contrast, as noted earlier, automatic-triggered atrial tachycardia has a more nonparoxysmal onset and termination.

PAROXYSMAL SUPRAVENTRICULAR TACHYCARDIA DUE TO ATRIOVENTRICULAR NODE REENTRY

Mechanism

Atrial or ventricular premature extrasystoles (AES, VES) can initiate PSVT as a result of AV nodal reentry (Fig. 9–14). The AV node is believed to contain functionally slow and fast conducting pathways, which begin and end at proximal and final common conducting pathways within the AV node or at its margins. With the *common form of AV node reentry*, PSVT is initiated by a premature AES (e.g., Fig. 9–14). The propagating impulse is blocked from anterograde conduction in the fast pathway because of longer refractoriness (Fig. 9–15). However, it propagates slowly in the slow pathway to excite the final common pathway. It also propagates retrogradely through the now recovered fast pathway to reexcite the atria via the proximal common pathway (Fig. 9–15). If this process perpetuates itself, PSVT due to the common form of AV nodal reentry has begun. With the common form of AV node reentry, if P waves are apparent, the ventriculoatrial (VA) interval is shorter than the AV interval. Premature VES do not commonly initiate PSVT due to the common form of AV nodal reentry. This is because they cannot easily enter the AV node because of refractoriness of the His bundle and right and left bundle branches. However, VES do initiate PSVT due to the *uncommon form of AV nodal reentry* (Fig. 9–16). In this case, the VES conducts retrogradely to the atria via the slow pathway and back to the ventricles to initiate tachycardia via the fast conducting pathway (Fig. 9–16). Only 5 to 10 percent of PSVT due to AV node reentry

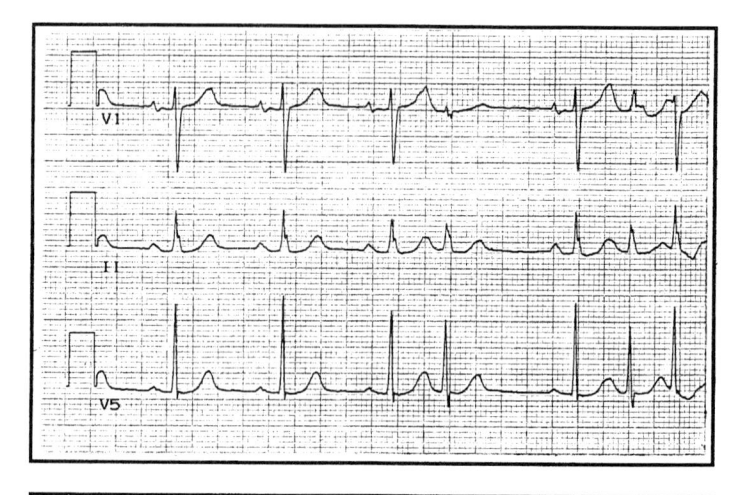

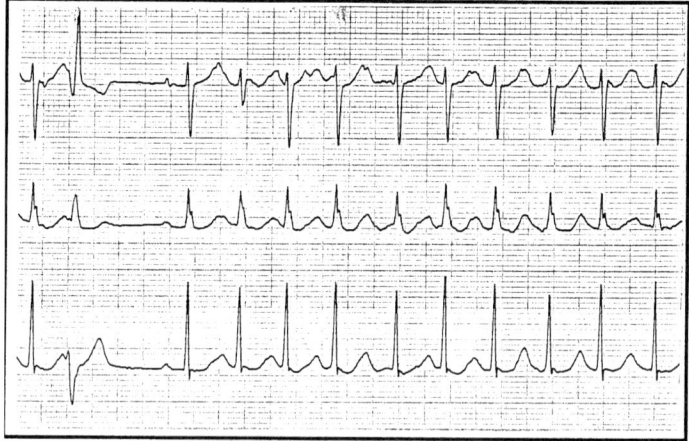

FIGURE 9-14 *Paroxysmal supraventricular tachycardia (PSVT) probably due to the common form of AV node reentry, but cardiac electrophysiologic evaluation is required to confirm this. The top and bottom tracings are contiguous. (Top) The third and fourth beats of normal sinus rhythm are followed by aberrantly conducted, premature atrial extrasystoles (AES). The second AES initiates three beats of PSVT and a short sinus pause. (Bottom) The sinus beat after the pause is followed by another AES with aberrant conduction and a run of PSVT. P waves during PSVT are nonapparent, and there is small variation in the R-R intervals, probably due to anterograde AV nodal conduction delay.*

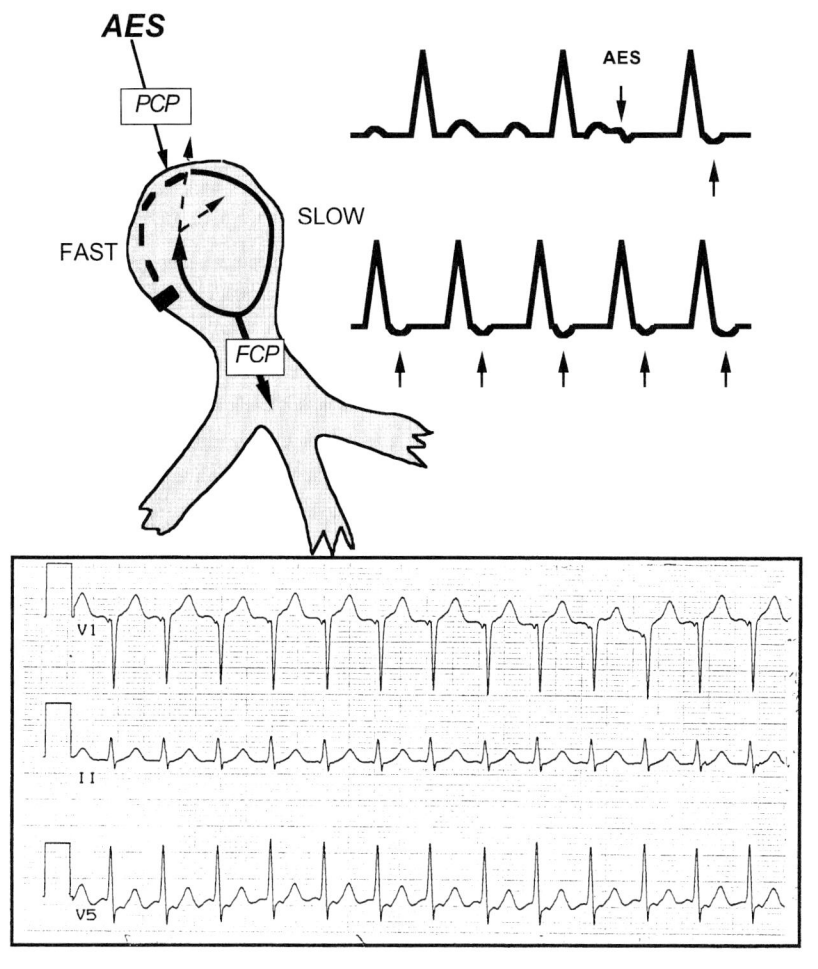

FIGURE 9-15 *Mechanism for initiation of paroxysmal supraventricular tachycardia due to the common form of AV nodal reentry. A single premature atrial extrasystole (AES) is responsible for initiating tachycardia. Anterograde conduction of the propagating premature impulse from the proximal common pathway (PCP) is blocked in the fast pathway (FAST). However, propagation is successful in the slow pathway (SLOW), and the impulse proceeds to excite the final common pathway (FCP). It also reenters the distal fast pathway and circles back to reexcite the PCP and cause a retrograde (negative) P wave (upward arrows). While the retrograde P wave is usually buried in the QRS complex, it sometimes occurs in the ST segment just at the end of the QRS complex (schematic) and rarely just at the beginning of the QRS complex (ECG tracings, lead V_1). If the impulse continues to circulate, sustained tachycardia due to AV node reentry occurs.*

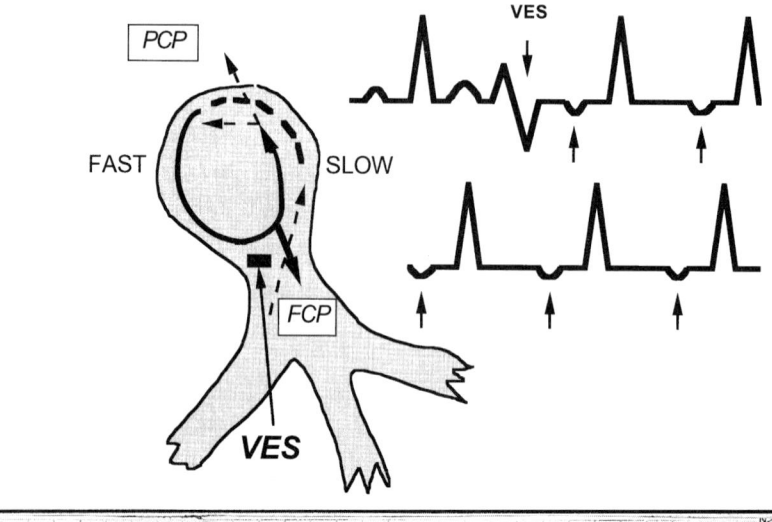

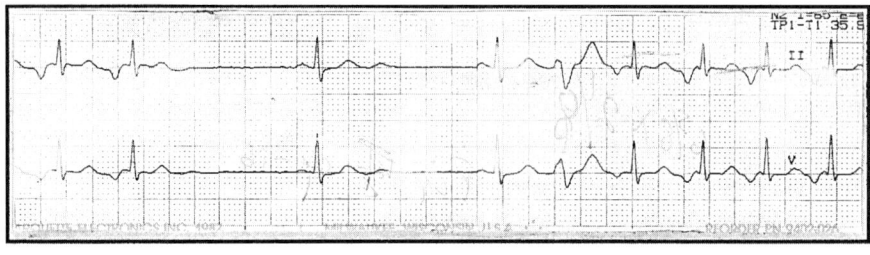

FIGURE 9-16 *Mechanism for initiation of paroxysmal supraventricular tachycardia due to the uncommon form of AV nodal reentry. A single premature ventricular extrasystole (VES) is responsible for initiating tachycardia. Retrograde conduction of the propagating premature impulse from the final common pathway (FCP) is blocked in the fast pathway (FAST). However, retrograde propagation is successful in the slow pathway (SLOW), and the impulse proceeds to excite the proximal common pathway (PCP). It also returns to excite the fast pathway in the anterograde direction, and circles back through the slow pathway to reexcite the PCP causing retrograde (negative) P waves (upward arrows) and tachycardia due to the uncommon form of AV node reentry. An ECG illustration of the termination and initiation of paroxysmal supraventricular tachycardia due to the uncommon form of AV nodal reentry is provided below.*

is of the uncommon variety.[3,24] With the uncommon form of AV node reentry PSVT, the VA interval is longer than the AV interval (Fig. 9–16).

Recognition

Atrioventricular node reentry PSVT is a narrow QRS tachycardia with a sudden onset and termination. Rates are between 140 and 250 beats/min, but are most commonly about 170 to 180 beats/min (Fig. 9–14). Retrograde P waves are "buried" in the QRS in 90 percent of cases (Fig. 9–14), and otherwise occur at the end of the QRS complex, but only rarely before it (Fig. 9–15).[1] AV nodal reentry PSVT recorded at the onset begins abruptly, usually following a premature atrial extrasystole that conducts with a prolonged PR interval. Abrupt termination is sometimes followed by a brief period of asystole or bradycardia (Fig. 9–16). The R–R interval may shorten over the first few beats of tachycardia and lengthen during the last few beats prior to termination. Variation in cycle length is usually caused by variation in anterograde AV nodal conduction time. Carotid sinus massage or edrophonium may slow AV node reentry PSVT prior to termination or, if the tachycardia fails to terminate, only slow it temporarily.

Management

Distinction as to the mechanism for AV node reentry PSVT (i.e., common vs. uncommon form) is moot, since acute management is the same for either variety. Initial treatment depends on hemodynamic status, the circumstances of PSVT, and available drugs or devices. With imminent hemodynamic collapse, immediate DC cardioversion is recommended. In the event that digitalis has been administered in large doses and DC cardioversion is contraindicated, atrial or ventricular pacing may be attempted, including atrial pacing from the esophagus. Otherwise, vagal maneuvers (carotid sinus massage), a Valsalva maneuver, or edrophonium is used. First-line antiarrhythmic drugs include adenosine (6 to 12 mg) and calcium-channel blockers (Table 9–5). Digitalis and beta-blockers may be tried if first-line drugs fail. Esmolol is preferred because of its shorter duration of action compared to other available beta-blockers. Use of vasopressors to cause a reflex increase in vagal tone is rarely done today.

ORTHODROMIC ATRIOVENTRICULAR REENTRY PAROXYSMAL SUPRAVENTRICULAR TACHYCARDIA

Atrioventricular reentry (also, AV reciprocating) PSVT requires a macroreentry loop that contains the atria, AV node, specialized ventricular conducting tissues, and ventricles, along with an anomalous or accessory pathway.[1,3,24] Ventricular activation during tachycardia may be via the normal (orthodromic PSVT) or accessory pathway (antidromic PSVT). Antidromic PSVT is discussed in Chapter 10 under Tachycardias with Ventricular Preexcitation (Wolff–Parkinson–White, WPW, syndrome). Orthodromic PSVT is discussed here since it is the mechanism for PSVT in patients with "concealed" accessory pathways.

Concealed Accessory Pathways

Normally, the atria and ventricles are separated by nonconductive connective tissue (i.e., annulus fibrosis), except for the AV node and His bundle. In an unknown percentage of persons, however, there are accessory pathways that bypass the AV node or portions of the specialized AV conduction system (Fig. 9–17). Accessory pathways are anomalous bands of conducting tissue that are electrophysiologically similar to atrial muscle. They can conduct rapidly from the atria to ventricles (anterogradely) or from the ventricles to atria (retrogradely), and participate along with the AV node in AV reentry SVT. When there

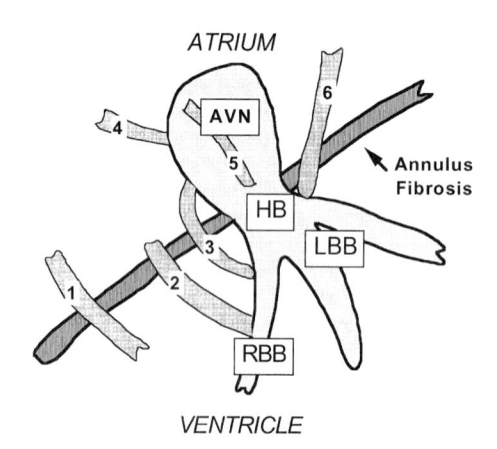

FIGURE 9–17 *Depiction of anomalous or accessory pathways that bypass portions of the normal specialized AV conducting system. 1, Accessory AV pathway (Kent bundle); 2, Atriofascicular; 3, Nodofascicular (Mahaim fiber); 4, Atrionodal; 5, Intranodal; 6, Atriohisian. AVN, AV node; HB, His (common) bundle; LBB, RBB, left and right bundle branches. See text for further discussion.*

is anterograde accessory pathway conduction during sinus rhythm, part of the ventricle is activated earlier than would have been the case had activation occurred via the normal (AV node–His bundle) pathway. This is the basis for the delta wave and short PR interval in patients with the WPW syndrome. However, up to one-quarter of accessory pathways conduct only retrogradely, so do not manifest as preexcitation during normal sinus rhythm. Hence, they are termed "concealed" accessory pathways. Concealed or manifest accessory pathways can participate in orthodromic PSVT.

Mechanism and Recognition

The mechanism for orthodromic PSVT with concealed (or manifest) AV pathways involves anterograde conduction over the normal pathway (atria → AV node → ventricles) and retrograde conduction over the accessory pathway back to the atria to cause an "orthodromic" AV reentry PSVT (Fig. 9–18). The tachycardia is orthodromic because ventricular excitation during PSVT is by the normal pathway, as opposed to by the accessory pathway with antidromic PSVT (see Chapter 10). Orthodromic PSVT is suspected when the P waves during PSVT are inverted and occur after the QRS complex in the ST–T segment. The P wave during orthodromic PSVT must follow the QRS complex because the ventricles are activated before the propagating impulse can enter the accessory pathway and excite the atria retrogradely, in contrast to the common form of AV node reentry in which the atria are excited just before or during ventricular excitation. While reentry tachycardia involving the other types of accessory pathways (Fig. 9–17) is possible, and has been described electrophysiologically,[1,3,22] such tachycardia appears to be extremely rare and is not distinguished clinically from other mechanisms for PSVT. Orthodromic PSVT involving the atria, AV node, ventricles, and a concealed AV accessory pathway is the mechanism for tachycardia in an estimated 30 percent of patients with PSVT referred for electrophysiologic investigation.[3] The rate of orthodromic PSVT is often faster ($\geq$ 200 beats/min)[3] than that of PSVT due to AV node reentry.

Treatment

The approach to management of orthodromic PSVT is similar to that described earlier for PSVT due to AV node reentry. It is necessary to block conduction of a single impulse from the atria to the ventricles, or vice versa. In general, the most successful approach is to use interventions or drugs to prolong AV nodal conduction time and

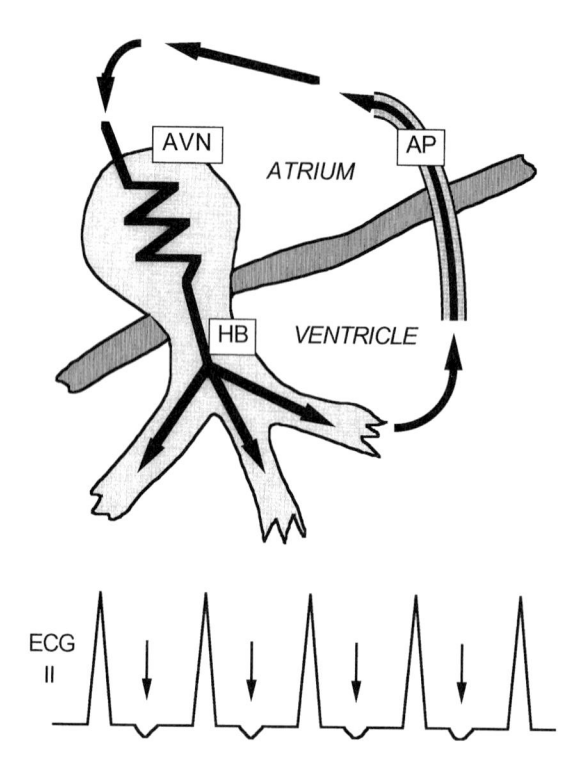

FIGURE 9-18 *Mechanism for orthodromic AV reciprocating (reentry) tachycardia in patients with concealed or manifest accessory AV pathways (AP). Anterograde conduction during tachycardia is over the normal AV pathway, namely the atria → AV node (AVN) → His bundle (HB) → bundle branches and ventricles. The distal AP is excited by the propagating impulse within the ventricles, which travels retrogradely over the AP to excite the atria. This process may perpetuate itself as orthodromic AV reentry tachycardia, the appearance of which in ECG lead II is depicted below. Note that the inverted P waves from retrograde atrial activation follow the QRS complex, in contrast to the common variety of AV node reentry PSVT (Fig. 9-15). Orthodromic AV reentry PSVT might be difficult to distinguish with surface ECG recordings from the uncommon form of AV node reentry PSVT (Fig. 9-16), except that inverted P waves may be more delayed (shorter PR interval) with the latter.*

refractoriness (adenosine, or drugs in Tables 9–3 and 9–5) as opposed to those that prolong accessory pathway conduction or refractoriness (procainamide). As with PSVT due to AV node reentry, with imminent hemodynamic collapse or myocardial ischemia, consideration should be given to immediate DC cardioversion. Also, following termination of tachycardia, there may be a period of sinus arrest or severe bradycardia due to suppression of sinus node automaticity during PSVT. Temporary pacing may be required, and we and others have used transesophageal atrial pacing for this purpose in anesthetized or sedated patients.

Atrial Flutter–Fibrillation

Persons with orthodromic PSVT and concealed accessory pathways are as prone as other people to develop atrial flutter–fibrillation. However, because the accessory pathway does not conduct anterogradely, it should not pose a problem with atrial flutter–fibrillation. In contrast, patients with manifest accessory pathways are at increased risk of extremely rapid ventricular rates during atrial flutter–fibrillation. With concealed pathways, AV conduction is over the AV node during atrial flutter–fibrillation, and the ventricular rate response is limited by prolonged anterograde refractoriness of the AV node compared to that of the accessory pathway. Therefore, drugs such as diltiazem, verapamil, and digoxin are not contraindicated in patients with concealed accessory AV pathways and atrial flutter–fibrillation. However, in some circumstances, such as with catecholamine stimulation, anterograde conduction in the apparently concealed accessory pathway can occur.[3]

SINUS NODE AND ATRIAL REENTRY PAROXYSMAL SUPRAVENTRICULAR TACHYCARDIA

Paroxysmal supraventricular tachycardia in 10 to 15 percent of cases may be due to sinus node (also, SA) or atrial reentry.[1,3] The onset of tachycardia is abrupt, the rate (typically 120 to 150 beats/min; range 90 to 200 beats/min) is usually slower than that of other PSVT, and the PR interval is a function of the tachycardia rate. The abrupt onset and termination of these tachycardias distinguishes them from sinus tachycardia or uniform automatic atrial tachycardia. Often, PSVT due to sinus node or atrial reentry appears as short bursts of regular PSVT. P waves with sinus node reentry are similar to those of normal sinus rhythm, while those of atrial reentry are different (Fig. 9–19). With sinus node or atrial reentry PSVT, in contrast to AV node reentry PSVT,

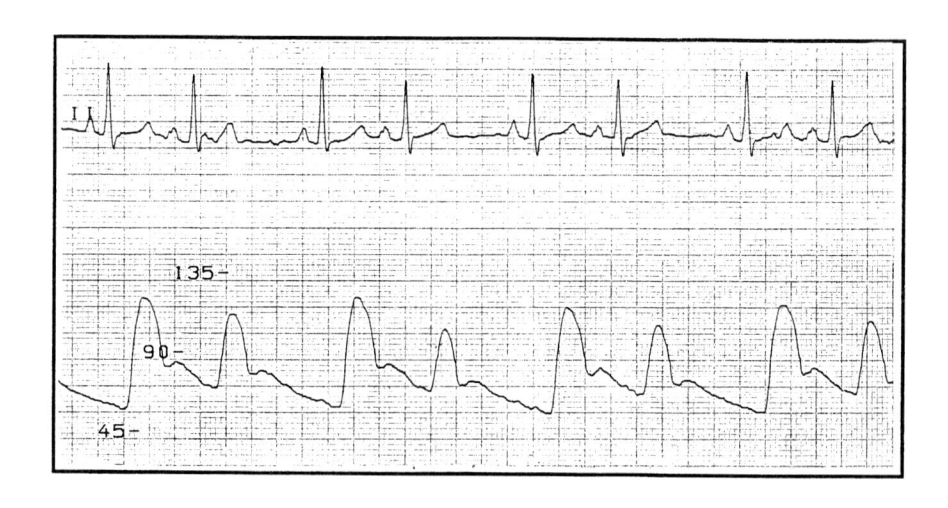

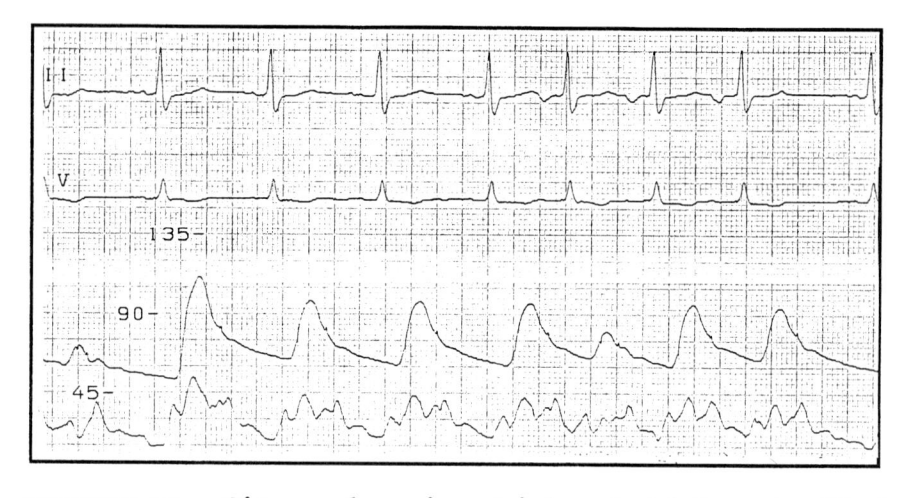

FIGURE 9-19 *Sinus node or sino-atrial, and atrial reentry. (Top) Atrial extrasystoles in a bigeminal pattern that are likely due to sinus node or SA reentry. SA block (3:2) is not likely because the longer P-P interval is not a multiple of that between bigeminal beats. Neither is sinus pause or arrest likely because ectopic and basic intervals recur on a regular basis. PSVT due to sinus node reentry could be initiated by one of these extrasystoles, and P waves of tachycardia would have a similar appearance to those of the extrasystoles. (Bottom) The basic rhythm (beats 1 to 4) is ectopic atrial rhythm at a rate of 71 beats/min. The fifth beat is premature, with a mainly negative P wave in lead II. This is followed by two more "premature" beats with similar P waves. The average rate of premature beats is 92 beats/min. A plausible explanation for the premature atrial beats is atrial reentry.*

AV block can occur without interrupting tachycardia. Treatment for PSVT due to sinus node or atrial reentry is the same as for that due to AV node reentry or orthodromic AV reentry with a concealed accessory pathway.

Atrioventricular Junctional Rhythm Disturbances

Secondary pacemakers found in the AV junctional tissues can assume control of the ventricles for one or more beats through *default* or *usurpation*. With default, the rate of the sinus node slows sufficiently to allow emergence of junctional pacemakers. With usurpation, the rate of junctional pacemaker discharge increases sufficiently to assume control of the ventricles from the sinus node. The mechanism for AV junctional rhythm disturbances could be altered normal or abnormal automaticity, or triggered activity. The term *AV nodal* rhythm is no longer used, since these rhythms most likely originate outside the AV node proper.

JUNCTIONAL PREMATURE AND ESCAPE BEATS

Recognition

Atrioventricular junctional *escape beats* occur with default of higher pacemakers (Fig. 5–20). The escape interval is equal to the intrinsic rate of the AV junctional pacemakers (35 to 60 beats/min). The pause between the dominant and escape beats is longer than the normal P-P interval. Junctional escape beats have narrow QRS complexes with absent or retrograde P waves that precede (PR ≤ 0.10 msec) or follow the QRS, along with nonconducted sinus or ectopic atrial P waves. Junctional *premature beats* are recognized by earlier than expected narrow QRS beats, unless there is functional QRS aberration (Fig. 9–20). A retrograde P wave may precede the QRS complex (≤ 0.10 second), be buried in the QRS complex, or occur after the QRS complex.

Management

Junctional escape beats occur with bradycardia due to SND or incomplete AV heart block. They are not treated per se, but the cause for escape is, if the bradycardia is disadvantageous. In perioperative settings, the imbalance causing junctional escape beats is often transient—perhaps vagally mediated or due to drugs. *Junctional*

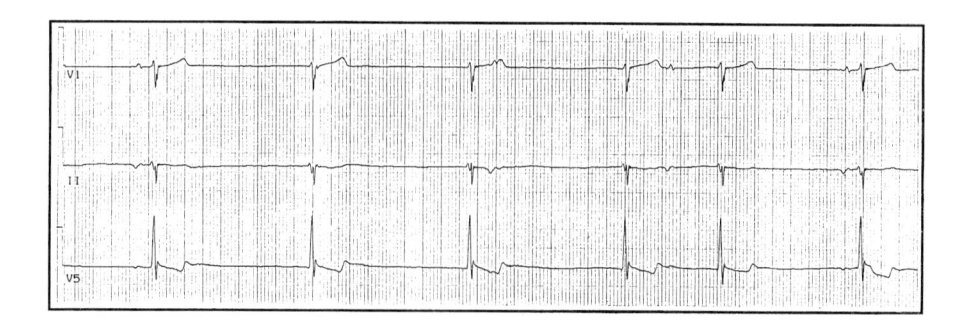

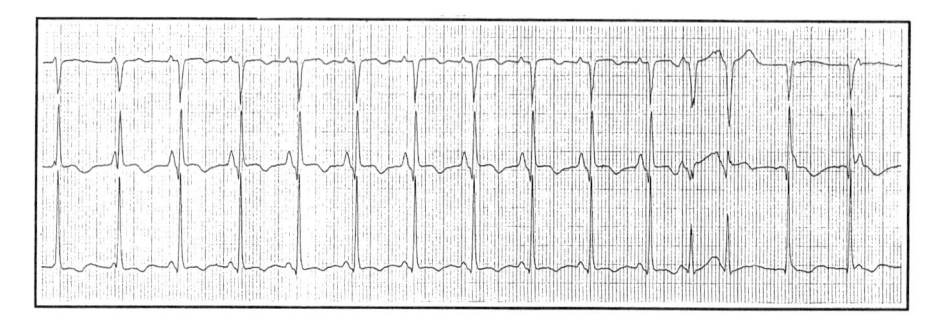

FIGURE 9-20 *AV junctional escape and premature beats.* **(Top)** *Escape beats. The first beat is a conducted sinus beat, followed by three AV junctional escape beats. Note the nonconducted atrial ectopic P wave superimposed on the T wave of the second junctional beat. The P wave following the fourth junctional beat is conducted with delay to cause the fifth QRS complex, and the last beat is a normally conducted atrial ectopic beat.* **(Bottom)** *Premature beats. The first two beats are AV junctional beats with isorhythmic AV dissociation (the P waves march through the QRS complex). The next nine beats are sinus beats, followed by two premature AV junctional beats conducted with ventricular aberration. These, in turn, initiate accelerated AV junctional rhythm with isorhythmic AV dissociation (last two beats).*

premature beats are not treated, unless they trigger worse arrhythmias. Treatment to suppress AV junctional premature beats associated with fast heart rates includes beta-blockers (esmolol) and lidocaine, similar to that for premature ventricular extrasystoles. For junctional premature beats associated with bradycardia, atrial overdrive pacing or chronotropes (Table 9-2) are used for suppression. However, pacing is preferred because of danger of worsening lower pacemaker instability and arrhythmias with chronotropic drugs.

ATRIOVENTRICULAR JUNCTIONAL RHYTHM

Recognition

Atrioventricular junctional rhythm (AVJR) is any sustained, narrow QRS rhythm with retrograde or nonapparent P waves at a rate between 35 and 70 beats/min (Fig. 9-21). AVJR in a patient with left or right bundle branch block and wide QRS complexes would be difficult to distinguish from idioventricular rhythm without intracardiac electrograms. AVJR is quite common during general anesthesia. For example, it was diagnosed in 6.5 percent of a representative population of 200 surgical patients.[19]

Mechanism

Why AVJR should be so common in patients under general anesthesia is not known, but may involve the interplay of several factors: (1) *accentuated antagonism*—effects of increased vagal tone are more pronounced against a background of high sympathetic tone or catecholamines;[25] (2) *anesthetic drugs*—with catecholamines, some potent volatile anesthetic agents do not depress, and may even stimulate AV junctional pacemakers compared to the sinus node or subsidiary atrial pacemakers;[13,14] (3) *vagal constraint*—vagal slowing is less for AV junctional compared to higher atrial pacemakers; (4) *predominant vagal tone*—this is presumably contributory to junctional rhythms during anesthesia in healthy, conditioned young adults; (5) *catecholamines and ischemia*—either may enhance the rate of junctional pacemakers to produce junctional rhythms in patients with ischemic heart disease.[12]

Significance and Management

Junctional rhythms, due to AV dyssynchrony, can produce severe hemodynamic compromise in some patients (Fig. 9-21). Patients at greatest risk appear to be those with noncompliant ventricles, since optimal filling requires effective and synchronized atrial contractions. Treatment is as outlined earlier for AV junctional escape beats. However, given that chronotropic drugs are often unreliable and may produce untoward effects, and AVJR is easily overdriven by atrial pacing (see Chapter 7), temporary atrial or AV sequential pacing is preferred treatment for perioperative AVJR with hemodynamic insufficiency.

ACCELERATED JUNCTIONAL RHYTHM

Recognition

Accelerated AVJR, also called nonparoxysmal AV junctional tachycardia, is recognized by narrow QRS complexes, nonapparent or

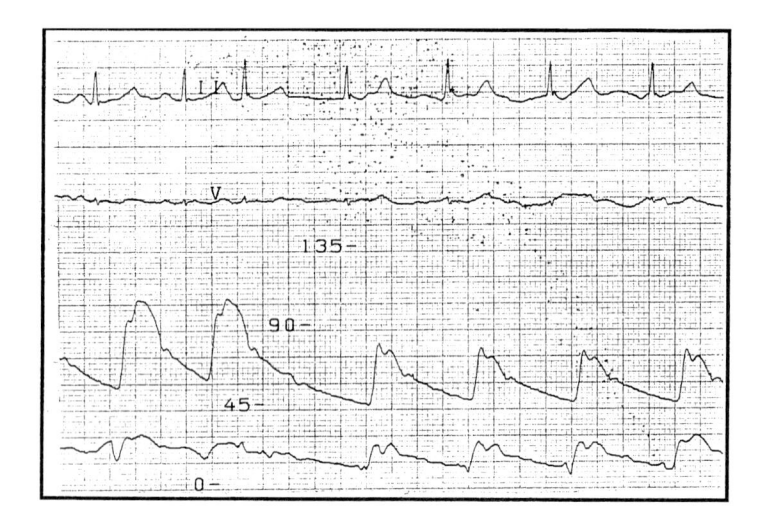

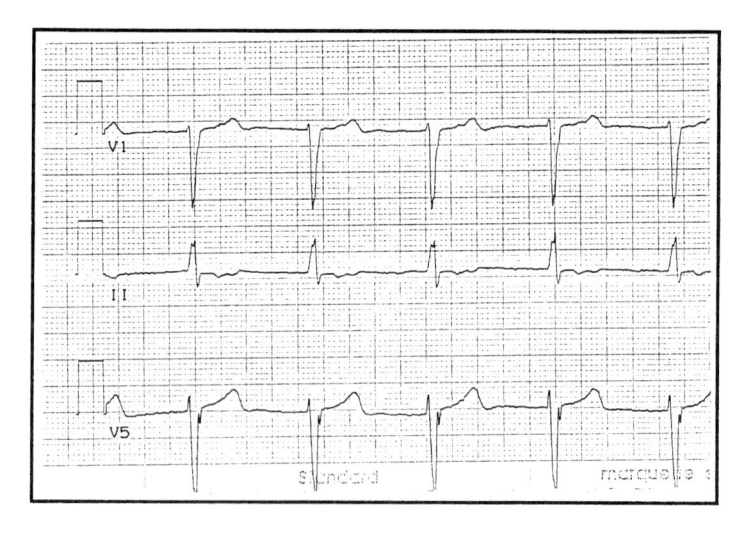

364 RECOGNITION/MANAGEMENT OF SUPRAVENTRICULAR ARRHYTHMIAS

FIGURE 9-21 *AV junctional rhythm (AVJR). (Top) AVJR at 75 beats/min initiated by a junctional premature beat (third beat) after two sinus beats. Note the immediate drop in systolic blood pressure from 103 to 80 mmHg. (Bottom) AVJR at 65 beats/min with retrograde, inverted P waves distorting the ST segment (lead II).*

retrograde P waves, and a rate typically between 70 and 130 beats/min (Fig. 9–22). The rhythm is fairly regular except when an atrial or ventricular pacemaker successfully competes for control of the ventricles (Fig. 9–22). ECG diagnosis can be complicated by the presence of entrance or exit blocks at the AV junction or incomplete AV dissociation. An example of the latter is "isorhythmic AV dissociation," where P waves march through the QRS complex (Fig. 9–23). Depending on the relation of atrial to ventricular systole, there can be beat-to-beat variations in stroke volume and pulse pressure, with stroke volume and pulse pressure greatest when the PR interval is nearly normal. Enhanced vagal tone or edrophonium can slow, while anticholinergics or beta-adrenergic agonists can enhance, the rate of accelerated AVJR.

Mechanism and Associations

Accelerated AVJR has the characteristics of an automatic or triggered as opposed to reentrant rhythm.[1,24,26] *First*, it is nonparoxysmal—namely, its onset and termination is gradual. *Second*, overdrive pacing at rates faster than rhythm can suppress it, but the disturbance returns after pacing if its causes are still present. *Third*, accelerated AV junctional rhythm is not terminated by DC cardioversion. *Fourth*, the rhythm cannot be initiated or terminated by programmed electrical stimulation. Accelerated junctional rhythm occurs most commonly in patients with underlying heart disease, including acute myocardial infarction, following open heart surgery (occurring in valve surgery more often than in coronary bypass grafting),[1] and acute rheumatic myocarditis.

Digitalis Toxicity

Probably the most important cause for accelerated AVJR is digitalis intoxication in association with severe underlying cardiac disease, since the rhythm disturbance does not develop in people with normal hearts following suicidal ingestion.[1] It is important to recognize slowing and regularization of ventricular rhythm due to development of AVJR in a digitalized patient with atrial fibrillation as an early manifestation of digitalis intoxication.[3] AV junctional escape rhythm develops in response to block of fibrillatory atrial impulses within the AV node by digitalis, as well as physiologic refractoriness created by junctional pacemaker discharge. As digitalis administration is continued, the ventricular rate increases, but still remains regular, because of the increased discharge rate of the AV junctional pacemaker. Further digitalis administration may cause accelerated AV junctional

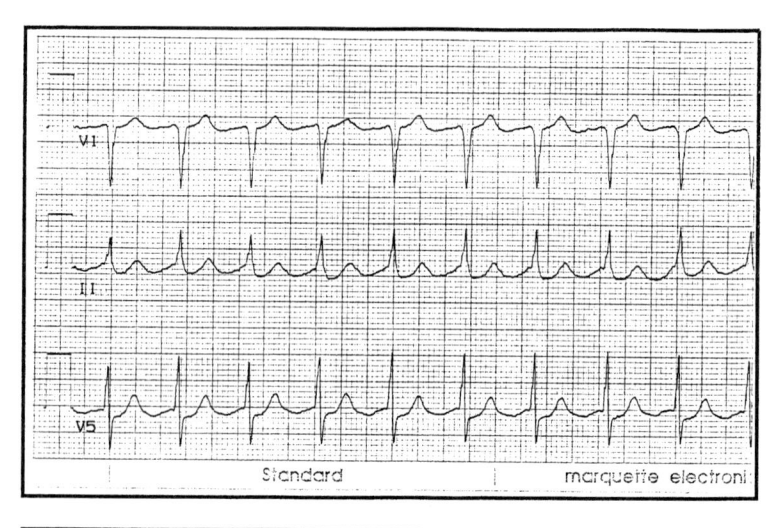

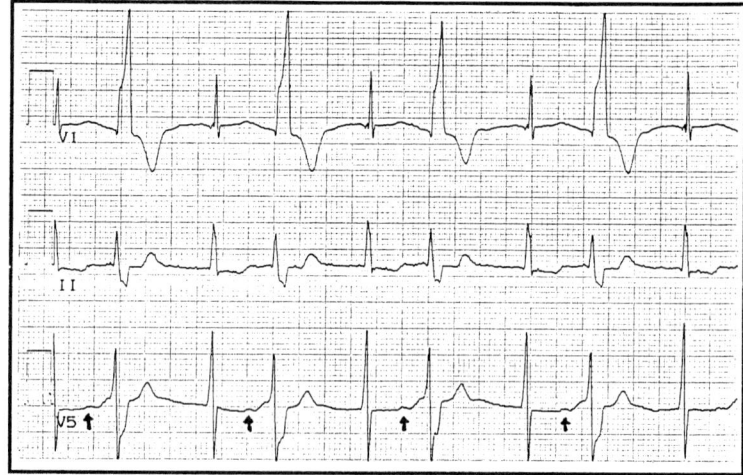

FIGURE 9-22 *Accelerated AVJR.* (Top) Accelerated AVJR at 107 beats/min. The rhythm is regular and there are no apparent P waves in any of the leads shown. (Bottom) Irregular accelerated AVJR due to frequent ventricular or atrial extrasystoles with ventricular aberration occurring in a bigeminal pattern. The presence of P waves in association with aberrant QRS complexes in lead V_5 (arrows) suggests the latter.

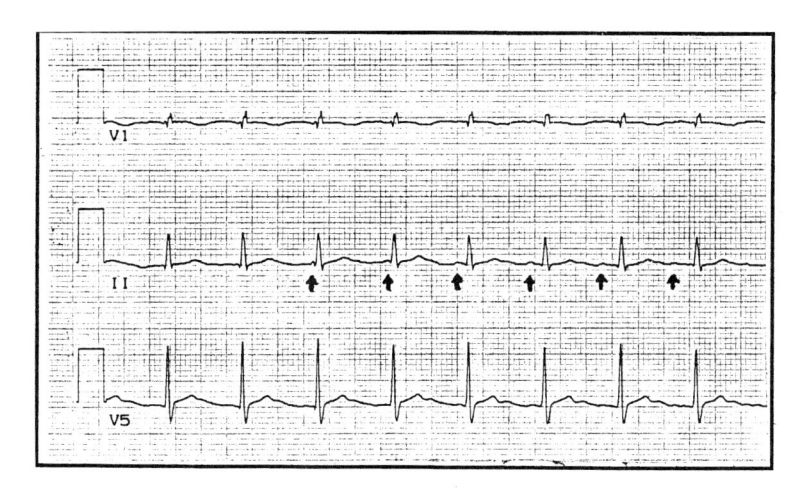

FIGURE 9-23 *Incomplete AV dissociation due to isorhythmic AV dissociation with accelerated AVJR. Note that sinus P waves in lead II (arrows) control the atria and "march" out of the QRS complex as the rhythm progresses. As these assume a more proper relation to the QRS complex, AV dissociation becomes incomplete from a physiologic perspective.*

escape rhythm to become slow and irregular because of varying degrees of AV junctional exit block, with the danger that this may be misdiagnosed as resumption of atrial fibrillation. With advanced intoxication, the ventricular rate increases, with the eventual development of ventricular tachycardia.

Management

If the patient tolerates accelerated AVJR, careful hemodynamic monitoring and supportive or corrective treatment for the underlying heart disease may be all that is required. If digitalis is or could be the cause, it should be withheld. Treatment for accelerated AVJR due to digitalis toxicity includes phenytoin, potassium administration, lidocaine, beta-blockers, and digitalis-specific antibodies. Otherwise, atrial overdrive pacing is preferred to chronotropic drugs for enhancement of sinus rate. The latter often only increase the rate of accelerated AVJR causing further hemodynamic deterioration. The rate of overdrive pacing may gradually cut back, with pacing terminated once hemodynamic stability is restored. Finally, as already noted, DC cardioversion is ineffective for accelerated AVJR.

JUNCTIONAL ECTOPIC TACHYCARDIA

Recognition, Prevalence, and Management

From the electrophysiologic perspective, junctional ectopic tachycardia and automatic ("ectopic") atrial tachycardia are similar.[1] They differ, however, in that AV dissociation is present with junctional ectopic tachycardia and absent in atrial automatic tachycardia. Junctional ectopic tachycardia is an automatic rhythm disturbance, similar to accelerated AVJR, only its rate is much faster (often > 200 beats/min). Junctional ectopic tachycardia is extremely rare in adults, and is the least common type of SVT in infants and children. It may occur in the absence of structural heart disease (congenital form) or following surgery for congenital heart disease. The atria are usually controlled by a sinus mechanism. P waves are present in almost all patients with congenital junctional ectopic tachycardia, but absent or more difficult to detect in those with the disturbance following cardiac surgery. AV dissociation and VA association (due to retrograde conduction) are present, so that PR intervals characteristically vary. QRS complexes have a supraventricular appearance (narrow as opposed to wide). Since junctional ectopic tachycardi ɩ usually occurs in severely ill patients with congestive heart failure and hypotension, primary treatment is directed at providing circulatory support. Specific antiarrhythmic treatment should be undertaken in all patients with congenital junctional ectopic tachycardia.[27] When the rhythm disturbance develops following surgery for congenital heart disease (acquired form), treatment should be instituted as soon as minimal acceleration of the junctional ectopic tachycardia is detected and before cardiogenic shock has developed.

Specific Treatment for Congenital Junctional Ectopic Tachycardia

Antiarrhythmic drugs rarely convert junctional ectopic tachycardia to sinus rhythm, but several of them may decrease the rate to improve hemodynamics. The combination of beta-blockers with digitalis may be particularly effective, with the former to reduce ventricular rate and the latter to improve cardiac function. Amiodarone, which possibly will be available in parenteral form by the time this work appears in print, is also effective for reducing the ventricular rate. Atrial pacing to overdrive the disturbance may temporarily increase cardiac output and improve hemodynamics by restoring AV synchrony, but the disturbance returns following cessation of pacing. DC cardioversion is ineffective against junctional ectopic tachycardia.

Specific Treatment for Acquired Junctional Ectopic Tachycardia

Potassium, calcium, and magnesium should be maintained in the normal to upper-normal range.[1] Exposure to sympathomimetic drugs and phosphodiesterase inhibitors (amrinone, milrinone) should be minimized. Vagotonia should be enhanced by use of opiates, but vagolytic drugs are avoided (e.g., meperidine, barbiturates). Vecuronium is preferred to relaxants that cause histamine release or pancuronium. Digitalis is administered to improve myocardial function, and atrial pacing used to restore AV synchrony. Junctional ectopic tachycardia usually resolves spontaneously within 48 to 72 hours following congenital heart surgery if the patient survives the operation.

Atrial Flutter

Prevalence, Mechanism, and Presentation

Atrial flutter is observed in approximately 1 percent of hospitalized patients.[1] Both clinical and experimental evidence point to reentry in the low right atrium as the mechanism for the disturbance.[1] There are two types of atrial flutter: type I or classical flutter, and type II or fast flutter. Type I flutter can always be interrupted by rapid atrial pacing and is characterized by atrial rates between 220 and 340 beats/min (Fig. 9–24). Type II flutter cannot be interrupted by atrial pacing, and is characterized by atrial rates between 350 and 450 beats/min (Fig. 9–25). Flutter–fibrillation, or "flitter",[3] occurs at a rate faster than pure flutter and with variability in the contour and rate of flutter waves (Fig. 9–25). In some instances, "flitter" may represent dissimilar atrial rhythms, i.e., fibrillation in one atrium and a slower, more regular rhythm resembling atrial flutter in the other atrium.[3] While the atrial rate with type I flutter may be slowed to 180 to 220 beats/min by drugs such as quinidine or amiodarone, the danger is that the ventricles may respond to the slower atrial rate on a one-to-one basis. Also, class 1A drugs such as quinidine increase the speed of AV node conduction by their vagolytic action. Catecholamines and anticholinergics have a similar action, except that the rate of atrial flutter remains unchanged. Drug effects on atrial flutter are illustrated in Figure 9–26.

Causes and Associations

There are no specific causes for atrial flutter, although it commonly develops in patients with chronic obstructive pulmonary

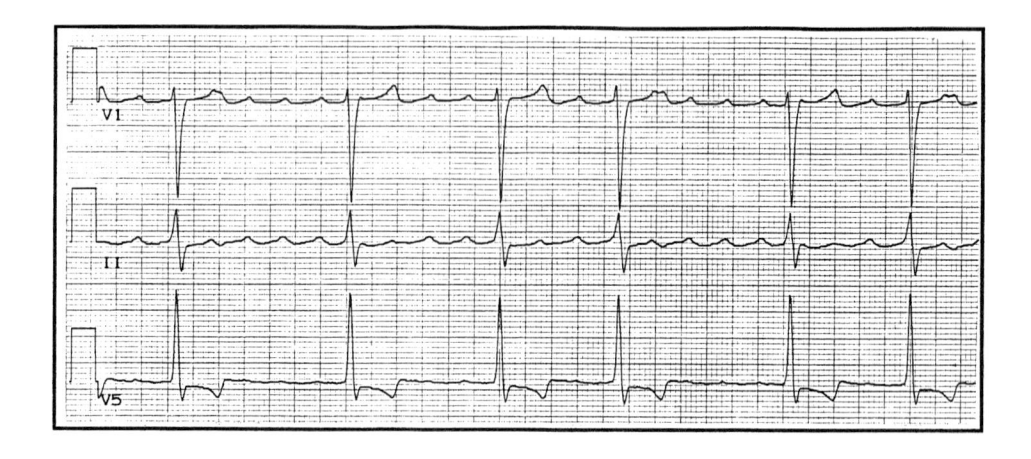

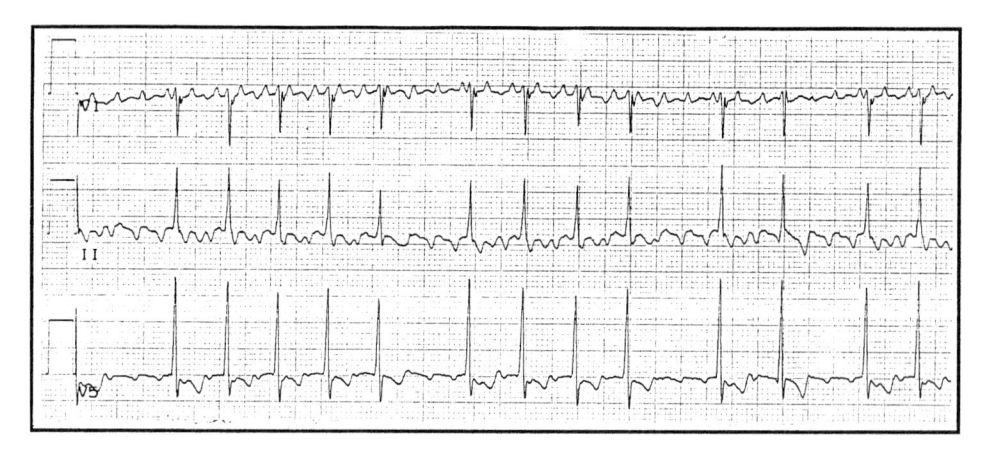

FIGURE 9-24 *Type I atrial flutter. (Top) Slow atrial flutter with variable (5:1, 4:1, 3:1) AV conduction. The atrial and ventricular rates are 214 to 231 and 51 beats/min, respectively. While this could be automatic atrial tachycardia with block, there is no stable isoelectric interval between flutter waves in lead II. (Bottom) Faster atrial flutter with variable (5:1, 4:1, 3:1 and 3:2) AV conduction. The ventricular rate is 127 beats/min.*

disease, AV valvular disease, following cardiac surgery, and with right atrial distension for whatever cause. Other conditions associated with atrial flutter include hyperthyroidism, ethanolism, pericarditis, myocarditis, rheumatic and ischemic heart disease, and dilated cardiomyopathy due to various causes.

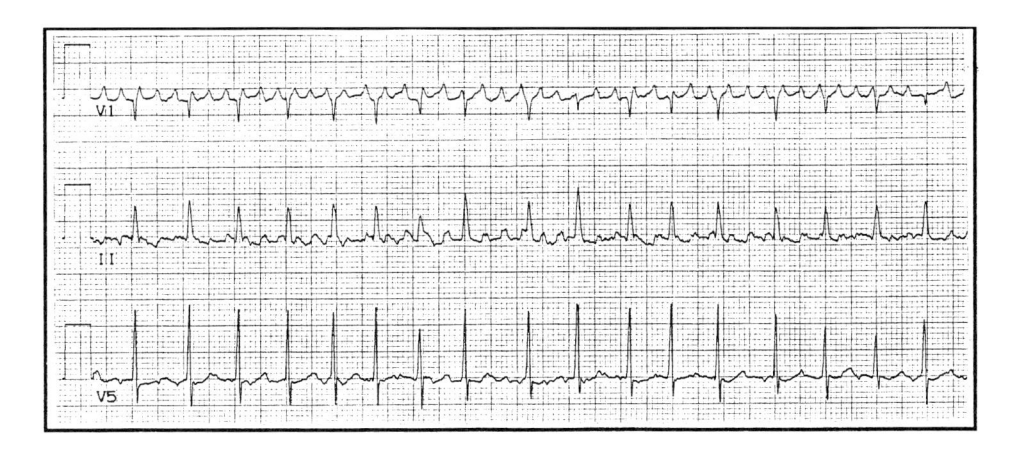

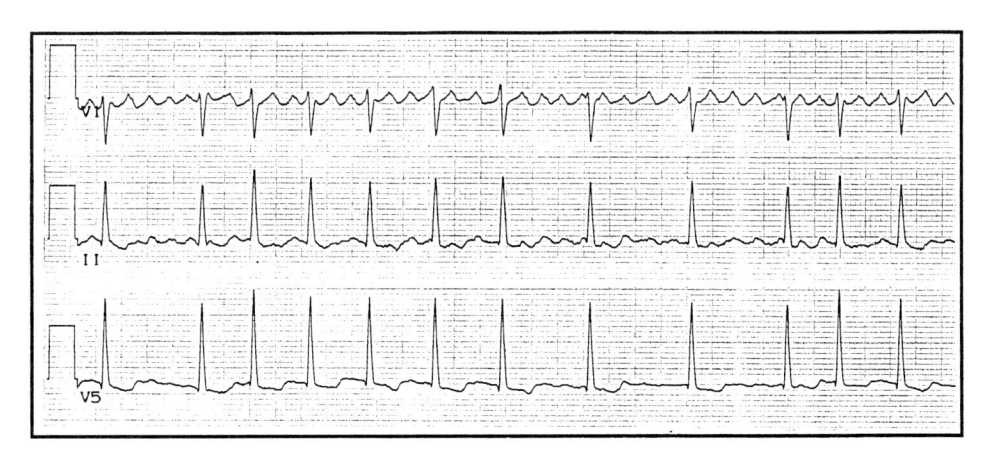

FIGURE 9-25 *Type II atrial flutter and flutter-fibrillation ("flitter").* (Top) Type II atrial flutter with a rapid ventricular response (152 beats/min). AV conduction is variable (3:1, 3:2, 2:1). (Bottom) Atrial flutter-fibrillation. Based on the contour of flitter waves in lead V_1, this would be diagnosed as atrial flutter, except that the F(f)-F(f) intervals vary from 160 to 200 msec, inconsistent with coarse atrial flutter. In lead II, the appearance of atrial activity is more consistent with coarse atrial fibrillation. The ventricular rate is 111 beats/min with variable AV conduction.

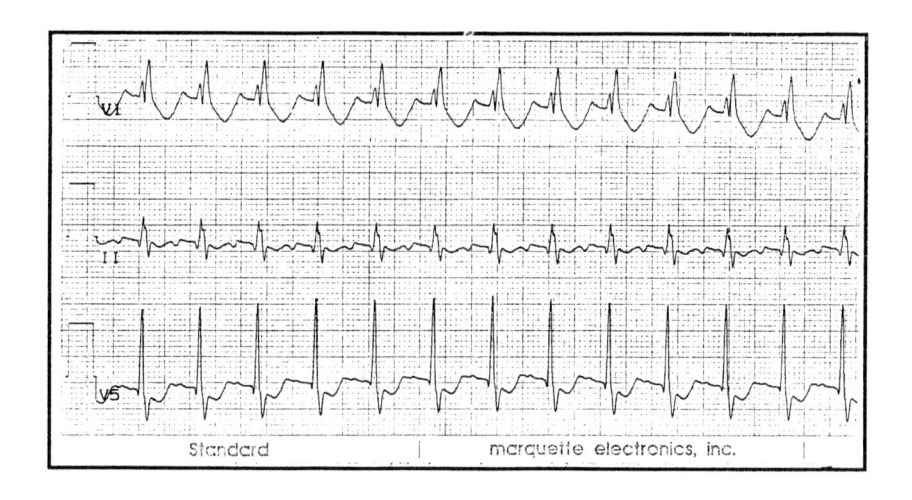

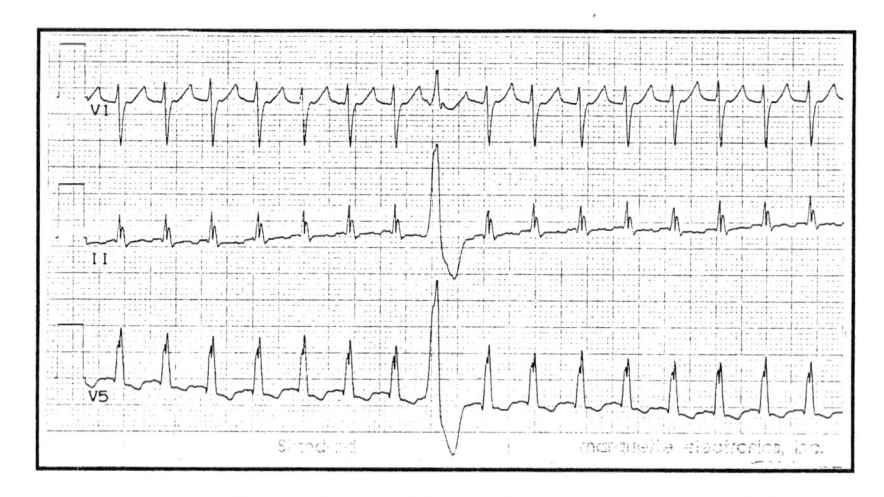

FIGURE 9-26 *Examples of how drugs and catecholamines affect atrial flutter. (Top) After administration of quinidine, the atrial rate is 270 beats/min with 2:1 AV conduction, whereas before it was 300 to 320 beats/min with variable, but slower AV conduction. While quinidine slows the flutter rate, its vagolytic action facilitates AV conduction. If the flutter rate slows further, there is the possibility of 3:2 or 1:1 AV conduction and extremely rapid ventricular rates. (Bottom) Type I atrial flutter (atrial rate 330 beats/min) with 2:1 AV conduction and a ventricular rate of 165 beats/min. While this ECG was recorded in a patient with heart failure and enhanced sympathetic tone, it is also an example of what can occur following atropine to increase slow ventricular rates with atrial flutter.*

Recognition

Atrial flutter is a paroxysmal disturbance, usually lasting for seconds to hours, but on occasion for days to months or even years. It terminates spontaneously, reverting to sinus rhythm or degenerating into atrial fibrillation (Fig. 9-27). Flutter (F) waves characteristically have a "sawtooth" appearance, and are best seen in the inferior leads (II, III, aVF) and right precordial leads (V_1). There is no isoelectric interval between flutter waves. The ventricular rate is regular with fixed AV conduction (Fig. 9-26), or regularly irregular with variable AV conduction (Figs. 9-24 and 9-25). By "regularly irregular" is meant recurring patterns of R-R intervals due to varying AV conduction.

Differential Diagnosis

Unless atrial flutter has produced life-threatening hemodynamic compromise or myocardial ischemia due to extremely fast atrial rates, it should be differentiated from other causes for regular or regularly irregular SVT before beginning treatment. Atrial fibrillation will be easily recognized by the totally irregular ventricular response ("irregularly irregular") and the absence of any organized atrial activity in the ECG. If flutter waves are not apparent, adenosine vagal maneuvers or edrophonium (5 to 10 mg) may be used to produce transient AV block to unmask flutter waves (Fig. 5-5). Leads that maximize flutter waves (inferior and V_1), and esophageal or invasive atrial leads should be recorded during these interventions.

FIGURE 9-27 *Degeneration of atrial flutter. Slow atrial flutter (250 beats/min) with variable (4:1, 6:1) AV conduction degenerates into coarse atrial fibrillation. This patient had repeated short paroxysms (≤ 10 seconds) of atrial flutter interspersed with coarse atrial fibrillation (not shown).*

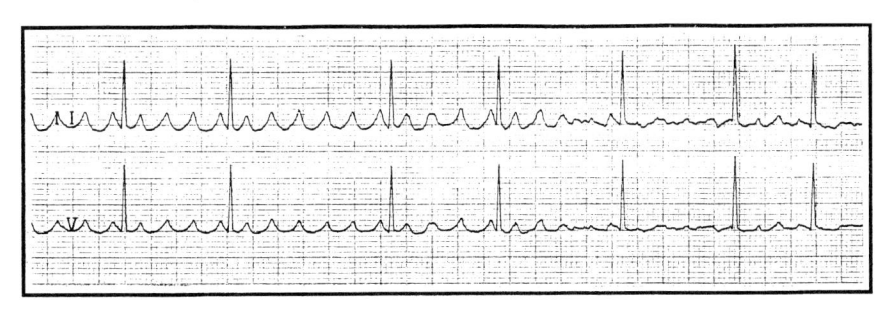

DC Cardioversion or Pacing

DC cardioversion and rapid atrial pacing are preferred to drugs for treatment of atrial flutter, especially with life-threatening circulatory compromise or ischemia. DC cardioversion usually requires relatively low-energy shocks (≤ 50 J). If this fails to convert the disturbance or converts it to atrial fibrillation, higher-energy shocks may be used or the patient may be left in atrial fibrillation. This may revert to atrial flutter or sinus rhythm, or ventricular rate reduction with drugs is easier with atrial fibrillation. If DC cardioversion fails, or the patient is not a candidate for cardioversion (i.e., digitalis has been administered), rapid atrial pacing may be attempted with type I atrial flutter. Pacing is not effective for type II flutter. A method for pacing termination of type I atrial flutter was outlined in Chapter 7.

Drug Treatment

Although DC cardioversion and pacing are preferred methods for treatment of atrial flutter, drugs may be used to slow the ventricular rate, enhance the efficacy of cardioversion or pacing, or reduce the likelihood of recurrences following conversion of atrial flutter. The author has found edrophonium to be reliable and useful for acute ventricular rate reduction with atrial flutter (Fig. 9–28) or atrial fibrillation.[28] In contrast to beta-blockers, which are also effective, edrophonium does not impair myocardial function, a distinct advantage for the patient with life-threatening circulatory compromise or reduced myocardial reserve. Verapamil and diltiazem can also be used for acute ventricular rate reduction, but may cause a paradoxical increase in ventricular rate due to systemic vasodilation and a reflex increase in sympathetic tone. Digitalis has been used in the past for ventricular rate reduction with atrial flutter, but is no longer recommended because edrophonium and esmolol are faster, more reliable, and safer. In fact, digitalis often has to be pushed to the point of toxicity to achieve adequate control of ventricular rate with atrial flutter. Finally, while not usually the responsibility of anesthesia or critical care practitioners, drugs used for suppression of recurrences of atrial flutter include class 1A (quinidine and related) and 1C (flecainide and related) antiarrhythmics, as well as amiodarone and sotalol (class 3 antiarrhythmics). Class 1C drugs are best avoided in patients with ischemic heart disease, since they may increase the risk of lethal ventricular arrhythmias.[29,30]

Time 18:57:31 - Edrophonium administerd

Time 18:59:07 - Maximum edrophonium effect

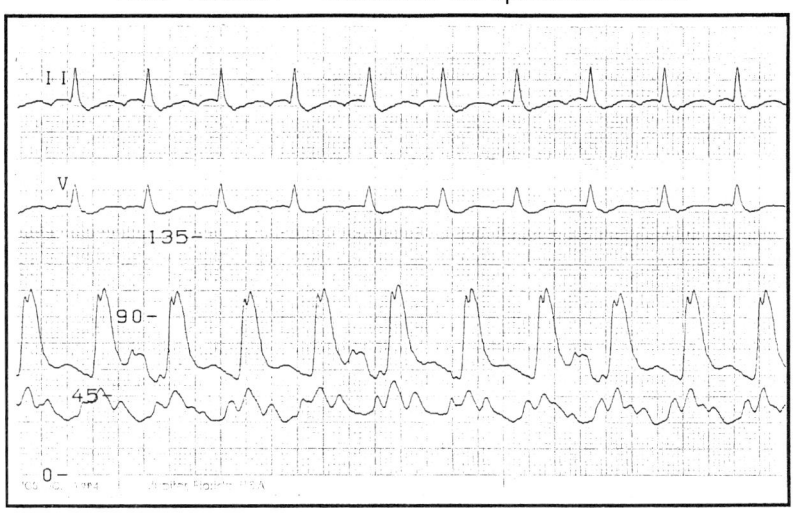

FIGURE 9-28 *Ventricular rate reduction with edrophonium. (Top) The patient probably has slow atrial flutter with mostly 1:1 AV conduction, so that the ventricular rate is between 170 and 200 beats/min, and blood pressure around 80 to 85 mmHg systolic. The bottom tracing is pulmonary artery pressure. (Bottom) Less than 2 minutes after edrophonium (10 mg), the ventricular rate is 105 beats/min with 2:1 AV conduction. Note the hemodynamic improvement following edrophonium.*

Atrial Fibrillation

Prevalence, Mechanism, and Presentation

Atrial fibrillation occurs in about 1 percent of persons older than 60 years of age, and in about 12 percent of hospitalized patients.[1,3] Its prevalence increases with age, so that 5 to 10 percent of people over 75 years of age are affected, aside from underlying condition that increases the likelihood of atrial fibrillation (discussed later).[1] It is rare in infants and young children, possibly because the atria are too small to sustain fibrillation.[1] The mechanism for atrial fibrillation is almost certainly microreentry involving multiple reentry wavelets.[22] Atrial fibrillation presents as a grossly irregular rhythm disturbance, with a ventricular rate between 100 and 200 beats/min (Fig. 9-29), except in patients with impaired AV impulse transmission or ventricular preexcitation (WPW syndrome), in whom ventricular rates may be quite slow (Fig. 9-30) or exceed 300 beats/min, respectively (Fig. 9-31). The cause for ventricular irregularity with atrial fibrillation is still uncertain, but atrial irregularity is certainly an important part of it. Other factors that could affect the ventricular rate with atrial fibrillation include changing AV node refractoriness, fast- and slow-pathway (AV node) dissociation, variation in autonomic tone, discharge of AV junctional pacemakers, retrograde conduction of AV junctional and ventricular beats, and concealed conduction. By concealed conduction is meant that some fibrillatory impulses are blocked within the AV node without reaching the ventricles. However, these same impulses can affect the conduction of subsequent fibrillatory impulses from above. Finally, atrial fibrillation can be intermittent or chronic. Chronic atrial fibrillation increases the risk of cardiovascular morbidity and mortality.

Causes and Associations

Most patients with atrial fibrillation have structural heart disease, including coronary artery disease, valvular and rheumatic heart disease, cardiomyopathy from various causes (e.g., ethanolism, amyloidosis, congestive heart failure, hypertrophic), atrial septal defect, chronic obstructive pulmonary disease, bacterial and viral myocarditis/endocarditis, cardiac tumors, and hypertension, or are recovering from cardiothoracic surgery.[1,3] Occult or manifest hyperthyroidism should be considered in patients with recent-onset atrial fibrillation. Patients without obvious heart disease are said to have "lone" or idiopathic atrial fibrillation.

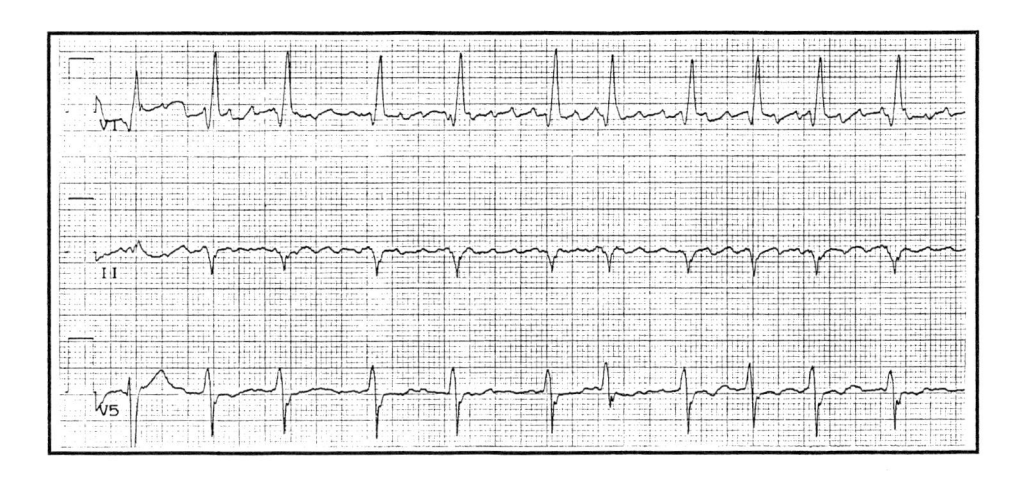

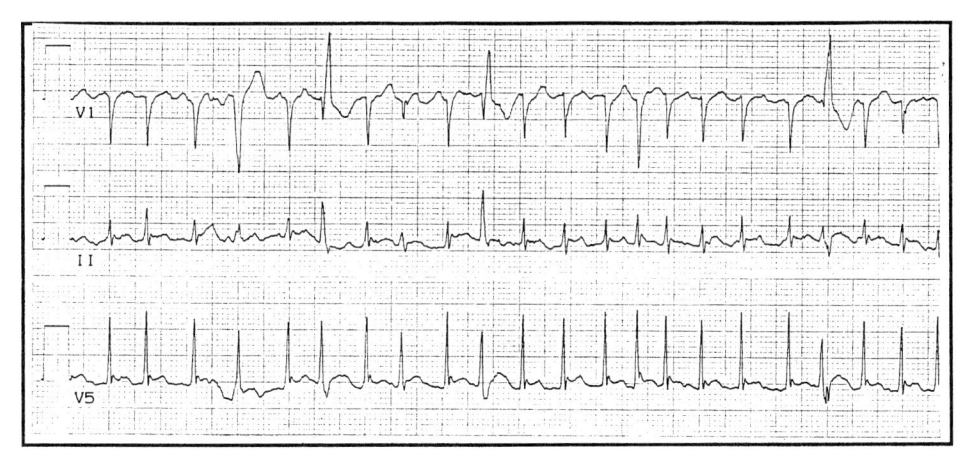

FIGURE 9-29   *Range of usual rates ventricular rates with atrial fibrillation.* (Top) *Coarse atrial fibrillation (some beats in V_1 consistent with "atrial flitter") with ventricular rate of 100 beats/min.* (Bottom) *Atrial fibrillation with ventricular rate of 195 beats/min. The patient was not known to have ventricular preexcitation, and the bizarre QRS beats (especially in lead V_1) are probably due to aberrant ventricular conduction (right bundle branch block pattern) as opposed to being ventricular extrasystoles.*

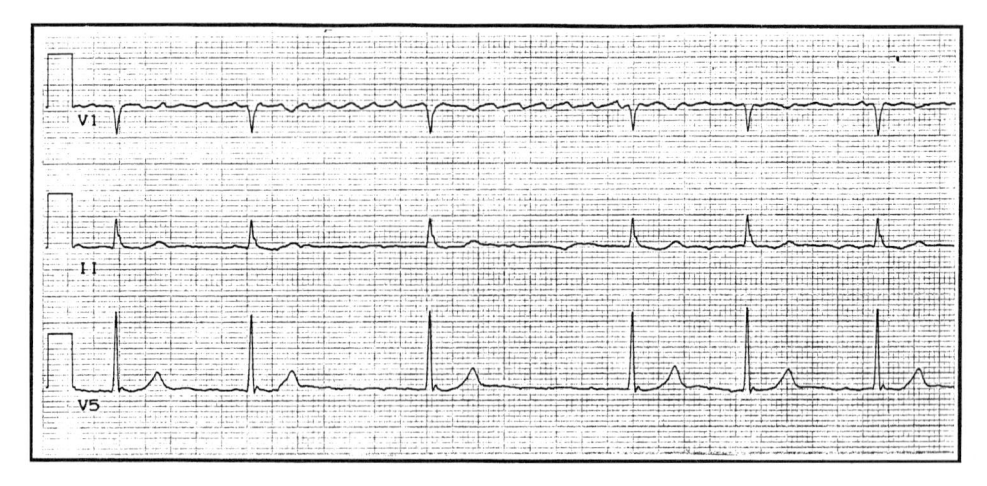

FIGURE 9-30 *Atrial fibrillation with a very slow ventricular response (53 beats/min). With circulatory insufficiency, this patient should be treated initially with temporary ventricular pacing.*

Electrocardiographic Recognition

The average ventricular rate in patients with atrial fibrillation decreases with age. Faster ventricular rates (≥ 160 beats/min) are likely with paroxysmal atrial fibrillation, but the rate of paroxysmal fibrillation spontaneously decreases as the rhythm continues.[1] Slower rates are characteristic of idiopathic atrial fibrillation, and in patients with impaired AV node conduction, whether due to drugs or disease. There are no P waves between T waves and QRS complexes, and the R–R intervals are grossly irregular. The fibrillating atria produce an undulating ECG baseline, with the amplitude, timing, and form of fibrillatory (f) waves constantly varying. These f waves may be barely discernible ("fine") or almost like flutter waves ("coarse"), and are usually best seen in lead II or the right precordial leads (Fig. 9–32). The coarseness of f waves tends to decrease with increased atrial size and duration of fibrillation, and patients with large f waves and a relatively small left atrium are more easily converted to sinus rhythm.[1] Other than f waves, the most characteristic ECG feature of atrial fibrillation is the irregularity of the QRS complexes (i.e., "irregularly irregular"). Namely, there is no recurring cycle length between successive QRS complexes.

RECOGNITION/MANAGEMENT OF SUPRAVENTRICULAR ARRHYTHMIAS 379

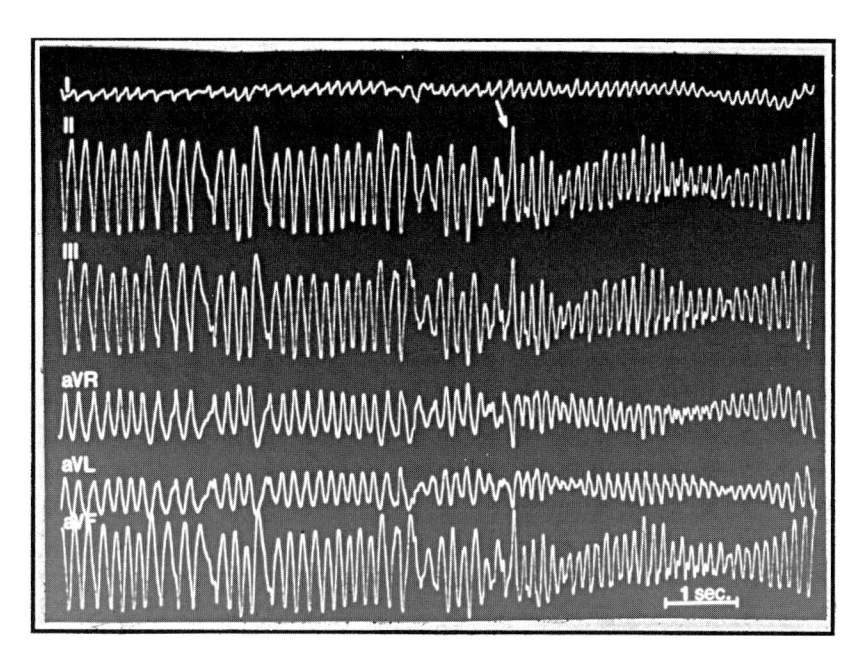

FIGURE 9-31   *Atrial fibrillation with an extremely fast ventricular response (180 to 360 beats/min) in a patient with a history of tachyarrhythmias and ventricular preexcitation (WPW syndrome). Atrial fibrillation soon degenerates into torsades de pointes VT or coarse VF* (arrow). *(Illustration kindly furnished by Dr. Fred Morardy, Director, Clinical Electrophysiology Laboratory, University of Michigan Medical Center, Ann Arbor, MI.)*

QRS Aberration

While the QRS complexes with atrial fibrillation are usually narrow (i.e., a supraventricular appearance), there may be beat-by-beat loss of conduction or coexisting conduction defects (i.e., bundle branch or fascicular blocks) that produce ventricular aberration. It is important to recognize ventricular aberration with fast atrial fibrillation to avoid misdiagnosis and mistreatment as ventricular tachycardia (Fig. 9-33). This problem is a common one, since anomalous beats can be found in approximately 60 percent of ECG's from patients with atrial fibrillation.[1] Causes and manifestations of QRS aberration were discussed in Chapter 4. Recall that usually (80 to 85 percent of cases) aberration has a right bundle branch block pattern due to longer refractoriness of the right bundle branch.[31] However, in patients with significant heart disease, left bundle branch block pattern aberration

(Coarse fibrillation)

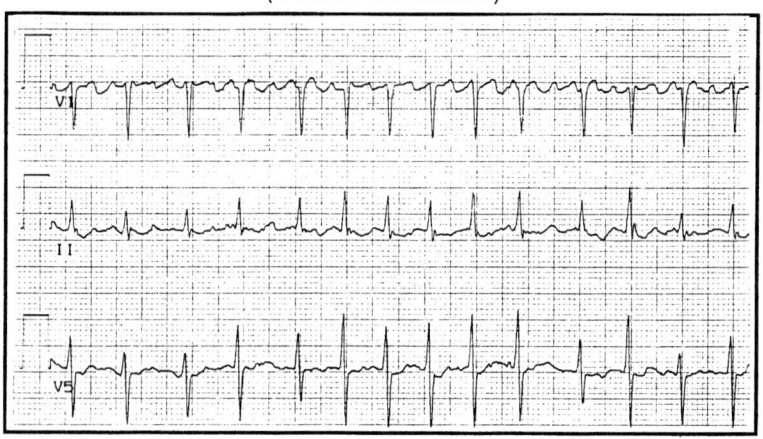

(Fine fibrillation)

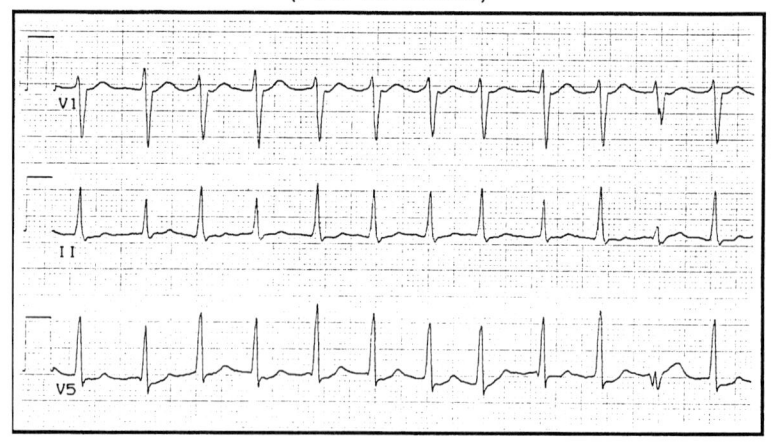

FIGURE 9-32 *Appearance of fibrillatory (f) waves with atrial fibrillation. (Top) "Coarse" atrial fibrillation. The f waves are easily recognized in all leads shown. (Bottom) Fine atrial fibrillation. In no lead shown are f waves unequivocally apparent. Nevertheless, the diagnosis of atrial fibrillation is fairly certain since there is beat-to-beat cycle length variation (400 to 520 msec) and most QRS complexes are normal, except that the second to last beat is conducted with ventricular aberration.*

(RBBB pattern aberration)

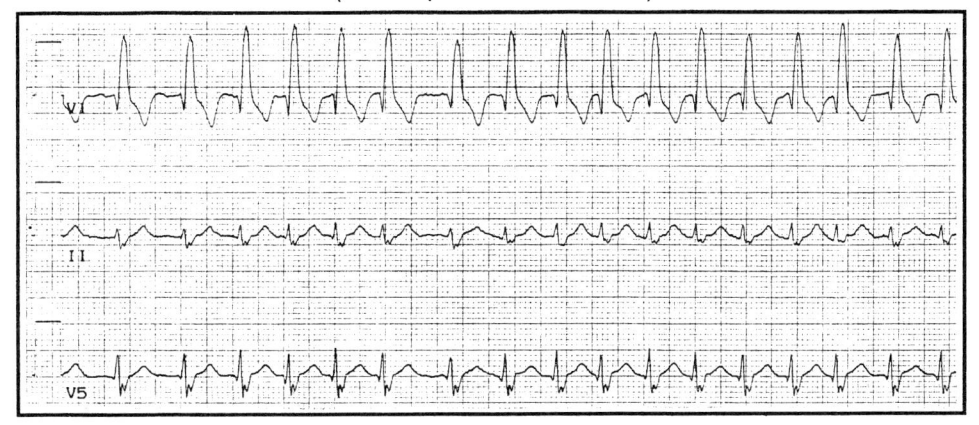

(LBBB pattern aberration)

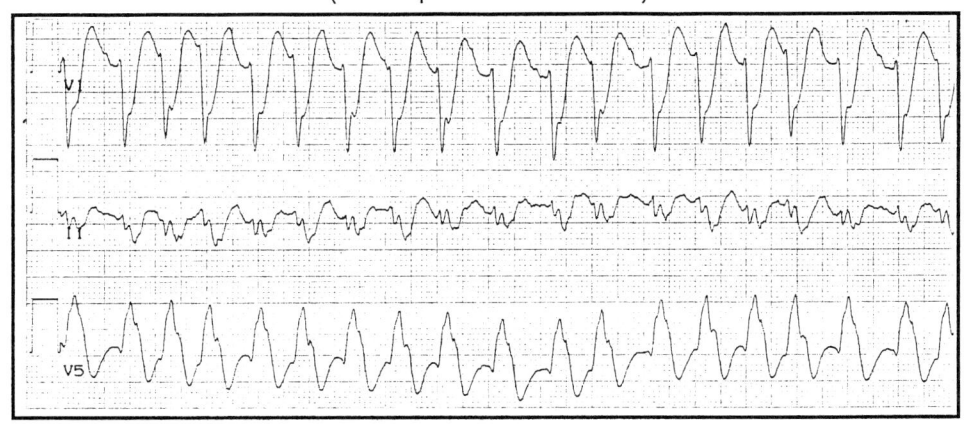

FIGURE 9-33 *Atrial fibrillation and anomalous tachycardia. Differentiation from VT.* (Top) *Atrial fibrillation with ventricular beats (rate 141 beats/min) conducted with right bundle branch block (RBBB) pattern ventricular aberration. The patient was known to have RBBB prior to developing atrial fibrillation. However, an important clue to the diagnosis of atrial fibrillation with ventricular aberration, in the absence of knowing that the patient had RBBB, is the irregularity of R-R intervals. Also, fine fibrillatory waves are recognized in leads V_1 and II between slower beats of tachycardia.* (Bottom) *Atrial fibrillation with ventricular beats (rate 152 beats/min) conducted with left bundle branch block (LBBB) pattern ventricular aberration. The patient was known to have LBBB prior to developing atrial fibrillation. Again, the irregularity of R-R intervals is an important clue to the diagnosis of atrial fibrillation in the absence of other patient history, and fine fibrillatory waves are seen in lead II. With both examples of wide QRS tachycardia, it would be highly unusual for monomorphic VT to show such R-R interval irregularity.*

assumes greater importance, accounting for up to one-third aberration in coronary care units.[31]

Differential Diagnosis

As for the differential diagnosis of ventricular aberration from ventricular ectopy with atrial fibrillation, much can be learned from close inspection of lead V_1 or MCL1 (see Chapter 4).[1] *First*, beats conducted with right bundle branch block pattern aberration tend to be triphasic, whereas ventricular ectopic beats are usually monophasic or biphasic (Fig. 9–34). *Second*, if the initial (0.02 second) QRS vector of anomalous beats is the same as that of normal beats, this strongly favors aberration as opposed to ectopy (Fig. 9–35). *Third*, aberrancy is more likely when one observes a progressive increase in the abnormality of the QRS complexes as the ventricular rate increases (Fig. 9–35).

Hemodynamics

Stroke volume and cardiac output are reduced in patients with atrial fibrillation because effective atrial contraction has been lost.[1] Also, atrial irregularity[32] and diastolic encroachment with fast ventricular rates contribute to beat-to-beat variation in stroke volume and cardiac output reduction. Right- and left-sided filling pressures, and systemic and pulmonary vascular resistance, decrease with restoration of sinus rhythm.

Cardiogenic Embolism

In addition to hemodynamic alterations, the risk of systemic embolization from the left atrial cavity or appendage is an important consideration in patients with atrial fibrillation.[1,3] Nonvalvular atrial fibrillation is the most common cardiac disease associated with cerebral embolism. Approximately 45 percent of cardiogenic emboli in the United States occur in patients with nonvalvular atrial fibrillation. The remainder occur with acute myocardial infarction (15 percent), chronic left ventricular dysfunction (10 percent), rheumatic heart disease (10 percent), prosthetic heart valves (10 percent), and other conditions such as bacterial endocarditis.[3] The risk of stroke in patients with nonvalvular atrial fibrillation is 5 to 7 times greater than in patients without atrial fibrillation, and about 15 percent of ischemic strokes are due to cardiogenic emboli. Patients with structural heart disease appear at greater risk of cardiogenic embolism than those with idiopathic atrial fibrillation. The risk of embolism following conversion to sinus rhythm varies from 0 to 7 percent, depending on associated

RECOGNITION/MANAGEMENT OF SUPRAVENTRICULAR ARRHYTHMIAS **383**

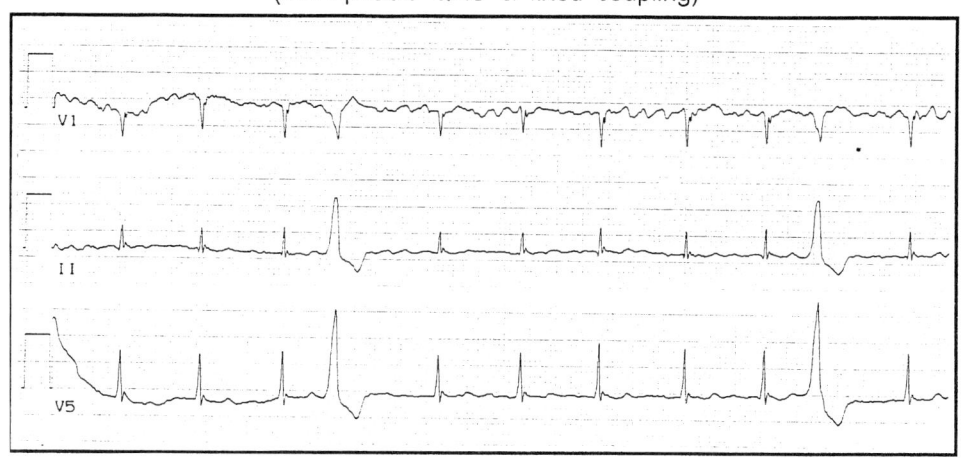

FIGURE 9-34 *Atrial fibrillation and anomalous beats. Differentiation from VES. (Top) Two anomalous beats interrupt atrial fibrillation with normal QRS complexes. These are conducted with right bundle branch block pattern aberration in lead V_1, and probably are due to deceleration-dependent aberrancy (see Chapter 4). (Bottom) Two anomalous beats again interrupt atrial fibrillation with normal QRS complexes. This time, however, the anomalous beats have a monophasic QRS complex and show fixed coupling to beats with normal QRS complexes. Also favoring VES is the uniform appearance of QRS complexes with anomalous beats.*

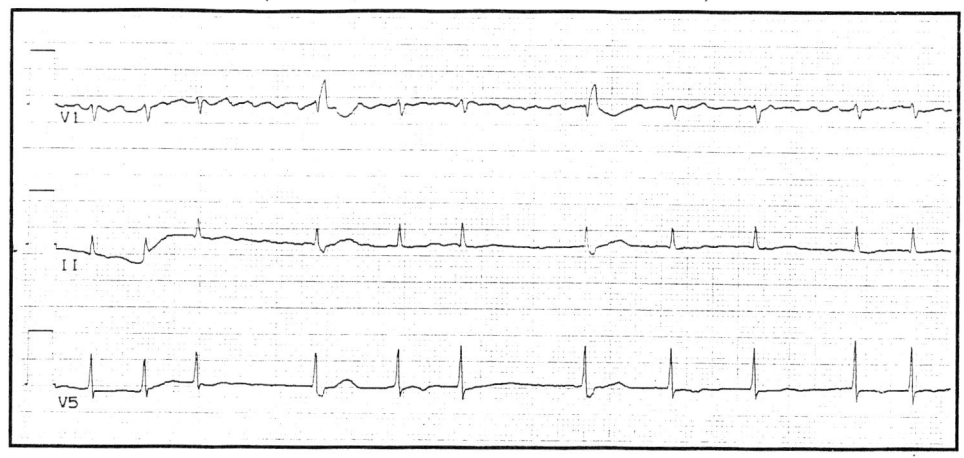

(Initial QRS Deflection)

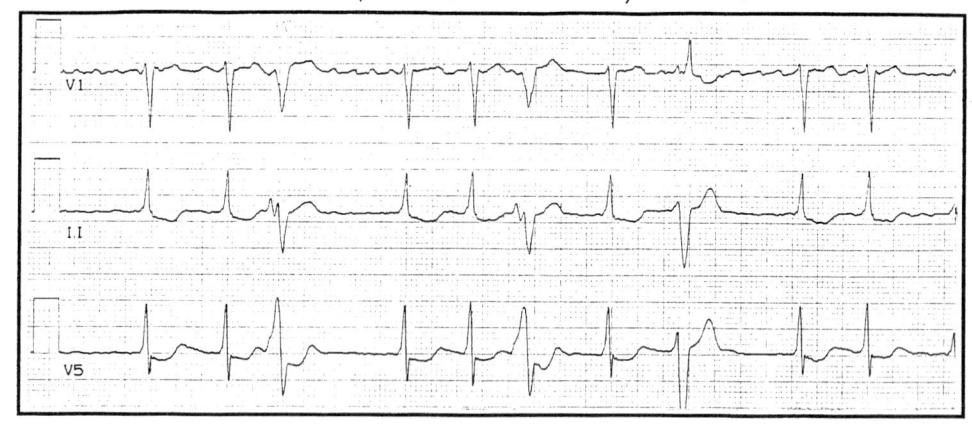

(Increased aberration with increased heart rate)

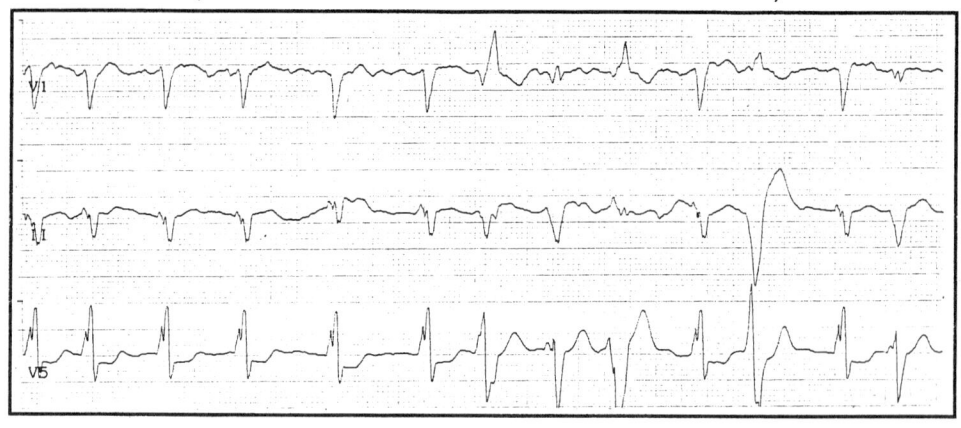

FIGURE 9-35 *Atrial fibrillation and anomalous beats. Differentiation from VES.* (Top) Atrial fibrillation with frequent anomalous beats. Note that the initial QRS deflection of anomalous beats has the same direction as normal beats, presumptive evidence for QRS aberration as opposed to VES. Also, there is variation in QRS aberration with anomalous beats, as well as in coupling intervals between normal and anomalous beats. (Bottom) The ventricular rate with atrial fibrillation suddenly increases after the sixth QRS complex, along with increasing QRS aberration with the three following beats. Anomalous beats are more likely due to ventricular aberration when there is an increase in the abnormality of QRS complexes when the ventricular rate increases. This is caused by functional (rate-dependent) QRS aberration.

risk factors.[3] Patients at highest risk are those with prior embolism, prosthetic valves, and mitral stenosis. Patients less than 60 years or with idiopathic atrial fibrillation are at lowest risk.

Anticoagulation

Patients at high risk of cardiogenic embolism or with known mural thrombi (by echocardiography) should receive anticoagulation, regardless of whether they will undergo elective cardioversion.[1,3] The American College of Chest Physicians has recommended that patients with atrial fibrillation longer than three days should receive warfarin to increase prothrombin time to 1.3 to 1.5 times normal for 3 weeks before elective cardioversion, and for 2 to 4 weeks afterward. Anticoagulation with heparin may be used in patients at high risk of embolization before emergency cardioversion. Long-term aspirin or warfarin is recommended for all patients with chronic atrial fibrillation and nonvalvular heart disease, with warfarin preferred for those at high risk for embolism or older than 75 years.[3]

Pacing and DC Cardioversion

Atrial pacing is *not* effective in patients with atrial fibrillation. Ventricular pacing may be required for patients with symptomatic bradycardia. Prophylactic dual-chamber pacing (DDD, DDI) is used to reduce episodes of paroxysmal atrial fibrillation in patients with the brady–tachy syndrome and SND. Cardioversion is the safest and most effective method for converting chronic atrial fibrillation to sinus rhythm (85 to 90 percent of cases),[1,3] and is at least twice as effective as quinidine for this purpose. Since the atria are often abnormal in patients with chronic atrial fibrillation (e.g., fibrosis; fibrous degeneration of the sinus node and perinodal tissues; chamber enlargement), maintenance of sinus rhythm following cardioversion is not guaranteed. Sinus rhythm remains for 1 year in only 30 to 50 percent of patients.[3] Patients with atrial fibrillation less than 12 months duration have a greater chance of remaining in sinus rhythm. Most patients can be converted (external paddles) with 100 to 200 J, and many with 50 J or less. If more current is required, patients are unlikely to remain in sinus rhythm for very long. While it is conventional practice to begin with 200 J, this also significantly increases the likelihood of postconversion arrhythmias.[1] Postconversion arrhythmias include atrial and ventricular extrasystoles, junctional and accelerated junctional rhythms, automatic and reentrant SVT, and ventricular tachyarrhythmias.[1] If the practitioner is particularly concerned about the possibility of inducing arrhythmias, initial shocks should be 25 to 50 J.

Drug Treatment

Drugs are no longer used to convert atrial fibrillation to sinus rhythm, but may be prescribed to help prevent recurrences following DC cardioversion. Class 1A, 1C, and III (amiodarone and sotalol) drugs are used, but no one drug, with the possible exception of amiodarone, appears superior for this purpose.[1,3] Anesthesia and critical care practitioners, however, are usually more concerned with drugs for acute ventricular rate reduction with atrial fibrillation than with drugs to help restore or maintain sinus rhythm following DC cardioversion. Beta-adrenergic (Table 9-3) and calcium-channel blockers (Table 9-5) are useful for this purpose, with esmolol usually preferred because of its prompt onset of action. Esmolol and other beta-blockers, in fact, may convert some patients with paroxysmal atrial fibrillation to sinus rhythm. Edrophonium is also useful for acute ventricular rate reduction in surgical settings, and has the added advantage that it has no adverse effects on circulatory dynamics in patients with impaired myocardial function.

References

1. Kastor J. Arrhythmias. Philadelphia: WB Saunders, 1994.
2. Waugh R, Ramo B, Wagner G, Gilbert M (eds). Cardiac Arrhythmias. 2nd ed. Philadelphia: FA Davis, 1994.
3. Zipes D. Specific arrhythmias: Diagnosis and treatment. In Braunwald E (ed): Heart Disease. 4th ed. Philadelphia: WB Saunders, 1992: pp. 667-725.
4. Atlee J. Anaesthesia and cardiac electrophysiology. Eur J Anaesth 1985;2:215-256.
5. Atlee J, Brownlee S, Burstrom R. Conscious-state comparison of the effects of inhalation anesthetics on specialized atrioventricular conduction times in dogs. Anesthesiology 1986;64:703-710.
6. Atlee J, Hamann S, Brownlee S, Kreigh C. Conscious state comparisons of the effects of the inhalation anesthetics and diltiazem, nifedipine, or verapamil on specialized atrioventricular conduction times in spontaneously beating dog hearts. Anesthesiology 1988; 68:519-528.
7. Atlee J, Yeager T. Electrophysiologic assessment of the effects of enflurane, halothane, and isoflurane on properties affecting supraventricular re-entry in chronically instrumented dogs. Anesthesiology 1989;71:941-952.
8. Atlee J, Bosnjak Z, Yeager T. Effects of diltiazem, verapamil, and inhalation anesthetics on electrophysiologic properties affecting

reentrant supraventricular tachycardia in chronically instrumented dogs. Anesthesiology 1990;72:889–901.
9. Laszlo A, Polic S, Atlee J, et al. Anesthetics and automaticity in latent pacemaker fibers: I. Effects of halothane, enflurane, and isoflurane on automaticity and recovery of automaticity from overdrive suppression in Purkinje fibers derived from canine hearts. Anesthesiology 1991;75:98–105.
10. Polic S, Atlee J, Laszlo A, et al. Anesthetics and automaticity in latent pacemaker fibers. II. Effects of halothane and epinephrine or norepinephrine on automaticity of dominant and subsidiary atrial pacemakers in the canine heart. Anesthesiology 1991;75:298–304.
11. Polic S, Atlee J, Laszlo A, et al. Anesthetics and automaticity in latent pacemaker fibers. III. Effects of halothane and ouabain on automaticity of the SA node and subsidiary atrial pacemakers in the canine heart. Anesthesiology 1991;75:305–312.
12. Laszlo A, Polic S, Kampine JP, et al. Halothane, enflurane and isoflurane on abnormal automaticity and triggered rhythmic activity of Purkinje fibers from 24-hour-old infarcted canine hearts. Anesthesiology 1991;75:847–853.
13. Woehlck H, Vicenzi M, Bosnjak Z, Atlee J. Anesthetics and automaticity of dominant and latent pacemakers in chronically instrumented dogs. I: Methodology, conscious state and effects of halothane during exposure to epinephrine with and without muscarinic blockade. Anesthesiology 1993;79:1304–1315.
14. Vicenzi M, Woehlck H, Bosnjak Z, Atlee J. Anesthetics and automaticity of dominant and latent pacemakers in chronically instrumented dogs II: Effects of enflurane and isoflurane during exposure to epinephrine with and without muscarinic blockade. Anesthesiology 1993;79:1316–1323.
15. Atlee JL. Perioperative Cardiac Dysrhythmias. 2nd ed. Chicago: Year Book Medical Publishers, 1990.
16. Atlee JL, Bosnjak Z. Mechanisms for cardiac dysrhythmias during anesthesia. Anesthesiology 1990;72:347–374.
17. Atlee JL, Pattison C, Mathews E, et al. Evaluation of transesophageal atrial pacing stethoscope in adult surgical patients under general anesthesia. PACE 1992;15:1515–1525.
18. Atlee J, Tscheliessnigg K, Gombotz H (eds). Perioperative Management of Pacemaker Patients. Berlin: Springer-Verlag, 1992.
19. Atlee JL, Pattison C, Mathews E, Hedman A. Transesophageal atrial pacing for intraoperative sinus bradycardia or AV junctional rhythm: Feasibility as prophylaxis in 200 anesthetized adults and hemodynamic effects of treatment. J Cardiothorac Vasc Anesth 1993;7:436–441.
20. Atlee JL. Cardiac pacing and electroversion. In Kaplan J (ed): Cardiac Anesthesia. 3rd ed. Philadelphia: WB Saunders, 1993: pp. 877–904.
21. Josephson M. Clinical Cardiac Electrophysiology. 2nd ed. Philadelphia: Lea & Febiger, 1993.

22. Zipes D, Jalife J (ed). Cardiac Electrophysiology. 2nd ed. Philadelphia: WB Saunders, 1995.
23. Hickey P, Wessel D, Reich D. Anesthesia for the treatment of congenital heart disease. In Kaplan J (ed): Cardiac Anesthesia. 3rd ed. Philadelphia: WB Saunders, 1993: pp. 681–757.
24. Ganz L, Friedman P. Supraventricular tachycardia. N Engl J Med 1995;332:162–173.
25. Levy M, Martin P. Neural control of the heart. In Berne R (ed): Handbook of Physiology. Section 2: The Cardiovascular System. Volume 1: The Heart. Bethesda, MD: The American Physiological Society, 1979: pp. 581–620.
26. Rosen M, Fisch C, Hoffman B, et al. Can accelerated AV junctional escape rhythms be explained by delayed afterdepolarizations? Am J Cardiol 1980;45:1272–1284.
27. Villain E, Vetter V, Garcia J, et al. Evolving concepts in the management of congenital junctional ectopic tachycardia. A multicenter study. Circulation 1990;81:1544–1549.
28. Atlee J. Adenosine, diltiazem, edrophonium, esmolol, magnesium sulfate, and other new antiarrhythmic drugs. Cardiothorac Vasc Anesth Update 1993;3:1–13.
29. The Cardiac Arrhythmia Suppression Trial (CAST) Investigators. Preliminary report: Effect of encainide and flecainide on mortality in a randomized trial of arrhythmia suppression after myocardial infarction. N Engl J Med 1989;321:406–412.
30. The Cardiac Arrhythmia Suppression Trial II Investigators. Effect of the antiarrhythmic agent moricizine on survival after myocardial infarction. N Engl J Med 1992;327:227–233.
31. Wagner G. Practical Electrocardiography. 9th ed. Baltimore: Williams & Wilkins, 1994: p. 434.
32. Gibson D, Broder G, Sowton E. Effect of varying pulse interval in atrial fibrillation on left ventricular function in man. Br Heart J 1971;33:388–393.

10

Recognition and Management of Arrhythmias Preexcitation, Ventricular Arrhythmias, and Heart Block

Abbreviations Used in Chapter Ten

AP	Accessory pathway
AV	Atrioventricular
AVIR	Accelerated idioventricular rhythm
AVJR	Atrioventricular junctional rhythm
CAD	Coronary artery disease
CPB	Cardiopulmonary bypass
CPR	Cardiopulmonary resuscitation
ECG	Electrocardiogram (-cardiography)
IVR	Idioventricular rhythm
LBBB/RBBB	Left/right bundle branch block
LGL	Lown–Ganong, Levine (syndrome)
PMVT	Polymorphic ventricular tachycardia
NSVT	Nonsustained ventricular tachycardia
PSVT	Paroxysmal supraventricular tachycardia
SND	Sinus node dysfunction

SVT	Supraventricular tachycardia
VES	Ventricular extrasystole
VT/VF	Ventricular tachycardia/fibrillation
WPW	Wolff–Parkinson–White (syndrome)

Ventricular Preexcitation

Ventricular preexcitation occurs when the supraventricular impulse activates a part of the ventricle earlier than would have occurred had the impulse traveled via the normal atrioventricular (AV) conducting system. In patients with preexcitation, muscular fibers outside of the normal specialized AV conducting system form connections between the atrium and ventricle or specialized AV conducting system (see Fig. 9–17). These are called accessory AV pathways (AP). The term ventricular *preexcitation syndrome* is used for patients with electrocardiographic (ECG) evidence of preexcitation and symptoms due to tachyarrhythmias. The most common type of tachyarrhythmia with preexcitation syndromes is AV reentry (reciprocating) tachycardia, in which the atria, ventricles, AV node, and AP participate in the reentry circuit.

TYPES OF ACCESSORY PATHWAYS

Nomenclature for AP with preexcitation syndromes is provided in Figure 9–17. With the Wolff–Parkinson–White (WPW) syndrome, discussed next, there is an *atrioventricular AP*, also termed a *Kent bundle.* Atrioventricular AP are by far the most common type of AP. Evidence to date does not support the involvement of *atriohisian bypass pathways* in AV reciprocating tachycardia in patients with the Lown–Ganong–Levine (LGL) syndrome.[1-6] Although such pathways exist anatomically, they or enhanced AV nodal conduction is believed responsible for the short PR interval (≤ 0.12 second) and normal QRS with LGL (Fig. 10–1). The major clinical significance of the LGL syndrome is the capacity for a rapid ventricular response during atrial flutter–fibrillation. *Nodoventricular* or *nodofascicular* pathways between the AV node and right bundle branch or right ventricular muscle (Fig. 10–2) are also known as *Mahaim fibers.* These do not necessarily shorten the PR interval, since the atrial impulse traverses at least a part of the AV node. Mahaim fibers do, however, produce ventricular

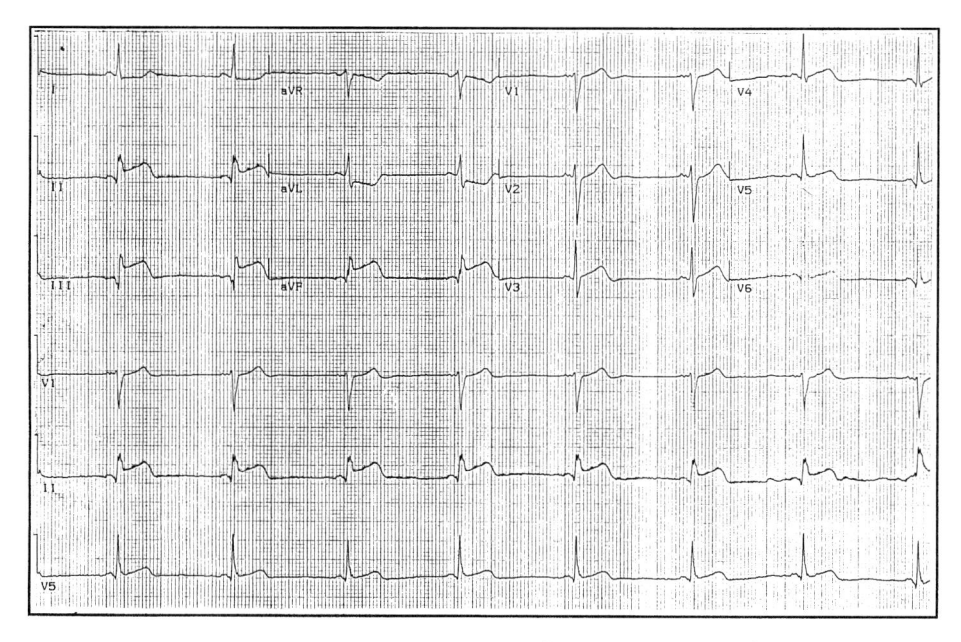

FIGURE 10–1 *Aside from marked sinus bradycardia (48 beats/min) and ECG changes of acute inferior wall infarction, the only other abnormal finding on this ECG is a short PR interval (0.10 second). Since the patient has no evidence of ventricular preexcitation, this ECG is consistent with the LGL syndrome.*

preexcitation and a delta wave (Fig. 10–2), and can participate in AV reciprocating tachycardia in which anterograde conduction proceeds over the accessory pathway. Because these pathways always enter the right ventricle or right bundle branch, the QRS complex during tachycardia has a left bundle branch block (LBBB) pattern, with the degree of preexcitation depending on the balance between the speed of conduction over the accessory pathway and that of the AV node and His–Purkinje system. Because the speed of AV node conduction is influenced by drugs and autonomic tone, manifestation of preexcitation can be intermittent (Fig. 10–3).

WOLFF–PARKINSON–WHITE SYNDROME

The Wolff–Parkinson–White syndrome is by far the most common preexcitation syndrome. The incidence of the WPW syndrome is estimated at between 0.1 and 0.3 percent of persons, with a 60 to 70

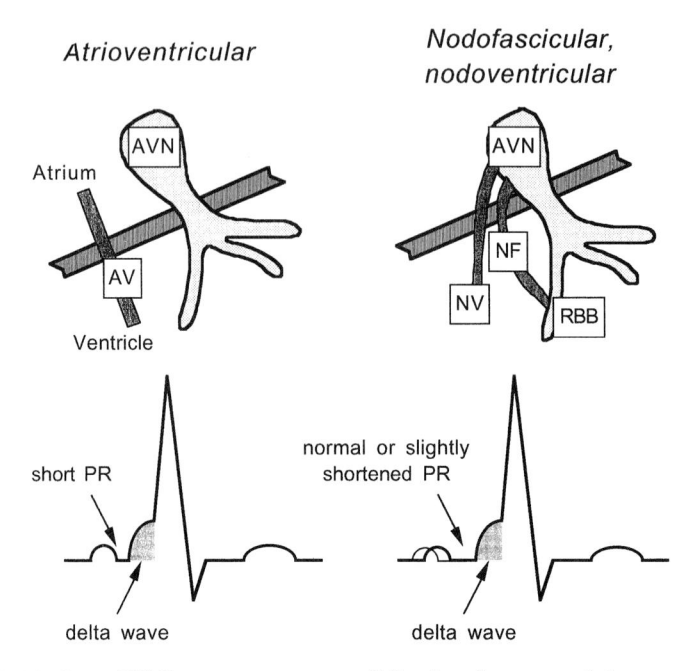

FIGURE 10-2 *ECG appearance of fusion beats with ventricular preexcitation.* **(Left)** *AV accessory pathway (Kent bundle). Accessory AV pathways, located almost anywhere in the circumference of the tricuspid or mitral annuli, including the interventricular septum (see Fig. 10-4), permit the propagating atrial impulse to completely bypass the AV node (AVN); hence, the short PR interval. Such preexcitation produces earlier than normal activation of some part of the ventricle, most commonly the left ventricle.* **(Right)** *Nodofascicular (NF) or nodoventricular (NV) accessory pathways. These connect the AV node to the right bundle branch (RBB) or right ventricular muscle. Because the AV node is involved in AV impulse transmission, the PR interval is normal or slightly shortened. However, a delta wave is present.*

percent male preponderance.[1,2,5] The incidence is difficult to estimate since the presence of preexcitation on the surface ECG can be highly variable, even on the same day in the same individual. In addition, AP express themselves at varying times during the life of an individual or conduct only in the retrograde direction (i.e., concealed AP) during orthodromic AV reentry tachycardia (discussed later). The incidence of orthodromic AV tachycardia in WPW syndrome patients increases from 10 percent in adults under 40 years to 35 percent or more in those over 60 years of age.

(During Halothane Anesthesia)

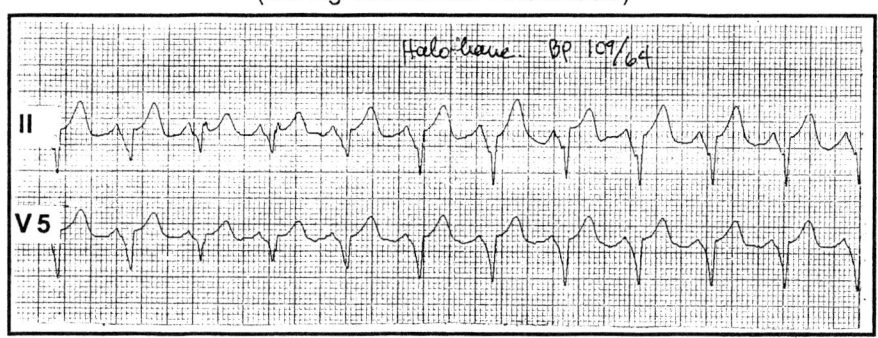

(During Isoflurane Anesthesia)

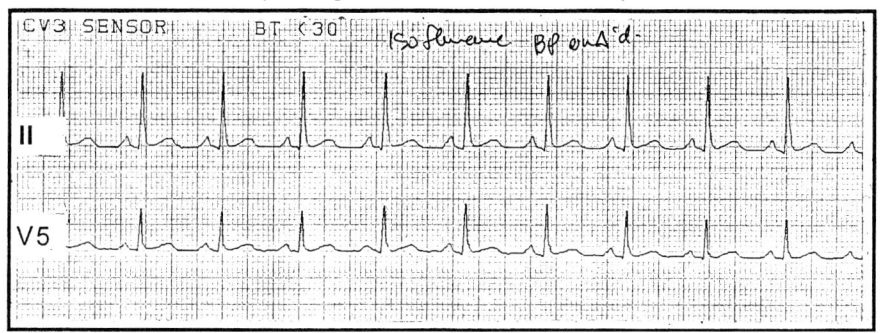

FIGURE 10-3 *Sinus tachycardia with apparent intermittent ventricular preexcitation in a patient not known to have preexcitation. (Top) During anesthesia with halothane, the patient has fusion or aberrant QRS complexes in association with sinus rhythm at 106 beats/min. In lead II, the PR interval is 0.10 to 0.12 second and the QRS duration 0.10 to 0.12 second. This was initially interpreted as slow ventricular tachycardia. However, there was no drop in blood pressure, so no treatment was offered. (Bottom) The anesthetic agent was changed to isoflurane. The rhythm remained sinus at 95 beats/min, but the PR interval and QRS duration normalized. The somewhat shortened PR interval with halothane could be explained by a nodofascicular or nodoventricular (Mahaim) fiber. Since either terminates in the right ventricle or right bundle branch, they are also expected to produce LBBB pattern ventricular aberration, since there is delayed activation of the left ventricle from the normal pathway and early activation from the right bundle branch or ventricle. The V_5 electrode is probably incorrectly positioned medial to V_5, since there should be no Q wave in V_5 or V_6 with LBBB (see Table 10-10). Note that the third and fourth QRS complexes (Top) have a more normal appearance. This might be due to changes in heart position with positive pressure ventilation.*

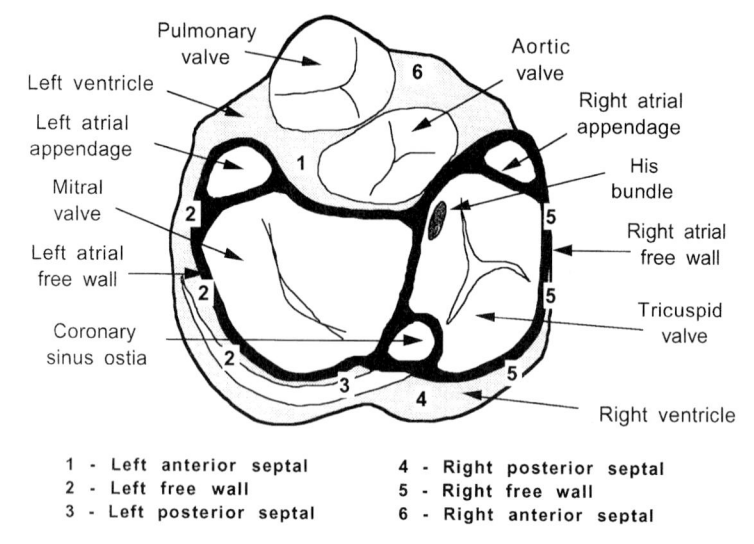

FIGURE 10-4 *Superior view of the heart with atria removed depicting the location of AP in patients with the WPW syndrome. AP may be found in one of four anatomic areas: left or right free wall, and the anterior or posterior septal space. Left or right free wall pathways may be further classified as anterior, lateral, or posterior.*

ELECTROCARDIOGRAPHIC APPEARANCE OF PREEXCITATION

The ECG with preexcitation includes a PR interval less than or equal to 0.12 second, anomalous QRS complexes equal to or greater than 0.12 second, slurred QRS onset (delta wave) in some leads, usually normal terminal QRS, and secondary ST–T-wave changes commonly directed opposite to the major delta and QRS vectors. ECG features can vary somewhat depending on the location of the AP (Fig. 10–4) and coexisting ECG abnormalities (Figs. 10–5 to 10–7).[7] Techniques to localize AP include careful inspection of the 12-lead ECG, rapid atrial pacing to increase the degree of preexcitation (Fig. 10–7)—since increased heart rate or prematurity of beats increases AV nodal delay—and electrophysiologic mapping.

TACHYARRHYTHMIAS WITH PREEXCITATION

The most common tachyarrhythmia with the WPW syndrome is characterized by a narrow QRS complex, ventricular rate between 150

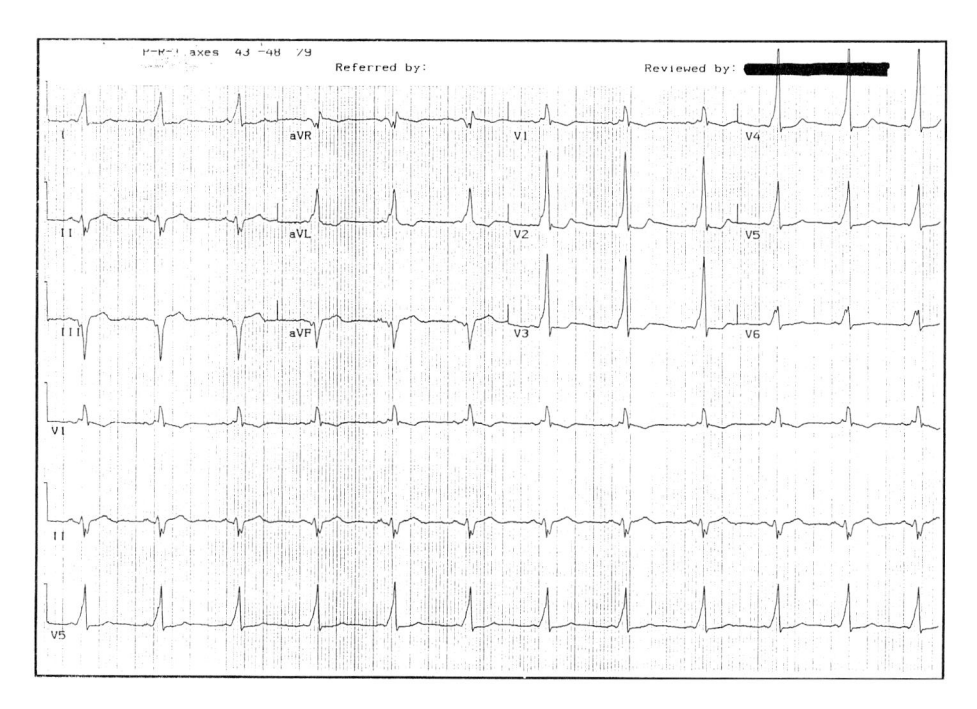

FIGURE 10-5 *ECG pattern consistent with a right or left posterior septal AP in a patient with the WPW syndrome. Note the positive delta wave and QRS in lead V_1, negative delta waves and QRS in leads II and aVF, and pronounced slurring of the QRS upstroke in leads I, aVL, and anterolateral precordial leads. The PR interval is 0.09 second in the leads with slurred QRS upstrokes.*

and 250 beats/min—usually faster than AV node reentry—and sudden onset and termination.[1-3,5-7] Such tachycardia, orthodromic AV reentry (reciprocating) tachycardia (Fig. 10-8), is for all intents and purposes the same as AV reentry paroxysmal supraventricular tachycardia (PSVT) in patients with concealed AP (see Fig. 9-18). Much less common (10 percent of AV reentry tachycardia) is antidromic (wide QRS) AV reentry tachycardia (Fig. 10-9). Orthodromic and antidromic AV tachycardia account for 70 to 80 percent of paroxysmal tachycardias in patients with the WPW syndrome, and atrial fibrillation (15 to 25 percent) or flutter (5 to 10 percent) for most of the remainder. Ventricular tachycardia is rare (< 1 percent), which is important to remember when confronted with a WPW syndrome patient with wide-QRS tachycardia. Of real concern for the WPW syndrome patient with atrial flutter–fibrillation is the capacity for anterograde conduc-

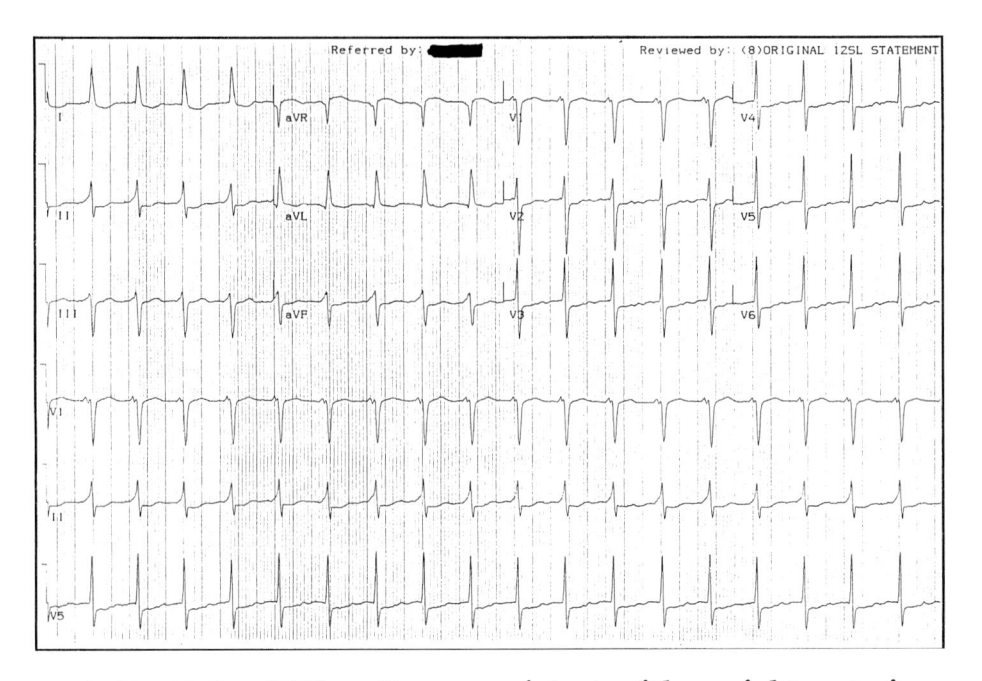

FIGURE 10-6 *ECG pattern consistent with a right anterior septal or anterior free wall AP in a patient with the WPW syndrome. The patient also has left axis deviation and change of inferior and lateral wall subendocardial injury or ischemia. Note the initially negative delta wave and QRS in lead V_1, positive delta waves in leads II, III, and aVF, and pronounced slurring of the QRS upstroke in leads II, III and aVF. Expected positive delta waves are not evident in the anterolateral precordial leads. The PR interval is 0.06 second (leads II and V_1).*

tion over the AP, with danger of extremely rapid ventricular rates and deterioration to ventricular tachycardia or fibrillation (see Fig. 9–31). Finally, it is possible that a patient may have several of the aforementioned rhythm disturbances or manifestations of preexcitation on a single occasion (Figs. 10–10 and 10–11).

MANAGEMENT OF ATRIOVENTRICULAR RECIPROCATING TACHYCARDIA IN WOLFF–PARKINSON–WHITE SYNDROME PATIENTS

Patients with the WPW syndrome may have infrequent tachyarrhythmias without significant symptoms. Such patients are not considered

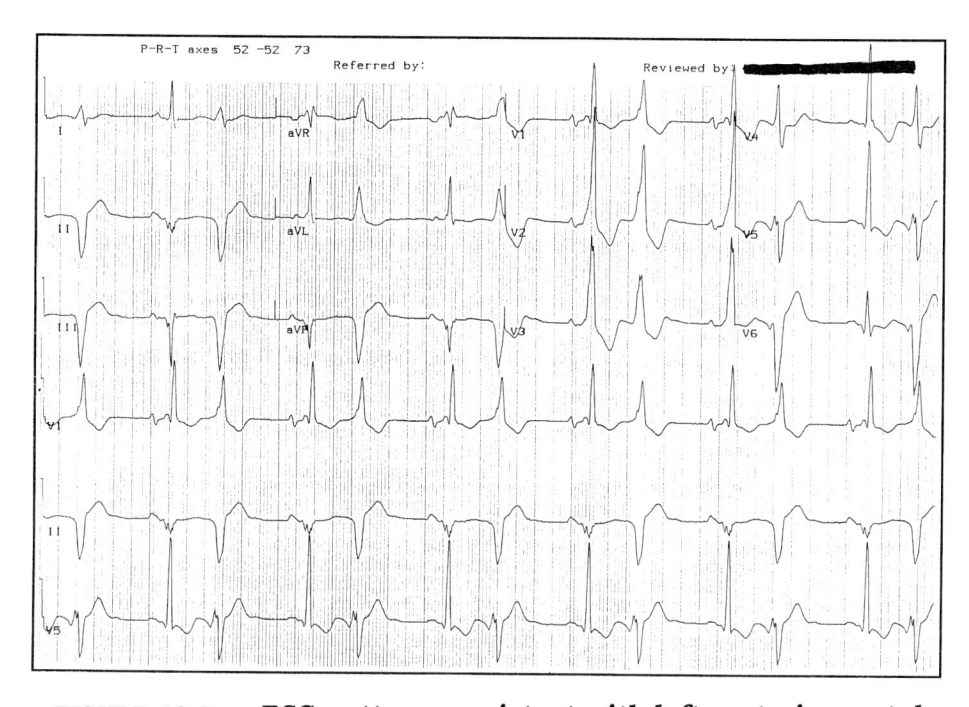

PREEXCITATION, VENTRICULAR ARRHYTHMIAS, AND HEART BLOCK **397**

FIGURE 10-7 *ECG pattern consistent with left posterior septal AP in patient with the WPW syndrome and anomalous premature beats. For normal beats, note the positive delta wave (initial 40 msec) and QRS in lead V_1, negative delta waves and QRS in leads II, III, and aVF, and pronounced slurring of the QRS upstroke in leads V_2 and V_3. The PR interval is 0.16 second in the latter leads. The longer than expected PR interval in a patient with preexcitation may be caused by drugs or intrinsic AV node conduction delay. Flattened T waves in the inferior leads, and inverted ones in the precordial leads, are consistent with infarction or repolarization abnormalities caused by preexcitation. The anomalous premature beats, although they occur in a bigeminal pattern and have wide QRS complexes, may in fact be premature atrial extrasystoles with increased preexcitation. Note the slurred QRS upstrokes (delta waves) in leads I, aVR, and V_1 to V_3.*

candidates for cardiac electrophysiologic studies and long-term drug or ablative (catheter, surgery) therapy.[2,5] Other patients may have frequent paroxysms of symptomatic AV tachycardia or atrial flutter–fibrillation, and preventive drug therapy should be instituted. Drugs are chosen based on their ability to increase conduction time and refractoriness in the AV node and/or AP (Table 10–1), except that

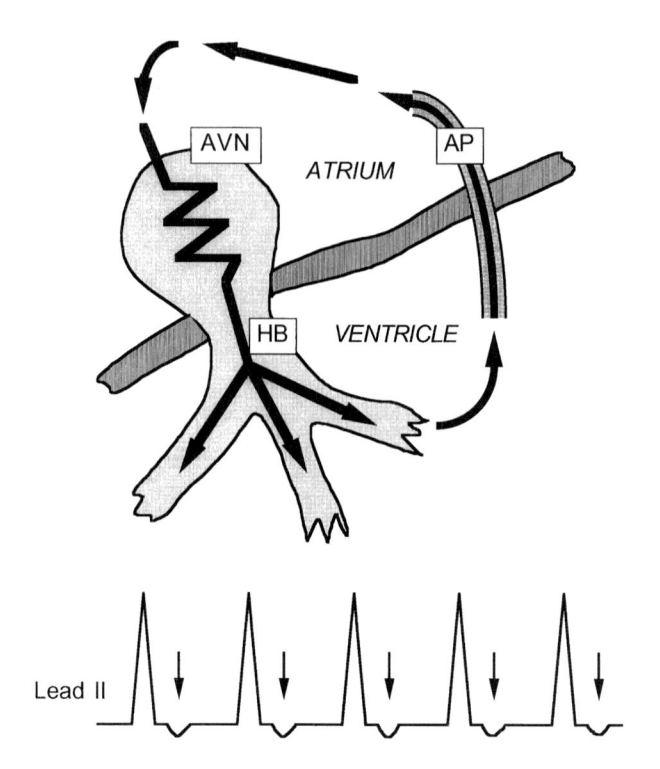

FIGURE 10-8 *Mechanism for and ECG appearance of orthodromic AV reentry (reciprocating) supraventricular tachycardia in patients with the WPW syndrome. The reentry loop includes the atrium, AV node (AVN), His bundle (HB), ventricle and accessory pathway (AP). During tachycardia, the ventricles are activated via the normal pathway (AVN → HB), and the atria by retrograde conduction through the AP. This sequence of myocardial activation explains the narrow QRS and retrograde P waves occurring following the QRS complex in lead II.*

digitalis is considered ill-advised given that it may increase the rate of AV tachycardia or the ventricular rate with atrial flutter–fibrillation, and better alternatives exist today. Patients with severe hemodynamic compromise from tachyarrhythmias should undergo electrophysiologic evaluation for ablative therapy, since the latter is curative. Ablative therapy is also indicated when drugs produce intolerable side effects, or they are only partially effective. The following discussion focuses on the acute aspects of management.

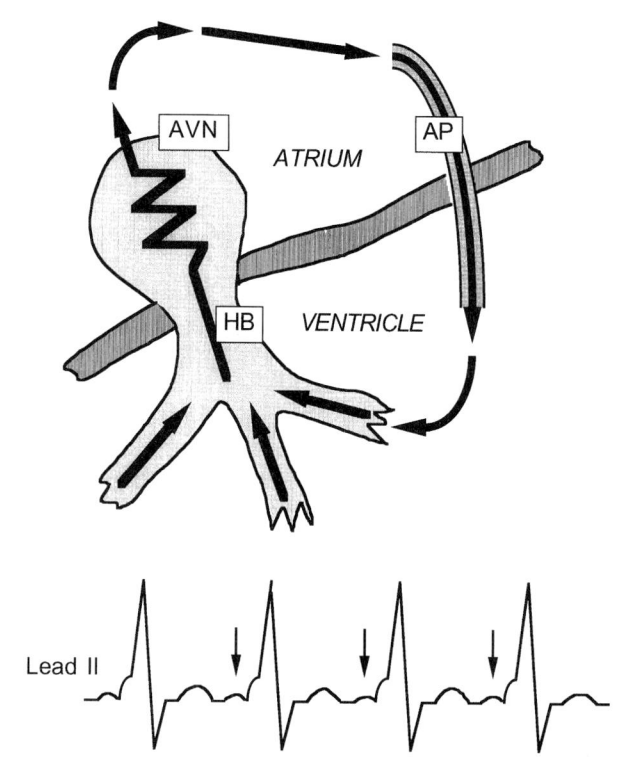

PREEXCITATION, VENTRICULAR ARRHYTHMIAS, AND HEART BLOCK **399**

FIGURE 10-9   *Mechanism for and ECG appearance of antidromic AV reentry (reciprocating) tachycardia in patients with the WPW syndrome. The reentry loop includes the atrium, AV node (AVN), His bundle (HB), ventricle, and accessory pathway (AP). During tachycardia, the ventricles are activated via anterograde conduction over the AP, and the atria by retrograde conduction over the normal pathway (HB → AVN). This sequence of myocardial activation explains the wide QRS complex and delta wave, with nearly normal P waves occurring just before the delta complex in lead II.*

Orthodromic Atrioventricular Tachycardia

Termination of an acute episode of orthodromic AV tachycardia is approached the same as for supraventricular tachycardia (SVT) due to AV node reentry. Vagal maneuvers are attempted first followed by drugs. However, with hemodynamic collapse, myocardial ischemia or inadequate cerebral perfusion, direct current (DC) cardioversion is the

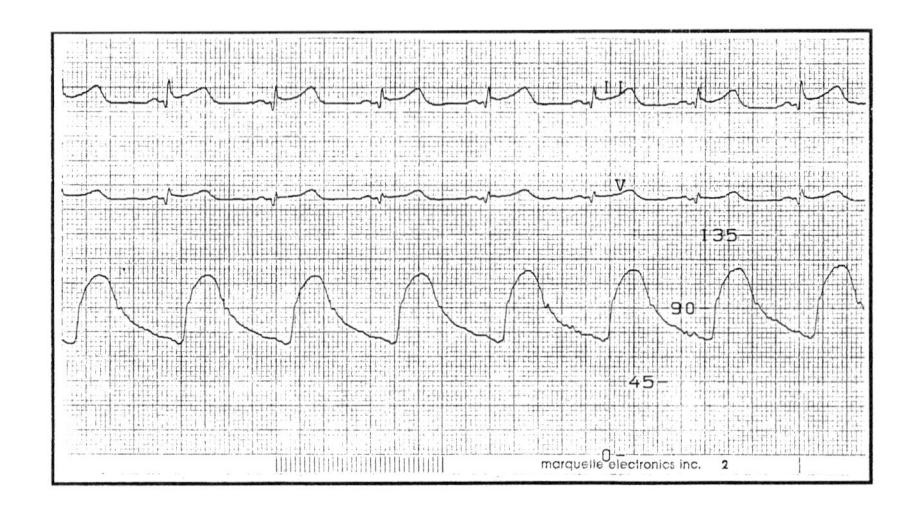

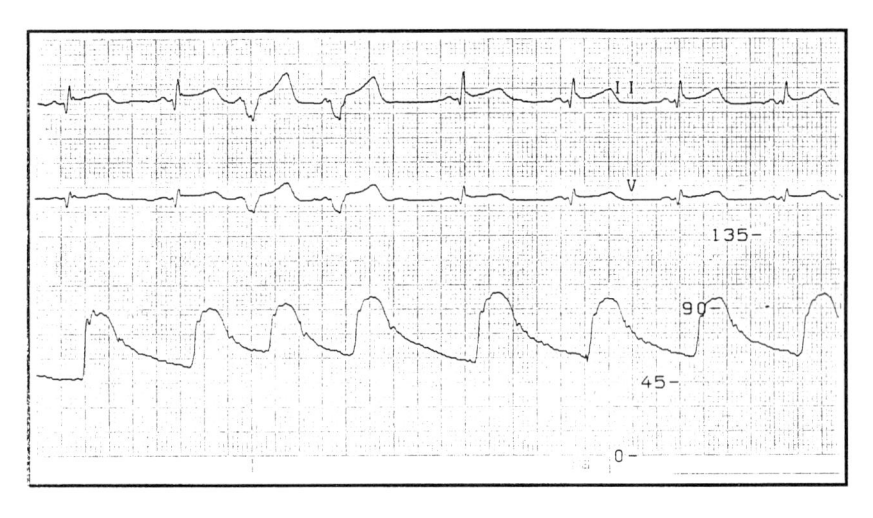

FIGURE 10–10 *ECG tracings from patient with the WPW syndrome undergoing catheter ablation of two left free wall AP, one of which conducted in both directions, and the other of which conducted only in the retrograde direction. (Top) ECG appearance during sinus rhythm without evidence of ventricular preexcitation. (Bottom) All beats are sinus, and most show normal ventricular activation. However, the third and fourth beats are preexcited, with the QRS morphology typical of that with a left free wall AP.*

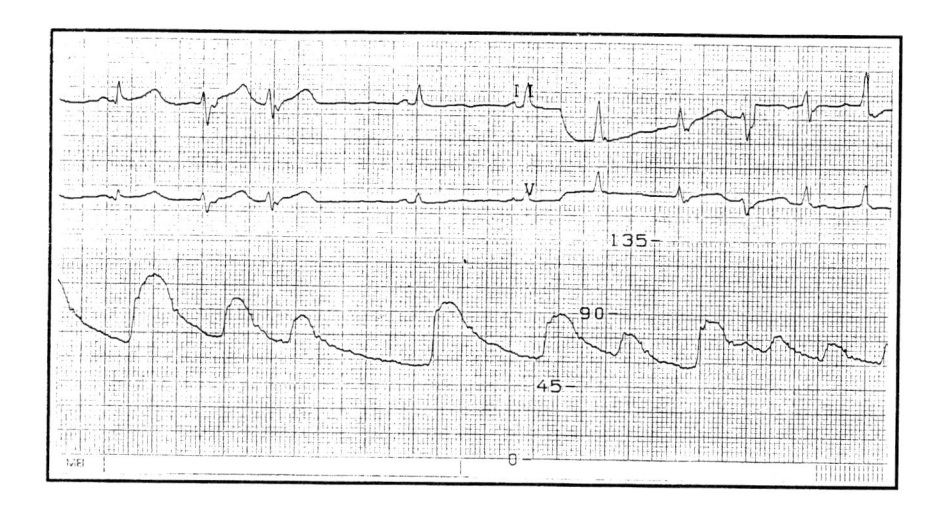

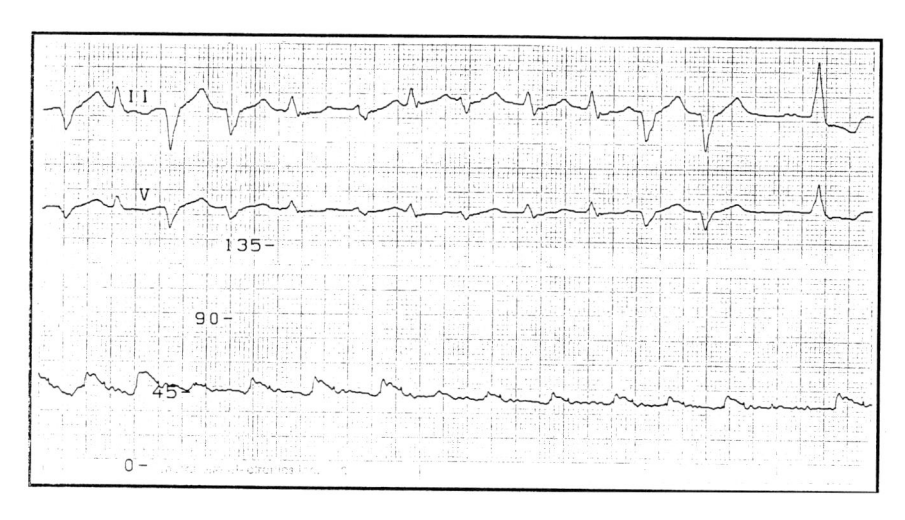

PREEXCITATION, VENTRICULAR ARRHYTHMIAS, AND HEART BLOCK **401**

FIGURE 10–11 *See legend on following page*

initial treatment of choice. Adenosine, edrophonium, esmolol (also metoprolol, propranolol), and verapamil or diltiazem are used to increase conduction time and refractoriness in the AV node. None of these drugs directly affects refractoriness in the AP, but verapamil or diltiazem may decrease AP refractoriness secondary to an increase in sympathetic tone with vasodilation. In fact, intravenous (not oral) verapamil can precipitate ventricular fibrillation when administered to WPW syndrome patients with atrial fibrillation.[5] While digitalis can convert orthodromic AV tachycardia by increasing refractoriness in the AV node, it is not particularly effective for this purpose. Furthermore, like verapamil, and probably also diltiazem, it can accelerate conduction and shorten refractoriness in the AP to increase the ventricular rate with atrial flutter–fibrillation, or the rate of orthodromic AV tachycardia. Therefore, it is advisable not to use digitalis as a single drug to treat orthodromic AV tachycardia or other types of SVT in WPW syndrome patients, especially if SVT is atrial flutter–fibrillation.[2,4,5] Procainamide, which increases AP conduction time and refractoriness, may be used in conjunction with beta-blockers to treat orthodromic AV tachycardia, especially with danger of atrial flutter–fibrillation. Catecholamines shorten AV node and AP refractoriness, expose WPW syndromes, and may reverse the effects of some antiarrhythmic drugs on the AV node or AP. Increased vagal tone has just the opposite effect.

FIGURE 10-11 *ECG tracing from the same patient as in Figure 10-10. (Top) The first beat is a sinus beat. It followed by two premature beats conducted with somewhat anomalous QRS complexes, but also associated with retrograde P waves early in the ST segment. These premature beats may be caused by orthodromic AV reciprocation. They are followed by two sinus beats. The final five beats also appear to have retrograde P waves, and may be the result of orthodromic AV reciprocation. Alternatively, they are partially preexcited during an ectopic atrial rhythm, since the R–R intervals (last four beats) are regular. (Bottom) The underlying rhythm is now atrial fibrillation (note R-R-interval variation), except for the last beat, which is ectopic atrial. The ventricular rate with atrial fibrillation is slow since one accessory pathway has been electrically ablated. QRS complexes during atrial fibrillation are normal or anomalous, showing varying amounts of preexcitation. The QRS complex with the last beat is anomalous. The positive delta wave and QRS complex in II and V_5 are consistent with preexcitation via a right free wall pathway.*

TABLE 10-1 *Site of action of drugs used to prevent AV reciprocation or reduce the potential for a rapid ventricular response with atrial flutter–fibrillation in WPW syndrome patients*

AV NODE	ACCESSORY AV PATHWAY	BOTH
Beta-blockers	Disopyramide	Amiodarone
Verapamil, diltiazem	Procainamide	Sotalol
Digitalis*	Quinidine	Class 1C

*Ill-advised because its potential to increase the rate of reciprocating tachycardia or ventricular rate with atrial flutter–fibrillation.

Antidromic Atrioventricular Tachycardia

The treatment for antidromic tachycardia in WPW syndrome patients is in all respects the same as for the orthodromic variety, only this tachycardia is far less common (as discussed earlier). Antidromic tachycardia is mentioned separately here only to call attention to the fact that it is easily mistaken for ventricular tachycardia (VT) and mistreated as such. For example, lidocaine might be administered, with the danger of accelerating antidromic AV tachycardia. Also, lidocaine, which has unpredictable effects on AP refractoriness, can increase the ventricular rate with atrial flutter–fibrillation.[1]

Atrial Flutter–Fibrillation

DIGITALIS.   *Digitalis is contraindicated.* While digitalis is still used for ventricular rate reduction with atrial flutter–fibrillation in patients without the WPW syndrome, it is contraindicated in patients with the syndrome. This is on account of possible dangerous ventricular rate acceleration and precipitation of ventricular fibrillation (VF).[1,2,4,5] Digitalis can increase the ventricular rate by any of the following mechanisms: (1) by shortening conduction times and refractoriness in atrial myocardium to increase the rate of flutter or fibrillation; (2) by shortening conduction time and refractoriness in the AP (which are essentially atrial fibers), increasing the number of atrial impulses conducted to the ventricles; (3) by blocking anterograde conduction in the AV node, so that there is a reduction in retrograde (concealed) conduction over the AP, but an increase in anterograde conduction; and (4) as digitalis is pushed in a futile effort to achieve ventricular rate reduction, increased central sympathetic tone further facilitates AV impulse transmission via the AV node or AP, as well as increases ventricular vulnerability to fibrillation.

INDICATED DRUGS FOR ATRIAL FLUTTER-FIBRILLATION. Instead of digitalis, drugs suitable for intravenous administration from those listed in Table 10-1 are used for acute ventricular rate reduction with atrial flutter–fibrillation in patients with ventricular preexcitation. However, a drug that increases AV nodal conduction time and refractoriness (esmolol, metoprolol, propranolol) must be coupled with one that has a similar effect on the AP conduction and refractoriness (procainamide). While edrophonium, a short-acting cholinesterase inhibitor, is expected to slow AV node conduction and refractoriness, it is possible that the effect of accumulated acetylcholine to shorten atrial refractoriness could increase the atrial reentry rate and also accelerate AP conduction. Therefore, edrophonium is not advised as a single drug for acute ventricular rate reduction with atrial flutter–fibrillation in patients known or suspected of having the WPW syndrome. Finally, in many if not most patients with the WPW syndrome and atrial flutter–fibrillation, the rapid ventricular rate response will produce severe hypotension or circulatory collapse (Fig. 10-11). Prompt (initial) DC cardioversion is the treatment of choice in these circumstances.

Ventricular Arrhythmias

OVERVIEW

Ventricular extrasystoles (VES) and nonsustained ventricular tachycardia (NSVT) are quite common in perioperative and critical care settings. NSVT is three or more VES in succession, but lasting less than 30 seconds. VES and NSVT are often the result of transient physiologic imbalance, which may be caused by the effects of drugs, dysautonomia, metabolic conditions, or medical intervention. It is not necessary that physiologic imbalance occur in association with structural cardiac abnormalities for VES or NSVT to occur. In contrast, sustained VT in perioperative or critical care settings is more likely to be a manifestation of structural heart disease in association with physiologic imbalance.

Just because new arrhythmias are VES or NSVT, they should not be presumed potentially malignant (life-threatening). Indeed, some supraventricular tachyarrhythmias are far more dangerous (see Chapter 9). Some factors to consider when determining the relative significance of VES or NSVT are listed in Table 10-2. Importantly, appearance and frequency of VES alone are insufficient criteria upon which to base the decision to treat, especially since there is risk of serious adverse effects with most drugs used to treat ventricular arrhythmias.

TABLE 10-2 *Relative significance of new or worsening ventricular rhythm disturbances*

	BENIGN	WORRISOME	MALIGNANT
Presentation	VES	VES, Couplet, NSVT	VES, Couplet, NSVT
Appearance	Uniform, multiform	Uniform, multiform	Any form, R-on-T
Heart Disease*	None	Present	Severe
Cardiomyopathy†	None	Present	Severe
LV Function	Normal	Impaired	Severely impaired
VES Frequency	≤ 5/min	6–10/min	> 10/min
Hemodynamics	Unaffected	Mild impairment	Heart failure
Coronary Disease	Absent	Chronic MI	Acute MI, ischemia
Setting–Cause	Mechanical, reflex	Ischemia	Acute MI
Anesthesia	Inadequate	Inadequate	Inadequate
COPD, Asthma	Mild impairment	Moderate impairment	Severe impairment
Stress, Anxiety	None, mild	Moderate	Severe, panic state
Imbalance‡	None, mild	Moderate	Severe
QT Interval	Normal	Prolonged	Prolonged + TDP§

*Coronary artery, hypertensive, valvular, idiopathic.
†Dilated or hypertrophic.
‡Physiologic imbalance (e.g., hypoxia, hypercarbia, potassium, magnesium, drug overdose or toxicity).
§History of torsades de pointes or in association with torsades.
LV, left ventricular; COPD, chronic obstructive pulmonary disease.

VENTRICULAR EXTRASYSTOLES

The term *ventricular extrasystole* includes both premature and postmature (escape) ventricular beats. Ventricular escape beats occur with bradycardia secondary to AV heart block, sinus node dysfunction (SND), or the hypersensitive carotid sinus syndrome. While ventricular escape and premature beats may have the same appearance, escape beats are not treated with drugs. Rather, they are suppressed by temporary or permanent pacing for the bradycardia that produced them, or chronotropic drugs (see Table 9-2) are used to accelerate the atrial rate. The following discussion concerns only premature VES, unless otherwise stated.

Electrocardiographic Appearance

Ventricular extrasystoles are characterized by a widened, bizarre QRS complex, distinctly different from those associated with supraventricular beats.[2,4,5,8] Usually the QRS duration is greater than 0.12 second, and the T wave large and opposite in direction to the major QRS deflection (Fig. 10-12). A broadly notched QRS > 0.16 second may be associated with a dilated, globally hypokinetic ventricle, whereas a shorter, smooth, narrow notched QRS may reflect a more normal-sized heart.[9] QRS complexes with two or more VES in the same lead may have the same *(uniform)* or dissimilar *(multiform)* appearance (Fig. 10-12). Because VES can arise in multiple sites in the ventricle, or in tissues with uneven refractoriness, they can show varying aberration or even a fairly normal appearance in different ECG leads (Fig. 10-13). While VES may be so premature as to occur during inscription of the T wave (R-on-T phenomenon), they may also occur so late as to fuse with the subsequent normal QRS complex, producing a fusion beat (Fig. 10-14). The QRS complex of VES is not preceded by a premature P wave. However, a sinus or ectopic supraventricular P wave occurring at its expected time may precede the QRS complex (Fig. 10-14). Intracardiac or esophageal ECG recordings may be required to ascertain the exact relationship of P waves to anomalous QRS complexes. Retrograde P waves with VES are common, but often obscured by the widened, bizarre QRS–T with the VES.

Compensatory Pause

Typically, a VES is followed by a *fully compensatory pause;* namely, the preceding normal beat–VES interval plus the VES–next normal beat interval is twice the normal beat interval (Fig. 10-12). This is because the VES collides with the normal impulse from above in the AV node. A more premature VES may conduct retrogradely to reset the timing of sinus node discharge before its full cycle of automaticity. Because of sinus node reset, the next normal beat will occur before the expected time to produce a *noncompensatory pause* (Fig. 10-15). Finally, a VES may be sufficiently premature so as to not affect the timing of sinus node discharge or conduction of beats during atrial flutter–fibrillation. If so, the normal beat–VES interval plus the VES–next normal beat interval is the same as the normal beat interval, and the VES is said to be *interpolated* (Fig. 10-15).

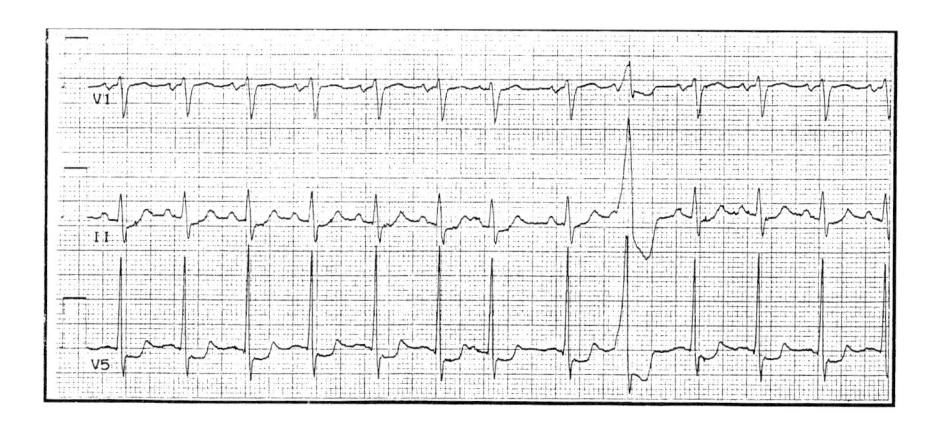

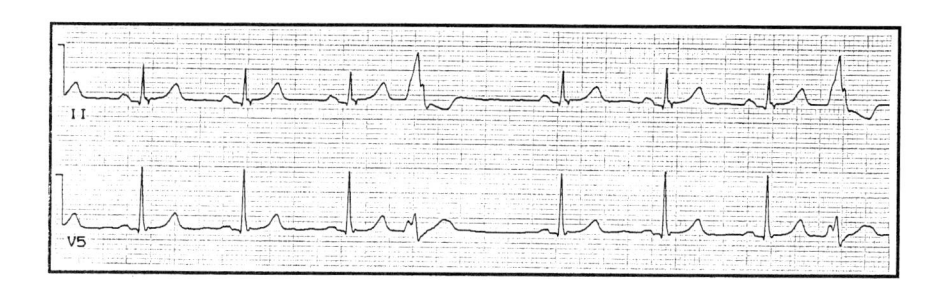

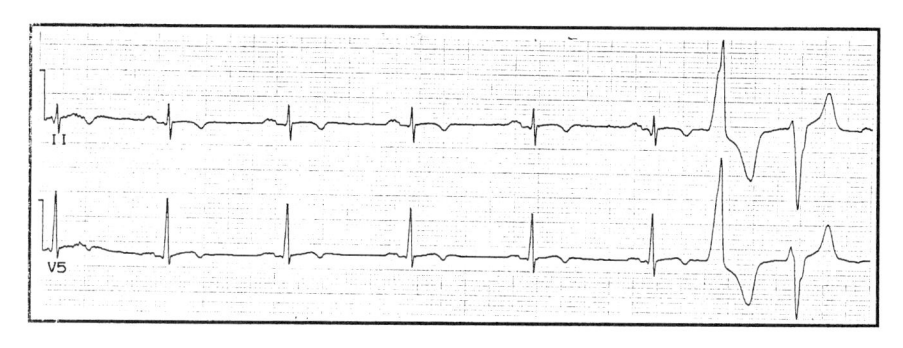

FIGURE 10–12 *Appearance of VES.* (Top) *Premature VES. Note the widened QRS (> 0.12 second) and large T wave that is opposite in direction to the major QRS deflection.* (Middle) *Uniform VES. The QRS complexes associated with VES are uniform in leads II and V_5. The first VES is followed by a fully compensatory pause (see text).* (Bottom) *Multiform VES. Successive VES (a couplet) with dissimilar appearance in the same lead.*

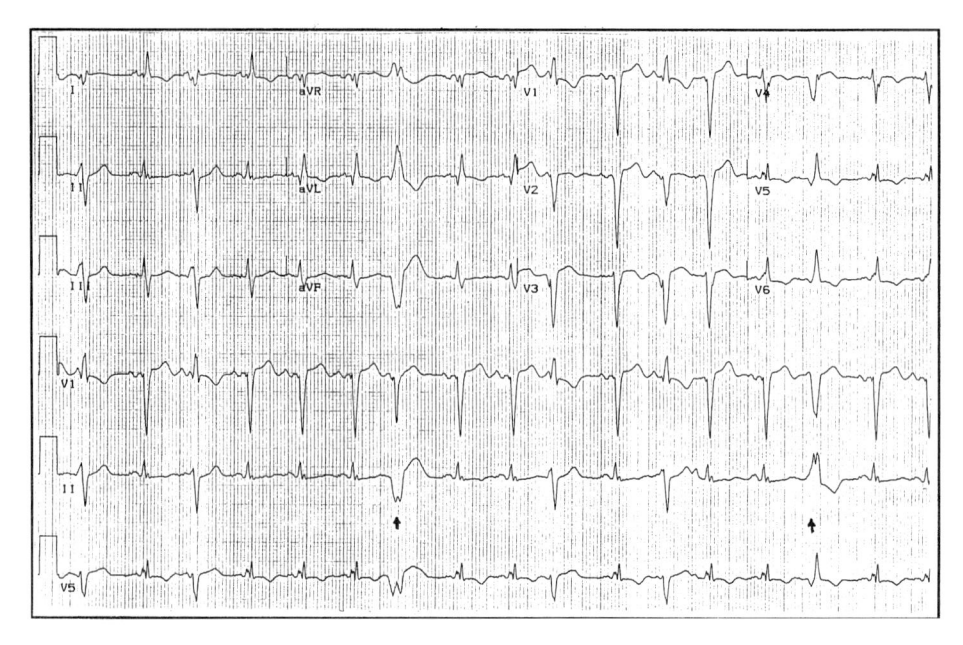

408 PREEXCITATION, VENTRICULAR ARRHYTHMIAS, AND HEART BLOCK

FIGURE 10–13 *Appearance of multiform VES in multiple leads. In the rhythm strip (V_1, II, and V_5—bottom tracings), beats 1, 3, 7, 10, 12, and 15 are VES. Beats 1, 3, 10, and 12 have the same QRS–T morphology in each of the leads. Note that in leads III and V_3 they appear similar to normal beats. The seventh wide-QRS beat (arrow) has an abnormal appearance in leads aVR, aVL, aVF, II, and V_5, but a normal appearance in V_1. The 15th wide-QRS beat (arrow) is clearly anomalous in leads II, V_1, V_4, and V_5, but nearly normal in V_6.*

Fixed and Variable Coupling

Fixed coupling between VES and preceding normal beats is usually considered a feature of reentry or triggering. However, if one carefully observes intervals between normal beats and VES for a sufficient period of time, there will be in all likelihood some subtle variation in coupling (≥ 0.06 second) between the preceding normal beats and VES.[2] More obvious variation is due to parasystole (discussed later), instability of a reentry circuit or multiple sites of origin, or variation in the rate of triggered automaticity.[2,5]

Patterns of Beating

When every other QRS complex is associated with a VES, the pattern is termed *ventricular bigeminy* (Fig. 10–16). When every third

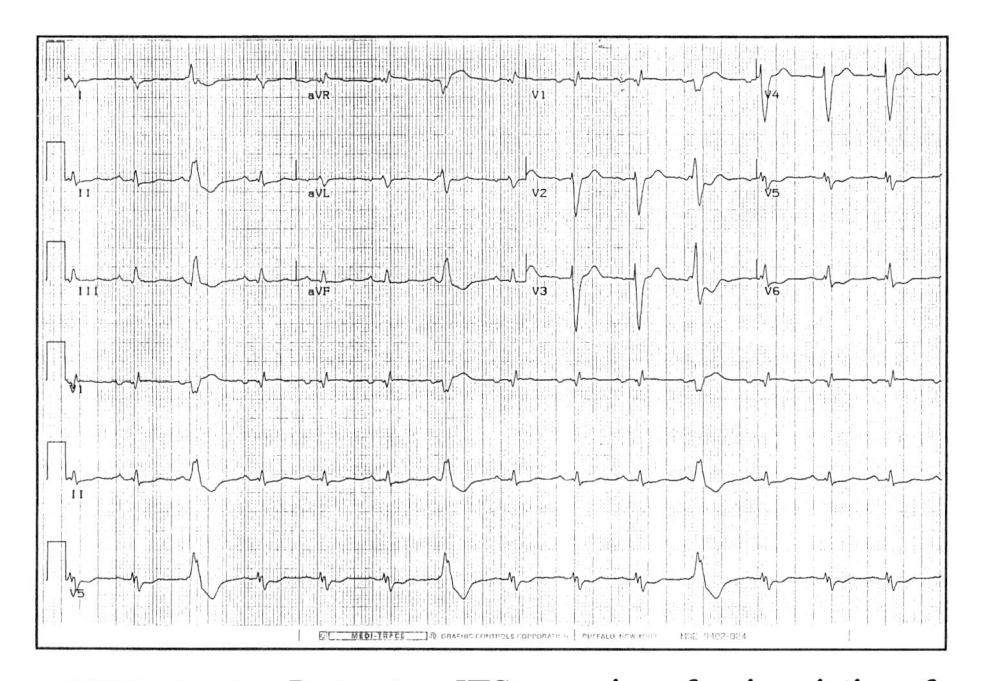

PREEXCITATION, VENTRICULAR ARRHYTHMIAS, AND HEART BLOCK   **409**

FIGURE 10–14   *Postmature VES occurring after inscription of the P wave (beats 3, 7, and 11 in leads V_1, II, and V_5—bottom tracings). Note that there is AV association between preceding P waves and wide QRS complexes of VES. The initial QRS deflection of VES is similar to that of normal beats, but the remainder of ventricular activation and repolarization (T wave) are not. Therefore, postmature VES are probably fusion beats, produced by simultaneous activation of the ventricles by impulses from the sinus node and ventricle.*

or fourth beat following normal beats is a VES, the pattern is *trigeminy* or *quadrigeminy*, respectively. Two successive VES are termed a *couplet*, and three successive complexes a *triplet* (Fig. 10–16). Arbitrarily, three or more successive VES are VT.

Ventricular Parasystole

Ventricular parasystole is an automatic rhythm originating in the His–Purkinje system that is reasonably independent of the dominant rhythm. Higher impulses are prevented by entrance block from discharging the parasystolic focus of automaticity. However, impulses can leave the parasystolic focus and discharge surrounding tissues, provided they are not refractory. Ventricular parasystole is recognized by VES recurring at regular intervals, which can be near or exact

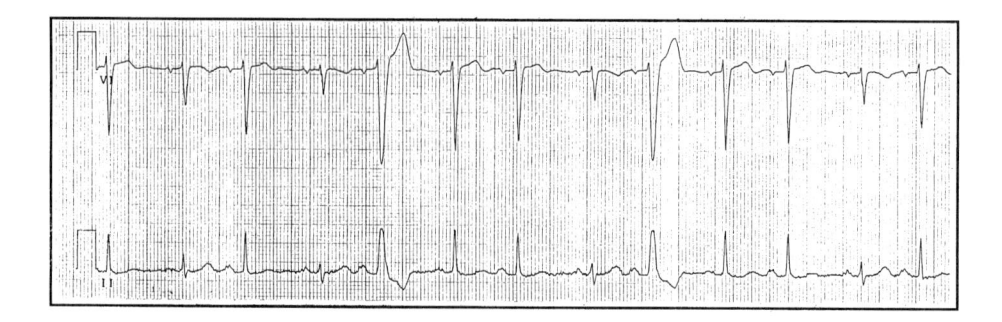

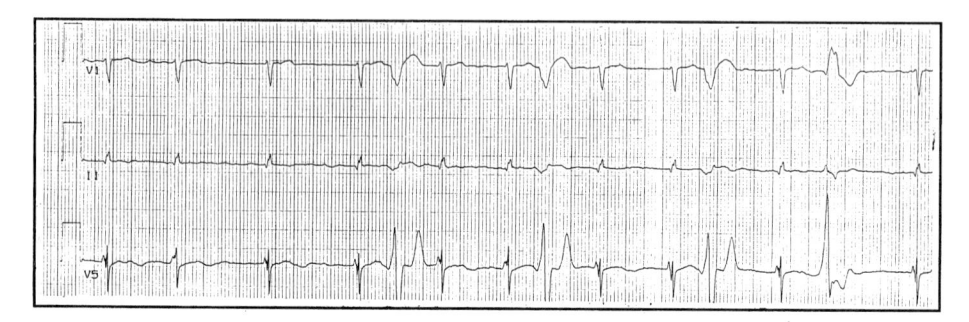

FIGURE 10-15 *Effect of ventricular extrasystoles on sinus rhythm. (Top) VES with noncompensatory pause (beats 5 and 9). The underlying rhythm is sinus with incomplete right bundle branch block pattern QRS aberration except for beats 2, 4, 8, and 12. The VES are probably fusion beats, since they are associated with P waves. These reset automaticity of the sinus node so that the next normal beat (P wave) occurs earlier than expected (0.84 second) had there been a fully compensatory pause (1.28 seconds—twice the interval between P waves preceding the VES). (Bottom) Interpolated VES. VES interrupt normally conducted beats during slow atrial fibrillation. These do not affect the R-R intervals during atrial fibrillation (i.e., cause a longer than expected conduction delay), so in a sense they are interpolated. Similarly, interpolated VES during sinus rhythm would not affect the timing of sinus discharge.*

multiples of each other (Fig. 10-17). In contrast to uniform VES, coupling between the parasystolic and preceding normal beats is quite variable, because the parasystolic focus is automatic (as opposed to reentrant or triggered) and unaffected by the dominant rhythm.

Idioventricular Rhythm

Idioventricular rhythm (IVR) is three or more successive, uniform ventricular beats with a rate below 60 beats/min (Fig. 10-18). If faster

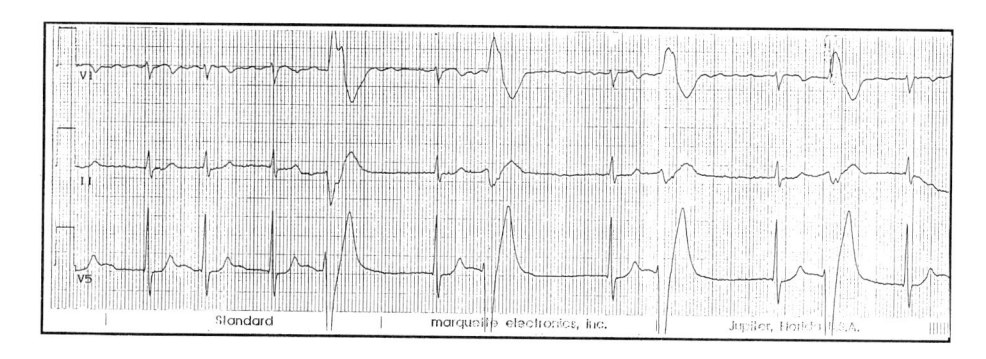

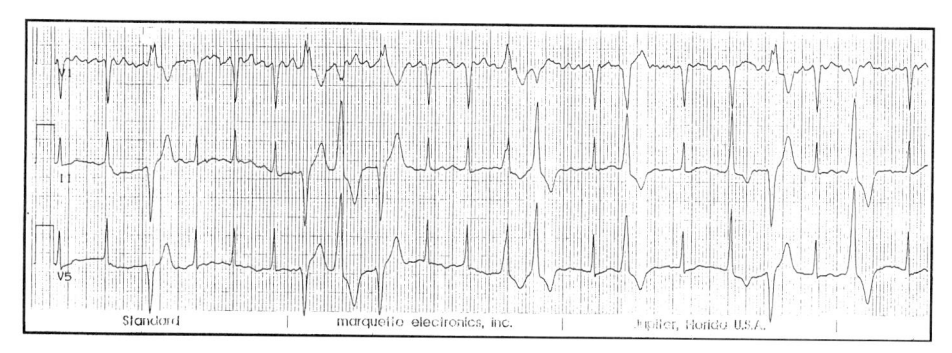

PREEXCITATION, VENTRICULAR ARRHYTHMIAS, AND HEART BLOCK **411**

FIGURE 10–16 *Patterns of beating with VES. (Top) Ventricular bigeminy in patient with atrial fibrillation. The interval between normal and anomalous QRS complexes is fairly constant. (Bottom) Frequent VES in pattern of couplets and triplets in patient with coarse atrial fibrillation.*

than this, it is termed *accelerated IVR*. AV junctional rhythm (AVJR) and IVR are the usual escape rhythms with complete AV heart block, sinus arrest, or sinoatrial block, unless a faster atrial ectopic rhythm emerges. Treatment for IVR associated with hemodynamic compromise is the same as for AVJR (see Chapter 9). Atrial or AV sequential overdrive pacing are preferred to ventricular pacing for the added hemodynamic benefit of atrial systole, and to reduce the risk of excess tachycardia or more dangerous arrhythmias with chronotropic drugs (see Table 9–2). Atropine is expected to have little effect on the rate of IVR because the His–Purkinje system receives little vagal innervation.

Classification of Ventricular Extrasystoles

Ventricular extrasystoles are observed in the majority of normal individuals continuously monitored for 24 to 48 hours.[2] They also

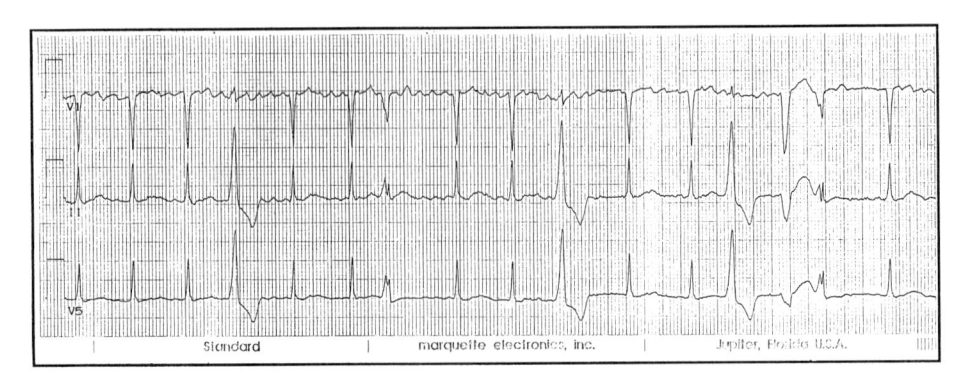

FIGURE 10-17 *Ventricular parasystole. Beats 4, 10, and 13 are VES, possibly originating in a protected focus of automaticity (i.e., a parasystolic focus). Note that the QRS complex has the same appearance in all the leads shown, which was also the case for other leads of the 12-lead ECG (not shown). The interval between beats 4 and 10 is 3.6 seconds, twice that between beats 10 and 13 (1.8 seconds). Note that parasystolic VES bear no constant relation to preceding normal QRS complexes. Coupling intervals between the preceding normal beats and parasystolic VES beats 4, 10, and 13 are 480, 520, and 400 msec, respectively. Presumably, the other VES (beats 7, 14, and 15) arise from ventricular foci unrelated to the parasystolic focus.*

occur frequently during anesthetic induction, airway manipulation and tracheal intubation, and emergence from anesthesia.[10] Many practitioners base the prognosis of VES primarily on appearance using the Lown–Wolf grading system (Table 10–3).[11] However, this system was developed in coronary care units, based on observations of ventricular arrhythmias in the setting of acute myocardial infarction. It does not take into account other circumstances of VES that also affect prognosis, and that are more applicable to patients in perioperative and critical care settings (Table 10–2). Consequently, high-grade VES based on Lown–Wolf criteria can be benign, worrisome, or malignant, depending on such factors as type of heart disease, physiologic imbalance, and cardiac function. For example, Lown–Wolf grade 3 to 5 VES (Table 10–3) with tracheal intubation under light anesthesia in a patient without heart disease rarely produce malignant ventricular tachyarrhythmias. However, grade 3 to 5 VES with QT-interval prolongation due to quinidine toxicity are.

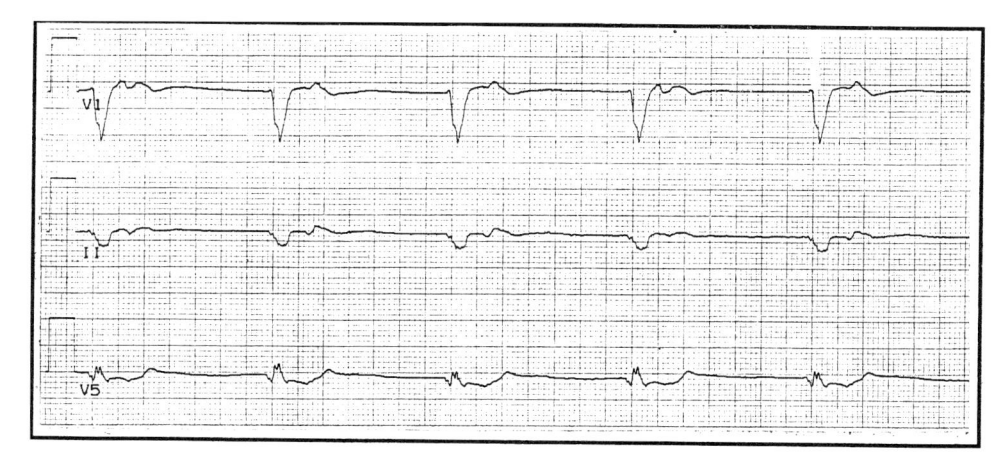

FIGURE 10-18 *IVR at 43 beats/min. Note retrograde (inverted) P waves in all leads shown.*

TABLE 10-3 *Lown–Wolf grading system for VES*

CLASS	CHARACTERISTICS
0	None or rare
1	Occasional (< 30 beats/hr)
2	Frequent (> 30 beats/hr)
3	Multiform beats
4	Couplets or triplets
5	Associated with R-on-T phenomenon

Hemodynamic Effects

As a rule, even when VES are frequent or occur in a bigeminal pattern, they do not cause significant hemodynamic effects. However, long runs of frequent VES in patients with significant heart disease may produce myocardial ischemia or hemodynamic deterioration. Also, frequent interpolated VES in effect double heart rate, and may compromise hemodynamics or cause myocardial ischemia.

Management

Especially in anesthesia and critical care settings, correction of causative or contributing factors, and appropriate treatment for the underlying heart condition, may be all the treatment required for VES, regardless of circumstances. Thus, such *remedial treatment* might be no more than providing adequate anesthesia, analgesia, or sedation, or improving oxygenation and correcting electrolyte imbalance. Whether or not more treatment should be provided depends both on the appearance and circumstances of VES (Table 10–2). Again, it is strongly emphasized that appearance and frequency alone provide insufficient information on which to base the decision to provide more specific treatment. However, a benign appearance with two or more risk factors in the malignant category (from Table 10–2) may provide sufficient reason for specific treatment. As a guide to the management of VES and nonsustained VT (NSVT) in anesthesia and critical care settings, but not necessarily out-of-hospital settings or emergency departments, where such arrhythmias are often caused by acute myocardial infarction or reperfusion of ischemic myocardium, the following recommendations are offered. VES with benign frequency and appearance, and in benign circumstances (Table 10–2), require only remedial treatment. Worrisome VES and NSVT, based on frequency, appearance, and surrounding circumstances, require remedial and in some instances, more specific treatment. Malignant VES and NSVT based or frequency and appearance invariably require both remedial and specific treatment. If the underlying heart rhythm is slow, and bradycardia contributes to VES, then consideration should be given to temporary pacing or chronotropic drugs to increase heart rate. We prefer to use noninvasive transesophageal or epicardial–endocardial atrial pacing (if available) for this purpose, provided AV conduction is intact and the patient is not in atrial flutter–fibrillation. Atropine and other chronotropes can also be used (Table 9–2). However, with chronotropes, there is the potential of worsening arrhythmias or causing excess tachycardia, which then requires further treatment. If VES are caused by or associated with sympathetic hyperactivity, a beta-blocker will often be effective for suppression. Otherwise, lidocaine is the initial drug of choice for treating VES that are worrisome or malignant based both on appearance and circumstances (Table 10–2). If maximal doses of lidocaine are ineffective, then procainamide may be tried. Phenytoin is effective for VES occurring in the setting of digitalis toxicity. Amiodarone, which may be available for intravenous dosing (see Chapter 5) by the time this book appears in print, should be reserved only for malignant VES after other treatment has failed.

VENTRICULAR TACHYCARDIA

Prevalence and Associations

At least 3 to 5 percent of patients who survive myocardial infarction will have at least one documented episode of sustained VT during the first year following infarction.[2,12,13] Arbitrarily, VT is sustained if it lasts longer than 30 seconds or requires termination because of circulatory collapse. An undefined number of patients may develop VT years later, and sudden cardiac death occurs at some time in 5 to 10 percent of survivors of myocardial infarction. Sudden cardiac death is usually due to rapid VT that degenerates into ventricular fibrillation (VF). At least 90 percent of patients with sustained, uniform VT have chronic coronary heart disease. Acute ischemia, which frequently causes polymorphic (multiform) VT and VF, seldom produces uniform VT. Sustained uniform VT, on the other hand, is most common in patients with chronic coronary artery disease. The likelihood of VT increases in patients with depressed left ventricular dysfunction (ejection fraction < 40 percent); it is also common in patients with other forms of heart disease, including dilated and hypertrophic cardiomyopathies and valvular heart disease, and following surgery for correction of congenital heart disease.

Electrocardiographic Appearance

REGULARITY. Uniform VT is the occurrence of three or more successive, similar, widened (QRS > 0.12 second) and bizarre QRS complexes at a rapid rate (≥ 100 beats/min), with the direction of T waves opposite that of the major QRS deflection.[2,4,5,8] While sustained uniform VT is usually a regular rhythm, a feature considered by many useful for distinguishing VT from atrial fibrillation with aberrant ventricular conduction, this is not always the case. In fact, the R–R intervals can vary by more than 20 msec in 20 percent of cases (Fig. 10–19), and is usually most pronounced at the beginning and spontaneous termination of VT.

P WAVES AND QRS COMPLEXES. P waves during VT have two possible origins. Either they are supraventricular (sinus, ectopic atrial) and dissociated from ventricular depolarization (AV dissociation; Fig. 10–19), or they are conducted retrogradely from the ventricles (ventriculoatrial, VA, association; Fig. 10–20). QRS widening ≥ 0.14 second is considered diagnostic of VT, whereas QRS duration between 0.12 and 0.14 second is consistent with either ventricular aberration or VT. QRS complexes during VT are more likely to be narrow in children, presumably because less ventricular tissue is available for depolarization compared to adults.[2]

QRS MORPHOLOGY. QRS morphology during VT is described as having a left (LBBB) (Fig. 10–19) or right (RBBB) bundle branch block morphology or configuration (Fig. 10–20). The former is ascribed to *VT*

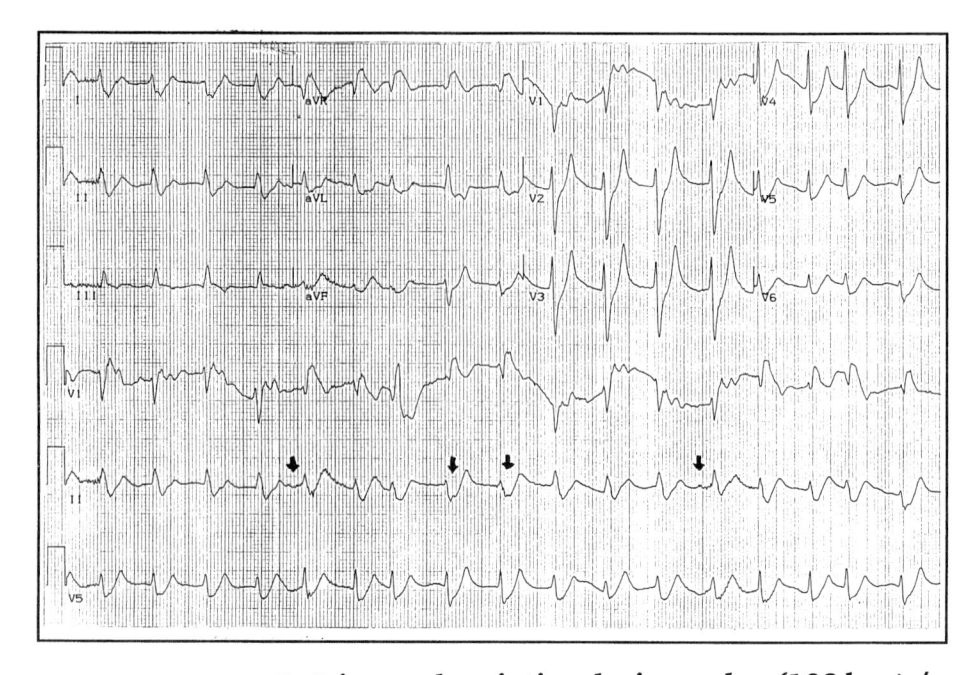

416 PREEXCITATION, VENTRICULAR ARRHYTHMIAS, AND HEART BLOCK

FIGURE 10-19 *R–R-interval variation during a slow (109 beats/ min) VT. QRS complexes with tachycardia have a LBBB configuration (see text), consistent with origin of VT in the right ventricle. The combination of LBBB pattern QRS configuration with right axis deviation strongly favors VT as opposed to atrial fibrillation with aberrant ventricular conduction as the mechanism for tachycardia in this patient, despite pronounced R–R-interval variation (420 to 600 msec) during tachycardia, although the R–R intervals are fairly constant for beats 1 to 4 and 8 to 13 of tachycardia. Also supporting the diagnosis of VT is the presence of AV dissociation. Dissociated P waves are indicated by arrows in lead II, and the first of these appears to produce a fusion QRS complex. Note also that the QRS in leads II and V_5 of the rhythm strip (bottom) is narrower and has a different morphology than in V_1.*

originating in the right ventricle, and the latter to *VT originating in the left ventricle.* However, LBBB or RBBB morphology differs from the respective patterns of QRS aberration with SVT or bundle branch block ([XXIV]Table 10–4).[2,4,5,8] By convention, the QRS complex in V_1 of VT with a LBBB configuration has a primarily negative deflection, and that of VT with a RBBB configuration a primarily positive deflection. With LBBB configuration VT, the negative deflections may also be deeper in

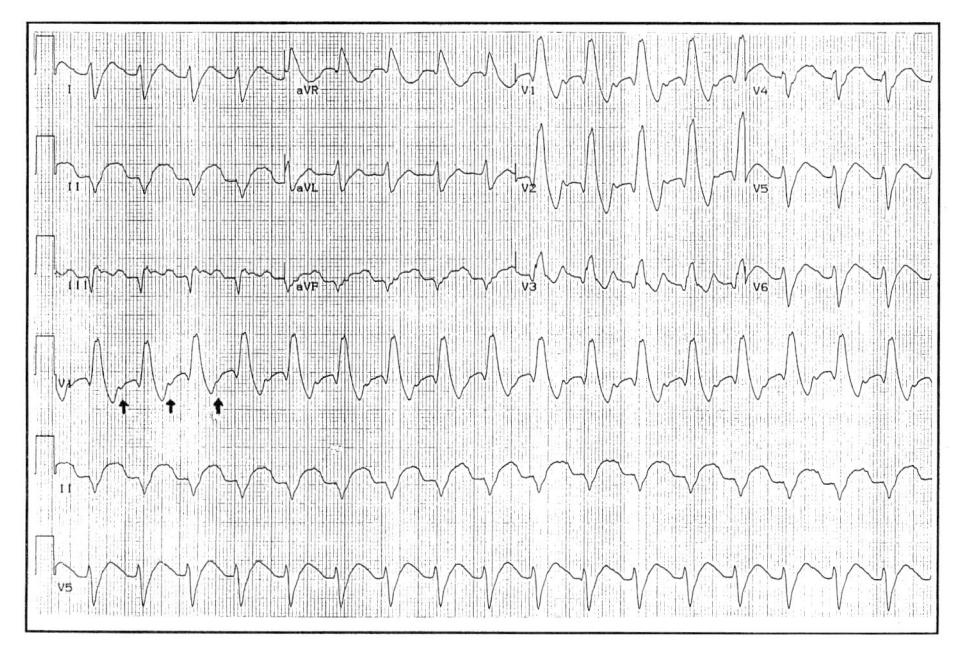

FIGURE 10-20 *VT with VA association. Note the appearance of P waves during VT. Inverted (retrograde) P waves are seen in the ST segment of all beats (leads III, aVF, V_1, V_2) during wide-QRS tachycardia. Such VA association strongly supports the diagnosis of VT. The RBBB configuration of QRS complexes in V_1 and V_6 is consistent with VT originating in the left ventricle (see text).*

TABLE 10-4 *LBBB or RBBB QRS morphology with VT Versus LBBB or RBBB aberration with SVT*

VENTRICULAR TACHYCARDIA		SUPRAVENTRICULAR TACHYCARDIA	
LBBB Morphology	RBBB Morphology	LBBB Aberration	RBBB Aberration
R wave > 0.04 sec in lead V_1 or V_2	QRS monophasic or biphasic in V_1	QS or rS in V_1 (r < 0.04 sec)	rSR' (qrSR') in V_1 and QRS < 0.14 sec
Notched downslope of S wave in V_1 or V_2	Early QRS deflection differs from NSR (V_1)	Monophasic R wave present in V_1	Sometimes a wide R or qR in V_1
Q wave in lead V_6 of any duration	R to S wave ratio < 1 or QS in V_6	No Q waves present in V_6	Wide S wave in lead V_6

NSR, normal sinus rhythm.

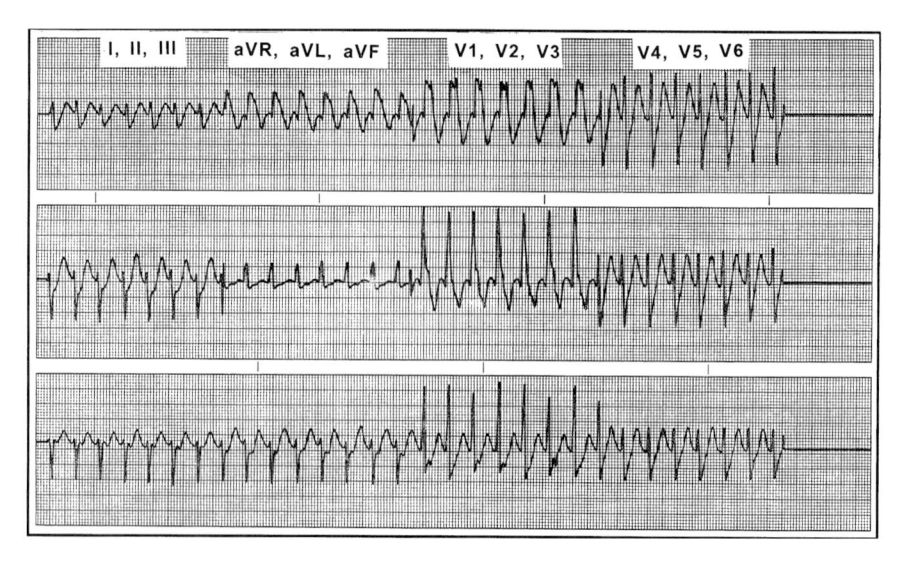

418 PREEXCITATION, VENTRICULAR ARRHYTHMIAS, AND HEART BLOCK

FIGURE 10-21 *Wide-QRS tachycardia with RBBB QRS configuration and positive QRS concordance in leads V_1 through V_6. The leads indicated are displayed from top to bottom in each quadrant. Note the QRS complexes in V_1 and V_2, and RS complexes in V_3 through V_6.*

the right compared to left precordial leads (Fig. 10-19). With RBBB configuration VT, there may be a small R and large S wave or QS pattern in V_6 (Fig. 10-20). While one authority states that 65 percent of spontaneous VT has a RBBB configuration compared to 35 percent with a LBBB configuration,[14] others suggest a more equal proportion.[4] *Positive QRS concordance* is present when all the QRS complexes are mainly upright in V_1 to V_6 (Fig. 10-21), and *negative concordance* when they are mainly negative in the same leads. Positive concordance is found in only 10 to 20 percent of VT, and in the absence of preexcitation indicates a left ventricular origin. Some consider negative concordance an unreliable criterion for VT,[4] while others consider it virtually diagnostic of right ventricular origin VT.[8] Brugada and coworkers developed to additional criteria for QRS appearance in the precordial lead for diagnosis of VT.[15] Either none of the precordial leads has an RS morphology, or with an RS morphology the interval from the onset of the QRS to the nadir of the S wave is > 0.10 second. When monitoring a right-sided lead such as MCL_1 or V_1 during wide QRS tachycardia with *QS morphology*, the nadir of the S wave is reached within 0.06 second during SVT with LBBB aberration, in contrast to > 0.06 second with right ventricular tachycardia and a LBBB pattern QRS configuration.[8] This is due to rapid activation of the right ventricle via the right bundle branch during LBBB pattern aberration compared to slower activation during VT originating in the right ventricle. Similar slow initial activation of the left ventricle during VT is indicated by a slow rise (to apex of R wave) or descent (to nadir of S wave) of the initial QRS waveform in V_6 (> 0.07 second).[8] Finally, extreme left axis deviation (–90 to –180 degrees) seldom occurs with aberrant conduction (exceptions: multiple infarction, congenital heart lesions), but commonly appears during VT arising from either ventricle. The presence of extreme QRS axis deviation during a wide-QRS tachycardia is considered strongly suggestive of VT.[8]

Capture and Fusion Beats

A hallmark of VT is the presence of capture or fusion beats. The sinus or ectopic atrial pacemaker may intermittently capture all of the ventricles during VT to cause capture beats (Fig. 10–22), or only a portion of the ventricles may be excited to produce fusion beats (Fig. 10–19). The presence of either capture or fusion beats during a wide-QRS tachycardia provides maximum support for the diagnosis of VT.

Differential Diagnosis of Wide-QRS Tachycardia

Some common sources of error in the differential diagnosis of wide-QRS tachycardias are listed in Table 10–5, and are discussed in more detail below.[2,8]

USE OF A SINGLE ECG LEAD FOR DIAGNOSIS. At least in perioperative settings, it is conventional practice to use ECG lead II for detection of P waves (arrhythmia diagnosis) and inferior wall myocardial ischemia, and lead V_4 or V_5 for detection of anterolateral ischemia. However, the QRS complex in lead II in patients with VT originating in the right ventricle (LBBB configuration) may have a similar appearance to the QRS with SVT and LBBB aberration or LBBB, and vice versa for VT originating in the left ventricle (Fig. 10–23). For this reason, a right precordial chest lead (MCL_1 or V_1) with a right-to-left orientation is better than an inferior (II, III, aVF) lead with a base-to-apex orientation. Alternatively, during anesthesia and surgery, since conventional five-lead ECG monitoring systems do not display two V leads, the left leg (positive) electrode can be relocated at the V_1 position (fourth intercostal space to right of the sternum), and lead III selected to provide a view similar to MCL_1, especially in patients considered at increased risk for tachyarrhythmias. This would provide a lead more suitable for detection of P waves and differential diagnosis of anoma-

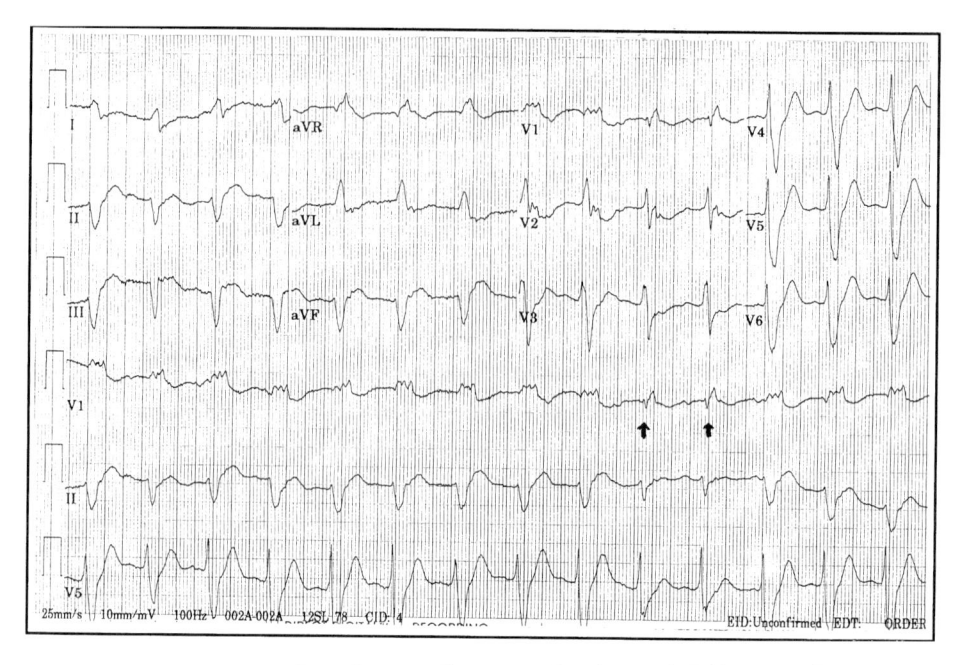

FIGURE 10-22 *Accelerated ventricular ("idioventricular") rhythm with capture beats. Note wide-QRS rhythm with RBBB morphology. Beats 10 and 11 (arrows) in the rhythm strip have a more normal appearance and are preceded by P waves, which are best seen in lead V_1. These beats are likely capture beats, possibly with minimal late QRS aberration due to fusion or an underlying intraventricular conduction defect.*

lous QRS complexes with VT or SVT, as well as a lateral precordial lead for detection of ischemia.

FIGURE 10-23 *ECG appearance of LBBB and RBBB, and VT with a LBBB or RBBB QRS configuration. (Top) Sinus rhythm with LBBB or RBBB. (Bottom) Right VT with LBBB QRS morphology (RVT-LBBB) or left ventricular tachycardia with RBBB QRS morphology (LVT-RBBB). In all panels, leads are II, III, and V_1 from top to bottom. Note that with both RVT-LBBB and LVT-RBBB, the QRS morphology in lead II is similar to that with LBBB or RBBB, respectively. This is also true for the QRS in lead III with LVT-RBBB and RBBB. However, with both RVT-LBBB and LVT-RBBB, the QRS morphology in leads V_1 differ from that of LBBB or RBBB, respectively.*

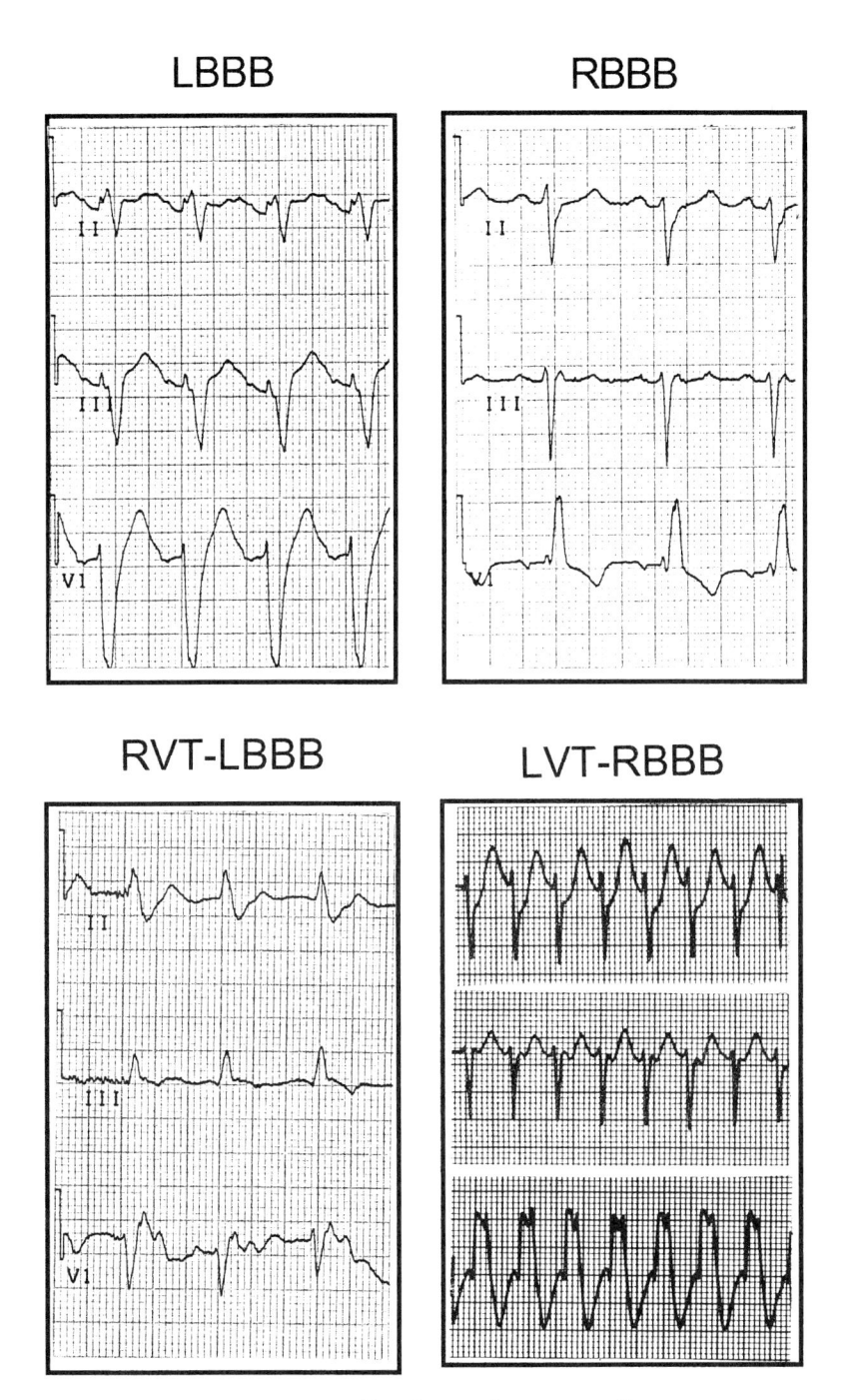

PREEXCITATION, VENTRICULAR ARRHYTHMIAS, AND HEART BLOCK **421**

LBBB

RBBB

RVT-LBBB

LVT-RBBB

FIGURE 10–23 *See legend on opposite page*

TABLE 10-5 *Errors in the differential diagnosis of wide-QRS tachycardias*

1. Relying on a single ECG lead to make the diagnosis, especially lead II.
2. Assuming that VT is hemodynamically less well tolerated than SVT.
3. Assuming that R–R-interval irregularity must be due to atrial fibrillation.
4. Depending on demonstration of independent supraventricular activity.
5. Failure to consider variations in the morphology of QRS complexes.

ASSUMPTION THAT VT IS HEMODYNAMICALLY LESS WELL TOLERATED THAN SVT. Just because a wide-QRS tachycardia is poorly tolerated does not mean that it is necessarily of ventricular origin. Both VT and SVT can be well tolerated or produce profound hemodynamic compromise. The single most important factor determining the amount of compromise is the rate of tachycardia. Even VT at 170 beats/min can be well tolerated, and some patients can withstand brief episodes of VT with rates up to 250 beats/min. However, slow VT (100 beats/min) can produce profound compromise in some patients with left severe ventricular dysfunction because of loss of AV synchrony and reduced diastolic filling. The significance of assuming that wide-QRS tachycardia is SVT, just because it is reasonably well tolerated, is that drugs used to treat SVT (verapamil, beta-blockers, adenosine) could be administered to a patient with VT, causing dangerous hemodynamic deterioration. In general, however, persistent VT in excess of 170 beats/min is likely to produce signs or symptoms of hemodynamic insufficiency, whereas SVT at the same rate may be tolerated for a longer period of time. Other factors that determine tolerance of tachycardia, regardless of whether it is VT or SVT, include the underlying heart disease, status of myocardial function, concurrent medications, and associated disease.

ASSUMING THAT R–R-INTERVAL IRREGULARITY MUST BE DUE TO ATRIAL FIBRILLATION. The R–R interval with VT may be irregular (Fig. 10–19). Although uniform VT is characteristically regular (< 20 msec cycle length variation), this is will not necessarily be the case if there is intermittent breakthrough of the atrial rhythm to produce fusion or capture beats. Also, varying discharge rates of automatic or triggered ventricular foci, functional changes in the reentry loop, autonomic factors, drugs, and physiologic imbalance might affect the cycle length of VT on a beat-to-beat basis. This applies to SVT as well, especially that caused by automatic or triggered (ectopic) foci. So, while an irregular wide-QRS tachycardia suggests underlying atrial fibrillation with aberrant ventricular conduction, or possibly ectopic atrial rhythm or atrial flutter with varying AV block, this is not invariably so. Nevertheless, beat-to-beat cycle length variation greater than 20 msec, especially with subtle changes in QRS morphology, strongly favors atrial fibrillation. With VT, on the other hand, there may be recurring, similar R–R intervals (Fig. 10–19).

DEPENDING ON DEMONSTRATION OF AV DISSOCIATION OR VA ASSOCIATION. The presence of dissociated P waves or associated retrograde P waves during a *wide*-QRS tachycardia excludes the diagnosis of SVT originating in the sinus node or incorporating an AP. However, it does not exclude SVT originating in the AV node in a patient with preexisting LBBB or RBBB fascicular heart block or an intraventricular conduction defect. However, since the aforementioned circumstances are quite unusual, and one would have to have on hand a previous ECG from the patient showing the conduction defect during sinus rhythm, it is highly probable that wide-QRS tachycardia with completely dissociated (i.e., AV dissociation) or associated (i.e., VA association) retrograde P waves *following* the QRS complex is VT. However, recall that *associated* retrograde P waves following (VA) or preceding (AV) a *narrow*-QRS tachycardia are due to the common or uncommon forms of AV node reentry (see Figs. 9–15 and 9–16), or orthodromic AV reciprocation with a concealed (Figs. 9–18) or manifest accessory AV pathway (Fig. 10–8).

FAILURE TO CONSIDER VARIATIONS IN THE MORPHOLOGY OF QRS COMPLEXES OR THEIR DURATION. It is necessary to distinguish SVT with aberration from VT if drugs such as verapamil or diltiazem are contemplated for the initial treatment of tachycardia, since these drugs have recognized potential to worsen VT or hemodynamic tolerance of VT. Electrophysiologic studies during induced tachycardia have confirmed that variations morphology with QRS aberration (Table 10–4, Fig. 10–23) can sometimes be more reliable than other criteria for differentiating aberration with SVT from VT. Also important is QRS duration > 0.14 second (Fig. 10–24), unless the patient already had impaired ventricular conduction during normal rhythm. QRS duration > 0.14 second is inconsistent with LBBB or LBBB pattern aberration.

Treatment of Ventricular Tachycardia

SUSTAINED VT. The treatment of acute episodes of VT is dictated by the degree of hemodynamic compromise and/or potential for producing VF. The sicker the patient and the greater the underlying

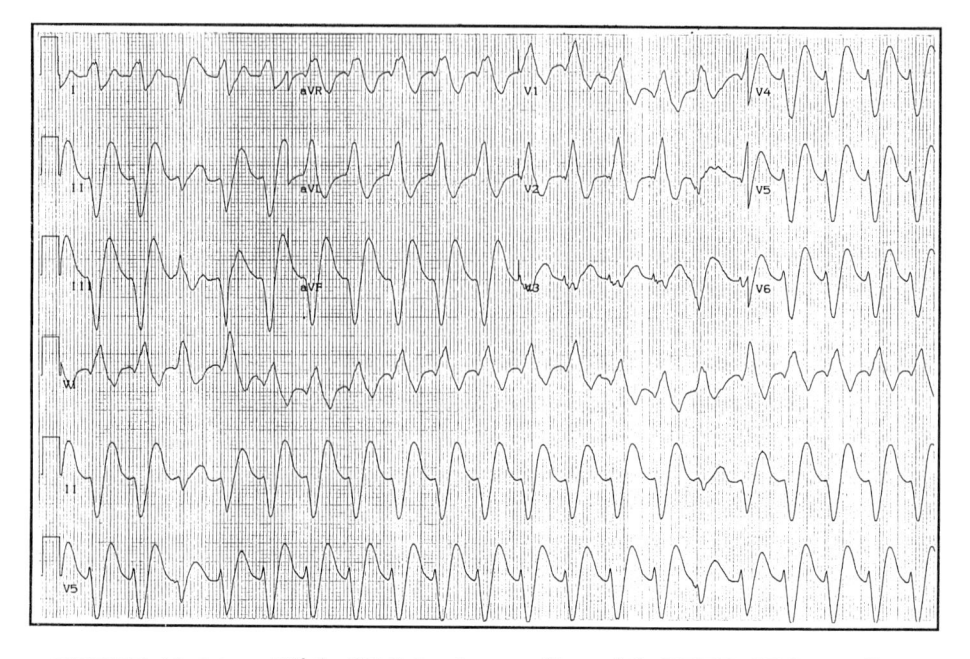

424 PREEXCITATION, VENTRICULAR ARRHYTHMIAS, AND HEART BLOCK

FIGURE 10-24 *Wide-QRS tachycardia with RBBB QRS configuration. In addition to probable fusion beats (beats 3 and 15, lead II and V$_5$ of rhythm strip), favoring the diagnosis of VT is QRS duration > 0.14 second, and near extreme left axis deviation of the QRS complex (− 83 degrees) in the frontal plane. Also note that with RS complexes in V$_4$ to V$_6$, the duration of the interval from the onset of the RS complex to the nadir of the S wave is 0.12 or 0.13 second, far greater than ≤ 0.10 second expected with aberration.[15] This too favors the diagnosis of VT.*

myocardial functional impairment, the greater the likelihood that VT will produce significant circulatory compromise or deterioration into VF. Prior to any intervention, intravenous access must be established if not available, and a working cardioverter–defibrillator obtained. Provision should also be made for tracheal intubation. While vagal maneuvers or edrophonium will not terminate or slow VT, they may convert or slow SVT with ventricular aberration. Therefore, they can be useful for differential diagnosis of wide-QRS tachycardia when there is reasonable doubt as to the mechanism. In no case should verapamil or diltiazem be administered to patients with wide-QRS tachycardia and hemodynamic impairment, unless it is certain that tachycardia is SVT. A precordial chest thump may convert some VT, most likely by stimulation of a low-energy depolarizing current.[2] If VT has produced significant hemodynamic impairment that threatens or compromises cardiac or cerebral perfusion, immediate DC cardioversion is indicated. If the patient is conscious but anxious because of dyspnea or angina with tachycardia, intravenous midazolam can be used for sedation prior to cardioversion. Time permitting, a 12-lead ECG should be obtained during tachycardia prior to conversion to assist in determination of the site of origin of VT. The initial shock should be 200 J, followed by 360-J shocks if 200 J is ineffective. Time should not be wasted with lower-energy shocks. If lower-energy shocks fail, valuable time is lost and the patient may receive more total delivered energy than is necessary. Lidocaine (Table 10–6) is effective for converting VT with myocardial ischemia or acute infarction, but not necessarily that with chronic infarction.[2] This is because tissue in the reentry loop with chronic infarction is electrophysiologically normal, and lidocaine has little effect on nondepolarized fibers (see Chapter 5). Lidocaine is also effective for VT with digitalis toxicity, catecholamines, anesthetic sensitization, and in association with cardiac surgery. For sustained VT in association with chronic infarction, intravenous procainamide (Table 10–6) is considered the drug of choice. For sustained VT with digitalis toxicity, digitalis-specific antibody fragments should be administered and are effective within minutes. Phenytoin, lidocaine, or beta-blockers are less effective.[2] Intravenous amiodarone (Table 10–6) may be effective against sustained VT, both in patients with acute or chronic myocardial infarction.[5] Amiodarone was not approved for intravenous administration in June, 1995. Bretylium (Table 10–6) is not used as a first-line drug for VT. It may worsen VT or cause VF as a result of initial catecholamine release. Finally, while ventricular extrastimuli or pacing may convert some VT, they are rarely used outside of the electrophysiology laboratory.

PREVENTION OF RECURRENCES. Deteriorating cardiac function from ischemia, hypotension, or congestive heart failure can exacerbate sustained VT. Treatment of these conditions often increases success with other treatment, and lessens the likelihood of recurrences. Hypokalemia and hypomagnesemia can also exacerbate VT, and should be corrected if identified. Some VT occurs in association with bradycardia and premature VES. Atropine, isoproterenol, or preferably temporary bradycardia pacing may be effective in preventing recurrences of bradycardia-dependent VT. Drugs prescribed for prevention of recurrences of VT are usually guided by invasive electrophysiologic studies. Drugs used for prevention of recurrences include class 1A (quinidine-like), 1C (propafenone, flecainide), beta-blockers, and amiodarone. Finally, catheter or surgical ablative therapy, or an implantable cardioverter–defibrillator may be used in patients who are refractory to drugs, or to reduce the requirement for drugs.[16]

TABLE 10-6 *Doses and adverse effects of drugs used in the acute management of VT*

DRUG	DOSE (IV)	ADVERSE EFFECT
Lidocaine	B: 1.0 mg/kg, then 0.5 mg/kg q 5–10 min up to 3.0 mg/kg total I: 1–4 mg/min	Paresthesias, tinnitus, dizziness, confusion, somnolence, seizures
Procainamide	20 mg/min to total of 1.0 g	Hypotension; QRS prolongation* and proarrhythmia (torsades)
Bretylium	B: 5–10 mg/kg over 2 min I: 1–2 mg/min	Hypotension; initial catecholamine release triggered VF
Amiodarone	5–10 mg/kg over 20 to 30 min; then 1.0 g/day for several days†	Bradycardia, hypotension, worsen congestive heart failure, ventricular proarrhythmia, interactions with inhalation anesthetics‡

B, bolus; I, infusion.
*Stop if QRS prolonged by more than 50 percent.
†Suggested dosing,[16] but was not approved for intravenous administration as of June 1995.
‡AVJR or complete AV heart block, low cardiac output syndrome, alpha-adrenergic blockade resistant to alpha-adrenergic agonists.

SPECIFIC VENTRICULAR TACHYCARDIA PATTERNS AND ASSOCIATIONS

Accelerated Idioventricular Rhythm

Idioventricular rhythm faster than 60 beats/min is accelerated idioventricular rhythm (AVIR). Usually, the rate is under 110 beats/min. While AVIR may begin with a premature ventricular beat, it commonly has a more gradual (nonparoxysmal) onset and termination than other VT, in keeping with its supposed mechanism—altered normal or abnormal automaticity. The slow rate and nonparoxysmal onset avoid the problems initiated by excitation during the ventricular vulnerable period, so that precipitation of more rapid VT is rarely seen in patients with AVIR.[5] The rate of AVIR may be nearly the same as the atrial rate, so that there may be competition between pacemakers for control of the ventricles (Fig. 10–22), particularly at the onset and termination of AVIR. AVIR is common in the setting of acute myocardial infarction, following cardiopulmonary bypass (CPB), with reperfusion of ischemic myocardium, and with digitalis toxicity. AVIR is almost invariably a transient rhythm disturbance. Other associations are with acute rheumatic heart disease and cardiomyopathy. Vagal stimulation may slow the rate of AVIR. AVIR is often hemodynamically well tolerated, so that no special treatment is required. Following reperfusion of ischemic myocardium or CPB, it may not be. In the latter circumstance, return to CPB for a period of time, and removal of obvious air from the heart and coronary arteries, may be all that is required to terminate AVIR. It is also necessary to correct any other obvious imbalance, including acid–base and temperature imbalance, hypokalemia, and hypomagnesemia. If these measures fail and AVIR is poorly tolerated, do not rely on atropine or other chronotropes (Table 9–2) to increase sinus rate or the rate of AVIR. Usually they don't, but accelerate the disturbance instead. Instead, temporary atrial or AV sequential overdrive pacing is used. Improved hemodynamics following restoration of AV synchrony, as well as rate optimization, usually prevent recurrence of AVIR following *gradual* weaning from pacing. This may take anywhere from several minutes to many hours.

Torsades de Pointes and Polymorphic Ventricular Tachycardia

The term *torsades de pointes* is reserved for VT that occurs in association with corrected QT-interval prolongation (≥ 0.50 second). It is characterized by QRS complexes of changing amplitude that appear to twist around the isoelectric line at a rate of 160 to 300 beats/min (Fig. 10–25).[2,5] VT that has the same appearance as torsades de pointes, but which occurs in patients without QT-interval prolongation, is classified as *polymorphic ventricular tachycardia* (PMVT) (Fig. 10–26). This distinction is important, because it has implications for therapeutics (below). The postulated mechanism for torsades de pointes VT is triggered automaticity from early afterdepolarizations, perhaps in association with ventricular reentry due to dispersion of repolarization. The mechanism for PMVT is likely ventricular reentry. Two forms of torsades de pointes VT are recognized. The first is *adrenergic-dependent torsades de pointes*, which is seen in patients with the congenital long-QT-interval syndrome. The second is *pause* or *bradycardia-dependent torsades*, which typically occurs in patients with acquired rather than congenital QT-interval prolongation. Potential causes for the acquired QT-interval prolongation and torsades de pointes are listed in Table 10–7.

ACUTE MANAGEMENT OF TORSADES DE POINTES OR PMVT. Acute management for these arrhythmias is similar, except that *antiarrhyth-*

428 PREEXCITATION, VENTRICULAR ARRHYTHMIAS, AND HEART BLOCK

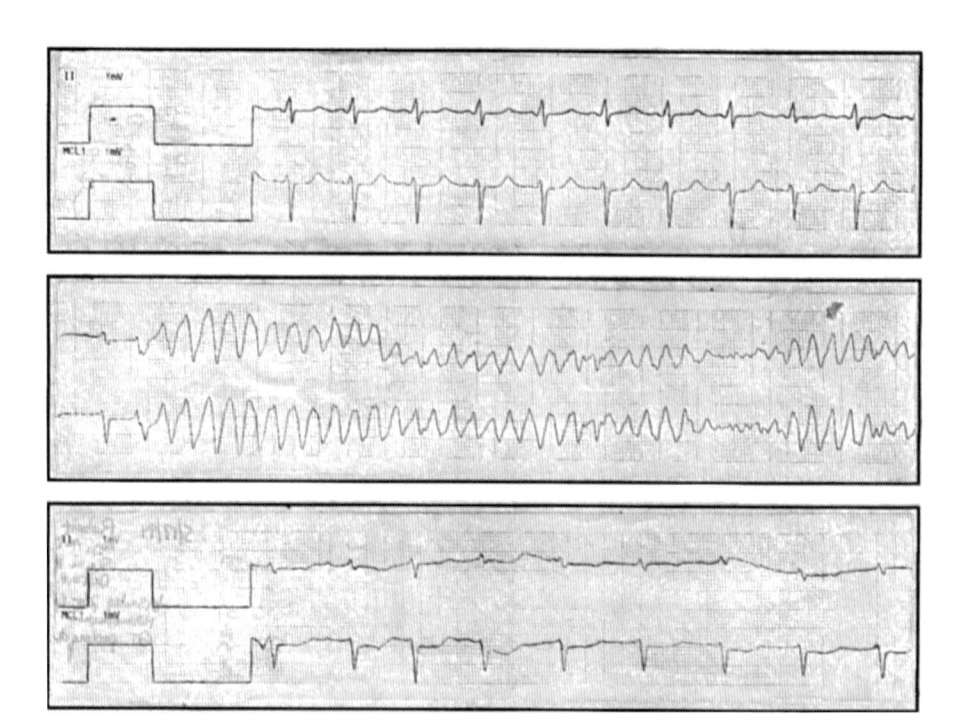

FIGURE 10-25 *Torsades de pointes VT in a male patient following CPB. (Top) The QT and QTc intervals in leads II and MCL$_1$ during ectopic atrial or sinus rhythm (68 beats/min) are 0.52 and 0.53 second, respectively. (Middle) Tracing contiguous with previous tracing. Torsades de pointes VT begins with a premature VES. The rate of torsades is between 230 and 300 beats/min. (Bottom) Later, the patient has returned to sinus rhythm. The QT and QTc intervals have shortened to 0.45 and 0.51 second, respectively. (Tracings supplied by Dr. Robert Murray, Sinai Hospital, Detroit, MI.)*

mic drugs that prolong the QT interval (Table 10-7) are withheld in patients with acquired QT-interval prolongation.[2,16]

Torsades de Pointes. Intravenous magnesium sulfate has become the initial treatment of choice for torsades de pointes, regardless of whether it occurs in the setting of acquired or congenital QT-interval prolongation. Lidocaine or phenytoin (not procainamide) might be tried if magnesium is ineffective. Pacing to increase the heart rate with either form of torsades may help prevent recurrences of tachycardia, and isoproterenol is sometime used to increase the heart rate until pacing can be instituted. Cardioversion or defibrillation may be required to

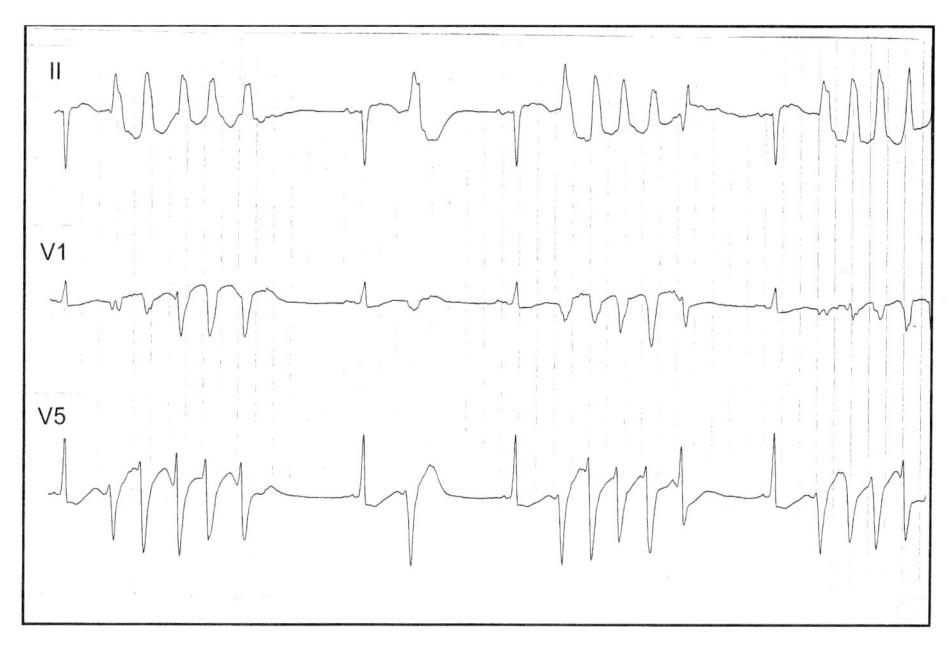

PREEXCITATION, VENTRICULAR ARRHYTHMIAS, AND HEART BLOCK **429**

FIGURE 10-26 *Nonsustained polymorphic VT in patient without QT-interval prolongation. In V_5, the QT and QTc intervals are 0.48 and 0.46 second, respectively.*

TABLE 10-7 *Some causes for acquired QT-interval prolongation and torsades de pointes*

ANTIARRHYTHMICS & CARDIAC	OTHER DRUGS	MISCELLANEOUS
Type 1A (quinidine-like)	MAO inhibitors	Weight loss and cachexia
Mexiletine (not other 1A)	Tricyclic antidepressants	Liquid-protein diets
Type 1C (flecainide-like)	Phenothiazines, lithium	Subarachnoid hemorrhage
Amiodarone, sotalol	Ampicillin, erythromycin	Stroke, encephalitis
Mitral valve prolapse, CAD	Alpha-blockers	Hypokalemia, hypocalcemia
Myocarditis, cardiomyopathy	Chloral hydrate	Hypomagnesemia

terminate torsades with congenital QT-interval prolongation. However, because torsades in patients with acquired QT-interval prolongation is recurrent and commonly terminates spontaneously, cardioversion or defibrillation are not usually required. Potassium-channel activators (e.g., pinacidil, chromakalim) may become useful for treatment or prevention of recurrences of torsades de pointes in the future.[5]

Polymorphic Ventricular Tachycardia. For PMVT, standard antiarrhythmic drugs for VT, including those that prolong the QT interval (Table 10–7), can be administered. However, in doubtful cases, where the QT interval is at the upper limits of normal, pacing and/or magnesium are preferred. Isoproterenol is contraindicated for increasing heart rate to prevent recurrences of bradycardia-dependent torsades or PMVT in any patient with coronary artery disease.

CHRONIC MANAGEMENT OF TORSADES DE POINTES OR PMVT. Chronic treatment for torsades de pointes differs for the congenital (adrenergic-dependent) and acquired (pause- or bradycardia-dependent) forms. Management PMVT is similar to that for prevention of recurrences of ventricular tachycardia in patients with coronary artery disease.

Congenital (Adrenergic-Dependent) Torsades de Pointes. With the congenital form of torsades de pointes, no therapy is recommended unless the patient has a history of syncope or complex ventricular arrhythmias, or a family history of sudden death.[5] For asymptomatic patients with complex ventricular arrhythmias or a family history of early sudden death, beta-adrenergic drugs are prescribed at maximally tolerated doses. These should be continued through the perioperative period. For patients with syncope, a class 1B antiarrhythmic may be added. If symptoms persist, despite maximum drug therapy, left stellate ganglionectomy is performed, sometimes along with permanent pacemaker implantation to increase heart rate. An implantable cardioverter–defibrillator is used to prevent sudden death in patients who are resistant to all of the preceding measures.

Acquired (Pause-Dependent) Torsades de Pointes. With torsades de pointes and acquired QT-interval prolongation, metabolic conditions or drugs that produce or aggravate the condition (Table 10–7) must be corrected, removed, or avoided. Since these provide a cure for torsades de pointes, no other special long-term treatment is needed.

Polymorphic Ventricular Tachycardia. Patients with PMVT often have coronary artery disease (CAD), and conventional drug, medical interventional, or surgical treatment for CAD is prescribed. Conventional antiarrhythmic drugs, including those that prolong the QT interval (Table 10-7), can be used for prevention of PMVT recurrences.

Nonsustained Ventricular Tachycardia

Nonsustained (< 30 seconds) VT (NSVT) usually occurs in patients with structural heart disease. It occurs in less than 5 percent of asymptomatic, apparently healthy individuals, and 5 to 10 percent of patients with CAD.[2] Also, 20 percent of patients with hypertrophic cardiomyopathy and 40 percent with idiopathic dilated cardiomyopathy have NSVT.[2] *Repetitive monomorphic ventricular tachycardia* is a term used to describe an incessant form of NSVT with only brief interludes of sinus rhythm.[5] The appearance, except for uniform QRS complexes, is similar to that of nonsustained polymorphic VT (Fig. 10-26). The rate of NSVT ranges between 100 and 200 beats/min, and sometimes higher. Blood pressure and cardiac output decrease during NSVT, with the amount of decrease dependent on the rate and duration of tachycardia and underlying myocardial function. Acute treatment is the same as for VT not occurring in association with QT-interval prolongation, but is reserved for patients with hemodynamic compromise or symptomatic arrhythmias. Preventive management includes beta-blockers or other antiarrhythmic drugs guided by electrophysiologic evaluation of effect on inducibility of NSVT.

VENTRICULAR FLUTTER AND FIBRILLATION

Prevalence

Ventricular fibrillation is the most common cause of sudden cardiac death, and accounts for 65 to 85 percent of out-of-hospital arrests.[2,5,12,13] Approximately 350,000 persons die from cardiac arrest each year in the United States. In cases reported in the literature where ambulatory monitoring recorded sudden death, VF developed in 62 percent of cases after VT, VF was the initial arrhythmia in 8 percent, and torsades de pointes in 13 percent.[17] Bradyarrhythmias accounted for the rest. Thus, primary or secondary VF might account for approximately 250,000 of those sudden deaths in the United States each year. In hospitalized patients, particularly those with impaired hemodynamics, VF accounts for a smaller proportion of deaths because of the fact that lesser arrhythmias are treated aggressively before they can evolve into VF. Patients who have acute myocardial infarction and VF have a 2 percent incidence of sudden death within the first year.[5] Some factors that increase the risk of sudden death from VF are summarized in Table 10-8, along with predictors of sudden death for resuscitated patients.[5]

TABLE 10-8 *Factors that increase the risk of sudden death from VF, or that predict death for patients who have been successfully resuscitated from VF*

INCREASE RISK SUDDEN DEATH	PREDICT SUDDEN DEATH
Persistent myocardial ischemia	Reduced LV ejection fraction
Reduced LV ejection fraction	Wall motion abnormalities
Spontaneous or inducible VT	History of congestive heart failure
Hypertension and LV hypertrophy	History of MI but not acute event
Smoking, obesity, male sex, increased age	Presence of ventricular arrhythmias
	Anterior MI complicated by VF*
Elevated cholesterol, excessive alcohol	

LV, left ventricular.
*Subgroup at especially high risk.

Electrocardiographic Appearance and Clinical Setting

Ventricular flutter and fibrillation are hemodynamically ineffective rhythms that terminate fatally within several minutes unless treated. Also, ventricular flutter almost invariably deteriorates into VF. Therefore, the distinction between ventricular flutter and fibrillation is moot and primarily of academic interest. Ventricular flutter presents as an orderly, wide-QRS, sine wave tachycardia at 150 to 300 beats/min, commonly about 200 beats/min (Fig. 10-27). P waves are absent or unidentifiable. With VF, there are irregular undulations of varying contour and amplitude, also without discreet P waves (Fig. 10-27). With coarse fibrillation, waveforms are > 0.2 mV, while with fine fibrillation they are < 0.2 mV.[2] The amplitude of waveforms with fibrillation is usually larger at the onset of the disturbance. Distinct ST segments and T waves are absent with both ventricular flutter and fibrillation. Hereafter, ventricular flutter-fibrillation are collectively referred to as VF. VF can be primary or secondary.[2] Primary VF develops because of specific electrophysiologic abnormalities (substrate) in the absence of hemodynamic factors severe enough to initiate the arrhythmia. However, other factors (e.g., hypoxia, reperfusion of ischemic myocardium, electrolyte imbalance, autonomic, drugs) may interact with the substrate to cause electrical destabilization and VF. Secondary VF is the result of severe cardiac damage producing unrelenting circulatory deterioration. The distinction between primary and secondary VF is important, since primary VF is often reversible with prompt treatment, while secondary VF is usually fatal because of the irreversible course of hemodynamic deterioration.

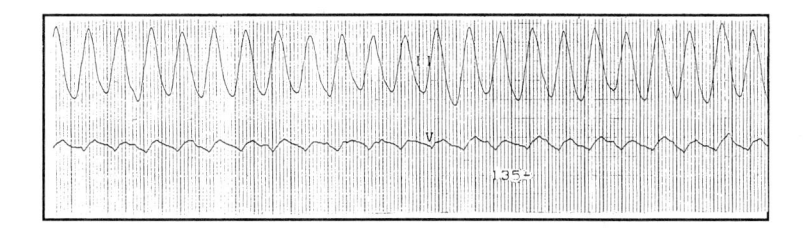

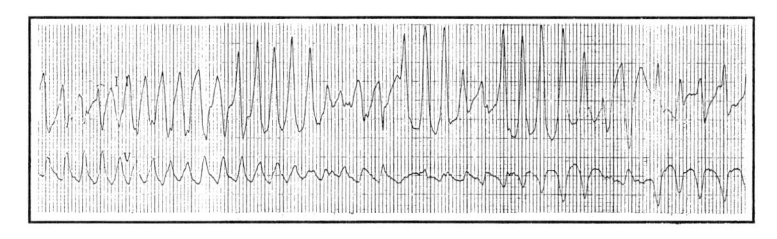

PREEXCITATION, VENTRICULAR ARRHYTHMIAS, AND HEART BLOCK **433**

FIGURE 10-27   *Ventricular flutter and fibrillation. (Top) Ventricular flutter at approximately 175 beats/min. Note orderly QRS complexes and the absence of distinct T waves and ST segments. (Bottom) Coarse ventricular fibrillation. In addition to the absence of distinct T waves or ST segments, QRS complexes vary in contour, amplitude and regularity.*

Treatment of Ventricular Flutter–Fibrillation

Once the diagnosis of VF has been made, immediate nonsynchronized DC shock (defibrillation) using 200 to 400 J is mandatory treatment for VF.[2,5] Cardiopulmonary resuscitation (CPR) is employed only until defibrillation equipment is readied. Time should not be wasted with CPR if electrical defibrillation can be done promptly.[5] Neither should time be wasted attempting to obtain an ECG to determine whether asystole or VF is present. Assume that VF is present and administer the shock as soon as possible. The longer one waits to deliver the shock, the less likely it is to be effective, or the more current will be required. DC defibrillation may cause the asystolic heart to resume beating, or it will terminate VF if the latter is present. If following conversion to sinus rhythm the circulation is inadequate, advanced life support should be instituted. Also, measures to prevent recurrences of VF (i.e., those for VT or other arrhythmias that precipitate VF) should be instituted. If VF is converted to a hemodynamically effective rhythm within 30 to 60 seconds, significant acidosis does not develop and sodium bicarbonate is not required. Intravenous calcium is generally reserved for hypocalcemia or calcium-channel blocker overdose, and sometimes for electromechanical dissociation. Antiarrhythmic drugs used to prevent recurrences of VF include lidocaine, bretylium, procainamide, and amiodarone (Table 10–6).

Heart Block

Heart block is a temporary or permanent disturbance of cardiac impulse propagation owing to functional or anatomic impairment.[2-5,8,18,19] It is distinguished from *interference*, a normal physiologic phenomenon, whereby impulse propagation is delayed or blocked as a result of persistent refractoriness from the previous impulse. Interference can occur anywhere impulses are conducted within the heart, but is most commonly recognized as occurring within the AV node. AV block may occur within the atria, AV node, His bundle, or bundle and fascicular branches. Demonstration of such localized block requires cardiac electrophysiologic study. Therefore, for clinical purposes, only two regions of abnormal conduction are usually recognized. These are within the AV node (intranodal block) or more distal tissues of the specialized AV conducting system (infranodal block). The diagnosis of intranodal or infranodal block can usually be made from the appearance of the surface ECG and clinical circumstances. However, in some cases, cardiac electrophysiologic study may also be required.

ATRIOVENTRICULAR BLOCK

Atrioventricular heart block is diagnosed when atrial impulses are conducted to the ventricles with delay (first-degree AV block), some atrial impulses are blocked (second-degree AV block), or all atrial impulses are blocked (third-degree AV block). With second-degree AV block, two patterns of conduction may be seen. With *type I (Wenckebach) block*, gradual PR-interval prolongation occurs prior to nonconducted atrial beats. With *type II (Mobitz) block*, the PR interval remains unchanged prior to dropped atrial beats. Type II block with two or more successive dropped beats is referred to as *advanced heart block*. For diagnosis of AV heart block, delayed or blocked impulse transmission must not result from interference caused by recovery from previous excitation. Causes or conditions associated with AV heart block are listed in Table 10–9.

TABLE 10-9 *Causes or conditions associated with AV heart block*

Idiopathic degeneration/fibrosis	Congenital complete AV bock
Coronary artery disease*	Atrial septal defect (secundum)
After aortic or mitral valve surgery	Following repair of TOGV
Lyme disease, bacterial endocarditis	Rheumatic heart disease
Chagasitic myocarditis†	Cardiomyopathies, tumors
Drug-prolonged AV conduction	Hyperkalemia, hypothermia
Hypothyroidism (myxedema)	Infiltrative processes‡
Rheumatoid nodules	Calcific aortic stenosis

TOGV, transposition of great vessels.
*Acute MI and chronic CAD.
†Common cause in Central and South America.
‡Sarcoidosis, amyloidosis, scleroderma.

First-Degree Atrioventricular Heart Block

With first-degree AV block, every impulse is transmitted to the ventricles, but with delay. The PR interval is longer than 0.21 second in adults and 0.18 second in children at resting heart rates, but rarely exceeds 0.30 second in asymptomatic persons (Fig. 10–28). PR intervals as long as 1.0 second have been noted with extreme first-degree AV block.[5] For diagnosis of *primary* first-degree AV block, the patient must not be receiving drugs that prolong AV conduction time, including digitalis, beta- and calcium-channel blockers, class IA and IC antiarrhythmic drugs, and amiodarone. Based on clinical reports and electrophysiologic investigation in chronically instrumented dogs with a conscious control, potent inhalation anesthetics, sedative hypnotics, or opiates alone or in combination are unlikely to produce appreciable AV conduction delay (> 0.05 second) with clinically useful doses at heart rates below 100 beats/min.[20–23] However with tachycardia in excess of 120 beats/min, and even normal heart rates with verapamil, diltiazem, beta-blockers, or high-dose opiate anesthesia, it is possible that there may be appreciable PR-interval prolongation due to AV nodal conduction delay, and even dropped beats (type I, second-degree AV block). Primary first-degree AV block can result from conduction delay in the atria (rare), AV node, His–Purkinje system, or both sites. With calcium-channel blockers, beta-blockers, and anesthetic drugs, however, delay is primarily at the AV node. Also, if the QRS complex has a normal appearance and duration in the surface ECG, AV delay almost always is in the AV node.

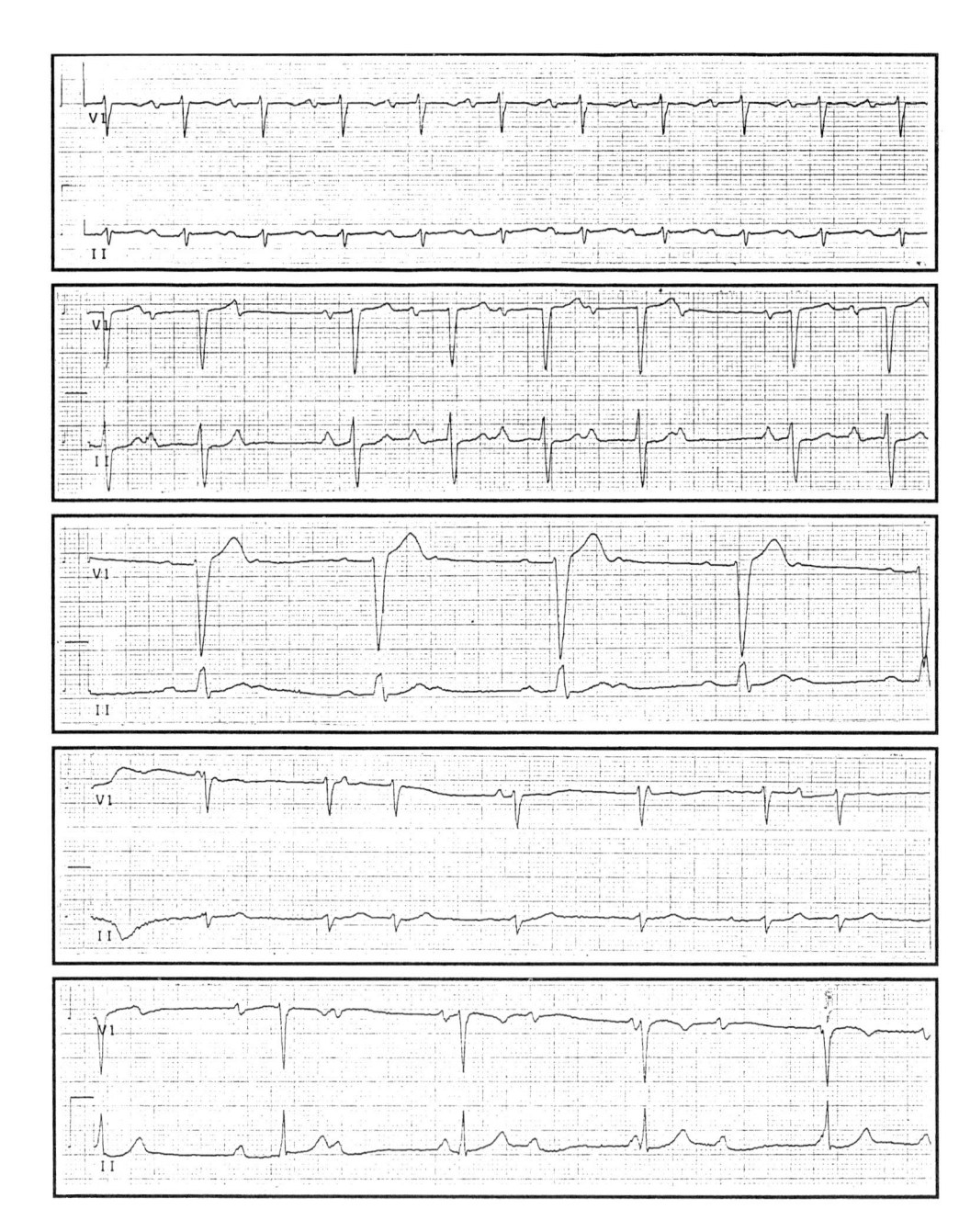

FIGURE 10–28 *See legend on opposite page*

With PR-interval prolongation and a widened QRS complex, there may also be disease in the His bundle or two of the three fascicular branches (discussed later), with delayed conduction in the remaining fascicle. The incidence of first-degree AV block can be as high as 2 percent in healthy young individuals.[8] In a 7-year follow-up study of 1893 males between 40 and 59 years of age, there was a 5.3 percent incidence of first-degree AV block unrelated to ischemic heart disease or the patient's prognosis.[24] First-degree AV block occurs in approximately 8 percent of patients with acute MI.[2]

Type I, Second-Degree Atrioventricular Heart Block

Type I, second-degree (Wenckebach) AV block with a normal QRS complex is almost invariably due to conduction delay within the AV node. The exception is the uncommon patient with infrahisian block, but this requires invasive electrophysiologic study to verify.[2,3,5] With type I, second-degree AV block, there can be as few as 3 to 10 or more conducted atrial beats prior to dropped beats. The more common P-to-QRS ratios with Wenckebach block are 3:2, 4:3, 5:4, 6:5 and 8:7. The second rhythm strip from the top in Figure 10–28 exhibits several characteristic features of type I, second-degree AV heart block: (1) there is progressive PR-interval prolongation prior to dropped beats; (2) the greatest increment in conduction time during progressive

---

FIGURE 10–28 *AV heart block.* **(Top)** *Sinus rhythm with first-degree AV heart block. The rate is 88 beats/min and the PR interval 0.28 second.* **(Top Middle)** *Sinus rhythm with type I, second-degree (Wenckebach) AV heart block. The greatest increment in conduction time is for the second beat of the Wenckebach grouping (beats 3 to 6). PR intervals for beats 3 to 6 are 0.23, 0.33, 0.37, and 0.41 second, respectively.* **(Middle)** *Sinus rhythm with type II, second-degree AV block, with 2:1 AV conduction. The PR interval is constant for conducted beats.* **(Bottom Middle)** *Advanced second-degree AV heart block. QRS complexes with short preceding R–R intervals are probably conducted atrial beats. Beats with long preceding R–R intervals are beats of junctional escape rhythm. Even though the fourth beat has a PR interval of 0.13 second, it is unlikely that it results from a propagated sinus impulse.* **(Bottom)** *Congenital complete (third-degree) AV block with AV dissociation. The atria are controlled by the sinus node, and the ventricles by a junctional pacemaker. Note the relatively constant R–R compared to P–P intervals.*

PR-interval prolongation is between the first and second beats of the Wenckebach grouping; (3) the duration of the pause produced by the nonconducted beat is less than twice the interval preceding the dropped beat; and (4) the cycle between the first two beats of the Wenckebach grouping is longer than the cycle preceding the dropped beat. In the patient with acute myocardial infarction, type I, second-degree AV block usually occurs with inferior wall and/or right ventricular infarction. This is not surprising, since in 83 percent of hearts, the AV node is supplied by a branch of the right coronary artery that arises proximal to the posterior descending branch.[2] In the other 17 percent, it is supplied by a branch of the left circumflex coronary artery. Also, in patients with right CAD, regardless of whether there has been a previous infarction, the AV node does not conduct as well as in patients without such disease.[25] Following acute inferior infarction, AV block usually develops within the first 48 hours and is transient, usually lasting only a few days, but occasionally up to several weeks. The long-term prognosis of patients with acute inferior wall infarction and type I or more advanced second-degree AV block is more related to the degree of ventricular dysfunction than to AV block itself. Finally, the incidence of second-degree AV heart block (type I or II) is much lower than for first-degree block.[2] It is rare in healthy adults, but Wenckebach periods may be observed in up to 10 percent of healthy children. Approximately 1 percent of hospitalized patients, and 3 percent of patients with heart disease have second-degree AV block. Second-degree AV block (type I or II) develops in approximately 5 percent of patients with acute myocardial infarction.

Type II, Second-Degree and Advanced Atrioventricular Heart Block

With type II, second-degree AV block, dropped atrial beats are not preceded by progressive PR-interval prolongation (Fig. 10–28). With advanced AV block (Fig. 10–28), there is block of two or more beats in succession (e.g., 3:1 or 4:1 conduction). Either type II or advanced second-degree block is more likely due to disease within the infranodal conduction system. Two-to-one and 3:1 AV block with narrow QRS complexes, in which Wenckebach periods are not seen, are produced primarily by conduction block within the His bundle.[2,3] With bundle branch block or fascicular QRS aberration, block is usually distal to the His bundle. While type II, second-degree AV block with a narrow QRS complex and 3:2 or higher atrial-to-ventricular conduction can be due to infrahisian AV block, it is more likely due to type I intranodal block, which exhibits small increments in AV conduction time.[5] Also, type II, second-degree or higher AV block with acute inferior myocardial infarction is associated with more myocardial damage and a higher mortality rate compared to patients without AV heart block.[5] Type II, second-degree AV block often antedates the development of Adams–Stokes syncope and third-degree AV heart block.[2,3,5] In contrast, type I AV block with a normal QRS has a more benign course, and does not progress to higher-degree AV heart block. However, in older persons with type I AV block, with or without bundle branch block, the clinical course may be more similar to that with type II AV block.

Complete Atrioventricular Heart Block

Complete or third-degree AV block occurs when no atrial beats are conducted to the ventricles, so that the atria and ventricles are controlled by separate pacemakers. The atrial pacemaker can be sinus, ectopic, AV junctional (with retrograde atrial activation), or the mechanism responsible for SVT (e.g., ectopic atrial tachycardia, reentry SVT, atrial flutter–fibrillation). The ventricles are controlled by a pacemaker just distal to the site of block, which may be the AV node with congenital third-degree AV block, or distal to the His bundle with acquired third-degree AV block. QRS morphology depends on the location of the pacemaker controlling the ventricles. If within or proximal to the His bundle, the QRS will be normal (narrow) in the absence of lower conduction defects. If distal to the His bundle, the QRS complex will be abnormal (widened). The rate of escape rhythm with third-degree AV block tends to be slower with more distal escape pacemakers. With acquired third-degree AV block, the ventricular rate is often 40 beats/min or less. With congenital third-degree AV block, since the pacemaker is commonly junctional, the rate is faster, often between 40 and 60 beats/min (Fig. 10–28). However, the junctional escape rate tends to be slower in adults than children. While the rate of the junctional or ventricular escape pacemaker is usually quite regular, it can vary as a result of changes in autonomic tone, pacemaker location, or the effect of premature beats originating in tissue distal to the site of AV block. Asymptomatic third-degree AV block is rare in normal adults (< 1 in 70,000).[2] Congenital third-degree AV block occurs in 1 in 15,000 to 25,000 live births.[2] Idiopathic, progressive fibrosis of the AV conducting system is the most common cause of acquired third-degree and other degrees of AV block. Other causes are listed in Table 10–9. Complete AV heart block develops in 12 percent of patients with inferior infarctions, and 2 percent of those with anterior infarctions.[2] It, and lesser degrees of AV block, rarely occur with non-Q-wave (subendocardial) infarction.

Treatment for Atrioventricular Heart Block

Indications for temporary or permanent pacing in patients with AV heart block were discussed in Chapter 6. In summary, AV heart block is generally not treated unless there are symptoms due to hemodynamic insufficiency, or vital organ perfusion is threatened or impaired by bradycardia and/or escape rhythms. For temporary management, chronotropic drugs (see Table 9–2) are sometimes used. However, if a means for temporary pacing (see Chapter 7) is available, or pacing can easily be instituted, pacing is usually preferred to chronotropic drugs. The exception is that chronotropes can be effective for temporary reversal of drug- or autonomic-related conduction defects at the sinoatrial margins or within the AV node. Anticholinergic drug efficacy will depend on the contribution of the vagus to delayed conduction, and beta-adrenergic efficacy to whether AV conduction or ectopic pacemaker automaticity is significantly influenced by the sympathetic nervous system. Therefore, chronotropic drugs are expected to have little effect on conduction or automaticity in His–Purkinje or ventricular tissue. Finally, with temporary or permanent pacing for AV heart block, modes that preserve atrial function should be used whenever possible.

FASCICULAR HEART BLOCK

Electrocardiographic Appearance

The infrahisian conduction system is trifascicular, composed of the right and left bundle branches, and the anterior and posterior divisions of the left bundle branch. If AV conduction is intact, *unifascicular heart block* is recognized as RBBB (Fig. 10–29), left anterior fascicular block (Fig. 10–30), or left posterior fascicular block (Fig. 10–31). *Bifascicular block* is LBBB (Fig. 10–32) or RBBB with left anterior (Fig. 10–33) or posterior (Fig. 10–34) fascicular block. ECG criteria for unifascicular and bifascicular heart block are summarized in Table 10–10.[8,19] Left posterior fascicular block is almost invariably associated with RBBB.[26] Left posterior fascicular block, alone or in combination with RBBB, is rare.[18]

Significance

Most patients with acquired complete AV heart block and idioventricular escape rhythm have reached this condition as a result of progressive disease in the bundle or fascicular branches of the infrahisian conduction system.[2,4,8] Support for this contention is that conducted beats have bifascicular QRS morphology in more than

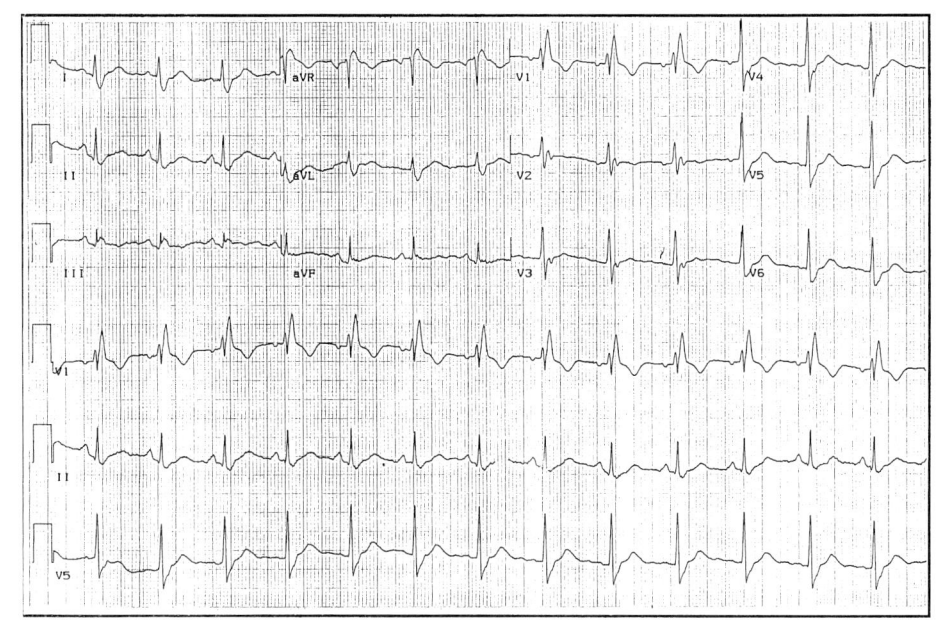

FIGURE 10-29 *Right bundle branch block. The QRS duration in V_1 is 0.15 second. Note the characteristic RSR′ complex in V_1 and wide S waves in leads I, V_5, and V_6.*

one-half of patients with transient or permanent complete AV heart block.[2] Most patients with RBBB and left axis deviation, and no symptoms attributable to bradycardia, do not develop advanced degrees of AV block, even during anesthesia and surgery. However, in patients with RBBB and left anterior or posterior fascicular block, high-degree AV block will *eventually* develop in from 6 to 30 or 10 percent of patients, respectively.[2] Few patients with LBBB and normal PR intervals develop complete AV block, although the likelihood increases as the PR interval lengthens. Bifascicular block is more likely to progress to high degrees of AV block in older patients and those with severe heart disease. Importantly, from the perspective of perioperative management, no study to date has shown that bifascicular heart block without PR-interval prolongation, including LBBB, is likely to progress to high-degree AV block during anesthesia and surgery. This is not to say that transient complete AV heart block might not occur during advancement of pulmonary artery catheters in the right ventricle in patients with LBBB. Therefore, prophylactic perioperative pacing does not appear warranted in asymptomatic patients with isolated fascicular or bifascicular heart block. This also assumes that

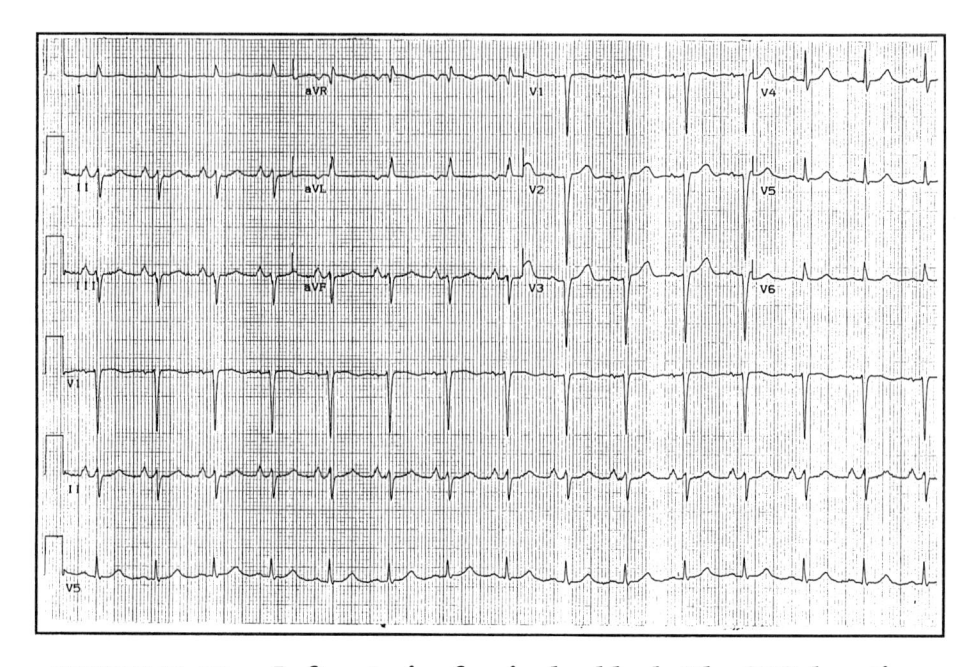

FIGURE 10-30 *Left anterior fascicular block. The QRS duration is 0.09 second. Note the rS complex in leads II, III, and aVF, and qR complex in I and aVL. The QRS axis in the frontal plane is − 65 degrees.*

the patient suffers no direct injury to the specialized conduction system during surgery or acute perioperative myocardial infarction. Finally, patients with preexisting bundle branch and fascicular blocks develop complete AV block more commonly during acute myocardial infarction than do patients with normal ventricular conduction.[2]

Atrioventricular Dissociation

Atrioventricular dissociation, independent or dissociated beating of the atria and ventricles, is *never* a primary rhythm disturbance.[5] Namely, one cannot make the diagnosis of AV dissociation. It must be stated that AV dissociation is present and due to one or a combination of the following causes: (1) default of a slower primary pacemaker, allowing escape of a secondary pacemaker; (2) usurpation of control of the ventricles from the primary pacemaker by a faster secondary

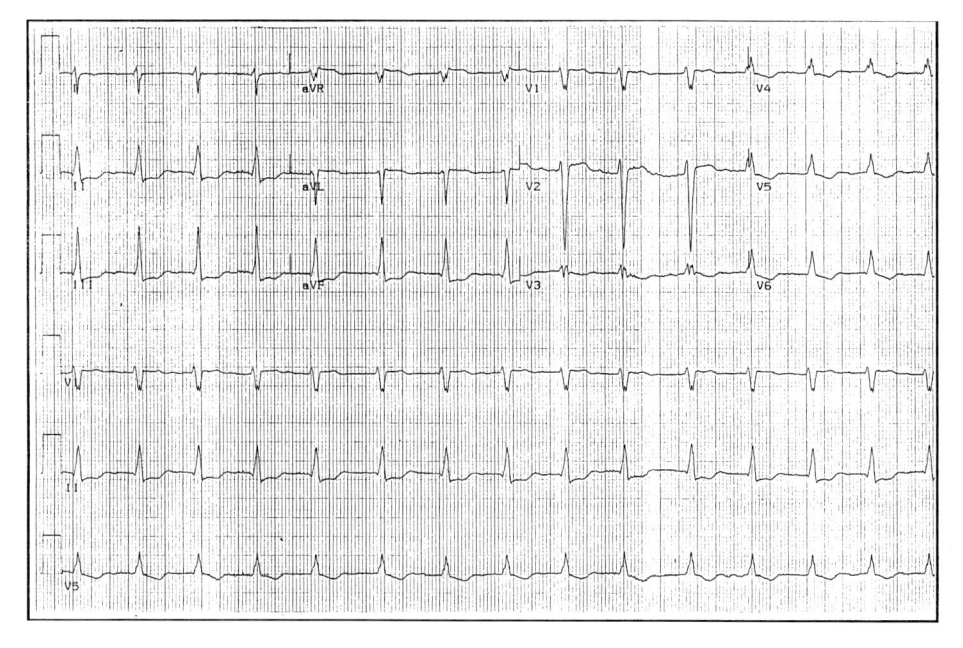

FIGURE 10-31 *Left posterior fascicular block and first-degree AV block (PR = 0.30 second). The QRS duration is 0.12 second. Note the qR complex in leads II, III, and aVF, and qRS and rS in I and aVL, respectively. The QRS axis in the frontal plane is + 118 degree.*

pacemaker; (3) physiologic interference due to AV nodal refractoriness caused by nearly simultaneous discharge of competing primary (sinus node) and secondary (AV junctional, ventricular) pacemakers (Figs. 4–22 and 9–23); or (4) atrioventricular heart block that permits the ventricles to be controlled by an AV junctional or ventricular secondary pacemaker. For example, there is complete AV heart block with dissociated sinus and IVR; or, sinus rhythm with a competing junctional pacemaker and AV dissociation by interference. AV dissociation can be complete or incomplete. The former means that all beats originate in the secondary pacemaker. The latter means that the primary pacemaker, or retrograde atrial activation from the secondary pacemaker with return ventricular activation, controls one or more beats. P-wave morphology during rhythms with AV dissociation depends on the location of the supraventricular pacemaker (sinus, atrial ectopic, AV junctional, fibrillation–flutter). With complete AV dissociation, P waves and QRS complexes appear regularly spaced, but have no temporal relationship to each other. With incomplete AV

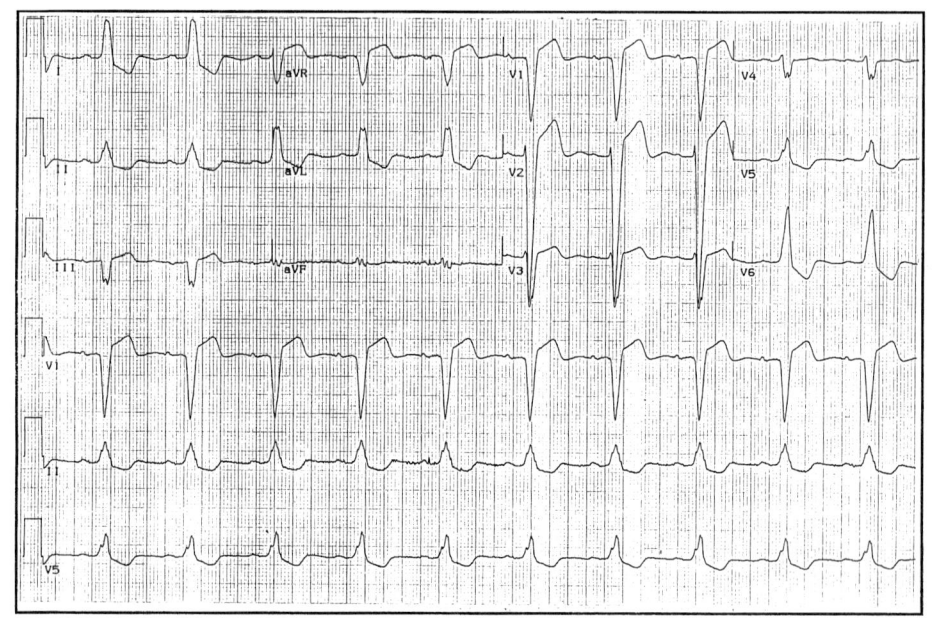

444 PREEXCITATION, VENTRICULAR ARRHYTHMIAS, AND HEART BLOCK

FIGURE 10-32 *Left bundle branch block. The QRS duration is 0.16 second. Note the QS complex in V_1. In leads V_5, V_6, and I, there are no q waves, only monophasic R waves.*

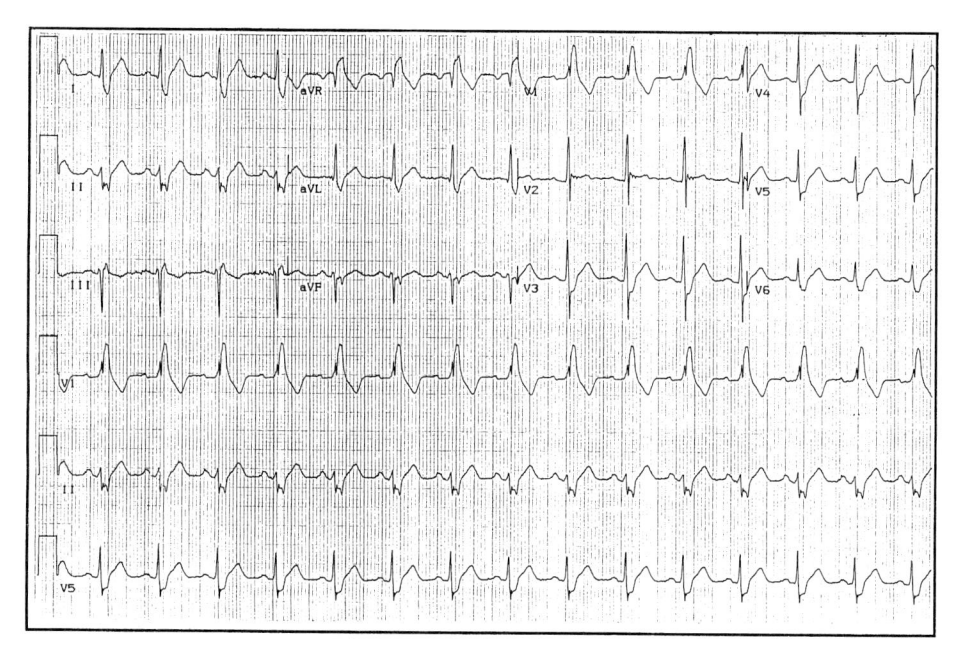

FIGURE 10-33 *Right bundle branch block (RBBB) and left anterior fascicular block (LAFB). The QRS duration is 0.14 second with RR′ morphology and a frontal plane axis of − 61 degrees. A wide S wave is seen in lead I and the lateral precordial leads, as expected with RBBB. The rS complexes in II, III, and aVF, and qRS complexes in leads I and aVL, are consistent with LAFB.*

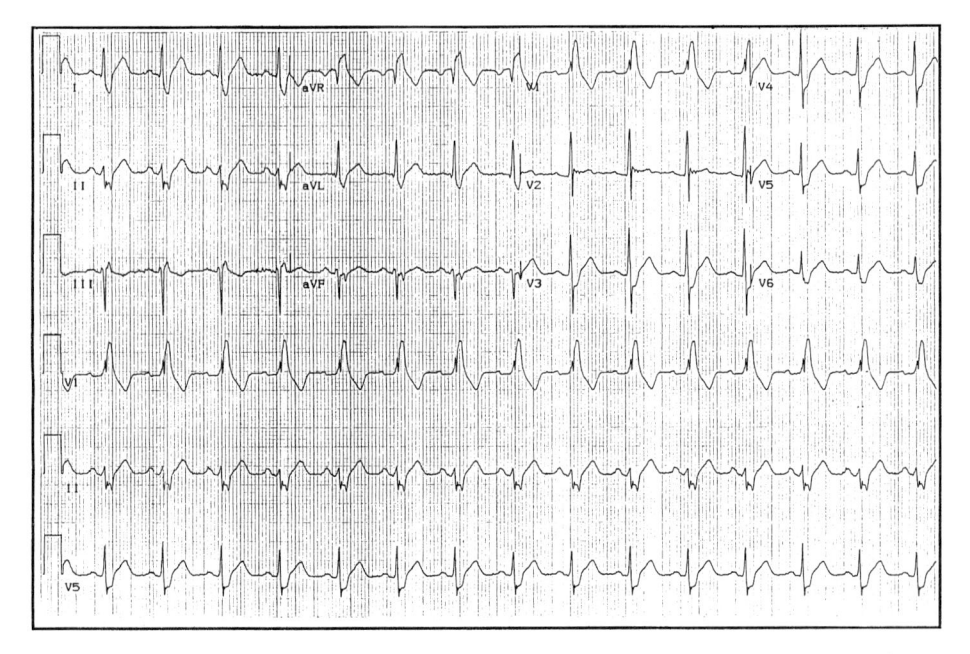

FIGURE 10-34 *Right bundle branch block (RBBB), left posterior fascicular block (LPFB) and first-degree AV heart block (PR + 0.23 second). The QRS duration is 0.13 second with wide S waves in leads I and V_5 and V_6. Because of low voltage, the QRS in V_1 is consistent with, but not typical of RBBB. The rS complexes in leads I and aVL, and q(tiny)R in leads II and III are consistent with LPFB, as is the QRS axis of + 117 degrees in the frontal plane.*

TABLE 10-10 *Summary of ECG criteria for the diagnosis of fascicular conduction block*

TYPE OF BLOCK	ECG CRITERIA*
Right bundle branch block (RBBB)	QRS > 0.12 sec; V_1-rSR' (wide R'); V_5, V_6 and I—possibly a small initial q wave, followed by R and wide S waves.
Left anterior fascicular block (LAFB)	QRS normal duration; left axis deviation (typically –60 degrees); small q and prominent R waves in I and aVL, and small r and prominent S waves in II, III, and aVF.
Left posterior fascicular block (LPFB)	QRS normal duration; right axis deviation (typically + 120 degrees); small r and prominent S waves in I and aVL, and small q and prominent R waves in I, III, and aVF; previous normal ECG for comparison to rule out right ventricular hypertrophy.
Left bundle branch block	QRS > 0.12 sec; V_1: QS or rS complex; V_5, V_6, and I: no Q, monophasic R wave.
RBBB + left anterior fascicular block	QRS > 0.12 sec; QRS axis typically between –45 and –120 degrees; prominent R' of RBBB in V_1 and initial r and prominent S waves of LAFB in II, III, and aVF.
RBBB + left posterior fascicular block	QRS > 0.12 sec; QRS axis at least + 90 degrees; prominent R' of RBBB in V_1; initial r and prominent S waves of LPFB in I and aVL.

*Lead V_1 is right ventricular epicardial complex, and leads V_5, V_6, and I the left ventricular epicardial complex.

dissociation, a narrow QRS occurs that is plausibly the result of supraventricular activation (PR interval > 0.12 second and within a conductible range). Similarly, a retrograde P wave following a QRS complex within a conductible range may indicate retrograde atrial capture from a junctional or ventricular secondary pacemaker focus. Treatment for arrhythmias or conduction disturbances with AV dissociation is that for the primary rhythm disturbance. This could be chronotropes for pacing for escape rhythms or AV heart block, or antiarrhythmic drugs or cardioversion for VT.

References

1. Benditt D, Benson DJ (eds). Cardiac Preexcitation Syndromes. Boston: Martinus Nijhoff, 1986.
2. Kastor J. Arrhythmias. Philadelphia: WB Saunders, 1994.
3. Josephson M. Clinical Cardiac Electrophysiology. 2nd ed. Philadelphia: Lea & Febiger, 1993.
4. Waugh R, Ramo B, Wagner G, Gilbert M (eds). Cardiac Arrhythmias. 2nd ed. Philadelphia: FA Davis, 1994.
5. Zipes D. Specific arrhythmias: Diagnosis and treatment. In Braunwald E (ed): Heart Disease. 4th ed. Philadelphia: WB Saunders, 1992: pp. 667–725.
6. Zipes D, Jalife J (eds). Cardiac Electrophysiology. 2nd ed. Philadelphia: WB Saunders, 1995.
7. Gallagher J, Pritchett E, Sealy W, et al. The preexcitation syndromes. Prog Cardiovasc Dis 1978;20:285—327.
8. Wagner G. Practical Electrocardiography. 9th ed. Baltimore: Williams & Wilkins, 1994.
9. Moulton K, Medcalf T, Lazzara R. Premature ventricular complex morphology: a marker for left ventricular structure and function. Circulation 1990;81:1245–1241.
10. Atlee J. Perioperative cardiac dysrhythmias in perspective. In: Perioperative Cardiac Dysrhythmias. 2nd ed. Chicago: Year Book Medical Publishers, 1990: pp. 1–13.
11. Lown B, Wolf M. Approaches to sudden death from coronary heart disease. Circulation 1971;44:130–142.
12. Gomes J, Winters S, Ip J. Post infarction high risk of sudden death. In Akhtar M, Myerburg R, Ruskin J (eds): Sudden Cardiac Death. Philadelphia: Williams & Wilkins, 1994: pp. 513–528.
13. Manolio T, Furberg C. Epidemiology of sudden cardiac death. In Akhtar M, Myerburg R, Ruskin J (eds): Sudden Cardiac Death. Philadelphia: Williams & Wilkins, 1994: pp. 3–20.
14. Wellens H, Bar F, Vanagt E, et al. The differentiation between ventricular tachycardia and supraventricular tachycardia with

aberrant conduction: The value of the 12 lead electrocardiogram. In Wellens H, Kulbertus H (eds): What's New in Electrocardiography. The Hague: Martinus Nijhoff, 1981: pp. 184–189.

15. Brugada P, Brugada J, Mont L, et al. A new approach to the differential diagnosis of regular tachycardia with a wide QRS complex. Circulation 1991;83:1649–1659.
16. Zipes D. Management of cardiac arrhythmias: Pharmacological, electrical and surgical techniques. In Braunwald E (ed): Heart Disease. 4th ed. Philadelphia: WB Saunders, 1992: pp. 628–666.
17. Manolio T, Furburg C. Anatomical features in victims of sudden coronary death: Coronary artery pathology. In Akhtar M, Myerburg R, Rushkin J (eds): Sudden Cardiac Death. Philadelphia: Williams & Wilkins, 1994: pp. 21–31.
18. Fisch C. Electrocardiography and vectorcardiography. In Braunwald E (ed): Heart Disease. 4th ed. Philadelphia: WB Saunders, 1992: pp. 116–160.
19. Goldman M. Principles of Clinical Electrocardiography. 12th ed. Los Altos, CA: Lange Medical Publications, 1986.
20. Atlee J, Brownlee S, Burstrom R. Conscious-state comparison of the effects of inhalation anesthetics on specialized atrioventricular conduction times in dogs. Anesthesiology 1986;64:703–710.
21. Atlee J, Yeager T. Electrophysiologic assessment of the effects of enflurane, halothane, and isoflurane on properties affecting supraventricular re-entry in chronically instrumented dogs. Anesthesiology 1989;71:941–952.
22. Atlee J, Bosnjak Z. Mechanisms for cardiac dysrhythmias during anesthesia. Anesthesiology 1990;72:347–374.
23. Atlee J, Bosnjak Z, Yeager T. Effects of diltiazem, verapamil, and inhalation anesthetics on electrophysiologic properties affecting reentrant supraventricular tachycardia in chronically instrumented dogs. Anesthesiology 1990;72:889–901.
24. Erikssen J, Otterstad J. Natural course of a prolonged PR interval and the relation between PR and incidence of coronary heart disease. A 7-year follow-up study of 1893 apparently healthy men aged 40–59 years. Clin Cardiol 1984;7:6–13.
25. De Soyza N, Bissett J, Kane J, Murphy M. Latent defects of atrioventricular conduction in right coronary artery disease. Am Heart J 1974;87:164–169.
26. Rosenbaum M, Elezari M, Lazzari J. The Hemiblocks. Oldsmar, FL: Tampa Tracings, 1970.

Index

Page numbers in *italic* refer to illustrations, page numbers followed by t refer to tables.

A

AAI (atrial-inhibited) pacing, in single-chamber mode pacemakers, 216, *217*, 218
AAT (automatic atrial tachycardia), 347, *348*, 349
Accelerated atrioventricular junctional rhythm (AVJR), 363, 365, *366–367*, 367
digitalis and, 365, 366
Acceleration-dependent QRS aberration, 139
Accessory pathway(s), atrioventricular, 390
in Wolff-Parkinson-White syndrome, 391–392, *394–397*, 395–396
catheter ablation of, *400–401*
nodoventricular, 390–391, *392*
preexcitation and, 135, *136*
ventricular, 390–391, *391–393*
(AP) action potential. See *Action potential (AP)*.
Action potential (AP), 29–30, 30t, *31–32*
current sink in, 39
in upstroke, 30t, *32*, 33–34
overshoot in, 30, *31*
propagation of, 38–40
safety factor of conduction in, 39–40
source of current for, 38–39
Adams-Stokes syndrome, and cardiac stimulation, 15–16
Adenosine, 167–168, 169t, *169–171*, 170–171
Adrenergic drug(s), mixed, 188–189, 189t
AES (atrial extrasystoles), 344, *345*, 346, 346t
Afterdepolarization(s), delayed, 43, *44*, 55t
early, 43, *44*, 45, 45t, 55t
experimental interventions and, 45t
Alcohol abuse, and arrhythmias, 93
Allergy(ies), to pacemakers, 297
Alpha-adrenergic blocker(s), 67
Amiodarone, 171–173
adverse reactions of, with pacemakers, 321
and implantable cardioverter-defibrillators, 324t
for atrial fibrillation, 386
for atrial flutter, 374
for junctional ectopic tachycardia, 368
for ventricular tachycardia, 425, 426t
Amyloidosis, and arrhythmias, 93–94
Analeptic drug(s), and arrhythmias, 87–88, 88t

Anaphylaxis, and arrhythmias, 94, 94t–95t
Anatomically defined circuit(s), in reentry, 48
Anesthetic(s), adverse reactions of, with pacemakers, 321
and arrhythmias, 76–88
and atrioventricular conduction time, 77–78, *79*
and atrioventricular junctional rhythm, 363
and atrioventricular refractory period, 79–80
and autonomic nervous system, 63–64, 64t
and ectopic rhythm disturbances, *78*
and latent pacemakers, 77, *78*
and myocardial infarction, 80
in catecholamine-induced arrhythmias, 67
Anomalous beat(s), atrial fibrillation and, *383–384*
Antiarrhythmic drug(s). See also specific types.
absorption of, 161–162
action of, 155–156, *156*
adverse reactions of, with pacemakers, 320–322, 321t
and reentry, 156
classification of, 157–159, 158t, *159*, 192–201, 199t–200t
limits of, *159*, 159–160, 160t
distribution of, 162–164, *163*
excretion of, 164–165
for polymorphic ventricular tachycardia, 429t, 430
indirect action of, 157, 157t
metabolism of, 164–165
oral, 192–201
parenteral, 167–192
adjunct, 187–192
pharmokinetics of, 160–165, *161*
vs. temporary pacing, for bradycardia, 248–253, 251t, *253–255*
Anticholinergic(s), and arrhythmias, 87, 88t
Anticholinesterase drug(s), and arrhythmias, 87
Anticoagulation, during cardioversion, 239
for atrial fibrillation, 385
Antidepressant(s), and catecholamine turnover, 69
Antidromic atrioventricular tachycardia, in Wolff-Parkinson-White syndrome, 403

451

452 INDEX

Antimuscarinic(s), action of, 249
Antitachycardia pacemaker(s), indications for, 227, 228t–231t, 229–234
Anxiolytic(s), and implantable cardioverter-defribillators, 324t
AOO (atrial asynchronous) pacing, in single-chamber pacemakers, 216, *217*, 218
Arrhythmia(s), 404–434, 405t
   after pacemaker implantation, 298, *299–300*, 300, 300t
   alcohol abuse and, 93
   amyloidosis and, 93–94
   anaphylaxis and, 94, 94t–95t
   and neuromuscular blocking drugs, 85–86, 86t
   anesthetics and, 76–88
   athlete's heart syndrome and, 95
   atrial transport dysfunction in, 8
   atrioventricular junction in, 4, *4*
   automatic, cardioversion and, 237, 237t
   autonomic dysfunction and, 97, 97t
   cardiomyopathy and, 62, 95–96
   conditions associated with, 61t, 61–63, *62*, 93–100
   conditions predisposing to, 2t
   coronary artery disease and, 96, 96t
   definition of, 3–4, *4*
   diagnosis of, electrocardiography for, 105–151. See also *Electrocardiography (ECG)*.
   errors in, 19
   diastolic encroachment in, 7
   drugs causing, 66–88, 88t. See also specific drugs.
   drugs for, disadvantages of, 16t
   electrocardiography in, 4–5
   electroconvulsive therapy and, 97–98
   electrolyte imbalances and, 88–93, 89t, *90*, 91t–92t. See also *Electrolyte imbalance(s)*.
   etiology of, 9–14
   extracorporeal shock wave lithotripsy and, 98
   from temperature imbalance, 64–66, *65*
   heart rate in, 3–4
   hemodynamic instability and, 6–9, 19–20
   incidence of, factors increasing, 10–11, *11–12*
   intravenous anesthetics and, 82–83
   lead selection in, 113, *115–116*
   left ventricular hypertrophy and, 98
   life-threatening, predisposition to, 5–6, *6–7*
   local anesthetics and, 83–85
   long QT interval syndrome and, 98–99, 99t
   management of, 19–20, *21*
   mitral valve prolapse syndrome and, 99–100, 100t
   Multicenter Study of General Anesthesia on, 11, *11–13*, 14t
   oculocardiac reflex and, 100
   pacemakers and, 14–18, 298, *299–300*, 300, 300t

Arrhythmia(s) *(Continued)*
   perioperative, adverse outcomes of, 13–14, *14–15*
   catecholamine surge in, *21*
   incidence of, 11, *11–12*, 12t
   temporary pacing for, 18
   physiologic imbalance in, 5, 5t, 60t, 60–61
   postulated mechanisms for, 55t, 55–56
   reported incidence of, 9, 10t
   right ventricular dysplasia and, 94–95
   role of cardiac conduction system in, 26, *27*
   significance of, 2t, 2–9
   susceptibility to, circadian variability in, 96
   triggered, cardioversion and, 237, 237t
Arrhythmia sensing function, of implantable cardioverter-defibrillators, 323
Arterial lead(s), placement of, complications of, 295
Artifact(s), in electrocardiography, 146, 147t, *148–151*
Ashman phenomenom, in electrocardiography, 139
Asynchronous atrial pulse generator(s), for epi-cardial pacing, *257*
   for transesophageal pacing, 275, *276*
Asynchronous pacing, 208–209
Asystole, ventricular, Lown-Wolf grading system for, 96, 96t
Athlete's heart syndrome, 95
Atrial asynchronous (AOO) pacing, in single-chamber mode pacemakers, 216, *217*, 218
Atrial capture, vs. ventricular capture, in trans-esophageal pacing, 282
Atrial extrasystole(s) (AES), 344, *345*, 346, 346t
Atrial fibrillation, 376, *377–381*, 378–379, 382
   and anomalous beats, *383–384*
   and embolization, 382, 385
   anticoagulation for, 385
   cardioversion for, 385
   catecholamines and, *21*
   causes of, 376
   coarse, *380*
   conditions associated with, 376
   diagnosis of, 376, *377–379*
   differential diagnosis of, 382, *383–384*
   drugs for, 386
   in Wolff-Parkinson-White syndrome, 403–404
   pacing for, 385
   QRS aberration in, 379, *381*, 382
Atrial flutter, 369–370, *370–373*, 373–374, *375*
   cardioversion for, 374
   catecholamines and, *21*, 372
   conditions associated with, 369–370
   diagnosis of, 369, *370–372*
   drugs for, 374, *375*
   in Wolff-Parkinson-White syndrome, 403–404
   pacing for, 374
   temporary, 286–287

INDEX **453**

Atrial flutter-fibrillation, in paroxysmal supraventricular tachycardia, 359
Atrial function, hemodynamics of, in physiologic pacing, 223–224, 224t
Atrial J catheter(s), for transvenous endocardial pacing, *262*, 263, *265*
Atrial myocardium, as reentry site, 51–52
Atrial pacemaker, wandering/shifting, 335, *337*
Atrial pacing, transesophageal, 274
Atrial pulse generator(s), asynchronous, for epicardial pacing, *257*
  for transesophageal pacing, 275, *276*, 277
Atrial reentry paroxysmal supraventricular tachycardia, sinus node reentry and, 359, *360*, 361
Atrial rhythm, chaotic, 349, *350*
  ectopic, disturbances in, 343–350, 344t
  multiform, 349, *350*
Atrial sensing refractory period(s), in artificial pacemakers, 213–214, *214*
Atrial systole, from cardioversion, 239
Atrial tachycardia, automatic, 347, *348*, 349
  ectopic, temporary pacing for, 288–289
  multiform, 349, *350*
Atrial transport dysfunction, in arrhythmias, 8
Atrial-inhibited (AAI) pacing, in single-chamber mode pacemakers, 216, *217*, 218
Atrial-triggered ventricular (VAT) pacing, for bradycardia, 218
Atrial-triggered ventricular-inhibited (VDD) pacing, in dual-chamber mode pacemakers, 219, *220*, 221, 222t
Atrioventricular (AV) accessory pathway(s), 390
Atrioventricular (AV) conduction system, autonomic innervation of, 40
Atrioventricular (AV) conduction time, anesthetics and, 77–78, *79*
Atrioventricular (AV) dissociation, 446–447
Atrioventricular (AV) heart block, 434–444, 435t
  advanced, *436*, 439–440
  complete, *436*, 441–442
  conditions associated with, 435t
  first-degree, 435, *436*, 437, *440*, *443*
  permanent pacemakers for, indications for, 227, 228t–230t
  second-degree, type I, 437–439
    type II, *436*, 439–440
  temporary pacing for, 283, *284*, 285, *286*
  third-degree, *436*, 441–442
  treatment of, 443–444
  Wenckebach, 437–439
Atrioventricular (AV) interval, and pacing rate, 209–210
Atrioventricular (AV) junction, in arrhythmias, 4, *4*
Atrioventricular (AV) junctional rhythm, accelerated. See *Accelerated atrioventricular junctional rhythm (AVJR).*

Atrioventricular (AV) junctional rhythm *(Continued)*
  disturbances of, 361–369
    diagnosis of, 363, *364*
  escape beats in, 361–362, *362*
  hemodynamic changes with, *225*
  premature beats in, 361–362, *362*
  vagal tone and, 363
Atrioventricular (AV) junctional tachycardia, nonparoxysmal, 363, 365, *366–367*, 367
  temporary pacing for, 287–289, 289
  in infants, 289–290
Atrioventricular (AV) nodal Wenckebach block, during epicardial pacing, *281*
Atrioventricular (AV) node, as reentry site, 53
Atrioventricular (AV) node reentry, paroxysmal supraventricular tachycardia from, 351, *352–354*, 355–359
Atrioventricular (AV) reciprocating tachycardia, in Wolff-Parkinson-White syndrome, 396–404, *398*, 403t
Atrioventricular (AV) refractory period(s), anesthetics and, 79–80
Atrioventricular (AV) sequential demand pulse generator(s), *257*
Atrioventricular (AV) synchrony, 4, *4*
  in physiologic pacing, 226
Atrioventricular (AV) tachycardia, in Wolff-Parkinson-White syndrome, 396–404, *398*, 403t
  antidromic, 403
  orthodromic, 355–359, *398*, 399, 402
  temporary pacing for, 287–288
Atropine, 187–188
  action of, 249
Automatic arrhythmia(s), cardioversion and, 237, 237t
Automatic atrial tachycardia (AAT), 347, *348*, 349
Automatic atrioventricular (AV) junctional tachycardia, temporary pacing for, 289
Automaticity, abnormal, 42t, 42–43, 55t
  altered normal, 42t, 42–43, 55t
  depolarization-induced, 42
  in pacemaker fibers, 35–38, *36*
  overdrive suppression of, 38
Autonomic dysfunction, and arrhythmias, 97, 97t
Autonomic nervous system, imbalance of, from anesthesia and surgery, 63–64, 64t
  in atrioventricular conduction system, 40
AV (atrioventricular). See entries under *Atrioventricular (AV).*

B

Baclofen, and arrhythmias, 74
Balloon flotation catheter(s), for transvenous endocardial pacing, *262*, 263, *265*

Barbiturate(s), and arrhythmias, 82
Battery(ies), for pacemakers, premature depletion of, 297
Benzodiazepine(s), and arrhythmias, 82
Beta-adrenergic agonist(s), 188–189, 189t
Beta-blocker(s), action of, 181t
　adverse reactions to, with pacemakers, 320–321
　and arrhythmias, 68
　and implantable cardioverter-defribillators, 324t
　for atrial fibrillation, 386
　for atrial flutter, 374
　for junctional ectopic tachycardia, 368
　for orthodromic atrioventricular tachycardia, in Wolff-Parkinson-White syndrome, 402, 403t
　oral, 197–199, 199t–200t
Bifascicular heart block, permanent pacemakers for, indications for, 228t, 230
Bigeminy, ventricular, in ventricular extrasystoles, 408–409, *411*
Bipolar esophageal lead(s), in intracavitary electrocardiography, 130, 132, *132–133*
Bipolar pacing catheter(s), for transvenous endocardial pacing, 262, 263, 265–266
Bradyasystolic arrest, transcutaneous pacing for, 273
Bradycardia, disadvantageous, definition of, 227
　drugs for, vs. temporary pacing, 248–253, 251t, *253–255*
　from cardioversion, 239
　in children, permanent pacemakers for, indications for, 230t
　pacing modes for, 216–221, *217*, 218
　sinus, 332, *333*, 334, 334t–335t, *336*. See also *Sinus bradycardia*.
　symptomatic, definition of, 227
　temporary pacing for, 283, 285, *286*
　　indications for, 234–235
　　vs. drugs, 248–253, 251t, *253–255*
Bradycardia-tachycardia syndrome, 340–341, *341–342*
Bretylium, 173–175
Bundle branch block. See *Left bundle branch block (LBBB)*; *Right bundle branch block (RBBB)*.

C

CAD (coronary artery disease). See *Coronary artery disease (CAD)*.
Calcium, imbalances of, 92–93
Calcium-channel blocker(s), and arrhythmias, 68–69, *70*
　for atrial fibrillation, 386
　for ectopic-reentrant supraventricular arrhythmias, 346t

Calcium-channel blocker(s) *(Continued)*
　parenteral use of, 175–177
Capture beat(s), 141–142, *143*
　in ventricular tachycardia, *416*, 419, *420*
Cardiac Arrhythmia Suppression Trials (CAST), 4–5
　and proarrhythmia, 165–166
Cardiac conducting system. See also *Conduction*.
　role of in arrhythmias, 26, *27*
Cardiac electrophysiology. See *Electrophysiology*.
Cardiac fiber(s), action potential characteristics of, 30t
　fast-response, *32*, 33
　　depressed, *41*, 41–42
　refractory, *32*, 35
Cardiac rhythm, in electrocardiography, 117, 119
Cardiomyopathy, and arrhythmias, 62, 95–96
Cardioversion, 235–240
　and automatic arrhythmias, 237, 237t
　and triggered arrhythmias, 237, 237t
　anticoagulation during, 239
　complications of, 239
　electromagnetic interference from, 312–314
　equipment failure in, prevention of, 237–238
　for atrial fibrillation, 385
　for atrial flutter, 374
　for ventricular tachycardia, 424–425
　indications for, 236t, 236–237
　monitoring during, 238
　pacemakers for, 205–244. See also *Pacemaker(s)*.
　position of electrodes for, 238
　procedure for, 237–240
　vs. drugs, for tachyarrhythmias, 236
　with implantable cardioverter-defibrillator, 238–239
Carotid sinus, hypersensitive, permanent pacemakers for, indications for, 229t, 231–232
CAST (Cardiac Arrhythmia Suppression Trials), 4–5
　and proarrhythmia, 165–166
Catecholamine(s), and arrhythmias, 67
　perioperative, 21
　and atrial fibrillation, 21
　and atrial flutter, *372*
　metabolism of, drugs affecting, 69
Catheter(s), for transvenous endocardial pacing, atrial J, 262, 263, 265
　balloon flotation, 262, 263, 265
　bipolar, 262, 263, 265–266
　flared, 262, 263
　pulmonary artery, 266, 267–268, 269
Catheter ablation, of accessory pathways, in Wolff-Parkinson-White syndrome, 400–401
Cell membrane(s), electrophysiology of, 29

INDEX **455**

Cellular connection sites, in unidirectional conduction block, 47
Central alpha-2 agonist(s), and arrhythmias, 67–68
Chaotic atrial rhythm, 349, *350*
Child(ren), bradycardia in, permanent pacemakers for, indications for, 230t, 233
Chronotrope(s), action of, 248
　and pacemaker function, 321–322
　for atrioventricular heart block, 443–444
　for ventricular extrasystole, 414
　intravenous doses of, for sinus bradycardia, 335t
Cimetidine, and arrhythmias, 74
Circuit(s), anatomically defined, in reentry, 48
Circus movement, 46
Coarse atrial fibrillation, 380
Cocaine, and arrhythmias, 73–74
Compensatory pause, in ventricular extrasystoles, 406, *410*
Computer electrocardiographic (ECG) analysis, 128–129
Conduction, concealed, in electrocardiography, 142–144, *144*
　drugs for increasing, 248–251
　retrograde, 142, *143*
　safety factor of, 39–40
　slowed, in unidirectional conduction block, 48
　ventriculoatrial, 142, *143*
Conduction block, unidirectional, 46–48
Conduction system, atrioventricular, autonomic innervation of, 40
　role of in arrhythmias, 26, *27*
Congestive heart failure, and arrhythmias, 62
Coronary artery disease (CAD), and arrhythmias, 96, 96t
Corticosteroid(s), and pacemaker function, 321
Couplet(s), in ventricular extrasystoles, 409, *411*
Coupling, fixed and variable, in ventricular extrasystoles, 408
Current, source of, in action potential, 38–39

D

DAD (delayed afterpolarization), 43, *44*, 55t
DDD (dual-sequential atrial-ventricular-inhibited) pacing, in dual-chamber mode pacemakers, 219, *220*, 221, 222t
DDD pulse generator(s), 257, *259*
Deceleration-dependent QRS aberration, 139–140
Defibrillation, 240–243
　equipment failure in, prevention of, 237–238
　for ventricular fibrillation, *242*, 433
　management algorithm for, *242*
　outcome of, factors affecting, 241, 241t

Defibrillation threshold(s), altered, of implantable cardioverter-defibrillators, 324, 324t
Delayed afterdepolarization (DAD), 43, *44*, 55t
Demand interval, in pacemakers, 210, *211*
　function of, assessment of, *311*
Demand rate, 210
Depolarization, automaticity inducing, 42
　on electrocardiography, 108–109, *110*
Depressed fast-response (DFR) fiber(s), *41*, 41–42
Desflurane, and arrhythmias, 76–77
DFR (depressed fast-response) fiber(s), *41*, 41–42
Diaphragm, stimulation of, by pacemakers, 302
Diastolic encroachment, in arrhythmias, 7
Diathermy, electromagnetic interference from, 316–317
Digitalis, 177–180, 178t, 180t
　and accelerated atrioventricular junctional rhythm, 365, *366*
　and arrhythmias, 69, 71, 72t
　for atrial flutter, 374
　for atrial flutter/fibrillation, in Wolff-Parkinson-White syndrome, 403
　for junctional ectopic tachycardia, 368
　for orthodromic atrioventricular tachycardia, in Wolff-Parkinson-White syndrome, 402, 403t
Diltiazem, 175–177
　and implantable cardioverter-defibrillators, 324t
　for atrial flutter, 374
　for ectopic-reentrant supraventricular arrhythmias, 346t
Direct current (DC) cardioversion, 235–240. See also *Cardioversion.*
Disadvantageous brachycardia, definition of, 227
Disopyramide, 193–194
Dobutamine, action of, 249–250
DOO (dual-sequential asynchronous) pacing, in dual-chamber mode pacemakers, 219, *220*, 221, 222t
Doxapram, and arrhythmias, 87–88
Dromotrope(s), action of, 248
　and pacemaker function, 321–322
　intravenous doses of, for sinus bradycardia, 335t
Droperidol, and arrhythmias, 83
Dual-chamber mode(s), in artificial pacemakers, 219, *220*, 221, 222t
Dual-chamber refractory period(s), in artificial pacemakers, 213–214, *214*
Dual-sequential pacing, in dual-chamber mode pacemakers, 219, *220*, 221, 222t
DVI pacemaker(s), ventricular oversensing with, *305*
Dysrhythmia, definition of, 3

E

Early afterdepolarization (EAD), 43, *44*, 45, 45t, 55t
ECT (electroconvulsive therapy), and arrhythmias, 97–98
Ectopic atrial tachycardia, temporary pacing for, 288–289
Ectopic rhythm, disturbances in, atrial, 343–350, 344t
    from anesthesia, *78*
    of pacemakers, 346–347
Ectopic tachycardia, junctional, 368–369
Ectopic-reentrant supraventricular arrhythmia(s), calcium-channel blockers for, 346t
Edrophonium, 189–191, 190t
    for atrial flutter, 374, *375*
    for atrial flutter/fibrillation, in Wolff-Parkinson-White syndrome, 404
    for noncompensatory sinus tachycardia, 340t
Effective contraction(s), definition of, 4
Electrocardiogram (ECG), interpretation of, 117t, 117–128
Electrocardiography (ECG), 105–151
    acceleration-dependent QRS aberration on, 139
    accessory pathways in, and preexcitation, 135, *136*
    applications of, 106t
    artifacts on, 146, 147t, *148–151*
    Ashman phenomenom in, 139
    computer-based analysis in, 128–129
    concealed conduction on, 142–144, *144*
    depolarization on, 108–109, *110*
    electrodes for, application of, 116–117
    epicardial leads in, 129–130, *131*
    for monitoring during cardioversion, 238
    heart beat patterns in, *134*, 135
    in arrhythmia incidence studies, 10–11, *11*
    in arrhythmias, 4–5
    in atrial fibrillation, 378, *380*
    in atrioventricular dissociation, 141, 141t
    in capture beats, 141–142, *143*
    in deceleration-dependent QRS aberration, 139–140
    in depolarization, 108–109, *110*
    in diffuse myocardial depression, 140
    in entrance block, 144, *145*, 146
    in exit block, 144, *145*, 146
    in fusion beats, 141, *142*
    in parasystole, 146, *147*
    in premature beats, 138
    in QRS complex aberrations, 135, *137–139*, 137–140, 139t
    in repolarization, *108*, 109
    in retrograde conduction, 142, *143*
    in ventricular aberration, 135, *137–139*, 137–140, 139t
    in ventricular extrasystoles, 406, *407–409*

Electrocardiography (ECG) *(Continued)*
    in ventricular flutter/fibrillation, 432, *433*
    in ventricular preexcitation, 394, *394–397*
    in ventricular tachycardia, 415, *416–418*, 417t
    in ventriculoatrial conduction, 142, *143*
    interference in, *140*, 140–141
    intervals in, 107–109, *108*
        normal values for, 109–112, *110–111*, 111t, *114*, 114t
    intracavitary, 129–132, *131*
        esophageal leads for, 130, 132, *132–133*
        intravascular leads for, 130, *131*
        transvenous endocardial leads for, 129–130, *131*
        unipolar epicardial leads for, 129–130, *131*
    leads for, 109, *111*, 128
        placement of, 115–116
        selection of, 112–113, *114*, 114t
    limitations of, 106–107
    normal sinus rhythm on, *116*, 333
    P waves on, 119, *120–121*, 126
    PR interval on, 111, 119, 122, 126
    QRS complex morphology on, *127*, 127–128
    QRS complex on, 122, *123*
    QTc interval on, 124
    R waves on, 108–109, *110*
    rate on, 117, *118*, 119t, 124, 126, *126*
    regularity on, 117, 119, 126, *126*
    rhythm on, 124–128, *126–127*
    S waves on, 108–109, *110*
    strip-chart recording in, 113
    T waves on, 124, *125*
    U waves on, 124
    waveforms on, 107–109, *108*
Electrocautery, electromagnetic interference from, 312–314
Electroconvulsive therapy (ECT), and arrhythmias, 97–98
Electrode(s), for electrocardiography, application of, 116–117
    for transesophageal pacing, 277, *278–279*
    positioning of, 277, *280*, 281
    position of, for cardioversion, 238
Electrolyte imbalance(s), 88–93, 89t, *90*, 91t–92t
    of calcium, 92–93
    of magnesium, 92, 92t
    of potassium, 88–92, 89t
Electromagnetic interference (EMI), 310–317
    from cardioversion, 312–314
    from diathermy, 316–317
    from electrocautery, 312–314
    from extracorporeal shock wave lithotripsy, 315
    from magnetic resonance imaging, 314–315
    from pulse generators, 313
    from radiofrequency catheter ablation, 317

INDEX 457

Electromagnetic interference (EMI) *(Continued)*
  from therapeutic radiation, 315–316
  from transcutaneous electrical nerve stimulation, 316
  pacemaker response to, 312
Electronic potential(s), in upstroke, 33
Electrophysiology, abnormal, 40t, 40–54
  automaticity in, 42t, 42–43
  and maximum diastolic potential, 29, 30t, *31*
  and transmembrane potential, 29, 30t, *31*
  definition of, 28
  normal, 28–40
  of cardiac cell membranes, 29
  phases of, 30, *32*, 33–35
Electroversion, 235–240. See also *Cardioversion.*
Embolization, atrial fibrillation and, 382, 385
EMI (electromagnetic interference), 310–317. See also *Electromagnetic interference (EMI).*
Emphysema, subcutaneous, from pacemaker implantation, 295
Encainide, 195t, 195–196
Endless-loop tachycardia, 298, 300
Endocardial lead(s), transvenous, in intracavitary electrocardiography, 129–130, *131*
Endocardial pacing, transvenous, 261–269, *262–268*. See also *Transvenous endocardial pacing.*
Enflurane, and arrhythmias, 12t, 77–80, 80–81
Entrance block, 144, *145*, 146
Ephedrine, 189, 189t
  action of, 250
Epicardial lead(s), in intracavitary electrocardiography, 129–130, *131*
Epicardial pacing, 253–261
  atrioventricular nodal Wenckebach block during, *281*
  disadvantages of, 252
  leads for, 255–256, *260*
  patient management during, 256
  pulse generators for, 254–255, *257–259*
  uses of, 256t, 261
Escape beat(s), atrioventricular junctional, 361–362, *362*
Escape interval, in pacemakers, 210, *211*
Escape rhythm(s), temporary pacing for, 283, 285
Esmolol, 180t, 180–182, 181t
  for noncompensatory sinus tachycardia, 340t
Esophageal lead(s), in intracavitary electrocardiography, 130, 132, *132–133*
ESWL (extracorporeal shock wave lithotripsy). See *Extracorporeal shock wave lithotripsy (ESWL).*
Ethanol abuse, and arrhythmias, 93
Etomidate, and arrhythmias, 82
Excitability, recovery of, in unidirectional conduction block, 46–47

Excitable gap, in reentry, 48, *50*
Exit block, 144, *145*, 146
  high pacing thresholds from, 296
Extracardiac stimulation, from pacemakers, 302
Extracorporeal shock wave lithotripsy (ESWL), and arrhythmias, 98
  electromagnetic interference from, 315
Extrasystole(s), atrial, 344–347, *345*, 346, 346t
  tip, 298
  ventricular. See *Ventricular extrasystole(s).*

F

Failure to capture, 271, *303*, 303–304, 304t
Fascicular heart block, *438–443*, 444, 445t, 446
  left anterior, 432, *439*, 445t
  left posterior, 440, 445t
  permanent pacemakers for, indications for, 228t
Fast-response fiber(s), *32*, 33
  depressed, *41*, 41–42
Fentanyl, and perioperative arrhythmias, 12t
Final rapid repolarization, 30, *32*, 34–35, 35t
First-degree atrioventricular (AV) heart block, 435, *436*, 437, *440*, 443
Fixed coupling, in ventricular extrasystoles, 408
Flared catheter(s), for transvenous endocardial pacing, *262*, 263
Flecainide, 195t, 196
  and implantable cardioverter-defibrillators, 324t
  for atrial flutter, 374
Flotation catheter(s), balloon, for transvenous endocardial pacing, *262*, 263, *265*
Free drug(s), distribution of, 162–163
Fusion beat(s), 141, *142*
  from improper sensing of pacemaker, *309*
  in ventricular extrasystoles, 406, *409*
  in ventricular preexcitation, *392*
  in ventricular tachycardia, *416*, 419, *420*

H

Halothane, and arrhythmias, 12t, 77–80, 80–81
Harrison subdivision, in antiarrhythmic drug classification, 158t
HCSS (hypersensitive carotid sinus syndrome). See *Hypersensitive carotid sinus syndrome (HCSS).*
Heart. See also entries under *Cardiac.*
  electrophysiology of. See *Electrophysiology.*
Heart beat(s). See also *Capture beat(s); Escape beat(s); Fusion beat(s); Premature beat(s).*
  patterns of, in electrocardiography, *134*, 135
Heart block, 434–446
  atrioventricular. See *Atrioventricular (AV) heart block.*

458 INDEX

Heart block *(Continued)*
  bifascicular, permanent pacemakers for, indications for, 228t, 230
  fascicular, *438–443*, 444, 445t, 446
    left anterior, 432, *439*, *445t*
    left posterior, *440*, *443*, 445t
    permanent pacemakers for, indications for, 228t
  intraventricular, 229, *232*
  trifascicular, permanent pacemakers for, indications for, 228t
Heart rate, 117, *118*, 119t
  in arrhythmias, 3–4
Hemorrhage, subarachnoid, and arrhythmias, 97, 97t
Hemothorax, from pacemaker implantation, 295
His-Purkinje system, as reentry site, 53
Histamine, and arrhythmias, 74
  drugs releasing, 95t
Hypercalcemia, 92–93
Hyperkalemia, 91–92
Hypermagnesemia, 92
Hypernatremia, 92–93
Hypersensitive carotid sinus syndrome (HCSS), 343
  permanent pacemakers for, indications for, 229t, 231–232
Hypertension, and arrhythmias, 62
Hyperthermia, and arrhythmias, 66
Hypocalcemia, 92–93
Hypokalemia, 89t, 89–91, *90*, 91t
Hypomagnesemia, 92, 92t
Hyponatremia, 92–93
Hypotension, from methyl methacrylate, 75t
Hypothermia, and arrhythmias, 64–66, *65*
  implantable cardioverter-defibrillators and, 324t
Hypothyroidism, and implantable cardioverter-defribillators, 324t
Hysteresis interval, in artificial pacemakers, 210, *211*

I

Identification code(s), for artificial pacemakers, 215–216, 216t
Idioventricular rhythm, 410–411, *413*
Implantable cardioverter-defibrillator(s) (ICDs)
  activation of, 324–325
  adverse reactions with pacemakers, 318–320
  altered defibrillation thresholds of, 324, 324t
  arrhythymia sensing functions of, 323
  cardioversion with, 238–239
  complications of, 294t, 322–325, 323t
    perioperative, 323t, 323–324
  deactivation of, 324–325
  drugs affecting, 324t
  history of, 14–16

Implantable cardioverter-defibrillator(s) (ICDs) *(Continued)*
  implantation of, patient management in, 327–328
  malfunction of, 322–325, 323t
  morbidity with, factors affecting, 323t
  prevalence of, 17–18
  use of, 243–244, 244t
Ineffective contraction(s), in arrhythmias, 8
Infant(s), atrioventricular junctional tachycardia in, temporary pacing for, 289–290
Infarction, chronic, anesthetics and, 80
Infection(s), from pacemaker implantation, 300–301
Interference, electromagnetic, 310–317. See also *Electromagnetic interference (EMI).*
  in electrocardiography, *140*, 140–141
Internal cardioverter-defibrillator(s) (ICDs). See *Implantable cardioverter-defibrillator(s) (ICDs).*
Interval(s), in electrocardiography, 107–109, *108*
  normal values for, 109–112, *110–111*, 111t, *114*, 114t
Intracavitary electrocardiography (ECG), 129–132, *131*. See also *Electrocardiography (ECG), intracavitary.*
Intravascular endocardial lead(s), in intracavitary electrocardiography, 129–130, *131*
Intravenous anesthetic(s), and arrhythmias, 82–83
Intraventricular heart block, 229, *232*
Ischemia, anesthetics and, 80
Isoflurane, and arrhythmias, 12t, 77–80, *80*–81
Isoproterenol, 188–189, 189t
  action of, 250

J

J catheter(s), atrial, for transvenous endocardial pacing, 262, *263*, *265*
Junctional ectopic tachycardia, 368–369
Junctional escape beat(s), in atrioventricular junctional rhythm disturbances, 361–362, *362*

K

Kent bundle(s), 390, *392*
Ketamine, and arrhythmias, 82

L

Latent pacemaker(s), anesthetics and, 77, *78*
  automaticity in, 37–38
Lead(s), arterial, placement of, complications of, 295
  for electrocardiography, 128
    placement of, 115–116
    selection of, 112–113, *114*, 114t, *115–116*
  for epicardial pacing, 255–256, *260*

INDEX **459**

Lead(s), arterial *(Continued)*
  for intracavitary electrocardiography, epicardial, 129–130, *131*
    esophageal, 130, 132, *132–133*
    intravascular, 130, *131*
    transvenous endocardial, 129–130, *131*
  for monitoring during cardioversion, 238
  for pacemakers, dislodgement and migration of, 297, 318
    insertion of, arrhythmias from, 298, *299*
    for transvenous endocardial pacing, 261, *262*, 263
    insertion of, 269
    positioning of patient with, 325
    transport with, 325
  insulation defects in, 296
  single, for diagnosis of wide-QRS ventricular tachycardia, 419–420, *421*
Leading circle reentry, 48, *51*
Left anterior fascicular heart block, *439, 442,* 445t
Left bundle branch block (LBBB), *441,* 445t
  in ventricular tachycardia, 415–419, *416,* 417t, *421*
Left posterior fascicular heart block, *440, 443,* 445t
Left ventricular hypertrophy, and arrhythmias, 98
Lidocaine, 182–185
  and implantable cardioverter-defribillators, 324t
  for ventricular tachycardia, 425, 426t
Lithium, and arrhythmias, 74–75
Lithotripsy, extracorporeal shock wave, and arrhythmias, 98
  elctromagnetic interference from, 315
LMP (loss of membrane potential). See *Loss of membrane potential (LMP).*
Local anesthetic(s), and arrhythmias, 83–85
Long QT interval syndrome, and arrhythmias, 98–99, 99t
Loss of membrane potential (LMP), 29, 30t, *31, 41,* 41–42
Lown-Ganong-Levine (LGL) syndrome, 390, *391*
Lown-Wolf grading system, for ventricular extrasystole, 96, 96t, 412, *413*

M

Macroeentry, 55t
Magnesium, imbalances of, 92, 92t
Magnesium sulfate, 191t–192t, 191–192
  and implantable cardioverter-defribillators, 324t
Magnetic resonance imaging (MRI), electromagnetic interference from, 314–315
Mahaim fiber(s), 390–391, *392*
Maximum diastolic potential (MDP), 29, 30t, *31*
Methyl methacrylate, and arrhythmias, 75, 75t

Methylxanthine(s), and arrhythmias, 69
Metoclopramide, and arrhythmias, 75
Microeentry, 55t
Mitral valve prolapse syndrome, and arrhythmias, 99–100, 100t
Mixiletine, 194
Monoamine oxidase (MAO) inhibitor(s), and catecholamine turnover, 69
Moricizine, 195t, 197
Motion artifact(s), on electrocardiography, 148–149, *151*
MRI (magnetic resonance imaging), electromagnetic interference from, 314–315
Multicenter Study of General Anesthesia, of preoperative and postoperative arrhythmias, 11, *11–13,* 14t
Multiform atrial rhythm, 349, *350*
Multiform atrial tachycardia, 349, *350*
Muscle relaxant(s), nondepolarizing, and arrhythmias, 86, *87*
Myocardial depression, diffuse, 140
Myocardial infarction (MI), acute, anesthetics and, 80
  permanent pacemakers for, indications for, 228t, 229
Myocardial ischemia, electrocardiography in, lead selection for, 112–113, *114,* 114t
  ST segment in, 112–113
Myocardial oxygen imbalance, in arrhythmias, 9, 9t
Myocardial oxygenation, factors in, 9t
Myocardium, as reentry site, 51–54
  atrial, as reentry site, 51–52
  perforation of, from pacemaker implantation, 295–296
Myopotential interference, with pacemaker function, 318

N

Naloxone, and arrhythmias, 88
NASPE-BPEG (North American Society of Pacing and Electrophysiology–British Pacing and Electrophysiology Group) code(s), 216t
NDMRs (nondepolarizing muscle relaxants), and arrhythmias, 86, *87*
Neonate(s), atrioventricular junctional tachycardia in, temporary pacing for, 289–290
Neuromuscular blocking drug(s), and arrhythmias, 85–86, 86t
Neurovascular syndrome(s), permanent pacemakers for, indications for, 229t
Nitrous oxide, and arrhythmias, 76–77
Nodoventricular accessory pathway(s), 390–391, *392*
Noncompensatory pause, in ventricular extrasystoles, 406, *410*
Noncompensatory sinus tachycardia, 340, 340t
  temporary pacing for, 289

460   INDEX

Nondepolarizing muscle relaxant(s) (NDMRs), and arrhythmias, 86, *87*
Nonparoxysmal atrioventricular junctional tachycardia, 363, 365, *366–367*, 367
Nonsustained ventricular tachycardia, *429*, 431
Normal sinus rhythm, *116*
North American Society of Pacing and Electrophysiology–British Pacing and Electrophysiology Group (NASPE-BPEG) code(s), 216t

O

Obesity, and arrhythmias, 63
Oculocardiac reflex, 100
Opiate(s), and arrhythmias, 83
Opioid(s), and arrhythmias, 87–88, 88t
  and implantable cardioverter-defibrillators, 324t
Ordered reentry, 48
Orthodromic atrioventricular tachycardia, in Wolff-Parkinson-White syndrome, *398*, *399*, 402
  paroxysmal supraventricular reentry, 355–359
Output failure, 304–306, *305*, 305t, *308*
  misdiagnosis of, 305–306
Overdrive suppression, of automaticity, 38
Oversensing, output failure from, 304, *305*, 305t, *308*
  ventricular, with dual-sequential pacemakers, *305*
Overshoot, in action potential, 30, *31*
Oxygen imbalance, myocardial, in arrhythmias, 9, 9t

P

P wave(s), 119, *120–121*, 126
  in ventricular tachycardia, 415, *416–417*
Pacemaker(s), adverse reactions with drugs, 320–322, 321t
  adverse reactions with implantable cardioverter-defibrillators, 318–320
  and arrhythmias, 14–18
  antitachycardia, atrial sensing refractory periods in, 213–214, *214*
  indications for, 227, 228t–231t, 229–234
  complications of, 294t, 294–302
    from allergic reactions, 297
    from arrhythmias, 298, *299–300*, 300, 300t
    from arterial lead placement, 295
    from extracardiac stimulation, 302
    from hemothorax, 295
    from high pacing thresholds, from exit block, 296
    from infection, 300–301
    from lead dislodgement and migration, 297
    from lead insulation defects, 296

Pacemaker(s), complications of *(Continued)*
    from myocardial perforation, 295–296
    from pneumothorax, 295
    from premature battery depletion, 297
    from pulse generator malfunction, 301
    from subcutaneous emphysema, 295
    from thromboembolism, 296
    from twiddler's syndrome, 297
  demand interval in, 210, *211*
  function of, assessment of, *311*
  design of, 208
    advances in, 206–207, 207t
  dual-chamber refractory periods in, 213–214, *214*
  electromagnetic interference with, 310–317. See also *Electromagnetic interference (EMI)*.
  escape interval in, 210, *211*
  function of, assessment of, 310, *311*
  history of, 14–16, 206
  hysteresis interval in, 210, *211*
  identification codes for, 215–216, 216t
  implantation of, patient management in, 325–326
  latent, anesthetics and, 77, *78*
    automaticity in, 37–38
  leads for, dislodgement of, 297, 318
    insertion of, arrhythmias from, 298, *299*
  malfunction of, 302–310
    and failure to capture, *303*, 303–304, 304t
    and inappropriate pacing rate, 307, 310t
    and output failure, 304–306, *305*, 305t, *308*
    misdiagnosis of, 305–306
    and oversensing, 304, *305*, 305t, *308*
    and undersensing, *306*, 306–307, 307t, *308*
  myopotential interference with, 318
  operation of, 208–223. See also *Pacing*.
  pacing threshold in, 211–212, 212t
  permanent, antitachyarrhythmia, indications for, 231t
    cardioversion with, 238–239
    for tachyarrhythmias, 222–223
    indications for, 227, 228t–231t, 229–234
    in adults, 228t–229t
    in children, 230t
  prevalence of, 17–18, 207
  pulse characteristics of, 210–211
  sensitivity of, 212
  stimulation of diaphragm by, 302
  system revision of, patient management in, 325–326
  temporary, for perioperative arrhythmias, 18
  use of, with concurrent conditions, 18
  uses for, 207–208
  ventricular refractory periods in, 212–213, *213*
  wandering/shifting, 335, *337*

INDEX **461**

Pacemaker fiber(s), automaticity of, 35–38, *36*
  latent, 26–28
Pacemaker rhythm, ectopic, 346–347
Pacemaker runaway, 298
Pacemaker syndrome, 301, 301t
Pacing, 208–223
  asynchronous, 208–209
    in single-chamber mode pacemakers, 216, *217*, *218*
  for atrial flutter, 374
  for tachycardia, indications for, 231t, 233–234
  in children, 230t, 233
  indications for, 227–235
  modes for, 216–221
    dual-chamber, 219, *220*, 221, 222t
    for bradycardia, 216–221, *217*
    NASPE-BPEG codes for, 216t
    physiologic, 224, 226
    single-chamber, 216, *217*, *218*
  paired, for atrioventricular junctional tachycardia, in infants, 289–290
  permanent, indications for, 227, 228t, 229–234, 230t–231t, 231t
  physiologic, atrial function in, 223–224, 224t
    atrioventricular synchrony in, 226
    hemodynamics of, 223–224, 224t
    modes for, 224, 226
    rate responsiveness in, 226
    ventricular function in, 224, *225*
  rate of, atrioventricular interval and, 209–210
    inappropriate, from pacemaker malfunction, 307, 310t
  synchronous, 208–209
  temporary, epicardial, 253–261. See also *Epicardial pacing*.
    for atrial fibrillation, 385
    for atrial flutter, 286–287
    for atrioventricular heart block, 283, *284*, 285, *286*
    for atrioventricular junctional tachycardia, 287–289
      in infants, 289–290
    for bradycardia, 283, 285, *286*
      indications for, 234–235
      vs. drugs, 248–253, 251t, *253–255*
    for ectopic atrial tachycardia, 288–289
    for escape rhythms, 283, 285
    for noncompensatory sinus tachycardia, 289
    for perioperative arrhythmias, 18
    for sinus bradycardia, 334, *336*
    for tachyarrhythmias, 221–222
    for ventricular extrasystoles, 414
    for ventricular tachycardia, 290
    perioperative indications for, 234–235
    transcutaneous, 270–274, 271t, *272*, 273t

Pacing, temporary, epicardial *(Continued)*
    transesophageal, 274–283. See also *Transesophageal pacing*.
    transvenous endocardial, 261–269, *262–268*. See also *Transvenous endocardial pacing*.
    transcutaneous, uses for, 256t
    ventricular, arrhythmias from, 298, *300*, 300t
    transesophageal, 275
Pacing threshold(s), 211–212, 212t
  high, from exit block, 296
Paired pacing, for atrioventricular junctional tachycardia, in infants, 289–290
Parasystole, 146, *147*
  ventricular, 409–410, *412*
Parenteral antiarrhythmic drug(s), 167–192. See also specific drugs.
  adjunct, 187–192. See also specific drugs.
Paroxysmal supraventricular tachycardia (PSVT), atrial fibrillation/atrial flutter in, 359
  atrial reentry, sinus node reentry and, 359, *360*, 361
  atrioventricular node reentry and, 351, *352–354*, 355–359
  orthodromic, 355–357, *358*, 359
  atrioventricular reentry, 355–359
Pectoral muscle(s), stimulation of, by pacemakers, 302
Pharmacokinetics, 162–164
  of antiarrhythmic drugs, 160–165, *161*
  two-compartment model of, 162, *163*
Phase 2. See *Plateau phase*.
Phase 3. See *Repolarization, rapid, final*.
Phase O. See *Upstroke*.
Phenytoin, 182–185
Physiologic imbalance, perioperative, causes of, 60t, 60–61
Physiologic pacing. See *Pacing, physiologic*.
Physostigmine, and arrhythmias, 88, 88t
Plateau phase, 30, *32*, 34–35, 35t
  refractoriness in, *32*, 35
Pneumothorax, from pacemaker implantation, 295
Polymorphic ventricular tachycardia, 427–431, *429*, 429t
Potassium, imbalances of, 88–92, 89t
  and hyperkalemia, 91–92
  and hypokalemia, 89t, 89–91, *90*, 91t
PR interval, 111, 119, 122, 126
Preexcitation, accessory pathways and, 135, *136*
  ventricular, 390–404. See also *Ventricular preexcitation*.
Premature beat(s), 138
  in atrioventricular junctional rhythm, 361–362, *362*
Proarrhythmia, 4, 165–167

462 INDEX

Probe(s), for transesophageal pacing, 277, 278–279
  positioning of, 277, 280, 281
Procainamide, 185–187, 187t
Propafenone, 195t, 196–197
Propanolol, for noncompensatory sinus tachycardia, 340t
Propofol, and arrhythmias, 83
Protein-bound drug(s), distribution of, 162–163
Pseudofusion beat(s), from improper sensing of pacemaker, 309
PSVT (paroxysmal supraventricular tachycardia). See Paroxysmal supraventricular tachycardia (PSVT).
Pulmonary artery catheter(s), for transvenous endocardial pacing, 266, 267–268, 269
Pulse, characteristics of, in pacemakers, 210–211
Pulse generator(s), and electromagnetic interference, 313
  for epicardial pacing, 254–255, 257–259
  for transcutaneous pacing, 272
  for transesophageal pacing, 275, 276, 277
  malfunction of, 301
Purkinje fiber(s), as cellular connection sites, 47
  in fiber automaticity, 37
  loss of membrane potential in, 41

Q

QRS complex, 110, 112, 122, 123
  aberrations in, 135, 137–139, 137–140, 139t
  in atrial fibrillation, 379, 381, 382
  in ventricular extrasystoles, 406, 407–409
  in ventricular tachycardia, 415–419, 416–418, 417t
  morphology of, 127, 127–128
    in Wolff-Parkinson-White syndrome, 127, 127–128
QT interval, 112
  prolonged, and arrhythmias, 98–99, 99t
QT interval prolongation, in life-threatening arrhythmias, 5–66
QTc interval, 124
Quadrigeminy, in ventricular extrasystoles, 409
Quinidine, 192–193
  for atrial flutter, 372, 374

R

R wave(s), 108–109, 110
Radiation, therapeutic, electromagnetic interference from, 315–316
Radiofrequency catheter ablation, electromagnetic interference from, 317
Random reentry, 48
Ranitidine, and arrhythmias, 74
Rate, in electrocardiography, 117, 118, 119t, 124, 126

Rate, in electrocardiography (Continued)
  of artificial pacemaker, 209–210
  responsiveness of, in physiologic pacing, 226
RBBB (right bundle branch block). See Right bundle branch block (RBBB).
Reciprocating tachycardia, 46
Reentrant excitation, 46–54
  unidirectional conduction block in, 46–47
Reentrant tachycardia, cardioversion for, 236t, 236–237
  supraventricular, 351–361. See also Supraventricular tachycardia (SVT), reentrant.
  paroxysmal, from atrioventricular node reentry, 351, 352–354, 355
  with anatomic obstruction, 49–51
Reentry, anatomically defined circuits in, 48
  antiarrhythmic drugs and, 156
  excitable gap in, 48, 50
  leading circle, 48, 51
  sites for, 49–54, 51t, 52
  types of, 48, 49–51
Refractoriness, and interference, 140, 140–141
  of cardiac fibers, 32, 35
Refractory period(s), atrioventricular, anesthetics and, 79–80
  in pacemakers, dual-chamber, 213–214, 214
  ventricular, 212–213, 213
  ventricular blanking, 213–214, 214
Regularity, in electrocardiography, 117, 118, 119, 126, 126
  in ventricular tachycardia, 415
Relative refractory period (RRP), 32, 35
Reperfusion injury, anesthetics and, 81, 81t
Repolarization, on electrocardiography, 108, 109
  rapid, final, 30, 32, 34–35, 35t
Resting membrane potential (RMP), basis of, 30–31, 32
Retrograde conduction, 142, 143
Rhythm, in electrocardiography, 124–128, 126–127
Right bundle branch block (RBBB), 438, 442, 443, 445t
  in ventricular tachycardia, 415–419, 417t, 417–418, 421, 424
  with sinus tachycardia, 115
Right ventricular dysplasia, arrhythmogenic, 94–95
RMP (resting membrane potential), basis of, 30–31, 32
R-R interval, in ventricular tachycardia, 416, 422–423
RRP (relative refractory period), 32, 35

S

S wave(s), 108–109, 110
Safety factor of conduction, 39–40

INDEX   463

Sarcolemma, electrophysiology of, 29
Second-degree atrioventricular (AV) heart
   block, type I, 437–439
   type II, *436*, 439–440
Sedative(s), and implantable cardioverter-
   defribillators, 324t
Sensing, improper, *306*, 306–307, 307t,
   308–309
Sensitivity, of artificial pacemakers, 212
Sensitization, 2
Sequential demand pulse generator(s), atrio-
   ventricular, *257*
Sevoflurane, and arrhythmias, 76–77
Shifting atrial pacemaker, 335, *337*
Shock wave lithotripsy, extracorporeal, and ar-
   rhythmias, 98
   electromagnetic interference from, 315
Sick sinus syndrome, and arrhythmias, 63
Single-chamber mode(s), in pacemakers, 216,
   217, 218
Sinoatrial (SA) block, *339*, 339–340
Sinoatrial (SA) node, anesthetics and, 77, *78*
   as reentry site, 49, 50, *52*
   in automaticity, 37
   sick sinus syndrome of, and arrhythmias, 63
Sinoatrial (SA) node reentry, and paroxysmal
   supraventricular tachycardia, 359, *360*,
   361
Sinus arrest, 335, *338*, 339
Sinus arrhythmia, 334–335, *337*
Sinus bradycardia, 332, *333*, 334, 334t–335t,
   336
   drugs for, 334, 334t
   perioperative, causes of, 334t
   temporary pacing for, 334, *336*
Sinus node dysfunction (SND), 331–343
   and bradycardia-tachycardia syndrome,
     341–342
   and hypersensitive carotid sinus syndrome,
     343
   and noncompensatory sinus tachycardia,
     340, 340t
   and sinoatrial block, *339*, 339–340
   and sinus arrest, 335, *338*, 339
   and sinus arrhythmia, 334–335, *337*
   and sinus bradycardia, 332, *333*, 334,
     334t–335t, *336*. See also *Sinus brady-
     cardia.*
   and sinus pause, 335, *338*, 339
   and wandering/shifting atrial pacemaker,
     335, *337*
   permanent pacemakers for, indications for,
     228t, 231
Sinus pause, 335, *338*, 339
Sinus rhythm, normal, *116*, 333
Sinus tachycardia, noncompensatory, 340,
   340t
   temporary pacing for, 289

Sinus tachycardia *(Continued)*
   with right bundle branch block, *115*
   with ventricular preexcitation, *393*
Slow-response fiber(s), *32*, 33
SND (sinus node dysfunction). See *Sinus node
   dysfunction (SND).*
Sodium-channel blocker(s), and arrhythmias,
   84t, 84–85, 85t
   autonomic effects of, 85
Sotalol, 199–201, 200t
   and implantable cardioverter-defribillators,
     324t
   for atrial flutter, 374
ST segment, in myocardial ischemia, 112–113
Strip-chart recording, in electrocardiography,
   113
Subarachnoid hemorrhage, and arrhythmias,
   97, 97t
Subcutaneous emphysema, from pacemaker
   implantation, 295
Succinylcholine, and arrhythmias, 85–86, 86t
   electrocardiographic artifacts from, *150*
Supraventricular arrhythmia(s), ectopic-
   reentrant, calcium-channel blockers for,
   346t
Supraventricular tachycardia (SVT), radiofrequency catheter ablationfor, electromagnetic interference from, 317
   reentrant, 351–361
   paroxysmal, from atrioventricular node re-
     entry, 351, *352–354*, 355
Sustained ventricular tachycardia, treatment
   of, 423–425
SVT (supraventricular tachycardia). See *Supraventricular tachycardia (SVT).*
Synchronous pacing, 208–209

T

T wave(s), 124, *125*
Tachyarrhythmia(s), cardioversion for, indications for, 236t, 236–237
   vs. drugs, 236
   pacemakers for, 221–223, 231t
   transcutaneous pacing for, 274
   with ventricular preexcitation, 394–396,
     398–401
Tachycardia, 7–8
   atrial, ectopic, temporary pacing for, 288–289
     multiform, 349, *350*
   atrioventricular, temporary pacing for,
     287–288
   atrioventricular junctional, temporary pacing
     for, 289–290
   atrioventricular reciprocating, in Wolff-
     Parkinson-White syndrome, 396–404,
     398, 403t
   ectopic junctional, 368–369
   endless-loop, 298, 300

464 INDEX

Tachycardia *(Continued)*
  pacing for, indications for, 231t, 233–234
  radiofrequency catheter ablation for, electromagnetic interference from, 317
  reciprocating, 46
  reentrant, cardioversion for, 236t, 236–237
    with anatomical obstruction, *49–51*
  sinus. See *Sinus tachycardia.*
  supraventricular, 351–361. See also *Supraventricular tachycardia (SVT).*
  ventricular. See *Ventricular tachycardia.*
Temporary pacing. See *Pacing, temporary.*
TENS (transcutaneous electrical nerve stimulation), electromagnetic interference from, 316
Third-degree atrioventricular (AV) heart block, 436, 441–442
Thromboembolism, from pacemaker implantation, 296
Tip extrasystole(s), 298
Tocainide, 194
Torsades de pointes, 427–431, *428*, 429t
Transcutaneous electrical nerve stimulation (TENS), electromagnetic interference from, 316–317
Transcutaneous pacing, 270–274, 271t, *272*, 273t
  uses of, 256t
Transesophageal pacing, 274–283
  atrial, 274
  disadvantages of, 252
  limitations of, 281, 283
  probes for, 277, *278–279*
    positioning of, 277, *280*, 281
  pulse generators for, 275, *276*, 277
  technique of, 280–281
  uses of, 256t
  ventricular, 275
  ventricular vs. atrial capture in, *282*
Transmembrane potential (TMP), 29, 30t, *31*
  afterdepolarizations in, 43, *44*, 45. See also *Afterdepolarization(s).*
Transvenous endocardial lead(s), in intracavitary electrocardiography, 129–130, *131*
Transvenous endocardial pacing, 261–269, *262–268*
  catheters for, atrial J, *262*, 263, *265*
    balloon flotation, *262*, 263, *265*
    bipolar pacing, *262*, 263, *265–266*
  disadvantages of, 252
  leads for, 261, *262*, 263
    insertion of, 269
    positioning of patient with, 325
    transport of patient with, 325
  pulmonary artery catheters for, 266, *267–268*, 269
  uses of, 256t, 269

Tricyclic antidepressant(s), and catecholamine turnover, 69
Trifascicular heart block, permanent pacemakers for, indications for, 228t
Trigeminy, in ventricular extrasystoles, 409
Triggered arrhythmia(s), cardioversion and, 237, 237t
Triplet(s), in ventricular extrasystoles, 409, *411*
Twiddler's syndrome, 297
Two-compartment model, of pharmokinetics of antiarrhythmic drugs, 162, *163*

U

U wave(s), in electrocardiography, 124
Undersensing, *306*, 306–307, 307t, *308*
Unidirectional conduction block, 46–48
Unipolar lead(s), in intracavitary electrocardiography, epicardial, 129–130, *131*
  esophageal, 130, 132, *132–133*
Upstroke, *32*, 34
  action potential in, 30, 30t, *32*, 33–34

V

Vagal tone, and atrioventricular junctional rhythm, 363
Variable coupling, in ventricular extrasystoles, 408
VAT (atrial-triggered ventricular) pacing, for bradycardia, 218
Vaughn Williams classification, of antiarrhythmic drugs, 157–159, 158t, *159*
VDD (atrial-triggered ventricular-inhibited) pacing, in dual-chamber mode pacemakers, 219, *220*, 221, 222t
Ventricular aberration, in electrocardiography, 135, *137–139*, 137–140, 139t
Ventricular arrhythmia(s), 404–434, 405t
  ventricular extrasystoles as, 405–414. See also *Ventricular extrasystole(s).*
Ventricular asynchronous (VOO) pacing, in single-chamber pacemakers, 216, *217*, 218
Ventricular asystole, Lown-Wolf grading system for, 96, 96t
Ventricular bigeminy, in ventricular extrasystoles, 408–409, *411*
Ventricular blanking refractory period(s), in artificial pacemakers, 213–214, *214*
Ventricular capture, vs. atrial capture, in transesophageal pacing, *282*
Ventricular demand pulse generator(s), 257
Ventricular diastolic dysfunction, physiologic pacing for, 224, *225*
Ventricular extrasystole(s), 3, 405t, 405–414
  beat patterns in, 408–409, *409*, *411*
  bigeminy in, 408–409, *411*
  classification of, 405t, 411–412, 413t
  compensatory pause in, 406, *410*
  couplets in, 409, *411*

INDEX **465**

Ventricular extrasystole(s) *(Continued)*
  electrocardiographic appearance of, 406, 407–409
  fixed and variable coupling in, 408
  from ventricular pacing, 300
  hemodynamic effects of, 413
  idioventricular rhythm in, 410–411, *413*
  Lown-Wolf grading system for, 96, 96t, 412, 413t
  management of, 405t, 413–414
  noncompensatory pause in, 406, *410*
  parasystole in, 409–410, *412*
  QRS complex in, 406, *407–409*
  quadrigeminy in, 409
  trigeminy in, 409
  triplets in, 409, *411*
Ventricular fibrillation, 431–434, 432t, *433*
  defibrillation for, *242*, 433
  from cardioversion, 239
Ventricular flutter, 431–434, 432t, *433*
Ventricular function, hemodynamics of, in physiologic pacing, 224, *225*
Ventricular oversensing, with dual-sequential pacemaker, 305
Ventricular pacing, arrhythmias from, 298, 300, 300t
  transesophageal, 275
Ventricular preexcitation, 390–404
  accessory pathways in, 390–391, *391–393*
  and Wolff-Parkinson-White syndrome, 391–404. See also *Wolff-Parkinson-White (WPW) syndrome.*
  electrocardiography in, 394, *394–397*
  fusion beats with, *392*
  sinus tachycardia with, *393*
  tachyarrhythmias with, 394–396, *398–401*
Ventricular proarrhythmia, 167
Ventricular refractory period(s), in pacemakers, 212–213, *213*
Ventricular tachycardia, 414–431
  capture beats in, *416*, 419, *420*
  electrocardiographic appearance of, 415, *416–418*, 417t
  fibrillation with, 431–434, 432t, *433*
  flutter with, 431–434, 432t, *433*
  fusion beats in, *416*, 419, *420*
  left bundle branch block in, 415–419, *416*, 417t
  nonsustained, *429*, 431
  P waves in, 415, *416–417*
  polymorphic, 427–431, *429*, 429t
  prevalence of, 414–415
  pulseless, defibrillation for, *242*
  QRS complex in, 415–419, *416–418*, 417t

Ventricular tachycardia *(Continued)*
  radiofrequency catheter ablation for, electromagnetic interference from, 317
  recurrence of, prevention of, 425, 427
  regularity in, 415
  right bundle branch block in, 415–419, 417t, *417–418*, *421*, *424*
  R-R interval in, *416*, 422–423
  sustained, treatment of, 423–425
  temporary pacing for, 290
  torsades de pointes in, 427–431, *428*, 429t
  treatment of, 423–427, 426t
  wide-QRS, differential diagnosis of, 419–423, 420t, *421*, *424*
Ventricular-inhibited (VVI) pacing, for bradycardia, 218
Ventriculoatrial conduction, 142, *143*
Verapamil, 175–177
  and implantable cardioverter-defibrillators, 324t
  for atrial flutter, 374
  for ectopic-reentrant supraventricular arrhythmias, 346t
  for orthodromic atrioventricular tachycardia, in Wolff-Parkinson-White syndrome, 402, 403t
VOO (ventricular asynchronous) pacing, in single-chamber pacemakers, 216, *217*, 218
VVI (ventricular-inhibited) pacing, for bradycardia, 218

W

Wandering atrial pacemaker, 335, *337*
Waveform(s), in electrocardiography, 107–109, *108*
Wenckebach atrioventricular (AV) heart block, 437–439
  during epicardial pacing, *281*
Wide-QRS ventricular tachycardia, differential diagnosis of, 419–423, 420t, *421*, *424*
Wolff-Parkinson-White (WPW) syndrome, accessory pathways in, 391–392, *394–397*, 395–396
  catheter ablation of, *400–401*
  atrial fibrillation in, 403–404
  atrial flutter in, 403–404
  atrioventricular tachycardia in, 396–404, *398*, 403t
    antidromic, 403
    orthodromic, *398*, 399, 402
  life-threatening arrhythmias in, 6, *7*
  QRS complex morphology in, *127*, 127–128
  reentry in, 52
WPW (Wolff-Parkinson-White) syndrome. See *Wolff-Parkinson-White (WPW) syndrome.*

ISBN 0-7216-5880-6

90038